SECOND EDITION

# EDUCATIONAL AND PSYCHOLOGICAL
# ASSESSMENT
# OF EXCEPTIONAL CHILDREN

*Theories, Strategies, and Applications*

**H. LEE SWANSON**

University of Northern Colorado

**BILLY L. WATSON**

University of New Mexico

MERRILL PUBLISHING COMPANY
A Bell & Howell Information Company
Columbus   Toronto   London   Melbourne

*To*
*Catherine, Randy, Ryan, Amy, Joshua, Joel, and Nathanael*
*and*
*Rose, Kim, and Tony*

Cover Art: Students at Southeast School, Columbus, Ohio

Published by Merrill Publishing Company
A Bell & Howell Information Company
Columbus, Ohio 43216

This book was set in Korinna.

Administrative Editor: Vicki Knight
Production Coordinator: Sharon Rudd
Art Coordinator: Gilda M. Edwards
Cover Designer: Cathy Watterson

Library of Congress Catalog Card Number: 88–63289
International Standard Book Number: 0–675–20651–1
Printed in the United States of America
1  2  3  4  5  6  7  8  9—92  91  90  89

# Preface

In this second edition, we have not lost sight of the original purpose with which we set out: "to link assessment practices to theory." The revised text is a clearly updated presentation of the state of knowledge on assessment. The presentation also has been considerably expanded to address the quickly developing assessment areas related to early childhood and neuropsychology, with the addition of two new chapters, 11 and 12. Furthermore completely new sections have been added related to curriculum-based assessment (chapter 2), the form, content, and use of language (chapter 5), new achievement measures (chapter 7), social competence (chapter 9), computer technology (chapter 14), and nondiscriminatory testing, to list a few. More than thirty additional new assessment instruments have been added to the previous summaries of tests. The reader will also note that two chapters from the earlier edition (social and legal issues in testing and a proposed intellectual assessment model) have been deleted, with the content of these chapters effectively integrated into other chapters.

Our intended audience includes school psychologists, special educators, and remedial educators, at various levels within the educational system. The book is intended to follow a basic foundation course that stimulates students to place assessment within a problem-solving or conceptual framework.

As noted in our first edition, there is immense frustration in the field of assessment in that most procedures exist in a theoretical vacuum. Although the majority of available texts provide thorough reviews of standardized measures, with several critiques of reliability and validity, they lack a conceptual model for testing. This separation of theory and measurement is apparent in the criticism of diagnostic and case-study workups of children in the public schools. Not only is testing under attack on ethical grounds because of its social consequences, but also, more recently, testing has been criticized on the grounds of the practitioners' inability to integrate a sound theoretical base for using the test instrument at all (see Messick, 1984). Sternberg (1979) capsulized this criticism more than a decade ago: "The theory thus dictates the choice of task(s) rather than the tasks being chosen more or less arbitrarily and then giving rise to a post hoc theory of task performance" (p. 218).

This lack of theoretical or strategic integration of tests in the field has been caused partly by "testing course instruction" that separates the theoretical orientation of the means by which children learn from the assessment instruments and procedures, and partly by instructors who feel compelled to focus exclusively on tests currently in use in local school districts, independent of their context in theory and human development. In this revised text, we have attempted to address the problem by establishing a comprehensive theoretical and developmental framework in which the reviewed tests can be used.

The revised edition differs significantly from the three basic types of books currently available in the field. Some texts focus primarily on major issues in measurement, and touch only briefly on assessment and testing. Others focus on the basic qualities of tests (for example, norm- and criterion-referenced, reliability, and validity) and extensively review test manuals. Still others focus on informal measures primarily in the field of education. In this text, we present major issues in the field of meaurement and information on the basic qualities of tests, but we also broaden the scope of the material to include social issues, such as the appropriate use of testing and assessment of minority children. We review educational and psychological tests, but we also attempt to place these tests in the context of theory and development, going beyond the manuals to the research literature.

As previously stated, the purpose of this text is to bring the process of testing into various theoretical perspectives. It can be considered traditional in that a multitude of tests are covered in terms of standardization, reliability, and validity; however, it breaks with tradition in that it entertains developmental, theoretical, and strategic formulations within the data base of each psychological domain (for example, intelligence, perception, language).

We have presented a balanced position on some less definitive or dogmatic issues (for example, Which IQ test is best? Do perceptual tests have any relation to academics? Are current IQ tests, such as the WISC-R, valid?) The controversy regarding these subjects results in large part from practitioners' lack of theoretical or strategic understanding of the assessment process. Although the psychological concepts of children as active learners are still being shaped, we have explored some conceptualizations within testing domains of assessment, such as intelligence, language, and perception, including discussion of some of the major theories viewing children as learners within each domain. We have deliberately avoided integrating all of the domains into one composite assessment model; we believe that this would further perpetuate a simplistic approach to assessment. Instead, we have developed strategies within chapters that view the child as a problem solver; these strategies allow practitioners to do some problem solving as well. So this text is *not* a "how to do it" book; rather, it provides a framework to guide the reader's own course of thought and action, step by step, piece by piece.

The book is divided into three parts. Part I provides an overview of assessment models, test construction, and social issues of testing. Chapter 1 provides a general perspective on assessment and briefly reviews some traditional testing issues. Specific attention is given to four assessment approaches: attribute, functional analysis, ecological, and decision making. A synthesis of these four models, in which test and decision-making phases are conceptualized into basic dimensions, is provided. The synthesized model is provided as a schema in which the reader may evaluate the strategic and theoretical limitations of each chapter. Chapter 1 helps the reader understand the text's purpose. Chapter 2 contends with the current issues of norm-referenced versus criterion-referenced assessment. Guidelines for selecting norm-referenced and criterion-referenced measures are accented, and the chapter includes a discussion of curriculum-based assessment. Introductory information on normal-referenced scores and elementary statistics for the novice are covered. To begin the discussion of reliability and validity, Chapter 3 emphasizes that a test is an indirect measure of a child's performance. Several variations of reliability and validity are discussed. The remainder of the chapter focuses on test selection and critical evaluation of a test's construction.

Part II encompasses the major portion of the the text. Special attention is given to the testing domains of intelligence, language, perception, academics, overt behavior, affective competence, and vocational assessment. Each chapter reviews major theoretical orientations, conceptual issues, and tests unique to that domain. Chapter 4 covers the extensive area of intellectual assessment. The chapter presents current conceptualizations of children's functioning and reviews major concepts in information processing. Several tests used to assess children's intelligence are reviewed. The chapter is nontraditional in that extensive attention is not directed to the Stanford-Binet or Wechsler Intelligence Scale; rather, the reader is given an information-processing basis of assessment. Chapter 5 covers the next major area of the assessment of exceptional children: the functions and meta-characteristics of language. The major theoretical explanations of language, as well as their components, are delineated. Chapter 6 provides an extensive review of perception research from a developmental approach. Attention is then given to the assessment of perceptual functioning, with critical reviews of the available tests. Chapter 7 reviews the major tests used to assess academic functioning. Because academic assessment is more pragmatic than theoretical in its orientation, available test instruments are the total focus of this chapter.

Chapter 8 reviews assessment from an applied, behavioral-analysis perspective, using a five-step model to illustrate the current research.

Several behavioral instruments are reviewed. Chapter 9 focuses on some critical concepts in the overall assessment of a child's affective competence. Some rather new conceptualizations (for example, ecological components of assessment) are blended with some traditional and nontraditional test measures. Chapter 10 extensively reviews current available test measures in vocational assessment and provides the reader with different levels of assessment.

Chapter 11 discusses the most widely used neuropsychological test batteries for collecting data for program planning. Chapter 12 reviews major tests and concepts related to preschool assessment. This chapter brings together current research in early childhood assessment with high-risk children, with a special focus on meaurement instruments.

Part III is concerned with the separate issues of minority assessment and futuristic trends. Chapter 13 covers historical background, test bias, test modification, equivalence in vocabulary, language dominance, local norms, culture-fair tests, and pluralistic assessment issues. Chapter 13 succinctly brings into focus the major social and legal issues in testing. The reader is also provided with a review of the major litigation leading up to enactment of PL 94-142. Chapter 14 speculates on the future of assessment. Some trends discussed are new theoretical concepts, computer simulations, criterion-referenced measures, legislative intervention, assessment of minorities, competency performance, and economics of test development.

We wish to thank numerous authors for allowing us to quote from their works. Specific scholars influencing our writing include Robert Sternberg, James Popham, Barbara Keogh, Klaus Wedell, and William Rhodes, to name but a few. Sincere thanks to the reviewers for their suggestions on updating and improving the second edition: Hyrum S. Henderson, Utah State University; Judy Olson, University of Central Florida; and Barbara Knight Given, George Mason University. For their help in preparing this text, we wish to thank Reid Lyon, University of

Vermont (chapter 11); Stan Scarpati, University of Massachusetts (chapters 10 and 12); Patricia Gillespie-Silver, University of Massachusetts (chapter 12); Eloy Gonzales, University of New Mexico (chapter 13); Patricia Tomlin, Red Rocks Community College (chapter 5); and Jane M. Flynn, Gunderson Medical Foundation (chapter 11), for their significant contributions.

H. Lee Swanson
Billy L. Watson

# Contents

# PART ONE

# AN ASSESSMENT PERSPECTIVE

# CHAPTER 1

# General Perspective on Assessment of Exceptional Children

## *Four Strategies*

## OUTLINE

Traditional questions
Narrow conceptualizations
Criticisms of testing
Testing: decline or upsurge
Assessment defined
Assessment goals
Locus of the assessment issue
Construct or attribute model
Functional model
Ecological model
Decision-making model
Synthesis of four models
Education potential
The list goes on
Summary and text perspective

**E**valuating and assessing a child's needs in an educational setting today are ambiguous and imprecise processes. Thus any conclusions are open to disagreement and can result in the child being re-evaluated. It is important, therefore, to understand how the concept of testing relates to the assessment process. Assessment, in contrast to testing, aims at discerning individual characteristics that are important to the establishment of a specific program relating to the child's educational needs. Assessment includes not only testing and systematically compiling a sampling of a child's behavior, but also such things as observation, interviewing, experimental teaching, and informal tests from multiple contexts. Various other methods, however, may be combined and utilized to communicate the information about the child. Although it would be helpful and indeed important to share some ideas and impressions about the nature and assessment of exceptional children, it would not be wise for this text to define and limit the meaning of assessment in a manner that would be too precise and perhaps even inflexible.

To explore the assessment process, this chapter will discuss (1) traditional assessment questions, (2) narrow conceptualizations of testing, (3) criticisms of testing, and (4) test use. Assessment will be defined, four assessment models will be reviewed, and a synthesis of the assessment process will be provided. This chapter emphasizes that the problems of assessment are related to the diagnosticians' lack of understanding of assessment theory and strategy.

## TRADITIONAL QUESTIONS

A traditional but still current image of assessment tends to restrict information to results obtained by standardized test batteries (systematic sample of performance). Selection of the particular test to be used may be based on answers to the following questions:

1. What questions do we wish to answer about the child?
   a. Is the child an exceptional learner?
   b. What norm-referenced instrument is needed for a decision to be made?
   c. What deficits (for example, emotional, intellectual) does the child have?
   d. What developmental levels are present in the child?
   e. What is the cause of the problem?
   f. What learning approach is necessary?
   g. What referral or recommendations are needed?
2. Is this test valid (i.e., does the test measure what it is supposed to measure) enough to provide answers to the preceding questions?
3. How practical is the test?
   a. Training needed by the examiner
   b. Time to administer
   c. Cost of test
4. Is the test suitable for the age and sex of the child?
5. What are the child's handicapping conditions (for example, sensory, language, cognitive) that affect test selection?
6. What type of evaluation is necessary?
   a. Placement evaluation (identify entry behavior)
   b. Formative evaluation (identify learning progress)
   c. Diagnostic evaluation (identify causes of learning problem)
   d. Summative evaluation (identify end of year or unit achievement)
7. What type of decision is necessary?
   a. Selection of individuals for placement in special education programs
   b. Placement—determine appropriate category or instructional setting
   c. Remediation
   d. Feedback—inform student, parents, and other involved persons about progress
   e. Program improvement—determine if linguistic or basal reading approach would be more effective

Data to provide answers to these questions are collected through group and individual tests, teacher-made versus standardized (general-referenced population) tests, power (test given with ample time) versus speed (how fast the children work) tests, and so on. Although some of these questions and activities would surely be included in the assessment process, they do have a decidedly narrow conceptualization (Dillon, 1980; Fuchs & Fuchs, 1986; Gresham, 1984; Synderman & Rothman, 1987).

Although no diagnostician would want to exclude any of these traditional questions from the assessment process, many might believe it either desirable or necessary to add some others (perhaps a reformulation of ideas about the original purpose of testing for exceptional children). Therefore an inclusive perspective on assessment should normally include virtually all the child's processes (for example, linguistic, intellectual, and achievement activities). Consequently, so that adequate assessment is provided, some theoretical understanding of various psychological domains is needed.

## NARROW CONCEPTUALIZATIONS

There are several kinds of assessment questions that need a theoretical or strategic perspective (see Keith, 1987, for a related discussion). Some perspectives are practical, others abstract, but all are related to placement of the problem within a theoretical or strategic framework. Practically speaking, suppose one accepts the notion that a child is retarded (or learning disabled, emotionally disturbed, or one of the other exceptionalities). What test should be used to assess the presence of retardation, without overrating or underrating the child's learning capacity? Overrating or extending our data would lead to a false positive diagnostic error: the child is not really retarded. A false-positive error results from falsely concluding, based on testing performance, that the child does possess, for example, the semantics of word knowledge necessary for regular classroom understanding. The child

could correctly answer on a vocabulary subtest, "What does nuisance mean?" without understanding what he has answered. It is often possible to administer a test in such a way that the probability of an accurate assessment is enhanced. Unfortunately, these very same conditions can increase the risk of underrating the child's performance. Underrating the child's performance would produce a false-negative conclusion that the child really does have some retardation. A false-negative error consists of the false conclusion, based on testing results, that a particular child has not yet acquired adequate word knowledge for regular classroom functioning. Although the child possesses this capability, he failed to perform because of selective attention, linguistic, perceptual, emotional, or other problems. Possibly the test demands more from the child than required in the educational context. The testing procedure may lead to incorrect conclusions based on inadequate or inaccurate information.

A theoretical strategic framework that will decrease the likelihood of both kinds of errors is needed. Of course, alleviation of a diagnostic error cannot be achieved by mere selection of another test.

## CRITICISMS OF TESTING

Careful consideration should be given to the problems and issues that educators and psychologists face in trying to assess or specifically test exceptional children. Unfortunately, students of the assessment process find problems that are many, varied, and very troublesome. Discussions of these problems and issues can be found in Chapters 4 and 12 and in Cronbach (1975), Reynolds and Brown (1984), and Reynolds, Gutkin, Elliott, and Witt (1984), to cite but a few references. Principal criticisms of formalized testing practices include these issues:

1. Testing practices are used to form homogeneous classroom groups that severely limit students' social, economic, and vocational

opportunities; testing thereby fosters undemocratic attitudes.

2. Testing practices foster expectations, such as a self-fulfilling prophecy, that may ensure low-level future achievement for children who score low on tests.
3. Tests are an invasion of privacy.
4. Norm-referenced tests are not useful for instructional or teaching purposes.
5. Test measurements rigidly shape school programming, and instruction limits innovative change.
6. Tests assess only a limited number of abilities, and can therefore impair the changes that schools should be interested in producing.
7. Tests and testing practices foster a notion of children having a fixed entity or ability (for example, intelligence).
8. Tests or assessment procedures are conducted incompetently by individuals who do not understand exceptional children or who lack the ability to elicit a level of performance that reflects the child's true ability.
9. Tests are biased against individuals of unique cognitive, linguistic, and affective learning styles.

We suggest that the basis of test criticism lies more specifically in the lack of theoretical or strategic understanding of assessment. Several authors support this contention (Adelman & Taylor, 1979; Cummings, Huebner, & McLeskey, 1986; Kaufman, 1980; Keith, 1987; Messick, 1984; Synderman & Rothman, 1987; and Wedell, 1970), but it was most appropriately expressed by Bersoff (1973) more than a decade ago:

> The purpose of assessment should be specified first. . . . The only legitimate reason for spending time . . . is to generate propositions which are useful in forming decisions to benefit persons under study. . . . Within that definitional framework . . . tests are generally not helpful in the acquisition of relevant knowledge to the accurate identification of potential talent nor the construction of intervention strategies for those assessed (p. 893).

Implicit within this statement is the idea that tests in themselves are not decision makers; they only represent a sampling device within a larger strategic framework. What is involved in the inappropriate or nonstrategic assessment of exceptional children is portrayed by Lumsden (1976) in his satirical portrayal of testing as a model T. The model T formula may be represented as $C = T + S$. For polemic purposes as applied to special education, $T$ = test, $S$ = same old test battery mentality of the diagnostician, and $C$ = cute little educational prescription. As suggested by Lumsden, this model T notion has been restated and variously applied to administrative as well as educational settings. In other words, the model T formula has been perpetuated by test publishers, school district administrators, and journal advertisements, for example. A casual view of the present state of affairs indicates that in-services, new tests, old tests criticized by individuals who have come up with their own new tests, and the same tests with different norms have all been espoused for the testing of exceptional children. If there has been some trend in the decomposition of the model T, it may be because the educational outcomes of testing or test interpretations are being doubted, but for the wrong reason. The latter represents the Nimzovitch dictum: "When there is no good move, a botch will come along to fill the breach." On the other side, critics of testing (Williams, 1972) note that there is little to be gained from prolonging the life of the platonic T of the formula. Perhaps test advocates have been too much interested in how tests are constructed (for example, how valid or reliable) rather than their usefulness.*

A casual review of the literature (Haertel, 1985; Messick, 1984; Smith & Knoff, 1981; Snow, 1980) suggests that progress in test methodology has been less than satisfactory in its applied settings. Some problems in educa-

---

*We are indebted to Donald Bersoff (1973) who suggested the analogy between test construction and decisional utility.

tional applications of testing information have been caused by the noncritical approach to the determination of appropriate tests to be used, but more specifically, practitioners lack a conceptual framework from which needed information can be derived. The only competing alternative to testing has been subjective or random decision, leading to inappropriate placement or remediation practices (Messick, 1980; Salvia & Ysseldyke, 1985).

## TESTING: DECLINE OR UPSURGE?

Whether the use of tests is declining is a question being raised in special education settings. Many educators and psychologists (Fuchs & Fuchs, 1986; Hogan, DeSoto, & Solano, 1977; Keith, 1987; Scott, 1980; Smith & Knoff, 1981; Synderman & Rothman, 1987) provide a degree of skepticism about the use of tests in the assessment process. Among the reasons given for this skepticism are (1) disappointing research findings, (2) irrelevance to remediation, (3) skepticism about tests' ability to identify traits and personality characteristics, (4) state and national laws restricting the use of testing, and (5) poor academic preparation in the use of tests. Even if there is apparent skepticism regarding public-school use of tests, it cannot be concluded that the use of tests in assessment practice is declining. A new focus on assessment demonstrates concern for the adequate sampling of situational domains, criterion-referenced measures (discussed in Chapter 2), and a critique of testing theory. An appropriate question to be asked now in our discussion is "What is assessment?"

## ASSESSMENT DEFINED

Educational and psychological assessment of exceptional children is a variable process that depends on the questions asked, the child involved, the classroom context, and a myriad of social and developmental factors. As such, as-

sessment cannot be reduced to a finite set of specific steps or rules. This chapter has suggested that assessment is a variable process, and we will consider assessment to be a strategic *problem-solving process* that uses educational and psychological measurements (tests) within a theoretical framework. Therefore this text will give some attention to theory. However, at this point it is appropriate to ask specifically, What is the relationship between tests and assessment procedures? Most educators, diagnosticians, and behavioral psychologists view testing as a tool to aid in the collection of relevant classroom data. Cronbach (1970) views a test as a "systematic procedure for observing a person's behavior and describing it with the aid of a numerical scale or category system" (p. 26). Therefore the theoretical structure underlying assessment can be delineated in the form of a theoretical model that reflects the assumptions that have been made regarding the nature of the data to be obtained (for example, which test to choose) and the uses to which the resulting data are put (for example, information used for educational remediation).

## ASSESSMENT GOALS

The remediation of perceptual, cognitive, linguistic, social, and behavior disorders, as well as related disabilities, is an ultimate goal of assessment. In the field of medicine, for example, it is traditional to speak of diagnosis and treatment as related to an illness or pathological condition. The illness model generally presupposes some cause of learning or emotional difficulties, a particular battery of diagnostic tests, some information about its prognosis, and knowledge of possible treatment. Contributions to prevention of learning and behavioral difficulties of exceptional children have come from all concerned professions and related scientific disciplines. However, attainment of the goal is not in sight, and there are many children for whom prevention is not possible, so for researchers there remains the task of developing assessment procedures. A variety of procedures from various conceptual frameworks must be reviewed, so that test data can be used accurately. New developments in assessment theory are likely to prompt impacts in areas of special-education testing where problems of measurement error, as well as inappropriate educational remediation, are hindering progress. One such area of development is the study of patterns of cognitive development.

## LOCUS OF THE ASSESSMENT ISSUE

If tests are simply tools and if the effectiveness of such tools can be assessed by means of sophisticated statistics (see Chapter 2), why is there so much controversy or criticism over a lack of assessment models? If psychologists and educators know the referral question they are attempting to answer, the kind of data to collect, and some notion of the problem's solution, then it would seem that an adequate assessment model can be utilized. If the data are ambiguous, one can utilize more tests whose validity and reliability are statistically unquestionable, and a fairly accurate representation of the child's functioning can be acquired. This logic seems straightforward, but *does not deal with the real problems.*

The real problems revolve around the use of tests and the conclusions drawn from them. This does not imply that tests are without fault, but they can be assessed statistically or empirically as to their efficacy. In contrast, assessment lacks precision and clarity in theory and strategy (see Adelman & Taylor, 1979; and Messick, 1984; for review). For example, as diagnosticians test children in relation to classroom competence, they confront several theoretical issues that are left untouched by a test instrument. Some of the legal and social issues will be discussed later in the text, but other "gaps" arise with regard to (1) the lack of an adequate taxonomy of classroom learning, which makes it difficult to compare results gathered in different situations or gauge those results in a specific

classroom, (2) the number of alternative theoretical perspectives from which diagnosticians can approach the complexities of children and their educational needs, and (3) the limited number of standardized tests available for observations of the behavior of children within naturally occurring settings. Ongoing attempts by educators and psychologists to confront these issues have provided some clarity in defining the role of testing in the assessment process (Messick, 1984). Special education assessment procedures have been directed and determined by four approaches: construct or attribute model, functional model, ecological model, and decision-making model.

## CONSTRUCT OR ATTRIBUTE MODEL

Traditionally, psychological and educational assessment of exceptional children has been conceptualized by the classic works of Galton (1883), Cattell (1890), Binet (1902), Goddard (1910), and Terman (1916), which are discussed in textbooks on the assessment of exceptional children (for example, Bush & Waugh, 1976; Sattler, 1988).

### Galton and Cattell

Sir Francis Galton was one of the first individuals to directly apply psychological techniques to the study of individual differences in human behavior. Galton's interests focused on heredity and its effects on individual differences. In 1883 he published *Inquiries into Faculty,* which was a series of separate essays, many of which had previously appeared in scientific journals. This publication included a discussion of mental imagery in which he suggested that people differ not only in their ability to recall scenes and objects vividly and in detail, but also in the devices they employ as aids to memory. His writings also included studies that concluded, for example, that genius had a tendency to run in families. Galton also believed that by measuring such characteristics as vision, hearing, reaction time, and physical strength, one could construct an estimate of an individual's mental ability. Galton made a significant contribution in the area of the application of statistical procedures to the analysis of data from tests and measurements. To validate some of his findings, he applied the statistical methods of Karl Pearson (correlations) and the Belgian statistician Quetelet (he first applied the normal probability curve of LaPlace and Gauss to human data). Galton's work dealt specifically with distinctions between individuals of different groups, and although he did not make a jump to exceptional children, his findings provide a basis for comparison of individual performance to a reference group.

In 1890 Cattell published an article in *Mind* that has since become a classic because it used the term "mental tests" for the first time in educational and psychological literature. The article describes tests as consisting of measurements of functions such as vision and hearing, sensitivity to pain, color preferences, reaction time, rote memory, and mental imagery. He noted that reaction time had little or no value in the estimation of intellectual abilities (college students served as subjects). The time variable alone played a minor role in most mental tests, except in those specifically devised to measure speed of performance for a specific purpose (for example, clerical aptitude). His conclusions from his simple tests were that they did not relate to students' grades and were not highly reliable.

Both Galton and Cattell, as well as many of their contemporaries, regarded motor and sensory manifestations as indicators of human intellect capabilities. They regarded sensory and motor tests as lower and higher rungs of the same intellectual sequence. This opinion sprung from their observations that "idiots" and "imbeciles" are usually slow and clumsy in their movements and are relatively slow in perceptual abilities such as response to pain. Cattell and his collaborators realized the need for measurement of the more complex mental processes

and the fact that further research was needed before adequate mental tests could be devised.

## Binet, Goddard, and Terman

From a historical point of view, Alfred Binet had a tremendous influence on the use of psychometric measures with exceptional children. As director of the Laboratory of Physiological Psychology at the Sorbonne, he laid the foundation for his involvement in the development of a measure of intelligence. This opportunity presented itself when he and Theodore Simon were commissioned by the Ministry of Education in France to develop a test that would distinguish normal children from those who were retarded. Binet and Simon did not follow the early example of Galton, but instead measured a variety of mental functions such as attention span, recall of digit sequence, identification of vocabulary words, and comprehension. The work of Esquirol (1772–1840), who suggested the importance of language rather than physical criteria, and Sequin (1812–1880), who suggested that sensory and motor-control abilities differentiated normal from retarded development, influenced Binet's test development. Thus a series of tests was developed (1905, 1908, 1917) that had several unique characteristics: (1) questions were arranged in a hierarchy of difficulty, (2) levels were established for different ages (establishment of mental age), (3) a quantitative scoring system was applied, and (4) specific instructions for administration were built into the test.

The Binet Scales were translated for use in the United States by H. H. Goddard (1910) and L. M. Terman (1916). At a training school in Vineland, New Jersey, Goddard applied the Binet Scale as a diagnostic instrument capable of distinguishing between those children who were to be regarded as normal and those of subnormal mentality, and between the different levels of subnormality among institutionalized children. He suggested that his new scale (Goddard, 1910) could identify children who could not be taught the ordinary subjects of school curriculum but needed an educational program especially adapted to their limited abilities. Terman's (1916) revision increased the length of the test by means of several new scales. Original tests were aligned to age levels according to new norms, and the concept of the intelligence quotient, identified by Wilhelm Stern, was added to that of mental age. Terman's revision, called the Stanford-Binet, has become a standard for measuring the intellectual performance of exceptional children. Some variations based on the Stanford-Binet Scale include the Cattell Infant Intelligence Scale (Cattell, 1940), constructed as a downward extension for younger subjects, Kohs Block Design Test (Kohs, 1923) for deaf and non–English-speaking children, and the Hayes-Binet Scale for blind children.

## Rorschach and Murray

Historically, the measurement of exceptional children has been entangled with the measurement of one complex function, intelligence. However, in 1921 Herman Rorschach, a Swiss psychiatrist, developed a projective technique utilizing amorphous, symmetrical ink blots. This test deviated from previous assessment procedures in that allowance was made for the individual being tested to express his or her own uniqueness as he or she perceived and organized amorphous stimuli. The most notable projective technique that followed Rorschach was the Thematic Apperception Test (TAT) developed by Murray (1943) at Harvard. Unlike the Rorschach, TAT cards contain photographs and drawings that are identifiable but ambiguous. Variations of personality measurements yielded newer methods of assessment, such as finishing incomplete sentences, responding to stimulus words, drawing persons, and manipulating and responding to culturally symbolic objects. By the 1950s, evaluation of exceptional children generally included personality as well as intellectual development.

## Guilford

Perhaps some of the most ambitious research in the measurement of human attributes, specifi-

cally as related to tests of intelligence, was done by Guilford (1967). His structural model was the result. Earlier models used factor analysis in their analysis of items (determination of correlation of every item with every other item) and viewed intellectual functioning as a composition of a general factor "G" and a specific factor "S" (Spearman, 1927; Vernon, 1960) or basic group factors such as verbal, numerical, special word fluency, memory, and vocabulary ability (Thurstone, 1938b). These models produced evidence in terms of discrete rather than parallel properties. Guilford's model includes a cross-classification of attributes with intersecting categories rather than discrete attributes within categories. Guilford's model (Figure 1-1) provides three major categories with subclasses in each. Guilford's theoretical model, called "structure of the intellect," contains five subclasses of operations, four classes of content, and six subclass products—a total of 120 different abilities ($5 \times 4 \times 6 = 120$). An intellectual factor is manifested in a child when any one of the five operations combines with any one of the six products and any one of the four contents. Each of the content, operations, and product categories is shown in Figure 1-2.

## Critique of the Construct or Attribute Model

The construct or attribute model as espoused by Galton, Binet, and more recently Guilford is based on the assumptions that (1) individuals can be characterized by attributes that can be placed at some point on a continuum, (2) children have different amounts or quantities of the same attribute, and (3) there is a true placement (score) on the continuum of attributes that can be approximated by test data. Implicit in this model, at least as carried out in special education, is a theory of child learning: that behavior is essentially determined by intraorganismic factors—constructs or traits. Contemporary application of the construct or attribute model is illustrated through what is popularly called "diagnostic-prescriptive teaching."

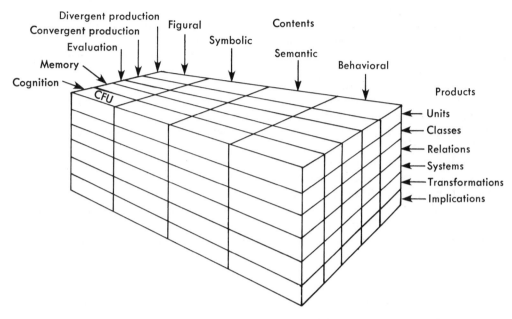

**Figure 1-1**
Guilford's structure of the intellect model in three dimensions. (Based on
material from Guilford, P. *The nature of human intelligence.* New York:
McGraw-Hill, 1967, p. 53.)

## Diagnostic-Prescriptive Teaching

Assessment from a diagnostic-prescriptive approach focuses on the identification of effective instructional strategies for children differing on any number of variables related to academic learning (Ysseldyke & Salvia, 1984; also see Deno, 1986, for a review). Newcomer (1977) suggests that the objective of assessment from this approach includes determination of (1) the cause of the learning handicap for purposes of classification, (2) diagnostic information about a child's style of learning and psychological processes, and (3) academic content needs for instructional purposes.

Cogent examples of such an assessment process would utilize standardized instruments to identify a child's strengths and weaknesses on subtest items, followed by extrapolation of the information to provide a plan for instruction. This approach stresses the diagnosis of specific constructs, such as form discrimination, audi-

tory sequencing, and anxiety, which are related to learning or affective processes, and the training and instruction in specific abilities, which are assumed to improve academic functioning.

Currently, diagnostic-prescriptive procedures are modus operandi for assessment of the various handicapping conditions, such as learning disabilities and mental retardation, in special education. Procedures for the development of a diagnostic-prescriptive assessment instrument can be logically broken down for classroom implementation as follows: (1) select a construct (for example, language, perception) on the nature of the learning process for consideration, (2) divide the construct into sequential, quantifiable, measurable categories, (3) administer a test(s) to evaluate performance in these categories, and (4) develop a program to remediate the deficit in the test-related skills. However, some

**Content:** Items of information grouped by virtue of their common properties. Emphasis is on attributes or properties of units of information.

*Figural:* Information in concrete form as perceived or recalled in the form of images. Different sense modalities such as visual, auditory, and kinesthetic may be involved.

*Symbolic:* Information in the form of symbols (for example, letters, numbers) that have no significance in and of themselves.

*Semantic:* Information in the form of meanings to which words have become attached.

*Behavioral:* Nonverbal information involved in human interactions. Awareness of the attitudes, needs, desires, moods, intentions, or perceptions of other people.

**Products:** Concerns how the individual conceives of information or forms information while attempting to know and understand it.

*Units:* Information conceived in such forms as things, segregated wholes, and figures on grounds.

*Classes:* Units that involve class membership by reason of common properties.

*Relations:* Connecting link between two things that have their own characters.

*Systems:* Structured items of information such as complexes, patterns, or organizations of interdependent or interacting parts.

*Transformations:* Information changed from one thing into another by revisions, redefinitions, or modifications.

*Implications:* Predicting information from given information.

**Operations:** Activities or processes involved in the handling of material that the organism discriminates.

*Cognition:* Immediate discovery or rediscovery, awareness, or recognition of information in various forms; comprehension or understanding.

*Memory:* Retention or storage of information in the same form in which it was committed to storage and connection with the same cues with which it was learned.

*Divergent production:* Productive thinking from given information, where the emphasis is on variety and quantity of output from the same source.

*Convergent production:* Generation of information from given information attempting to achieve better or unique outcomes.

*Evaluation:* Procedure for deciding worth of information in terms of criteria such as identity, similarity, satisfaction of class membership, and consistency.

**Figure 1-2**
Guilford's structure of the intellect model.

authors (Newcomer, 1977) have raised some questions as to whether this procedure can be used to determine what a child does or does not know, and under what conditions a child can learn within the context in which the problem behavior was manifested. Some criticisms are directed at traditional test construction theory (Anastasi, 1982; Carew, 1981; Kaufman, 1980), while others demonstrate the social ramifications of the misuse of tests (Haney, 1984; Messick, 1984; Reynolds, 1984).

Some evidence suggests that psychoeducational diagnosis does not provide adequate individualized educational instruction because of the failure of its constructs, interpretations, and assumptions. For example, Ysseldyke (1973) reviewed forty-seven representative studies designed to demonstrate the effectiveness of differential instructional programming, and concluded that there is little empirical support for the diagnostic-prescriptive model. He focused on the methodological problems related to major research designs (descriptive and aptitude-treatment research) typically used to assess diagnostic accountability. Because diagnostic-prescriptive teaching is the current strategical modus operandi for the assessment of exceptional children, a brief review of three issues is necessary.

*Construct Issue.* Debates on the usefulness of univariate, psychological constructs have taken place for some time. For example, the model of the Illinois Test of Psycholinguistic Abilities (discussed briefly in Chapter 5), which had considerable influence in the area of learning disabilities, was severely criticized (Hammill & Larsen, 1974a; Newcomer & Hammill, 1976). Psycholinguistic assessment is based on the assumption that the cause of the learning problem is a failure within the child and that strengthening the weak area will improve learning. Hammill and Larsen's (1974a) review of studies on the efficacy of psycholinguistic training concluded that this assumption has not been proved effective. Investigations of academic performance of learning-disabled children indicate that problems are not unequivocally perceptual-, psycholinguistic-, or verbal-based difficulties.

Analyses of the school achievement of other exceptional children have indicated that several components and constructs are involved in their learning processes. Assessment procedures could be rendered more effective for programming if many aspects (constructs) of behavior within several instructional contexts were considered. A comprehensive task of this nature is beyond the scope of univariate diagnostic-prescriptive testing because test responses are translated, according to the theoretical orientation of the diagnostician, into single constructs (for example, psycholinguistic, perceptual, language). Such information viewed singularly tells us little concerning actual skills possessed by a student but instead focuses on relative abilities (Deno, 1986; Hodge, 1985; Messick, 1984). One may *safely conclude, then, that for some children, testing instruments might not be totally*

*appropriate for providing information about learning problems or for prescribing instructional activities.* Some tests simply are not related closely enough to classroom activities to be used as designators of specific teaching activities for special education students. In summary, an educational prescription based solely on test information should be viewed with caution. As suggested earlier, assessment is a process leading toward a problem's solution, and tests are only one of several methods for the collection of data. When test data are relevant to the problem's solution, the attribute or construct model is equated with the process itself.

*Interpretation Problems.* Testing procedures assume that within the child are several relatively independent, underlying construct processes that can be assessed separately. Causes of the learning problem are believed to lie within the child. Even if empirical data within the classroom could substantiate an unequivocally deficient trait(s), the next problem becomes one of interpretation. For example, Huelsman (1970), in his review of some twenty studies using the Wechsler Intelligence Scale for Children (WISC), found that children with reading disabilities usually had low scores on the subtests of information, arithmetic, digit span, and coding. Unfortunately, these patterns are meaningless unless one can provide a logical rationale for their existence and one interpretation that excludes all others. Hallahan (1975) has found no fewer than twelve interpretations in WISC pattern performance of learning-disabled children.

Sternberg (1985; in press) stated that a strict testing approach has not been helpful in the acquisition of knowledge relevant to the construction of intervention strategies for those assessed. Individual educational programs based on interpretive test data focus on internal processes instead of on influencing what the child is doing, that is, the product. Earlier, Mann (1979), in reflecting his concerns about the interpretation of diagnostic ability tests, noted, "Let us free ourselves from the spurious belief

that tests directly measure organismic processes, and avoid the danger of developing
prematurely narrow programs committed to the
training of reifications" (p. 12). Thus analysis of
the learning processes of children within the
diagnostic-prescriptive framework has not en-
abled us to make rigorous interpretations or
inferences about their academic performance.

*Failure of Assumptions.* The tacit assumption
behind this diagnostic procedure is that the
classroom teacher will be able to translate these
evaluations and recommendations into effective
individual programming. The teacher receives
statements that reveal, for example, that the
child has auditory receptive difficulties, along
with further comments from other tests on the
child's visual discrimination, oral reading, comprehension, and phonetic abilities. However,
these statements seem at least one step removed from the direct programming task of the
regular or special education teacher (Deno,
1986; Howell, 1986). Mischel (1968) suggested
earlier evidence that, contrary to predictions of
construct theorists, behavior is situation specific.
Thus behaviors generated in a testing situation
might not be similar to the behavior generated in
the classroom. Even within a single classroom,
behavior varies as the situation varies. Behavior
that is appropriate during seat work might not
be appropriate during instruction. Because test
constructs describe a contextual behavior, removed from the setting in which the disturbance
occurred as the basis for referral, it is highly
possible that teacher judgments are in conflict
with those of the testers. (See Ellis, 1980; Fuchs
& Fuchs, 1986; Lentz & Shapiro, 1986; Nelson
& Hayes, 1979, for further discussion.) Another
issue being raised is, Are the individual constructs being assessed (for example, sound
blending) essential to a child who is engaged in
a program of learning to read, write, spell, and
perform mathematical calculations? Earlier,
Wedell (1970) and Keogh (1971) stated that
school learning required a minimal level of
competency in a number of areas and a sound

development in others. This is a rejection of a
single-factor assessment based on the assumptions that (1) there is no single best method of
task mastery, and (2) there is no direct one-
to-one causal relationship between disturbance
in a single underlying process and a learning
problem. Performance levels under particular
conditions are but fragmentary indicators of
capacity.

In summary, it can be concluded that the
construct or attribute model is limited by the
narrowness of its underlying theory and that it
encourages reification of proposed attributes.
On the other hand, there is much to commend
in the approach, including emphasis on test
validity and reliability, focus on individual variations in responses, and provision of a theory of
child behavior. Despite these positive features,
however, if special-education assessment procedures are to be adequately conceptualized when
the influence of interactive variables on child
behavior is considered, additional assessment
models must be reviewed.

## FUNCTIONAL MODEL

The functional analysis approach to assessment
of exceptional children is quite recent and broad
in scope (Craighead, Kazdin, & Mahoney, 1981;
Ellis, 1980; Greenwood, Delquadri, & Hall, 1984;
Gresham, 1984; Lentz & Shapiro, 1986; Nelson
& Hayes, 1979). An important characteristic of a
functional behavioral model, as viewed from a
general perspective, is that it attempts to consider attributes or constructs, stated in observable terms (for example, attention, amount of
eye contact to task), and the situational (environment) determinants of behavior. Although it
has perhaps been systematically developed
from a behavioral perspective by Bijou and
Peterson (1971), other individuals (Craighead,
Kazdin, & Mahoney, 1981; Goldfried & Kent,
1972; Haring & Gentry, 1976; Howell, 1986;
Lovitt, 1967; Meichenbaum, 1976; Nelson &
Hayes, 1979) have been involved. Extensions of
this approach have also included a focus on the

task analytical process (Ysseldyke & Salvia, 1974); this focus was intended to broaden the diagnostic-prescriptive approach as well as to generalize to the child's ecosystem (Lentz & Shapiro, 1986).

Within the functional model, no general class of exceptional children's behavior is likely to be sufficient for the description of a particular child's behavior. The classifications are described functionally, not in terms of attributes or underlying deficiencies. Although no single summary describes functional assessment, some authors (Kanfer & Grimm, 1977; Kanfer & Nay, 1982) suggest that assessment should focus on five categories: (1) deficiencies in information or required behavior, (2) behavioral excesses, (3) inappropriate environmental stimulus control, (4) inappropriate self-generated stimulus control, and (5) problematic reinforcement contingencies. For each category, Kanfer and Grimm have delineated particular behavioral problems, which are discussed in Chapter 8 (also see review by Powers, 1984).

## Assessment Perspective

McReynolds (1971) has delineated four aspects of the functional model as conceptualized for assessment:

1. Identification and description of behaviors and behavior settings. This aspect focuses on applying reliable techniques for given behaviors (for example, visual perception, anxiety, auditory discrimination, conceptual, aggression, nasality) delineated in the environmental context in which they occur.
2. Assessment of incidence and generalization of the behavior. This includes both a behavioral and a sociological idea. It focuses on obtaining answers to questions such as: Does the behavior occur in other situations besides the regular or special classroom? To what environmental events is the behavior related? What event and what context set the occasion for the behavior? What is the rate or frequency of this behavior?
3. Assessment of behavior determinants. This aspect focuses on behavioral classes such as the relationship between behaviors or behavior set-

tings and their long-term consequences (for example, the relationship between special education placement and later regular classroom functioning) or control and modification of behaviors by programmed patterns of immediate consequences (reinforcers).
4. Assessment of the consequences of behavior. A behavior is assessed by the degree to which it is under the control of consequences. Assessment involves the identification and description of the consequent behavior (p. 8).

## Functional Versus Attribute Model

Although the functional and construct or attribute assessment approaches share some of the main concerns in their attempts to produce reliable, valid, and useful data, the methods vary considerably in their assumptions of how children learn. Goldfried and Kent (1972) provide three major differences between the assumptions of functional and traditional attribute assessments. First, the attribute model views test behavior as a sign of a hypothetical construct that accounts for the consistency in an individual's behavior, whereas the functional model is less inferential in postulating underlying factors to account for problem behaviors. As Mischel (1968) indicates regarding the latter approach, "Emphasis is on what a person does in situations rather than about inferences about what attributes he has" (p. 10). This functional-analytical approach is more likely to look at test results as the relationship between behavior and specific environmental factors (e.g., Ollendick & Hersen, 1984).

Second, the selection of test items or situations differs for the two approaches. The attribute model assumes that behavior will be quite stable regardless of the specific situational context. Therefore minimal efforts are made in departing from the use of standardized instructions or test items. In certain cases an attempt is made to gather peripheral information (that is, with informal testing procedures, further probing of the child's response is made after his response has been evaluated from the standardized procedures). The functional model is concerned with the relationship between behavior and specific environmental contexts and, therefore, makes an attempt to sample these situations thoroughly. The concern for adequate sampling of various social and educational settings has been interpreted as demonstrating the importance of content validity in behavioral social assessment (Kanfer & Grimm, 1977).

The third assumption relates to the sign versus sample interpretation of test responses. The sign approach, characteristic of the attribute model, assumes that a test response is an indirect manifestation of some underlying educational or psychological construct. The sample approach, characteristic of a functional model, on the other hand, assumes that test responses constitute only a subtest of actual behaviors that occur in the classroom.

In a discussion of the functional model, several authors have outlined a procedure for establishing content validity of child functioning (Goldfried & D'Zurilla, 1969; Kanfer & Grimm, 1977; Lentz & Shapiro, 1986; Meichenbaum, 1977). Goldfried and D'Zurilla view the first step as situational analysis, or the sampling of typical situations in which a behavior of interest is likely to occur (for example, classroom, home, community center). The second phase consists of response enumeration, which suggests a sampling of typical responses to each of the relevant situations generated during the situational analysis. Both of these phases are carried out through direct measurement of behaviors as they occur within these natural settings. The third and final phase, criterion analysis, includes a response evaluation with regard to competency level. In the measurement of competence, these judgments can be made by significant individuals who would typically label the behavior as inappropriate or maladaptive. These judgments can be made in relation to standardized test performance or in terms of generally how well the child fits the definition of behavioral capability of interest to the individual doing the assessment. Each situation may have associated with it a variety of different responses that can be grouped functionally, according to the

demand of the context (for example, classroom) (Figure 1-3). This three-stage analysis may be used during the selection of items to be used in one's testing instrument; it can also provide content validity (see Chapter 3) for the child's test performance.

As noted previously, the primary limitation of using tests within a diagnostic-prescriptive framework is that the framework reduces opportunities for interaction of other extraneous variables that might be affecting the child's performance. This is true when tests are seen as a basis for special education evaluation. Kratochwill (1977) suggests that if tests are used for administration purposes (for example, ability assessment), they must (1) outline strategies that contribute sophisticated educational recommendations, (2) outline populations that can best be served by these procedures, (3) indicate how diagnostic information will generalize across different task situations, and (4) develop a theoretical orientation through which systematic assessment can be directed. Perhaps the most well-known application of a functional model is task analysis.

## Task Analysis

Task analysis focuses on a child's level of skills in relation to a particular task. Using the assumption that successful learning outcomes are based on prerequisite skills, this analysis assesses the skills that the child can demonstrate at various points along the way toward the achievement of learning objectives. Through the use of a variety of formal and informal assessment techniques, the teacher determines at what point the child will enter the continuum of academic skills. Task analysis identifies the component or prerequisite tasks a student must ultimately be able to do, if he or she is to perform a desired behavior. The basic philosophy of the skill development approach places little emphasis on discovering abilities or deficits within the child but places major emphasis on the specific educational tasks to be taught (Craighead, Kazdin, & Mahoney, 1981). The

**Figure 1-3**
Problem situation with varying levels of effective responses. (Based on material from Goldfried, M., & D'Zurrila, T. A behavioral analytic model for assessing competence. In C. Spielberger [Ed.], *Current topics in clinical and community psychology.* New York: Academic Press, 1969, p. 161.)

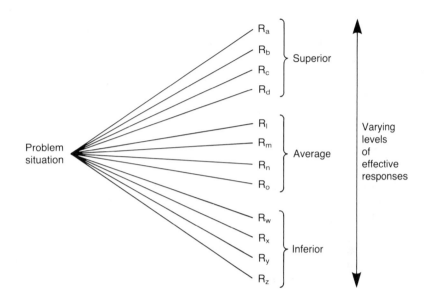

important questions for assessment using this approach are (1) What specific educational tasks are important for the child to learn? (2) What are the sequential steps in the learning of this task? (3) What specific behaviors does the child need to perform this task? In summation, task analysis involves a sequential series of many small steps. If any of these steps are "short circuited" or missed, the desired result might not come about and the child fails to become a learner. Analysis of the learning task may reveal to the teacher the problem area in which the learning difficulty occurs. Task analysis logically follows the writing of performance objectives. The objective tells "what is being learned." Task analysis then suggests the sequential learning steps involved in students' developing the skill to perform a particular objective. Because task analysis is learner oriented, the following components are necessary.

*Behavioral Objective.* Stating the task in behavioral or performance terms is one component of assessment. For example:

**Math:** The learner will write the correct response to multiplication problems given in the form of mathematical sentences or story problems in which each of the two factors is less than ten.

**Reading:** Given words containing the /ē/ sound, represented by -e in the CV pattern, in lists of other words, the child will identify, by circling, the known -e pattern words as rhyming words.

Stating the task simply means saying what the learner should do.

*Prerequisite Skills.* Another component of task analysis is testing the prerequisite skills. The teacher evaluates the prospective learner to see if he or she possesses the required skill. For example, in a reading task, the prerequisite skills for a child to visually discriminate single consonants in the initial word position would include the ability to

1. Follow directional drills
2. Verbalize differences in geometric forms
3. Do sequential geometric form drills
4. Demonstrate likenesses in abstract figures
5. Demonstrate position of body in space
6. Demonstrate laterality—right from left
7. Visually discriminate between objects
8. Demonstrate visual discrimination for details in pictures
9. Complete pictures
10. Demonstrate visual discrimination of gross symbols

11. Perform perceptual constancy drills
12. Discriminate differences in form and position of objects
13. Demonstrate perceptions of spatial relationships
14. Compare contrasting configuration of words and letters
15. Perform figure-ground perception
16. Perform visual-motor drills
17. Discriminate differences in gross symbols
18. Discriminate differences in the horizontal and vertical lines and curves that make words
19. Discriminate likenesses and differences in word configurations
20. Perform matching drills with initial letters
21. Discriminate between small symbols
22. Perform word pattern matching drills

*Scope and Sequence.* After the component of readiness has been assessed through tasks that determine prerequisite skills, an analysis of the task for its sequential learning steps is done. A general scope and sequence must be followed for test development. Analyzing the skills means listing the steps necessary to complete a long-range task. Before tasks are assessed, an outline of the assessment procedure is necessary. For example, a terminal program objective in phonetic analysis would be for a child to read difficult words that in some cases have no letter sounds:

*b* before *t*—doubt
*d* at the end of a syllable preceding another consonant—Wednesday
*c* after *s*—scene
*g* before final *m* or *n* and before *n* at the beginning of a word—sign, gnaw
*h* in certain words—honest
*k* before *n* at the beginning of a word—know
*l* in certain words—would
*n* after *m*—hymn
*s* in certain words—isle
*p* in certain words—cupboard
*t* in certain words—listen
*w* before *r*—write

A program outline to meet this objective might include assessment of the child's knowledge of

1. Important single consonants in the initial position: *b*, *c* (hard sound only); *d*, *f*, *g* (hard sound); *h*, *j*, *l*, *m*, *n*, *p*, *r*, *s* (soft *c* sound); *t*, *w*. Omit *k*, *v*, *x*, *y*, *z*, and *q*
2. Speech consonants in the initial position: *ch*, *sh*, *th*, *wh*
3. Consonant blends in the initial position: *sk*, *sm*, *sn*, *sp*, *st*, *sw*, *tw*, *bl*, *br*, *gl*, *fl*, *pl*, *cl*, *fr*, *tr*
4. Single consonants in the initial position: *v* and *y*
5. Consonant blends: *bl*, *cl*, *fl*, *gl*, *pl*, *sl*, *br*, *cr*, *dr*, *fr*, *gr*, *pr*, *tr*, *scr*, *str*, *thr*
6. Preparation for learning the short sounds of vowels; using familiar words, have pupils note the constant short sound of the vowel in the medial position in monosyllabic words.
7. Short sounds of vowels: *a*, *e*, *i*, *o*, *u*
8. Long sounds of vowels: *a*, *e*, *i*, *o*, *u*
9. Speech consonants in the final position: *ch*, *sh*, *th*
10. Consonant blends in the final position: *sk*, *sp*, *st*
11. Vowel blends: *ow*, *ou*, *oi*, *oy*, *au*, *aw*, *oo*
12. Long sounds of the vowels as discovered in familiar long vowel endings
13. Double vowels as they occur within words and as the endings of words in which the first vowel is long and the second is silent; teach within words: *ai*, *ae*, *oa*, *ui*, *ee*; teach as endings: *ie*, *ow*, *ue*, *ay*, *ea*, *ee*
14. Soft sounds of *c* and *g*
15. Single consonants in the final position only: *x* and *z*
16. Letters that sometimes have no sound
17. Sound groups: though, although, dough; ought, bought, brought
18. Rule that a vowel usually is short when it is the only vowel in a word and is followed by a consonant
19. Rule that a vowel usually is long when it is the only vowel and is the last letter in the word

20. Rule that when two vowels are side by side the first is usually long and the second is silent
21. Rule that in a short word that has two vowels, one of which is at the end of the word (for example, *e*), usually the first vowel is long and the *e* has no sound

Once an outline from the assessment has been determined, all performance steps involved in each subcomponent of each part of the outline are listed in sequence. Following is an example of performance objectives for a sequence to be assessed and taught. The same procedure would be followed for all the long vowel sounds.

1. Given a list of one-syllable words, the child will circle the vowel combination that has the long sound of /ā/ -ai- (sail, coat).
2. Given words containing the -ea- /ē/ pattern, the child will be able to select from a list of written words and circle the words having the same sound.
3. Given words containing the -ee- /ē/ pattern, the child will be able to select from a list of words and circle the word having the same sound.
4. Given words containing the long /ō/ pattern, the child will select from a list of words and circle the words having the same vowel sound.

For each step, one or more performance behaviors are assessed in the process. In the preceding example, assessment would include not only having the student circle the correct responses but also verbalize, write, orally recall, match, and underline the correct response.

## Critique

The task analysis approach places little emphasis on standardized tests but focuses on the enabling objectives or skill level of the child. (This concept will be developed in Chapter 2.) Eaves and McLaughlin (1977) criticized task analysis proponents for syllogistic reasoning in their de-emphasizing the use of standardized tests. Task analysis assumes that because certain tests are structurally unsound within the classroom context, all standardized tests are useless to the development of educational objectives. Such an argument, according to Eaves and McLaughlin, obscures the point of standardized testing, in that the value of testing is not the specification of objectives, but is "in deciding whether or not the diminutive objective needs to be specified at all" (p. 100). The task analysis model ensures that the situation can be generalized to the classroom, but special arrangements are needed to measure the variety of setting characteristics that may relate to task achievement. An ecological approach, such as arrangement of desks or community expectations, can prove relevant. Although task analysis provides measures from which learning outcomes can be determined as related to the classroom context, it does not provide a schema for the conceptualization and choice of independent variables (for example, teacher characteristics or peer interactions) related to classroom objectives.

## ECOLOGICAL MODEL

Another assessment perspective has been developed within the last decade and has been described as an ecological approach. The model incorporates behavioral and ability assessment measures, although most of its literature focuses on behavioral and social interaction (see Scott, 1980). The gathered assessment data pertain, for example, to academic needs, school-community intervention, natural-community intervention, family environmental intervention, and architectural intervention (such as residential and home living centers built for therapeutic purposes). The focus of the approach is on socializing, or teaching the child to perform socially competent or adaptable behavior.

## Assessment Process

The actual assessment process involves several activities: (1) identifying the child's microecology (components of various environmental contexts), (2) establishing a task inventory of each social setting within the child's microecology, (3) assessing the child's competency to perform each task, (4) assessing characteristics judged deviant within each social setting, (5) assessing the child in each social setting, (6) assessing tolerance of individuals interacting significantly within the child's ecosystem, and (7) analyzing data on the child's competency, deviance, and tolerance for differences. This model specifically extends the role and objectives of assessment. For example, Sundberg (1977) suggested a three-dimensional model involving the interactions of (1) methods (interviews, projectives, observational techniques, biophysical techniques), (2) levels (child, group, organization, community, state), and (3) functions (child selection, training and education, remediation, program evaluation, and theory building). From this perspective, the assessment of an individual child can require complex interactions of the various methods, levels, and functions.

## Objectives and Roles

The goal of assessment is to determine the adaptation of individuals to the demands of their environment. It is not sufficient to state that evaluation roles are merely to identify elements in the school system that impair or are incongruent for the child's functioning. The role of assessment becomes one of identifying elements in the child's ecosystems as well as the demands from program elements in the school context. The evaluation has the following focal points:

1. Accountability—to determine if information from the child's evaluation is directed to each individual or group concerned with child–school-related performance

2. General needs assessment—to determine if the child arrives at goals and objectives for the classroom/community

3. Individual needs assessment—to determine how the child's instructional needs can be met

4. Strategies for providing instruction—to determine the most advantageous way to facilitate school learning:
   a. Curriculum—to assess quality of program planning and organization for classroom/community
   b. Classroom—to assess the extent to which educational programs are being appropriately implemented
   c. In-class evaluation—to assess the extent to which criterion-referenced or formative evaluations have occurred
   d. Learning locus of control—to assess the extent to which the student perceives his or her own efforts as necessary for academic success
   e. Materials—to assess whether specific material or stimulus improves the student's performance
   f. Teacher—to assess the ability of the personnel within the educational context to achieve the goals of the community and objectives of the school
   g. Environment—to assess the extent to which the classroom contingencies encourage the child to meet educational/community objectives
   h. Staff training—to assess the extent to which teachers are being trained to meet individual children's needs
   i. Administrative support—to assess the extent to which the school's staff members make decisions that result in successful child performance

5. Instructional outcome—to assess the extent to which a child is becoming competent in the goals and objectives provided

6. Resources—to assess the extent to which there is adequate funding to meet all individual needs

## Ecological Interactions

Perhaps the most ambitious attempt to systematize human exchange within an ecological framework was the earlier work of Barker (1968). Although Barker is not interested in assessment, many of his concepts have been applied by his associates. According to Barker, behavior settings (for example, the classroom) exert a great deal of influence over the behavior of their occupants. Thurman (1977) has referred to this phenomenon as "child-environment congruence." To understand Barker's view on how behavior congruence occurs with exceptional children, one must consider an important question: How are behavior settings (for example, classrooms) and children related to one another? That is, what are the exchanges (or as Barker calls them, "circuits") that link the child in the behavior setting to the setting itself?

Barker suggests that the following circuits occur between the setting and individuals: (1) goal circuits, (2) program circuits, (3) deviation-counter circuits, and (4) vetoing circuits. Applied to assessment, goal circuits involve the child's perception of goals within a setting, ways to achieve these goals, and the type of satisfaction achieved from these goals. For example, if a child fails to see the teacher as possessing skills that satisfy his or her goals, the child will prefer to avoid that setting. If the classroom is frustrating for the child in terms of the means to meet a goal or if the child does not recognize classroom goals as valuable, it would not be surprising to see the child performing poorly in that context.

Program circuits specify how the setting (in this case the classroom) works. They specify fairly precisely how transactions between child and teacher are to take place. For example, the focus is on reading or math during certain periods of the day, and a particular sequence of activity is required. The child and teacher carry on a transaction related to this program according to classroom rules. An incongruence or aggravated exchange can occur when a system-atic program or structure is unclear from the child's perspective.

Deviation-counter circuits are the inadequacies in the exchange that prevent the child and teacher from achieving satisfactions they seek. This refers more directly to the stability of the setting and the child's behavior. Deviation-counter circuits can assess not only the behavior of the child, but also the physical (for example, lighting, weather, seating arrangement) aspects of the environment. Barker describes these circuits as being characterized by the individual's ability to sense the presence of conditions that prevent the program from being carried out. An intervention is made to alter or to modify setting conditions.

Vetoing circuits specify the mode of relationship between the setting and the child, and involve eliminating or removing the deviant component of the setting. An example is the removal of the child from the classroom. Barker (1968) gives this example: "Oran was acting silly. Miss Rutherford said, 'Evidently, you do not wish to play in our band, Oran.' She took the cymbal away and gave it to Selma Bradley. Miss Rutherford put Oran on the far side of the piano away from the class" (p. 15). Although this exchange typically is not seen as an assessment procedure, the human exchange factor removes a component from the setting that threatens its stability.

Figure 1-4 provides a schematic representation of the ecological approach to child assessment and remedial intervention. At the center is the child's intervention program (demands of the classroom). This program is accessible to all members of the child's ecological system; the main priority is coordination of the community activities and utilization of effective community resources. The upper part of the diagram represents an assessment system that serves to identify competencies expected of the child. Made with an ecological approach, the adaptation of social context relies on ecological assessment of the child. Assessment focus is on (1)

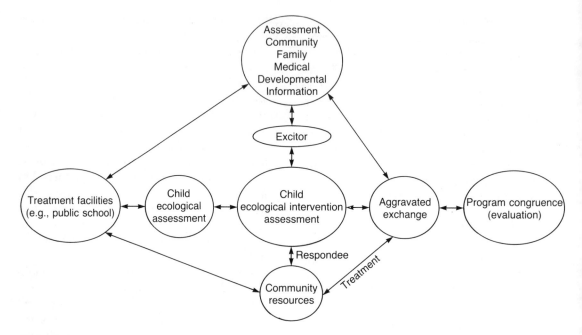

**Figure 1-4**
Ecological assessment model.

delineating the parameters of the child's ecosystem and (2) developing measures to quantify the competency of the child's behaviors within that specific ecosystem. The assessment system primarily serves to direct the intervention; this focus is consistent with Rhodes' (1970) goal of identifying the "point of convulsive encounter between the child and the surrounding human community" (p. 313). Data sources include the family's resources, stresses, expectations, and levels of understanding and accepting the child's problem, plus medical, developmental, psychological, and educational information.

The bottom of the diagram in Figure 1-4 shows that ecological assessment and intervention are achieved through a *feedback* relationship with community services. These services include counseling, parent involvement programs, in-school interventions, medical services, and a wide range of community-based family support systems.

Treatment facilities (on the left in Figure 1-4) depend on the social context in which the child operates. Change in any one aspect causes a shift in other parts of the child's ecological system. Obviously, discerning signs of adaptation in the child in relation to assessment is difficult in every contextual environment. Yet within microecologies, adaptive behaviors are assessed. Table 1-1 provides a distinction between specific ecological strategies and other assessment strategies based on classroom applications.

Assessment progression is to first identify congruence within the family, then gradually progress toward identification of congruence with the community. The primary assessment goal (shown on the right in Figure 1-4) is established by finding a goodness-of-fit between the child and the microecology. Once the child's ecosystem has been defined, assessment categories are determined and parameters are selected. Then the teacher must select relevant measurement instruments.

**Table 1-1**
Comparison of ecological with traditional assessment.

| Nonecological strategies | Ecological strategies |
|---|---|
| Responsive only to child crisis | Responsive to child, adaptive to classroom context |
| Deals in specific assessment measures | Concern with comprehensive assessment and individually adapted measures |
| Requires consent from social system for assessment and intervention | Requires participation from child's social system for assessment intervention |
| Assesses conflict in classroom | Asesses conflict of child in all natural settings |
| Assessment information provides short-range classroom planning | Assessment information provides long-range community planning |
| Standardized and formalized classroom assessment | Innovative classroom assessment |
| Separate ancillary assessment for child and community | Coordinated assessment services for child and parent |

A "valid" instrument in other systems may be totally irrelevant for a given child's ecological system. It is important to find and develop instruments sufficiently sensitive to record the child's and the community's changes.

Whatever the focus in the community-and-child interaction process, the measurement of program outcomes involves two basic issues: (1) the selection of outcome variables for ecological adaptation and (2) the appropriate points of measurement. Outcome variables can include such aspects as adaptive school performance data as measured by standardized and informal tests, behavior ratings, and systematic classroom observations by teachers; behavior at home (for example, parent evaluation forms, adaptive behavior ratings); behavior in the community as measured by social services, mental health, and other relevant community organization services; and attitude changes as measured from inventories or sociometric questionnaires directed to all significant individuals in the child's ecosystem. The appropriate point of measure refers to the measure that is meaningful to the teacher, parents, and salient members of the community, and refers

directly to behaviors exhibited by the child with low community tolerance. One method of measurement is attitude assessment. A wide range of attitude assessments has been described in several texts and is beyond the scope of this chapter. One simple approach is a self-report procedure administered to parents or significant community individuals as illustrated in the following example:

**Instructions:** Most people think stealing is very wrong, while something like bragging may be considered a little wrong. You can show how wrong you think something is by circling a number from 0 to 9 (0 = not wrong; 1, 2, 3 = a little bit wrong; 4, 5, 6 = wrong; and 7, 8, 9 = very wrong).

0 1 2 3 4 5 6 7 8 9  To be tardy to school
0 1 2 3 4 5 6 7 8 9  To not listen in class
0 1 2 3 4 5 6 7 8 9  To disobey teacher
0 1 2 3 4 5 6 7 8 9  To swear or use vulgar
                        language
0 1 2 3 4 5 6 7 8 9  To fight with peers
0 1 2 3 4 5 6 7 8 9  To disobey parents
0 1 2 3 4 5 6 7 8 9  To read below grade level

When items of community toleration are developed, special focus is placed on items for intervention that yield the greatest intolerance.

## Summation

Making the assessment of ecological competence requires the assessor to assume a number of social responsibilities. Among those obtained from several reviews (Scott, 1980; Thurman, 1977) are (1) development of a child-context framework in which labels that arise from intelligence testing and psycho-orientation are avoided, (2) recognition of pluralism of cultural background, (3) determination of appropriate opportunities for the whole range of measured competencies, (4) assessment of child without assessment of past and present environments. An ecological perspective implies a greater emphasis on adaptation than on selection. This emphasis may include ultimately a criterion-referenced analysis but more specifically a general, intensive analysis of decisional systems.

## DECISION-MAKING MODEL

Several authors (Adelman, 1979; Cronbach & Gleser, 1965; Haertel, 1985; Wagner & Sternberg, 1984; Wedell, 1970) suggest that neither attributes, functional assessment, nor ecological

models are adequate for the assessment of exceptional children because those models lack a basis for decision making. A premise of the decision-making model is that testing is not only gathering information and summarizing results, but also systematically using the obtained data to arrive at decisions. This model concerns itself with strategies for the making of those decisions. In contrast to the attribute model, which focuses on a static procedure or series of tests, the decision-making model is a problem-solving approach.

Historically, Cronbach and Gleser (1965) view decision theory as a "general model for stating any particular testing problem" (p. 139). The investigations of problems characteristically lead to either a terminal decision or an investigatory decision. A final or terminal decision completes the diagnostic process (Figure 1-5). The investigatory process, information gathering, and decision making continue until a terminal decision is made. A function of the model is to provide a rule or strategy for the utilization of test information. Cronbach and Gleser suggest that when a strategy is being utilized, the following questions be asked:

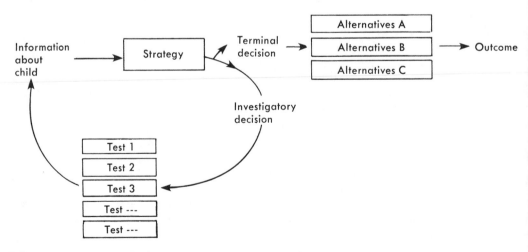

**Figure 1-5**

Decision-making model for diagnostic procedures. (Based on material from Cronbach, E., & Gleser, B. *Psychological test and personnel decisions* [2nd ed.]. Urbana, Ill.: University of Illinois Press, 1965, p. 140.)

1. Would additional information (for example, test data) permit better decisions?
2. Does this strategy provide the best remediation possible with this body of information?
3. Does the existing data conform to an evaluation and prediction of possible outcomes?

The practical uses to which a test is put and the resulting strategies should not be separated. When decisions are based on test scores, it is the accuracy of assessment that matters; precision of measurement is valuable in that it enhances the quality of the assessment and reduces the amount of information that is irrelevant to classroom functioning.

## Decision Principles

McReynolds (1971) stated that the decision-making model developed from concepts of game theory and modern decision theory. Four heuristic principles were developed for this assessment model. First, the child should be given the opportunity to operate in various learning environments. The child should not be viewed simply as a passive recipient of information from the school environment, but as an active problem solver adapting to all aspects of the environment. Second, test information should represent diverse goals and sources of information, not just the means to an end (for example, placement into special education). Therefore assessment is seen as autotelic (see Moore, 1965, for development of this principle for the deaf); that is, the best way to assess a child is to place that child in an environment in which different tasks can be tried with no consequences for performance outcomes. Third, the child should be assessed under a general theory of probable inference. Because there are several ways in which children can learn the same information, the most productive method, as well as the problem strategy that will lead to greatest independence from special programs, must be determined for each child. Fourth, assessment should be responsive to learning activities and provide a structure for

the child not only to learn whatever is to be learned, but also to learn about himself as a learner. That is, responsive assessment observes the child trying to spell "cup" and allows him to spell it "kup." There is no rule or consequence for this performance; rather, this performance provides strategies for the achievement of success in the environment (the obtaining of a satisfactory response from the environment) and insight into how the information in the environment was devised to help the child learn.

## Test Tailoring

One distinct advantage of decision theory is that it indicates the precise level of difficulty that is optimal for testing a child of any given competence. This is in sharp contrast to the static attribute model that treats precision of measurement as if it were independent of a child's level of functioning.

According to decision theory, the efficiency of a test can be improved if items are chosen to be optimal for the child's level of functioning, as estimated from his response to previous test items (Skaggs & Lissitz, 1986). This procedure of adapting a test to an individual has been called "tailored testing" (Lord, 1969). Two notions about the use of tailored testing within a decision theory framework are proposed. First, a system of rules governing the testing strategy is mapped out; the system portrays branching (which shows inefficiencies on certain tests lead to assessment on others) and step sizes (which demonstrate how test items vary in difficulty) are delineated. An example of this approach by Wedell (1970) is discussed later in this chapter. A second approach to tailored testing is to not use static test frameworks (for example, intelligence test, followed by achievement, followed by personality) but to perform a selection of tests during the interview period. Such a procedure requires extended time for interaction between the tester and the child. A Bayesian procedure may provide a basis for test selection.

## Bayesian Estimation

Recent trends in decision-making models have included a Bayesian theoretical base. Several articles (e.g., Haney, 1984; Mercer & Lewis, 1978) have called attention to the weak conceptualizations of what constitutes referral for testing, what variables yield poor academic performance, and whether a test score is a true evaluation according to observations in the classroom and other settings. In the context of decision making, no inference about a child's true functioning can be made from observed performance unless the distribution of performance by other children with similar difficulties is specified. Thus the problem becomes one of estimating a distribution of ability among a population of children from a random sample of exceptional subjects. This would be considered an empirical, Bayesian estimation problem. Because Bayesian theory is rather technical and there are so many different applications, we shall restrict ourselves here to a few general remarks. Bayesian theorists (see Cronbach, 1978, for review) believe that classical attribute or psycho-educational assessment fails because it neglects information about deficient performances between children, and instead chooses to estimate deficits within (subtest analysis) test performance. Accordingly, to improve the understanding of a child's performance involves use of relevant information gathered about diagnosed comparable children (for example, mentally retarded, physically handicapped, learning disabled) of an appropriate reference group. Such knowledge is utilized in tailored testing on the grounds that if little is known about a child's abilities, the best initial guide is the test performance of other children like him. As data accumulate about the child, there is less need to rely on group performance. The child's score can be regarded as an independent realization of a score whose true function is inferred from a known (theoretically) sample. Test performance of children is taken to be a random sample, the degree of confidence one places in the child's score as related to the general population is not an issue, only that the score is one that should be in the range of the distribution suggested by assumptions of exceptional child functioning.

In decision-making models, the Bayesian rationale accommodates the parameters to be tested. A postulation is made on the ability of exceptional children, and test items are chosen that will maximize the discrepancy of successful classroom functioning to maximize information gained. In summary, Bayesian formation as applied to assessment of exceptional children is best in the fetal stage, but it may provide a basis for the termination or redirection of certain test data, with the aim of maximizing overall prediction (see Cronbach and Gleser, 1965; and Wissink, Kass, & Ferrell, 1975; for discussion).

## Sequential Strategy

Wedell (1970) views assessment not necessarily as an attribute or functional analysis procedure, but as a strategy of cognitive and educational features of children's learning. Such a strategy is based on assumed factors that contribute to successful educational performance—not necessarily the validity of those assumptions. Factors contributing to a child's level of functioning are (1) sensorimotor function (physical condition), (2) acquisition of cognitive concepts (for example, conservation of volume, reversibility, socialized speech), (3) acquisition of cognitive skills (for example, language), (4) application of concepts and skills to education tasks, (5) motivational base, and (6) differential opportunities in acquiring the preceding factors. Sequential strategies, when considering these variables, depend on a number of component skills or processes.

Wedell's proposed strategy consists of four successive stages (Table 1-2). Stage 1 focuses on screening to isolate factors that seem to be contributing to the child's problem. Mechanical skills of the child are gathered by abbreviated tests, observation checklists, anecdotal records, and surveys of information. After screening information has been collected, the diagnostician evaluates screening information (Stage 2). If the

**Table 1-2**
Wedell's sequential strategy (pp. 27–29).

| Stages | Number for areas of further investigation |
|---|---|
| **Stage 1: Screening assessment** | |
| *Observation and conversation* | |
| Attention, responsiveness, educational motivation | 44 |
| Social adjustment—classroom | 37–39 |
| Adjustment beyond educational context | 35–38, 41, 42 |
| History | |
| Personal | 40 |
| Medical | 42 |
| Educational | 41 |
| Sensorimotor state | 24–27, 29–31 |
| Health | 42 |
| Speech (primarily expressive language) | 28 |
| *Testing* | |
| General abilities (abbreviated individual intelligence test) | |
| Verbal | 10–13, 22, 23 |
| Nonverbal | 18–23 |
| Educational achievement | |
| Reading (e.g., word recognition) | (+)1, 4–6 |
| Spelling (e.g., word spelling) | (+)2, 4, 6, 7 |
| Math (oral problem with explanation of method) | (+)3, 8, 9 |
| **Stage 2: Evaluation of screening assessment** | |
| *Possible outcomes* | |
| Rapport too poor for reliable evaluation | |
| Discontinue testing and observe | 44 |
| Build rapport for subsequent testing | |
| Formulate hypothesis | |
| No problem: discontinue assessment | |
| Problem not psychoeducational; re-refer | |
| Screening indicates areas for further investigation (Stage 3) | |
| No hypothesis possible | |
| **Stage 3: Hypothesis testing** | |
| *Testing* | |
| Educational skills (assessment leading to 44, 45 where required) | |
| Adaptive skills: | |
| 1 Reading (comprehension) | 10–13 |
| 2 Spelling (composition) | 10–13 |
| 3 Math (problems) | 12–14, 1 |
| Basic skills: | |
| 4 Reading: knowledge of letter sounds | 14–16, 18, 19 |
| 5 Blending | 14, 18, 19 |
| 6 Knowledge of spelling patterns | 14–17 and rules, 22 |
| Spelling: | |
| Knowledge of letter sounds | 14–16, 18, 19 |
| Spelling patterns | 14–17 and rules, 22 |
| 7 Handwriting | 19, 20, 33 |

Based on material from Wedell, K. Diagnosing learning difficulties: A sequential strategy. *Journal of Learning Disabilities,* 1970, *3,* 313–314.

**Table 1-2**  *continued*

| Stages | Number for areas of further investigation |
|---|---|
| Math: | |
| 8 Written sums | 20 |
| 9 Basic operations | 22, 31 |
| Cognitive skills (assessment leading to 44, 45 where required) | |
| Language: | |
| Expressive: | |
| 10 Vocabulary | 14, 18, 26, 28 |
| 11 Syntax | 14, 15, 18 |
| Receptive: | |
| 12 Vocabulary | 14, 15, 18 |
| 13 Syntax | 14, 15, 18 |
| Memory: | |
| 14 Auditory: Verbal | 18 |
| 15 Nonverbal: Rhythm | 18 |
| Visual: | |
| 16 Simple | 19 |
| 17 Sequential | 19 |
| Perception: | |
| 18 Auditory | 26, 27 |
| 19 Visual | 24, 25, 31 |
| Perceptual/motor: | |
| 20 Pencil copying | 19, 21, 29, 31 |
| 21 Three-dimensional copying | 19, 29, 31 |
| Concept development and reasoning | |
| 22 e.g., Piagetian analysis (seriation, conservation, and reasoning) | 12, 13, 19, 44 |
| 23 e.g., cognitive style | 44 |
| Sensory screening | |
| Vision: | |
| 24 Acuity | 42 |
| 25 Eye movement | 42 |
| Hearing: | |
| 26 Speech sounds | 42 |
| 27 Pure tone | 42 |
| Motor function screening | |
| 28 Articulation | 43 |
| 29 Fine motor skills | 39, 40–42 |
| 30 Gross motor skills | 39, 40, 42 |
| 31 Awareness of body coordinates | 41 |
| Lateral preference | |
| 32 Eye | 40–42 |
| 33 Hand | 40–42 |
| 34 Foot | 40–42 |
| Adjustment | |
| 35 Personality | 40–42 |
| 36 Attitudes | 40–42 |

**Table 1-2** *continued*

| Stages | Number for areas of further investigation |
|---|---|
| 37 Family relations | 40 |
| 38 Peer group relations | 40, 41 |
| 39 Social adequacy | 40, 41 |
| *Consultation* | |
| 40 Family and personal history (e.g., social worker) | |
| 41 School behavior: Peer and teacher-pupil relations, study habits (class teacher, counselor) | |
| 42 Medical information | |
| 43 Speech (speech pathologist) | |
| *Experimental investigation (cognitive and behavioral)* | |
| 44 e.g., Response to graded clues; brief instruction and rewards in free-field or structured situations | |
| **Stage 4: Diagnostic formulation** | 45 |
| *Provisional diagnosis* | |
| 45 Recommend experimental action (e.g., in classroom), retesting, serial testing | |
| Problem not primarily psychoeducational; transfer case as appropriate | |
| *Full diagnostic formulation and recommendation for action, including provision for report back on adequacy of diagnosis* | |

diagnostician can formulate a tentative hypothesis, Stage 3 provides an immediate check on the assumptions, the main focus of educational assessment and, in particular, makes use of standardized assessment procedures. Several outcomes are possible, as shown in Stage 4. Assessment at Stage 4 is an ongoing process of hypothesis verification. Wedell's model is not only concerned with the gathering of certain kinds of data, but also with the systematic use of these data to arrive at a decision. Wedell's model represents a different approach from the attribute model, but as suggested by McReynolds (1971), the decision-making model should be seen as a supplement to the attribute model.

Swanson (1982) extended Wedell's model to incorporate Mercer and Ysseldyke's (1976) analysis of diagnostic intervention programs. According to Mercer and Ysseldyke, a complete diagnostic intervention process consists of (1) historical-etiological information, (2) currently assessable characteristics, (3) specific treatments or interventions, and (4) a particular prognosis. To obtain a comprehensive assessment of exceptional children, one must use a combination of assessment techniques.

Swanson (1982) suggested that a team effort be a part of the assessment process. Team members essential to the process are parents, teachers, school administrators, and consultants who provide appraisal data through observation and formal testing. The various aspects of a comprehensive assessment include (1) intellectual, (2) adaptive behavior, (3) educational, (4) observational, (5) medical and developmental data, (6) personality, (7) sensorimotor/psycholinguistic, (8) language dominance, and (9) ecological assessment. It is possible to formulate a model utilizing these concepts. The following format is in harmony with the four diagnostic-intervention processes suggested by Mercer and Ysseldyke (1976) and Wedell (1970). The classroom teacher is responsible for team leadership.

As shown in Figure 1-6, a suggested evaluation sequence can begin after a referral is made by the regular classroom teacher (Intervention 1). Intervention 1 requires the special education teacher to act as a consulting teacher. The objective at this point is to gather objective data within the child's learning environment as related to the behavioral and instructional objectives of the classroom. Observational data follow

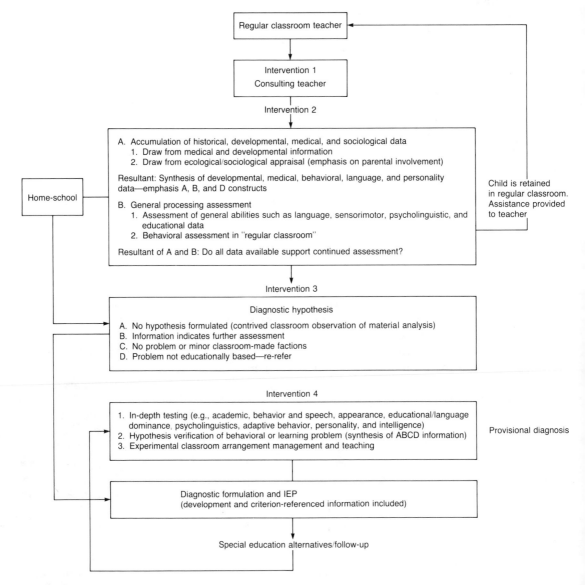

**Figure 1-6**
A sequential strategy for diagnostic procedures.

the functional analytical approach (for example, time-sampling, continuous recording, criterion-referenced testing) with no attempt at labeling the child's difficulty. An informal survey might be used at this point. A functional analysis approach (discussed earlier) would provide an overall framework for the observation process by quantifying behaviors to be measured. A functional approach provides a systematic process for observation, instructional objectives, task analysis, class structure, and reinforcement factors. Sample questions for assessment might include:

1. Observation
   a. Is the behavior observable?
   b. Can it be reliably measured?
   c. Is the behavior repeatable?
2. Instructional objectives
   a. Are objectives stated in terms of the terminal behavior you want the child to perform?
   b. What are the stated standards of performance desired of the child (level of allowable error)?
   c. Is the objective within the child's capability?
3. Task analysis
   a. Are the current instructional objectives stated as a series of specific tasks for this student?
   b. Is every concept needed for the task noted for successful performance?
   c. Are the tasks that teach these concepts specific enough for the student?
4. Class and student structure
   a. What is the child's preferred seating and which is to his best advantage?
   b. Do movement patterns within the room interfere with the child's work?
   c. Is the child in proximity to the materials, activity centers, and storage centers that will be needed?
5. Reinforcement
   a. Does the child respond positively to direct reinforcements?
   b. To what type of reinforcement does the child respond most readily (for example, tangible items, tokens, one-to-one teach-

ing, verbal reinforcement for task completion, knowledge of results)?
   c. At what task and learning level is the child (in terms of, for example, attention, response, order, exploratory, social mastery, achievement)?

Although the observation or functional analysis approach is often thought to be incongruent with the psychological constructs approach, contextual assessment can be made within both schools of thought (see Meichenbaum, 1977). Theories on assessment techniques and remediation programs have often been based on assumptions about the child's information processing abilities (see Chapter 4). Attributes of attention, perception, language, and integration of information perceived in different modalities, can all be placed in the general category of information processing. The study of information processing places an emphasis on the acquisition, storage, and utilization of information within a mediational model. Simply stated, in the information processing model, the child's responses are influenced by his information processing, that is, by the way the child mediates stimulation.

One assumption made in information processing is that the crux of the child's difficulty is a breakdown in the information processing component. Another assumption is that the more specific the identification of the breakdown, the more useful the analysis. A third assumption is that effective treatment can be initiated when an information processing deficiency has been identified. Although these assumptions underestimate the complexity of information processing, various information processing constructs can be observed within the classroom. Four categories are delineated for observation.

1. *Attention.* This category deals with the selective orientation toward and assimilation of specific stimuli. Sample questions include,
   a. Does the child pay attention to learning tasks?

b. Does the child engage in repetitive behavior that interferes with learning?

c. Is the child's interest age appropriate?

2. *Mode of input (encoding).* This category involves the symbolic means by which stimuli are encoded according to various factors, such as modality features and semantics. Sample questions include,

a. At what point do intermodal or intramodal tasks break down (for example, how do writing performances of copying and writing from memory compare)?

b. At what point in the auditory hierarchy is the child functioning (for example, gross sounds, speech sounds, single words, multiple words, single directions, multiple directions)?

c. At what point in a visual hierarchy is the child functioning (real objects, replica, photograph, line drawing, abstract picture, picture missing parts, symbols)?

3. *Input and output processing variables.* Although information about stimulus input and output performance is employed in the interpretation of mediational activities, the information-processing viewpoint invokes a variety of different mediators to relate these two events. Cognitive and perceptual development research are generous contributors to information processing analogs. Gibson (1969), Neisser (1967), and Piaget and Inhelder (1969) have contributed findings that can be used as references for teachers' observations. Sample questions relating to cognitive development include,

a. Is the child capable of mentally returning to a point so that he or she can overcome perceptual contradiction (reversibility; what percentage of responses is correct for orally presented words)?

b. Can the child see that objects with common features are able to form a class of objects (class inclusion-matching tasks)?

c. Does the child have a language of quantity (for example, can say more than or less than and match objects)?

Sample questions relating to perceptual development include,

a. Can the child differentiate one object from another (for example, match identical pictures, designs, shapes, letters)?

b. Can the child recognize or identify an object despite the fact that the total stimulus is not present?

c. Can the child blend single phonic elements or phonemes into a complete word?

4. *Mode of response.* Also called "retrieval," this category involves the subsequent utilization of stored information that guides performance. Sample questions include,

a. At what level verbally does the child prefer to respond (yes or no, labeling, phrase, sentence, sequence of labels, sequence of ideas)?

b. At what level physically does the child prefer to respond (gross motor, point, imitation, trace, copy, match object, completion, multiple choice, sequential order, write from recall)?

c. What output channel does the response require (verbal, vocal, nonverbal, motor, manipulative, pointing, gesture, more than one)?

Because functional assessment is performed within the context of instructional procedures and methods, the following sample questions could be asked.

1. Procedures

a. What is the child's most effective way of encoding? (Does he perform better on word recall if he hears things rather than sees them, or sees rather than hears? What motor activity is involved?)

b. What is the child's preferred response channel (for example, what frequency or percentage of times does the child write instead of saying an answer)?

c. What level of response does the child need after performance of a specific task?

2. Methods
   a. What are the alternative methods of presentation that might be useful for the child?
   b. Can the child choose the method that he would like to use in learning?
   c. Can you learn the child's interests and strengths to get him interested in the work?

As can be seen from these questions, special emphasis is placed on collaborating information from the classroom teacher and the diagnostician. Special emphasis is placed on keeping the child in the least restrictive environment: behavior management techniques are implemented and instructional procedures are modified.

As shown in Figure 1-6, if Intervention 1 is unsuccessful, because of the severity of the child's problem, Intervention 2 is implemented. Emphasis is placed on a multidisciplinary information-gathering process. Information to be gathered includes medical history, development, school history, language dominance, personality, and ecological and psychoeducational testing information. Special emphasis is also placed on adaptive behavioral ratings. Home-school conferences are scheduled.

After all pertinent data have been gathered, the process moves to Intervention 3. The parents or guardians are presented with the team's findings and recommendations, which, as shown in Figure 1-6, include several choices. An individual program can be developed to make certain that the child receives appropriate school services.

If further verification is necessary, Intervention 4, which includes more in-depth testing, is implemented. Unique to this stage is experimental teaching as suggested by Wedell (1970). The goal here is not to remediate the child's problem, but to restructure and simulate the regular classroom situation and to reassess that situation so that an appropriate program can be developed. The simulated classroom provides experimental teaching, and at the end of four weeks, a comprehensive instructional program is developed. The teacher's observations at this stage are made specifically for children within a self-contained setting, for a 3-hour period.

Intervention 4 is necessary to (1) verify the reliability and validity of diagnostic intervention, (2) seek additional information concerning specific aspects of student behavior under different conditions, (3) study the consistency of behavior patterns under typical and atypical conditions, (4) "try out" instructional and management procedures to serve as a basis for Individual Educational Program (IEP) development, and (5) establish a baseline for the measurement of IEP progress. Data are accumulated strategically from all diagnostic-intervention processes. The appropriate placement of the child has been established. By incorporating all available data on the child, the team has sought to reduce bias in educational programming and placement through all four interventions.

## SYNTHESIS OF FOUR MODELS

The four assessment strategies that have been reviewed can be characterized in terms of two basic dimensions: (1) trait or construct (for example, cognitive, affective versus behavioral forms of transactions) as inferred from tests versus situational (behaviors in various contexts) transactions and (2) passive (static) versus active (problem-solving or decision-making) phases of test transactions. These dimensions essentially concern the extent to which abilities of the child are inferred from test performances and behavioral performances, and how social features of the environment are assessed through a standard or problem-solving battery.

Figure 1-7 shows the four models used in the assessment of child-environment interaction: (1) interpretative (passive construct), (2) opera-

|  | **Trait-construct** | **Situational** |
|---|---|---|
| **Passive** | *Interpretative*\* <br> Standardized and informal test <br> Representation of intellectual, perceptual, language, emotional, academic performance <br> Static battery | *Operative*[†] <br> Functional assessment <br> Behavioral observations of class-relevant behaviors <br> Theoretical orientation for classroom function |
| **Active** | *Decision making* <br> Problem-solving battery | *Context generalizing* <br> Ecological variables <br> Generalization of behavior in natural and simulated settings |

\*Interpretative refers to intermediate variables involved in explaining test performance.
[†]Operative refers to situational variables that contribute to the interpretation of test performance.

**Figure 1-7**
Test information transaction.

tive (passive behavioral), (3) decision making (active interpretative), and (4) context generalization (active behavioral). The first model involves the diagnostician's theoretical construct for exceptional children and is characterized by a static battery approach. The second model involves a functional analysis orientation against predefined objectives of the classroom. The third model involves an experimental decision processing for possible explanations of behavior. The fourth model involves the extent of behaviors outside the school context.

The combination of the models represents major areas of assessment of exceptional children. For instance, the attribute approach emphasizes mode 1: the impact of outcomes is based on tests of the evaluation battery; whereas ecological orientations place greater emphasis on mode 4. One implication of the proposed representation is that a single mode of child-environment interchange has been the focus of most testing (in some cases two—Ysseldyke and Salvia, 1984; or three—Thurman, 1977, but rarely all four). Consequently most theoretical orientations of testing tend to overemphasize partic-

ular aspects of interchange while ignoring or downplaying the possibility that the form, situations, and directionality of child-environment relationships vary. Thus important directions in testing are to link conceptually the various modes of children's assessment and to describe patterns of occurrence across different settings.

*The proposed categorization of test transaction modes is presented simply as a preliminary schema by which forthcoming chapters can be evaluated.* Assumptions are made about the order in which sequences should occur (modes 3 and 4 are given preference in the extant literature). It should be recognized that the boundaries between the various modes are not always clear and distinct. For example, intellectual functioning in the classroom can also affect active behavioral functioning in various settings. Also, Wedell's sequential strategy can be seen as an extension of attribute testing. With these qualifications, this text will consider the following areas of testing: conduct behaviors, cognitive development, language, perceptual/motor development, academic skills, affect, and vocational education.

## EDUCATION POTENTIAL

The theme that seems to underlie research on the assessment of exceptional children is the need for a strategy to assess educational potential. An assessment strategy may be based on cyclical feedback concepts (as suggested by functional assessment procedures) and/or learning and behavior transactions that occur in the school environment or some other ecological unit. Of course, an assumption is that children ideally strive to achieve success in school. In actuality (as suggested from an attribute model), children are forced to adapt to situational constraints (for example, classrooms) resulting from cognitive, affective, or motor deficits, to which tests might be only partially sensitive. Although a child's potential is never realized in its ideal forms, the notion of potential ability is heuristically useful in emphasizing children's performances on tests and in suggesting certain processes by which transactions with their environment occur.

Specifically, the assessment of children's potential for learning, as suggested by several test theorists (Adelman, 1979; Anastasi, 1982; Berk, 1986; Keith, 1987), is defining their adaptation to the environment (for example, classroom) in terms of existing information, goals, and expectations. Children interact with the environment in an effort to achieve their goals and maintain desired levels of satisfaction by society. Children are directly affected by external and covert contingencies (for example, classroom supports, cognitive constraints). They are evaluated in relation to their potential within a learning context or social goal. These concepts, unlike the attribute model, emphasize the child's environmental interactions, but, unlike the functional analytical model, focus on developmental domains or attributes.

## THE LIST GOES ON

Within the issue of assessment approach, there is a long list of needs for special children. Practically speaking, some special children do not treat words or letters as belonging to the same dimension, cannot on their own generate mediators when memorizing, cannot deal in part-whole relations, do not ignore irrelevant information. The list of incompetencies that can be found with standard testing is long, although it contains some equivocal documentation. Depending on one's assessment bias, one might say that the child is unable to think logically or symbolically, fails to use a language system, has poor skills in various microecologies, lacks adaptive behaviors, or lacks nonverbal mediators. Regardless, there is an overriding tendency to treat test information on exceptional children in light of children who are functioning adequately in the regular classroom. Children of various motor, affective, and cognitive styles are given the same task, which is assumed to be well suited for testing a given competence. The child who performs well is said to possess that skill or capacity, and the child who fails is viewed as deficient in the content of the task. There is an implicit assumption that the task is an accurate assessment of the skill or capacity in question.

A review of the ecological, functional, and decision models does much to challenge this assumption. *When diverse tests are used, standard tests are modified, or experimental training, testing, and teaching are introduced, educators begin to glimpse what a child can do.* Standard tests underscore the fact that some children, when compared with their norm-referenced group, seem to differ in their ability to negotiate a particular domain (for example, affective, cognitive, motor). This cannot be denied. But to the extent that a diagnostician makes it possible to determine what a typical learner can do, assessment can then consider test differences with a view to determining what might underlie the child's difficulty on test performance. From there, we can begin to determine an educational program.

## SUMMARY AND TEST PERSPECTIVE

The concept of assessment favored in this text is a broad and inclusive one covering much more than the traditional or more narrowly defined view. Each chapter is written from existing theoretical bases within each psychological domain. The chapter provides a basis on which the strengths and weaknesses of models can be judged. Before various domains of testing are discussed, the basics of testing construction, use, and implications will be discussed in Chapters 2 and 3.

In summary, this text has a twofold purpose. First, an attempt will be made to place tests and testing in a theoretical and strategic (for example, developmental, problem-solving) perspective. Each chapter will review research and pertinent references to unique areas (for example, intelligence). Assessment instruments applicable to each area will be considered. Within the data of each chapter a strategic orientation will be presented. It is hoped that the overview of assessment presented in this chapter will help the reader to note strengths and weaknesses of these testing approaches and perspectives. The second purpose is to consider some of the unique aspects of psychological and educational tests that can be used to provide a sampling of the child's performance.

# CHAPTER 2

# Norm-Referenced, Criterion-Referenced, and Now, Curriculum-Based Tests

*Determining What to Use When*

## OUTLINE

The usage of a particular test depends on the purpose of the testing. Tests are usually given for the purposes of screening, diagnosis and placement, or instructional planning. They can also be used to determine progress in the curriculum, or for program evaluation (Berdine & Myer, 1987; Paget & Nagle, 1986).

Norm-referenced tests are measures that examine a given student's performance in relation to the performance of a representative group. Criterion-referenced tests and curriculum-based assessments gauge an individual's skill in relation to a domain of knowledge or to some subdomain incorporated in a specific curriculum. These types of measurement have been the subject of extensive and heated discussion in the measurement literature. Unfortunately this polarized approach has not been helpful in fostering the use of each type of measurement in the way that would be most useful.

Who or what is referenced is the key to the determination of the primary use of the measurement. In norm-referenced testing, the norm refers to the test performance of a sample of subjects with characteristics similar to those for whom the test was designed (e.g., a sample in proportion to the 1989 U.S. Census update in the following areas: ages eight–twelve years, race, ethnicity, sex, geographical area, and socioeconomic status). This fact dictates that norm-referenced tests are most useful for the discrimination of one group of individuals with a given set of traits from another group of individuals who share many but not all of those traits; that is, the norm-referenced tests are most useful for screening and for diagnosis and placement.

Who or what is referenced in criterion-referenced tests? There has been some confusion on this point. Some commercial tests have been advertised as criterion-referenced because the test constructors have set a criterion (usually on some totally arbitrary basis) that they say separates the masters from the nonmasters. This

claim has probably been made because of the close historical relationship between criterion-referenced measures and instructional (behavioral) objectives, and because of the fact that Mager (1962), a major proponent of such objectives, listed a criterion as one of three characteristics of a well-written objective. However, the criterion to which Mager referred and the criterion in criterion-referenced measurements are two different things. *The latter criterion refers to the domain of information, skill, or affect being measured by the test. A better label for this type of test would be domain-referenced tests.* This description has occurred in the literature, but many graduate students in educational diagnosis classes believe (before instruction, of course) that domain-referenced tests and criterion-referenced tests are two different procedures. From the beginning of the concept of criterion-referenced measurement, the domain of information being assessed was very often the behavioral objectives of a specific curriculum (Tucker, 1985); in such a case a criterion-referenced test is a curriculum-based test. However, some criterion-referenced tests are purported to deal with broader domains not unlike those considered by norm-referenced achievement tests (Whitely, 1971).

Tucker (1985) noted that there is nothing new in curriculum-based assessment and commented that "it is unfortunate that good practice in education is often cast within the framework of 'new' theories and 'new' terms used to describe what has been a tried-and-true approach to teaching since the dawn of educational history" (p. 199). Another unfortunate event is that most researchers of curriculum-based assessment have not taken advantage of the advances made in procedures for the selection of appropriate test items, the evaluation of item responses, the determination of test length, or the selection of appropriate cutoff scores.

Criterion-referenced measurement and curriculum-based assessment, because they are historically and functionally rooted in instruction, are most useful for instructional planning and the determination of progress through the curriculum. Because these measurement procedures are best for these purposes does not mean that they serve no purpose in the other aspects of assessment, and despite Glass's (1983) contention otherwise, anyone who has done a careful analysis of correct and incorrect items of a norm-referenced test knows that information useful for planning instruction can be obtained from the process. In the same way Pecyna and Sommers (1985) found that criterion-referenced tests of receptive language skills of severely handicapped preschool children could serve a diagnostic function. Each of the types of tests has a primary use, but available data should not be discarded because it was obtained in less than the optimum way.

Another term frequently encountered and often confused in discussions of these two types of tests is "standardized test." The confusion arises when a standardized test is automatically inferred to be a norm-referenced test. As Popham (1978) noted, a criterion-referenced test can be standardized in the same way that a norm-referenced test is. In fact, many commercial criterion-referenced tests are standardized. Any test with uniform directions is a standardized test.

The basic distinctions between criterion-referenced and norm-referenced tests are straightforward. For example, some students are sufficiently advanced in motor skills to warrant the formation of a special gymnastics class and there just happens to be a gold medal gymnast in the community who has agreed to teach a class for the ten most motorically efficient students. But the teachers have identified forty-five students who they think would benefit from the class. The solution—a reliable norm-referenced, motor-skills test that predicts with great accuracy those youngsters who are most motorically proficient. When the task is to determine the relative position (high or low) of a youngster's given skill in relation to similar characteristics of other youngsters, a well-constructed norm-referenced test is the appropriate instrument. On the other hand, if the teachers want to improve their instruction or perhaps the accuracy with which they report their students' competency in motor skills, a criterion-referenced test is the preferred instrument. The criterion is the domain of motor skills, or more precisely, their motor-skills curriculum. They want an accurate measure of what their students can do in the motor area, of how they are progressing through their curriculum; they are not primarily interested in whether ten of their students are better than 99% of the youngsters in the group on which the test was normed.

In the rest of this chapter we will focus on a review of the statistics used in norm-referenced and criterion-referenced test construction and evaluation, how these tests are constructed, what kinds of scores they use, and how to tell a "good" one from a "bad" one.

## NORM-REFERENCED TESTS

### Statistics

If we assume that almost all, if not all of the characteristics and behaviors we are interested in measuring are normally distributed, a review of statistical procedures starts with an introduction to the normal curve (in which scores are distributed symmetrically about the mean).

*Measures of Central Tendency.* Figure 2-1 shows three terms—mean, mode, and median—represented by the same line. These are the names of the measures of central tendency, and they can be represented by the same line only when there is a perfect match between the sample distribution and the normal curve distribution. All of these terms refer to the typical or average performance. Use of the word *average* here must not be confused with *mean.* The best way to understand these terms is from examination of an example. Figure 2-2 is a set of ten fictional scores that will be used as data for the discussion of the various statistics; these data do not have a normal distribution.

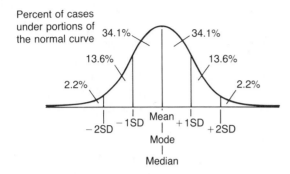

$$M = \frac{\Sigma x}{N} = \frac{440}{10} = 44$$

$\Sigma x$ is the sum of scores in the distribution; in this case, 440. N represents the number of scores. As occurred with the median, no student obtained a score of forty-four, which is the mean of the distribution. This is an example of one way in which measures of central tendency are often misinterpreted: any time a distribution, even one with only a few scores, is described by a single term, the interpreter must be aware that such a term is appropriate to describe the *group,* but not necessarily any individual group member.

**Figure 2-1**

Normal curve showing mean, mode, median, and percentage of individuals falling within each standard deviation.

Generally, when teachers have a large set of test scores, they want to have a general idea of how well the group performed. One simple way to determine this is to identify the mode, which is the score that occurs most frequently. In the distribution in Figure 2-2, the score forty-one occurs three times, forty-two twice, and forty-seven twice. This is a good example of why the mode is often not very useful in describing central tendency. If two more students had scored forty-seven, the mode would have shifted almost the entire length of the distribution.

A more helpful way to represent the central tendency of a distribution is to determine the median, which is the point in a distribution at which half the scores are higher and half are lower. In the distribution in Figure 2-2, forty-three is the median. As sometimes happens, no student actually scored forty-three. In other instances, to divide a group into two equal halves it is necessary to interpolate between two numbers, and the result is also a score that no student obtained. The median is especially useful in describing central tendency of a distribution that has atypically high or low scores.

The mean (M) is simply the arithmetic average of a distribution:

*Measures of Variability.* Another way of describing a distribution is to show how much the scores vary from one another. There are several ways of doing this, but we will discuss only the one most useful in educational diagnosis. The standard deviation (SD) is a unit of measurement based on the degree to which the scores deviate from the mean. For example, we can refer to scores as being a certain number of standard deviations above ( + ) or below ( − ) the mean, depending on whether the score is greater than or less than the mean. Standard deviation is calculated in five steps (Figure 2-2):

1. The mean of the distribution is determined.
2. Each score is subtracted from the mean. Scores less than the mean are given a negative sign, scores greater than the mean are given a positive sign.
3. The deviations are squared (multiplied by themselves) so that the negative signs are eliminated.
4. The squared deviations are summed and divided by the number of scores. The result is a statistic called "variance" ($s^2$ or $\sigma^2$). Although it is very useful in determining the contributions of different factors in individual differences (Anastasi, 1976), its primary use at this point is in calculations of the standard deviation.

| Score (X) | (2) Deviation from the mean (x) [Score − mean = deviation] | (3) Deviation squared (X²) |
|:---:|:---:|:---:|
| 48 | +4 | 16 |
| 47 | +3 | 9 |
| 47 | +3 | 9 |
| 46 | +2 | 4 |
| 45 | +1 | 1 |
| 42 | −2 | 4 |
| 42 | −2 | 4 |
| 41 | −3 | 9 |
| 41 | −3 | 9 |
| 41 | −3 | 9 |
| $\Sigma x = 440$ | | (4) $\Sigma x^2 = 74$ |

(1)  Mean $= \dfrac{\Sigma x}{N} = \dfrac{440}{10} = 44$

(Median = 43)

(5)  Standard deviation $= \sqrt{\dfrac{\Sigma x^2}{N}} = \sqrt{\dfrac{74}{10}} = \sqrt{7.4} = .72$        Variance ($s^2$ or $\sigma^2$) $= \dfrac{74}{10} = 7.4$

**Figure 2-2**
Example of central tendency and variability.

5. Obtain a square root of the arithmetic average of squared deviations from the mean (variance). The result of this final calculation is the standard deviation.

A review of the distribution in Figure 2-2 shows that one SD is equal to 2.7 raw score points. Because the M is 44 and the SD is 2.7, and 44 + 2.7 = 46.7, scores greater than 46.7 are more than one standard deviation above the mean (+1SD). Conversely a score of 41 is more than one standard deviation below the mean (−1SD).

Such findings take on additional meaning when they are made in regard to distributions that approximate the normal curve, because the normal curve has a precise relationship between the SD and the proportion of cases (Figure 2-1). For any normal distribution, 68.2% of the cases will be between +1SD and −1SD. For example, the normalized IQ on the WISC-R is 100 and the SD is 15. This indicates that 68.2% of the standardization sample obtained IQs of between 85 and 115. For persons to be considered mentally retarded (on the intellectual component of the definition of mental retardation), they must receive an IQ approximately 2SDs below the mean (Grossman, 1983). On the WISC-R this means a score of seventy or below. The percentages shown in Figure 2-1 demonstrate that only 2.2% (−2SD) or less of the population could be considered mentally retarded by this definition.

Is an SD of fifteen points a large SD? In this context, the question is relevant only when the test in question is considered against other carefully constructed tests. For example, test A has an SD of thirty and test B has an SD of five. Relative to test A, an SD of fifteen is not large; relative to test B, an SD of fifteen is large. The answer to this question of appropriate size also depends on what the individual scores represent. Say that one distribution represents the number of minutes of instruction necessary for a subject to master a given task. If that distribution had an SD of eight, we might regard that as a small standard deviation. However, if the same set of numbers represented the number of weeks of instruction a subject required to master the task, an SD of eight could be considered large.

***Measures of Relationship.*** Educators often want to know whether pupils who scored well or poorly on one measure are likely to score well or poorly on a second measure. For example, a school administrator would be greatly assisted in planning if it were known whether high teacher ratings of students at the kindergarten level were correlated with reading success at the first-grade level. However, the more immediate relevancy of correlation to our discussion is the fact that procedures for the evaluations of norm-referenced tests are largely based on correlational procedures. In educational measurement, correlation

coefficients are the most frequently encountered indices of relationship between two variables.

Correlational coefficients calculated by the Pearson method are designated by the symbol $r$. They can range between 1.00 and $-1.00$. A perfect positive relationship is indicated by $r = 1.00$. Conversely, a perfect negative relationship is designated by $r = -1.00$. Two variables that have no relationship are described by $r = 0.00$. The Pearson procedure was designed to quantify only linear (straight line) relationships. Examples of these three extremes are shown in Figure 2-3 ($A$–$C$).

Descriptively, a correlation coefficient of $r = 1.00$ means that people who scored low on variable $Y$ (Figure 2-3, $A$) also scored low on variable $X$, and those who scored high on variable $Y$ also scored high on variable $X$. Because of the statistical requirements for a perfect positive correlation, such an occurrence is rare to the extreme. Figure 2-3 $D$–$F$ show a much more common occurrence in the world of real data.

A statistically perfect positive relationship indicates that every individual score is exactly the same *relative* distance above or below the mean for variable $X$ as it is for variable $Y$. "Relative

**Figure 2-3**
Examples of distributions of scores for representative values of correlation coefficients.

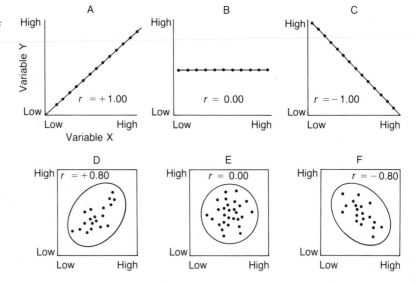

**Table 2-1**
Perfect positive linear correlation.

| Subject | Raw score ($X$) | z score ($X$) | Raw score ($Y$) | z score ($Y$) |
|---|---|---|---|---|
| John | 2 | −1.4 | 13 | −1.4 |
| Terry | 4 | −0.71 | 16 | −0.71 |
| Kim | 6 | 0.00 | 19 | 0.00 |
| Tony | 8 | 0.71 | 22 | 0.71 |
| Tomas | 10 | 1.4 | 25 | 1.4 |
| TOTAL | 30 | | 95 | |
| Mean | 6 | | 19 | |
| SD | 2.8 | | 4.2 | |

$rxy = 1.00$

distance" means the distance in terms of SD units (Popham & Sirotnik, 1973). Consequently, the scores themselves do not have to be identical; they only have to be the same distance from their respective means in SD units. Scores expressed in such units are called "standard scores." The specific standard score in which we are interested at this point is the z score. The formula for z scores is:

$$z = \frac{X - M}{\sigma}$$

where $X$ is the raw score, $M$ is the mean, and $\sigma$ is the standard deviation. Table 2-1 shows a positive linear correlation between variables $X$ and $Y$. Even though the means and standard deviations of the two groups are different, the distance from their respective means expressed in standard deviation units (z scores) is the same. For example, John's raw score of 2 on the $X$ variable is −1.4SD from the $X$ variable mean of 6, and his raw score of 13 on the $Y$ variable is also −1.4SD from the $Y$ variable mean of 19. John's identical relative position on the $X$ and $Y$ distribution is shown graphically in Figure 2-4, as are the scores of the other students.

Figure 2-3, $C$, describes a perfect negative relationship; that is, persons scoring high on variable $Y$ scored low on variable $X$. Described in

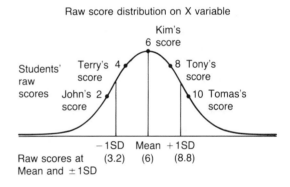

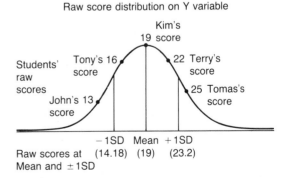

**Figure 2-4**
Equivalent distributions with different raw scores.

a more technical way, the scores on the two variables are the same distance from the mean, but the $Y$ score is in the positive direction from the mean and the $X$ score is in the negative direction from the mean. If the data on the $Y$ variable in Table 2-1 were reversed, it would be an example of a perfect negative correlation. John's $z$ score on the $X$ variable would be $-1.4SD$ below the mean, and his $Y$ variable score would be $1.4SD$ above the mean. Again, a more common occurrence in the world of negative linear correlations is shown in Figure 2-3, $F$; that is, subjects who score high on variable $Y$ tend to score low on variable $X$.

A correlation of coefficient, $r = 0.00$, means that the variables have no relationship to one another. The distances from the mean cancel one another and the horizontal line shown in Figure 2-3, $B$, results. Although $r = 0.00$ correlations are as rare as perfect positive and perfect negative correlations, the no-correlation data is much more likely to look like the scatter diagram in Figure 2-3, $E$, than Figure 2-3, $B$.

A major misinterpretation of the concept of correlation is that correlated variables are also causally related. Obviously causally related variables are correlated, but the reverse is not necessarily true. A story goes that in some years in the midwestern states there is a high correlation between deterioration of highways made of macadam (variable $1$) and the size of the corn crop (variable $2$). Few people would be willing to argue that variable $1$ caused variable $2$ or vice versa. However, most farmers from that area would guess that a third variable, the heat of the sun, would account for the correlation between variable $1$ and variable $2$. In educational measurement this example is similar to the relationship reported in studies of criterion-related validity, as, for example, when a new test in mathematics is related to an older, widely accepted measure of mathematical ability. That a correlation exists is obviously a result of the fact that they are tapping the same latent trait and not that one is causing the other. However, in studies of construct validity, in which a so-called

aptitude measure is correlated with an achievement measure, there is a great temptation to conclude that the aptitude caused the achievement. Such a conclusion is indefensible when based only on a correlational study.

## Norm-Referenced Test Construction

To understand how a norm-referenced test is constructed, one must review the purpose of such tests. A norm-referenced test is designed to determine an individual's rank-order position in relation to the performance of peers (a norm group) who have also taken the test. So that the individual's relative position can be determined accurately, the norm group must include a wide range of performances.

A 100-item test on which all the examinees scored between forty-two and fifty-eight would not tell much about relative position because the range of scores is only sixteen and there would of necessity be many ties. Consequently, to produce the desired variability, authors of norm-referenced tests attempt to develop items that are answered correctly by between 40% and 60% of those taking the test (Popham, 1978).

With this need in mind, authors of norm-referenced tests first select a topic around which test items are developed. One of the major shortcomings of many such tests is the inadequate description of that topic. The items developed around a vaguely defined domain of knowledge tend to be at least equally vague and general. Ebel (1972) noted that "more and more the offerings of test publishers have tended to concentrate on tests of general fields of knowledge rather than on specific course content" (p. 469). Test publishers often argue that tests of general knowledge are more appropriate measures of educational outcomes than are tests in specific knowledge of a subject area. Ebel contended, however, that this was not the case because "in most walks of life where knowledge is used, general knowledge is not adequate" (p. 469).

Assume, however, that the test domain has been adequately described. The next step in test construction is the development of unambiguous test items from the domain description. Anyone interested in improving his skills in this area should consult Ebel (1972) and Popham (1978).

Once the items are written, they must be tried out on a sample of people representative of those for whom the test is designed. The key word is representative. If the test is to be used with boys and girls, both must be included in the field tests. If the test is to be used with different racial or ethnic groups, they, too, must be included in the sample, ideally to the extent that they make up part of the general population. Such statements could continue with variables such as socioeconomic status, age, school experience, and geographic region.

Individuals with handicaps should also be included in the norming process and in the determination of reliability and validity, if the test is to be used with handicapped individuals. Fuchs, Fuchs, Benowitz, and Barringer (1987) found in a review of twenty-seven aptitude and achievement tests that most test developers had either not included handicapped individuals in the norming process or had not specified the characteristics of such individuals if they had included them. These omissions clearly violate the *Standards for Educational and Psychological Tests* (American Educational Research Association, American Psychological Association, & National Council on Measurement in Education [AERA, APS & NCME], 1985), P. L. 94-142 (1975 Education for All Handicapped Children Act) and Section 504 of the Rehabilitation Act of 1973, which forbids discrimination against handicapped persons.

The next step in the construction of a norm-referenced test is to analyze the results, item by item, from the field testing. Remember that because the purpose of norm-referenced testing is to compare individual performance with a normative sample's performance, the best items are judged to be those that produce the greatest variance in scores. Note that the goal of item selection has shifted from items that best measure performance in the domain of knowledge, to items that provide the greatest diversity in scores. Items answered correctly or incorrectly by too many students tend to be eliminated.

Popham (1978) analyzed the effect of this strategy in test construction. He noted that test items on which pupils tend to do best are likely to be those that have received the greatest emphasis in classroom instruction. Items answered incorrectly by most students are probably not emphasized in instruction or are inappropriate for the age or grade of subjects; hence, those items should be discarded. The result of this procedure might well be that norm-referenced tests do not include items that measure the major instructional emphases of the schools. This effect would tend to be enhanced with every revision of the test. Jenkins and Pany (1978) also questioned the adequacy of many achievement tests' sampling of the curriculum in which students are instructed, and Floden, Porter, Schmidt, and Freeman (1980) pointed out that among four major group achievement tests there is considerable variability in content tested. On the other hand, Mehrens and Phillips (1986) found that neither the particular textbook series used by students nor the extent of curricular match as judged by school district personnel had a significant effect on the standardized test scores.

Once the item analysis has been completed and the final list of items is formulated, the test is administered to a (norm) group also representative of those for whom the test was designed. At this point, it is even more critical that the norm group be representative in all the ways discussed previously in regard to field testing.

The final step is to conduct studies of reliability and validity with the final version of the test. These studies must also include a representative sample of subjects like those for whom the test was designed. This requirement is rarely met despite its importance. These topics will be discussed extensively in the next chapter.

## Test Scores

The raw score, or number of correct answers, is the basic score for both norm- and criterion-referenced tests. Raw scores for norm-referenced tests are made meaningful by a comparison with the scores of persons in the norm group. The type of score obtained by this comparison is called a "norm," but one must remember that it is only a description of the performance of that specific group. A norm is not a standard of achievement (Hagen, 1961).

Thorndike and Hagen (1969, pp. 212–213) suggest three important properties that should be characteristic of norms:

1. Uniform meaning from test to test, so that the basis of comparison is provided through which we may compare different tests, for example, different reading tests, a reading test with an arithmetic test, or an achievement test with a school aptitude test
2. Units of uniform size, so that a gain of 10 points on one part of the scale signifies the same thing as a gain of 10 points on another part of the scale
3. A true zero point of "just none of" the quality in question, so that we can legitimately think of scores as representing "twice as much as" or "two-thirds as much as."

Thorndike and Hagen noted that significant progress has been made toward obtaining scores with the first two properties, but that the third probably lies forever beyond our reach, for those traits with which educational measurement is primarily concerned.

In the discussion of measurement statistics the normal curve was presented. The types of scores to be discussed are shown, in Figure 2-5, in relationship to one another and to the normal curve.

*Percentile Norms.* A percentile indicates the percentage of a norm group that falls at or below a particular score. If a person received a raw score of 25, which is better than that re-

ceived by 49% of the norm group, that person's percentile is forty-nine.

There are several advantages to using percentiles. First, they are easily understood. In the example just cited, parents can easily understand that a percentile of forty-nine indicates average performance in comparison with the norm group. Again one can see why adequate norms are critical to the correct understanding of what a given performance level means. If the test involved aptitude in physics and the norm group consisted of people with Ph.D.s in physics, a raw score of 25, percentile of forty-nine, by a high-school student would certainly not represent average performance in the usual sense.

A second advantage of percentile scores is that they meet the first criterion described by Thorndike and Hagen: they can be used in the comparison of performances across various topics. Referring again to our example, the forty-ninth percentile on a physics aptitude test and the forty-ninth percentile on an algebra aptitude test have the same meaning in regard to relative performance on the two tests.

A third advantage of percentile norms is that the reference point is usually closely related to the characteristics of the person taking the test. For example, on wide-range (K to twelfth grade) achievement tests, the score of a fourth grader is generally based on a comparison with other fourth graders, not with second or sixth graders. For each group with which the test is to be used, a set of different percentile norms is required.

The major disadvantage of percentile norms is that they do not provide the second of Thorndike and Hagen's desired characteristics of test norms: a percentile norm does not have equal units at all points on the scale. If the scores on the distribution approximate normality, percentiles of forty-eight on reading and fifty-three on arithmetic represent very similar raw scores, whereas the same five-point difference at the ninety-third and ninety-eighth percentiles represent rather large differences. This clustering of scores toward the middle of the distribution is shown in Figure 2-5. In fact, however, the distri-

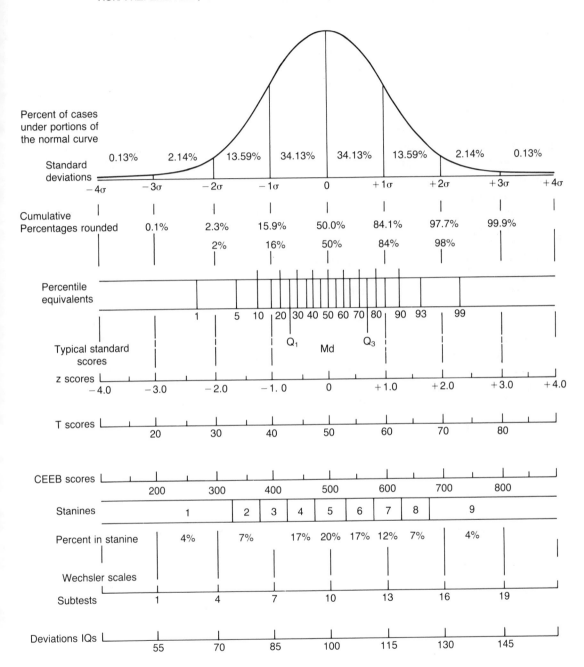

**Figure 2-5**
Relationship of the normal curve to various types of scores.

bution of scores on many tests does not fit this pattern. This discrepancy indicates the extent to which the test performance of the norm groups deviates from the normal (curve) distribution.

***Standard Score Norms.*** Standard score norms describe, in terms of standard deviation units, the distance between a particular score and the mean. Standard scores can be derived from linear or nonlinear conversions of the original raw scores. An example of a linear conversion or transformation is shown in the formula for deriving a $z$ score. In such linear transformations, the standard score maintains the same numerical relations as the original raw scores. Unfortunately, $z$ scores are sometimes negative and involve decimals that cause a high incidence of errors and confusion. However, this difficulty can be corrected by further linear transformations.

One such conversion results in a normalized standard score: a standard score that has been transformed to fit the normal curve or distribution —a $T$ score. Additional transformations eliminate the negative signs. The $T$ score has a mean of 50 and a standard deviation of 10. A $T$ score of 40 is equal to a $z$ score of $-1$ (Figure 2-5). Likewise, in the distribution of scores of Scholastic Aptitude Test (SAT) or the College Entrance Examination Board (CEEB), the mean is 500 and the standard deviation is 100. A score of 400 is thus equivalent to a $T$ score of 40 and a $z$ score of $-1$.

Another standard score commonly used in educational and psychological tests is the "stanine scale." Developed by the United States Air Force, the stanine is a single-digit standard score with a mean of five and a standard deviation of approximately two. The standard deviation is probably its major shortcoming. In recent years, the stanine has become widely used in the reporting of group test results in education.

The various types of standard scores meet two characteristics that Thorndike and Hagen (1969) indicated as desirable in test scores: their

meaning is uniform from test to test and their units are of uniform size. Unfortunately, the scores in no way deal with the problem of a true zero point in educational measurement. Overall, standard scores are among the most useful available. However, one note of caution: sometimes standard scores are contaminated by other variables. For example, on the Wide Range Achievement Tests (discussed in Chapter 7), the scores are grouped by age rather than grade placement. Consequently, the standard scores of youngsters who have been retained will appear unduly low because they are being compared with students who have had an additional year of more advanced school experience. On the Peabody Individual Achievement Test, standard scores are based on percentile ranks, which in turn might have been derived either from grade or age data. Unfortunately, the label *standard score* does not ensure that it is free from interpretation difficulties. For example, a comparison of age-based and grade-based standard scores for children who have repeated a grade and hence are older than their grade peers, will show that the age-based standard scores are lower than the grade-based scores. The difference is especially important since one frequently used criterion for identifying individuals with learning disabilities is a discrepancy between the intelligence standard score (IQ) and achievement standard scores. An individual might qualify for services as learning disabled if age-based standard scores were used, but not qualify if grade-based standard scores were used.

It is important again to note the equivalency of various types of scores that are based on the normal curve. If a ruler is laid along a $+2SD$ and a $z$ score of $+2$ in Figure 2-5, the reader can see that these are the same as a percentile rank of 98, a CEEB score of 700, and a stanine of 9. Figure 2-5 can also clarify the meaning of statements such as, "All scores were more than 1.5SD below the mean." This statement means that the scores were in the second stanine or lower, below about the 7th percentile, and less than a $T$ score of 35.

*Developmental Norms.* Some test scores are meaningful because they indicate a person's progression along the normal developmental continuum. Often these norms are used to describe highly specific functions, as in the Denver Developmental Screening Test subscales of Personal-Social, Five Motor-Adaptive, Language, and Gross Motor (Frankenburg & Dodds, 1967). Such scales can indicate that a four-year-old youngster's current behavior is about like that of other four-year-old children in the personal-social area, more like five-year-old children in the language area, but more typical of three-year-old children in the gross motor area.

However useful that scale can be, a problem arises in the comparison of mental ages. Growth from four to five years of age is not equivalent to growth in mental age from twelve to thirteen, because mental functions develop more rapidly at early than at late ages.

Developmental norms are found almost exclusively in tests for young children and severely handicapped individuals. Among such tests are the Bayley Scales of Infant Development (Bayley, 1969) and Developmental Activities Screening Inventory (DASI-II) (Fewell & Langley, 1984). These norms are especially useful in clinical case studies, screening, and longitudinal research, but they are not exact enough for many types of statistical treatment (Anastasi, 1976).

*Age Score Norms.* The scores in the Denver Scale are age scores. Another type of age score is mental age. This type of score became well known because of its use on the Binet-Simon scales and their various revisions. In the standardization, items answered correctly by a majority of persons in a given age group were assigned to that age group on the test. The process was continued until there were sufficient items at each age level. Consequently, a six-year-old child who passes a majority of items appropriate for eight-year-old children is said to have a mental age of eight.

Age scores are sometimes used in achievement tests. However, because age and educational experience often do not go hand in hand, age scores can sometimes be misleading. "Because progress in school achievement does *not* depend upon chronological age, but exposure to the learning situation in the classroom . . . age norms should not be used for achievement tests" (Hagen, 1961, p. 12). However, most currently available tests provide both age and grade norms.

*Grade Equivalent Norms.* One of the most popular ways in which educational achievement test results are interpreted is in the form of grade equivalent scores. What could be more obvious than to describe a child's performance in comparison with his grade-level peers?

Unfortunately, the popularity of grade equivalent scores is probably based on a misunderstanding of what such scores actually reveal. One often hears a parent say happily, "My child was at grade level in all areas." Teachers, generally with much satisfaction, inform their principal that their students were at grade level in reading. The only problem with this is that grade level scores cannot be taken as a standard of excellence. The norms generally are taken from many different school districts, some with good programs and some with very poor programs. Consequently, performance that is only at grade level could mean poor student effort and poor instruction.

Furthermore, grade equivalent scores are in most cases median scores; that is, 50% of the scores of the norm group are higher and 50% are lower. This means that if half the students in a class score above grade level and half score below grade level, their performance is similar to the norm group. Most teachers would be unhappy with such a performance by their class. Because grade equivalent scores are not standards of excellence, neither happiness nor unhappiness is justified.

Another problem is that grade norms are appropriate only for subject matter studied throughout the grade levels covered by the test. For example, students who take more history, English, and fine arts courses than science and mathematics courses in high school are not likely to do well on achievement tests in the latter two areas. Students who took no courses in mathematics and science past the tenth grade would probably not score higher than tenth grade on an achievement test in these areas, even though they could be seniors in high school. The testing would reflect their exposure to the subject, but there is a tendency to interpret the results as though the students had had twelve years of instruction in mathematics and science.

Also, scoring three grades higher than their actual grade placement does not mean that children have mastered the academic material at that higher grade level. Most likely they did extremely well on material at or slightly above their grade placement, and thereby accrued raw score points similar to those of youngsters at the higher placement. These students are *probably* competent at their grade level, but there is no basis for assumptions that they are ready for material three grade levels above their current placement.

Still another problem is that grade equivalent scores of 3.4 in reading and mathematics do not mean that the performance in reading and math is equivalent. If the child is in third grade, it is likely that the mathematics score represents a higher percentile ranking than does the reading score. Typically, mathematics and spelling scores are closely related to the school curriculum, whereas reading, language arts, and social studies tend to reflect more directly a combination of out-of-school experience plus the school curriculum (Hagen, 1961).

Because of these numerous shortcomings, many school districts are discontinuing the use of grade equivalent scores in favor of percentiles and standard scores. Obviously, grade equivalent scores do not meet any of the three characteristics of test scores proposed by Thorndike and Hagen (1969). Consequently, they are of limited use in educational measurement.

## Guidelines for Excellence

Through the efforts of the American Psychological Association, the American Educational Research Association, and the National Council on Measurement in Education, the *Standards for Educational and Psychological Testing* was published first in 1966 and revised in 1971 and 1985. No other single factor has contributed so much toward the improvement of tests and testing practices. It is the bible for test developers and test users.

The *Standards* covers three broad categories of testing instruments: "constructed performance tasks, questionnaires, and to a lesser extent structured behavior samples.... It will generally not be possible, however, to apply the standards with the same rigor to the broad range of unstructured behavior samples that are used in some forms of clinical and school psychological assessments and to instructor-made tests that are used to evaluate student performance in education and training" (AERA, APA, & NCRE, 1985, p. 4).

Because no test manual can include all the optimal information, the standards are grouped into two levels: primary and secondary. Primary standards should be met by all tests before they are made available for general use; these standards should also be met by all test users unless there are compelling professional reasons why they have not been or cannot be met in a particular case. Secondary standards are worthy as goals but are "beyond reasonable expectations in many situations" (AERA, APA, & NCRE, 1985, p. 3). Some standards are designated as conditional; that is, they should be treated in some situations as primary and in others as secondary. The trade-off in such situations is between the potential consequences for a significant number of test takers and the feasibility of meeting the standards.

Specific application of the standards must involve professional judgment based on a knowledge of psychometrics, behavioral science, and the field in which the application is being made. The first time the standards are applied to a test the process will seem long and tedious; but after they have evaluated several tests and testing practices, educational diagnosticians with appropriate training will be able to use the standards readily.

On some occasions the test user will not require the detailed information that is provided by a complete and systematic use of the standards. In such cases, a helpful source on published tests is *The Ninth Annual Mental Measurements Yearbook* (Mitchell, 1985). This publication provides factual information on the tests, "candidly critical test reviews," and extensive bibliographies. The test reviews are most helpful because they often are written by persons who use the test and who are authorities in the particular content field.

Another source for test evaluations is the series of publications from the Center for the Study of Evaluation, University of California, Los Angeles (1971, 1974, 1976). The series includes tests at the preschool and kindergarten, elementary, and secondary levels. The last is divided into three volumes, covering tests for grades seven and eight, nine and ten, and eleven and twelve. The series uses the *MEAN* evaluation procedures. MEAN is an acronym that refers to the four general areas in which the tests are evaluated: measurement validity, examinee appropriateness, administrative usability, and normed technical excellence. Each subcategory within these areas is rated along a numerical scale. This rating system makes it possible for a test user who needs a measure with a very high reliability or a measure that is very easy to administer, to identify such a test within a given area. A total score, which has a specific meaning, is also given. An elementary test with a total of twelve to fifteen points is endorsed by the Center for general use and specifically for use in its projects.

Another unique aspect of this series is that the tests are organized in categories based on a taxonomy of goals for that grade level. For example, one goal in the language arts area is language construction. In that category is still another subcategory, grammar and usage, under which are listed two subtests from tests of language. A carefully constructed index helps users find the references to specific tests, if that is their need. Unfortunately, these books are out of print and are available only through libraries.

With the help of the *Standards, The Ninth Annual Mental Measurement Yearbook* and the Center for the Study of Evaluation series, test users have available whatever level of evaluation they need. The latter two are especially useful for the prospective test buyer, because to use the aids, the buyer does not have to have the test.

## CRITERION-REFERENCED TESTS

Glaser and Klaus (1962) were the first to use the term "criterion-referenced measures." They stated: Underlying the concept of proficiency measurement is a continuum of skill ranging from no proficiency at all to perfect performance. ... The degree to which his proficiency resembles desired performance at any specified level is assessed by *criterion-referenced measures* of proficiency.

Proficiency measures which reflect a continuum of attainment usually imply cumulative level achievement, in that a master machinist is also proficient at the tasks required at the apprentice and journeyman levels. Knowledge of an individual's score on a criterion-referenced measure provides explicit information as to what an individual can or cannot do. ... In this sense, criterion-referenced measures indicate the content of the behavioral repertoire and the correspondence between what an individual does and the underlying continuum of proficiency. Measures which assess performance in terms of a criterion standard thus provide information as to the degree of competence attained which is independent of the performance of others. [pp. 421–422]*

Glaser further elaborated his ideas on criterion-referenced measurement, and more precisely distinguished it from norm-referenced measurement, in an essay published in 1963, which was the stimulus for the deluge of articles that started to appear after a period of six years had passed. In 1978 Popham stated, "... In 1968 Ted Husek and I were so frustrated with our measurement colleagues for not moving faster that we wrote an article to get our friends off their tails and interested in the field of criterion-referenced testing" (p. 17). Since the Popham and Husek (1969) article was published, very few issues of journals in educational research have appeared without at least one article on criterion-referenced measurement. Gray (1978) reviewed the different uses of the term and cited almost forty authors and co-authors who gave more than fifty descriptions of criterion-referenced measurement.

In a Johns Hopkins National Symposium on Educational Research in 1978, Berk (1980) treated domain-referenced and mastery tests as two types of criterion-referenced measurement. Domain-referenced tests were thus identified in Popham's definition of criterion-referenced testing: "A criterion-referenced test is used to ascertain an individual's status with respect to a well-defined behavioral domain" (Popham, 1978). Berk (1980) described a mastery test as one

> ... used to classify students as masters or non-masters of an objective in order to expedite individualized instruction. Empirical item analysis procedures are recommended to determine whether the items are instructionally sensitive or discriminate between instructed and uninstructed groups. Methods for setting absolute performance standards for mastery and the estimation of classification errors are particularly important (p. 5).

*From *Psychological Principles in System Development,* edited by Robert M. Gagné. Copyright © 1962 by Holt, Rinehart and Winston, Inc. Reprinted by permission of Holt, Rinehart and Winston.

In an effort to systematize the burgeoning body of knowledge, Nitko (1980) developed a taxonomical classification that integrates the various concepts of criterion-referenced testing. Interestingly, some of his categories are exemplified by tests whose authors would deny that they are criterion-referenced; some tests were developed more than fifty years before the term was first used. Nitko's two-dimensional classification system, which covers only achievement tests, is shown in Table 2-2. Tests are grouped according to their domains, as well-defined, ill-defined, or undefined. Nitko considers a domain to be well-defined when it is clear to both the test developer and the test user those types of tasks that could or could not be considered to be part of the domain. The well-defined domain is further subdivided into ordered and unordered domains.

In the well-defined categories are such tests as those measures of proficiencies to which the original Glaser and Klaus article (1962) referred. In another category are tests of Gagné's learning hierarchies (1977). The Key Math Test, which is frequently used by educational diagnosticians, is listed as an example of ordering based on an empirically defined latent trait.

The "well-defined but unordered" category includes tests in which the stimulus properties of the items are verbally described; these tests include Ebel's Content Standard English Vocabulary Test (1962). "To focus on defining and sampling from a domain of words is to focus on stimuli, rather than centering attention on a stimulus-response complex or focusing on abstractions or constructs used to explain and/or interpret several stimulus-response complexes" (Nitko, 1980, p. 473). Also included in this domain are tests such as those based on Hively's (1973) Item Forms and Popham's (1978) criterion-referenced tests.

The category of ill-defined domains includes those tests based on behavioral objectives that are so ambiguous that it is impossible for any agreement of what should or should not be included in the domain to be obtained. Another type of test included in this category is one in which the items define the domain and thus preclude further generalization.

Within the undefined domain are those tests in which no attempt was made to define a body of knowledge to which the test performance could be referenced. Nitko also included in this category those tests labeled criterion-referenced whose authors confused Glaser's (1963) and Mager's (1962) use of the word "criterion." A cutoff score for these tests is set without any attempt being made to define the domain of behavior being assessed.

Nitko noted that the scheme is not exhaustive. However, it does bring into clear focus major similarities and differences among several types of criterion-referenced tests. Perhaps the most important function of the taxonomy is the emphasis on well-defined domains of behavior. The essence of a criterion-referenced test is the knowledge of what is and is not included in the referenced domain. This knowledge is necessary for the person who must develop the specific items on the test, for the diagnostician who must decide which test to administer and how to interpret the results, and for the person who receives the interpretation.

## Test Construction

The construction of criterion-referenced tests involves a series of steps that are at least as complex as those required in development of a norm-referenced test. First the domain specifications must be developed and items constructed that conform to these specifications. Popham (1978, pp. 138–140) gives an example of test specifications "for those whom time-telling passed by" (Figure 2-6). According to this procedure, the first task is the development of test specifications that communicate to the user what the test is measuring and that describe the procedure by which "functionally" homogeneous items can be generated. According to Popham, test specifications should include five components: general description, sample items, stimulus attributes, response attributes, and specification supplement. The specification supplement, which is not always included, usually consists of a list of possible additional content. After the items are developed they must be field tested and revised as is necessary, and the revised items must be field tested. From these items, test forms are developed (Haladyna & Roid, 1983; Hively, 1973; Roid & Haladyna, 1982).

The development of test forms is a very involved process. The first task is to decide which items should be included. To determine the method of item selection that minimized the error of measurement, Haladyna and Roid (1983) compared a random selection of items with a stratified, adaptive testing procedure. The latter procedure, which is based on item response theory, is a method by which items are first grouped into strata according to their level of difficulty; items are then selected from the resulting difficulty level that matches the examinees' level of ability. These authors' comparison revealed that although the random sampling approach "guarantees a moderate but controllable amount of measurement error," adaptive testing "provides a chance for superior precision provided there is an accurate means of assigning each student the test of appropriate difficulty level" (p. 279). In regard to test length they found that "satisfactory precision" can be obtained with tests containing between twenty and thirty items. They concluded "that the use of item response theory to calibrate items can result in what is called a curriculum referenced scale (Rentz, 1982; Woodcock, 1982) if items can be shown to have adequate model-data fit" (p. 279).

Harris and Subkoviak (1986) examined three statistical methods for the selection of items for what they called "mastery tests." The first method was the pretest-posttest method proposed by Cox and Vargas (1966). The second was the latent trait method recommended by van der Linden (1981), and the third was a method, developed by the authors, that they called the *agreement statistic*. Harris and Subkoviak (1986) found that the pretest-

**Table 2-2**

Classification system for criterion-referenced test (characterization of domains of behavior for achievement testing).

| Well-defined and ordered domains | | Well-defined but unordered domains | | | Ill-defined domains | Undefined domains |
|---|---|---|---|---|---|---|
| Basis* for scaling or ordering the defined domain of behavior | Examples† | Basis for delineating behavior domain‡ | Area of emphasis during test development | Examples† | | |
| Judged social or esthetic quality of performance | Thorndike's Handwriting Scales (1909) | Stimulus properties of domain and sampling plan of test | Defining content and content strata | Ebel's Content Standard English Vocabulary Test (1962) | Poorly articulated behavioral objectives; defining the domain only in terms of the particular items on the test | No attempt to define a domain to which test performance is referenced: using a cutoff score but not defining a performance domain |
| Complexity or difficulty level of subject matter | Cox and Graham's Arithmetic Scale (1966) | | Specifying stimulus properties of item domains | Hively's Item Forms (1966, 1968, 1973) | | |
| Degree of proficiency with which complex skills are performed | Glaser's Criterion-Referenced Measures II (1962–1963) | | Specifying precise relationship between instructional content and item domain | Bormuth's Transformational Rules (1970) | | |
| Prerequisite sequence of acquiring intellectual and psychomotor skills | Gagné's Learning Hierarchies (1968) | Verbal statements of stimuli and responses in domain | Behavioral objectives with or without the cutoff score (criterion) specified | Popham and Husek's Criterion-Referenced Testing (1969) | | |
| Location on empirically defined latent trait | Connolly, Nachtman, and Pritchett Key Math Arithmetic Tests (1976) | | Elaborated descriptions of behavior and stimuli | Popham's Criterion-Referenced Tests (1978) | | |

| Diagnostic categories of performance | Identifying entry-level behaviors | Hunt and Kirk's Tests of School Readiness (1974) |
| | Identifying behavior components missing from a complex performance | Tests built on Resnik's Component Analysis (1973) and Gagné's Two-State Testing (1970) |
| | Identifying and categorizing erroneous responses | Nesbit's CHILD Program (1966); Hsu's Computer-assisted Diagnostic Tests (1972) |
| | Identifying erroneous processes | Beck's Blending Algorithm (1972); interview to determine what processes were used in responding |
| Abstractions, traits, or constructs | Specifying specific behaviors or categories of behaviors that delimit the abstraction, trait, or construct | Tests based on the Taxonomy of Educational Objectives (Bloom, 1956); certain basic-skills surveys |

Adapted from Nitko, A. J. Distinguishing the many varieties of criterion-referenced tests. *Review of Educational Research*, 1980, *50*, 461–485. © 1980, American Educational Research Association, Washington, D.C.
*Other bases for scaling or ordering the defined domain of behavior exist.
†Examples are illustrative, not representative or exhaustive.
‡Other bases for delineating exist.

GENERAL DESCRIPTION: When presented with sketches of various types of clock faces depicting different times, the examinee will be able to select from numerical alternatives the time coinciding with that presented in the pictorial clock.

SAMPLE ITEM: For the clock pictured at the left, circle the letter of the time at the right that is represented by the clock.

*Stimulus attributes*

1. The clock faces should be round or square, approximately the size of a U.S. quarter. The clock faces, roughly sketched, may represent any temporal moment as long as the time depicted is in five minute units.
2. Arabic or roman numerals may be used, or no numerals whatsoever. In the latter instance, dots or a similar designator may be employed to represent some or all of the numbers 1–12.
3. The minute hand will only be directed at points on the clock representing five minute increments in time (e.g., 5:10 or 5:15), never at points between these five minute markers (e.g., 5:17 or 5:06). The hour hand should accurately reflect, at least approximately, a position between hour markers consistent with the location of the minute hand.
4. No digital clock faces will be used.

*Response attributes*

1. Four answer options will be presented, one of which corresponds to the time depicted by the clock, with hour(s) first, followed by a colon, then minutes. All answer options will reflect five minute intervals.
2. Incorrect answers may be:
   a. The time that would be depicted by the clock if the minute and hour hand had been reversed.
   b. A time of five minutes earlier or later than the correct time.
   c. The transposal of the correct time, for example, 15:3 instead of 3:15.
   d. Only the even-numbered hour, 4:00, instead of the pictured 4:20.
   e. A time with the correct minutes but an hour figure one hour earlier or later than the correct time.
   f. A time randomly selected.
3. The order of correct and incorrect answer options will be random.

**Figure 2-6**
For those whom time-telling passed by. From W. James Popham,
*Criterion-referenced measurement.* © 1978, pp. 138–140. Reprinted by
permission of Prentice-Hall, Inc., Englewood Cliffs, N.J.

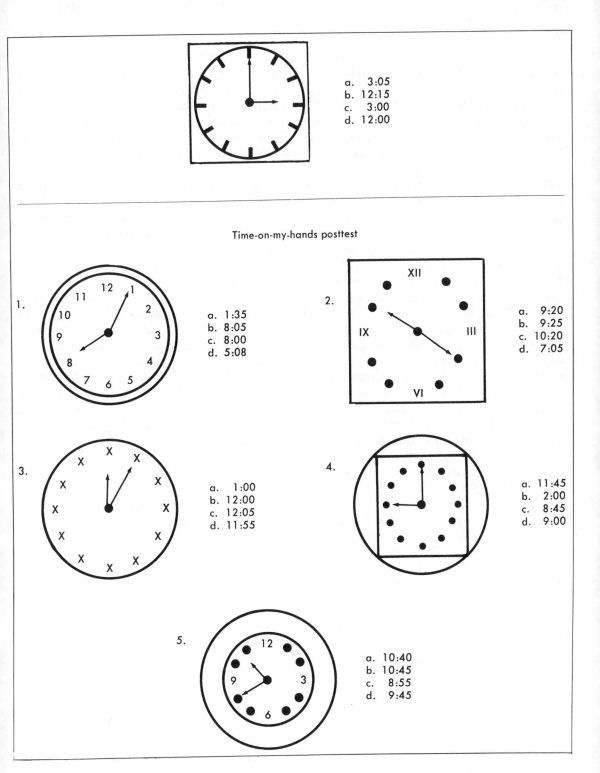

a. 3:05
b. 12:15
c. 3:00
d. 12:00

Time-on-my-hands posttest

1.
a. 1:35
b. 8:05
c. 8:00
d. 5:08

2.
a. 9:20
b. 9:25
c. 10:20
d. 7:05

3.
a. 1:00
b. 12:00
c. 12:05
d. 11:55

4.
a. 11:45
b. 2:00
c. 8:45
d. 9:00

5.
a. 10:40
b. 10:45
c. 8:55
d. 9:45

**Figure 2-6** *continued*

57

posttest method had several serious limita- tions, although it has the advantage of being computationally simple. The latent trait statis- tic, based on the concept of a specific item characteristic curve, "assesses the power of an item to discriminate at a given cutoff point" (Harris & Subkoviak, 1986, p. 497). A simplifi- cation of the equation that defines the item characteristic curve is known as the Rasch (1960, 1966) model. This model (Wright & Stone, 1979) is the basis of item selection procedures for a number of widely used tests, such as the Woodcock Reading Mastery Test-Revised (Woodcock, 1987). Use of the latent trait statistic can result in appropriate item selection, but its calculation requires a computer and appropriate software.

The agreement procedure is similar in many ways to the latent trait statistic, but the agree- ment procedure is easier to calculate. "Items selected by the agreement statistic were found to overlap to a large extent with items selected by the latent trait statistic" (Harris & Subkoviak, 1986, p. 505), but of the two, the agreement statistic is much simpler to calculate.

Also involved in the assembling of test forms is the problem of determining appropriate cutoff scores, the score that separates masters from nonmasters. In his work, van der Linder (1984) ar- gued that decision theory offered an adequate ap- proach to the setting of cutoff scores, because "tests are more often used for decision making than for measurement purposes" (p. 9). Decision theory involves the definition of classes of deci- sion rules and the evaluation of their properties against "certain criteria of optimality" (p. 10). However, de Gruijter and Hambleton (1984) pointed out five problems that can arise when de- cision theory is used to set cutoff scores. On the other hand, Glass (1980) reiterated a position he stated in 1976, that "To my knowledge, every at- tempt to derive a criterion score is either blatantly arbitrary or derives from a set of arbitrary premises." He concluded, " 'Goodness' and 'bad- ness' must be replaced by the essentially compar- ative concepts of 'better' and 'worse.' " This notion

seems compatible with the way educators view progress in learning; because scholars cannot agree on other methods by which cutoff scores should be set, repeated measures that will help the test-maker evaluate better and worse might be the best procedure at this time.

Although criterion-referenced tests do have some unique characteristics—such as the fact that they assess level of knowledge or skill in a domain rather than comparing the individual's performance with that of the norm group—there are similarities to norm-referenced test con- struction. When multiple-choice, true-false, or other common formats are used, the same item-writing rules apply regardless of whether the test is norm- or criterion-referenced. In what Popham (1978) referred to as a "bit of heresy," he suggested that the collection of normative data for criterion-referenced tests is desirable. He stated, "Without comparative data, criterion- referenced measures will never win acceptance of the many citizens, legislators, and educators who are properly asking, 'Is the schools' perfor- mance good enough?' " (p. 171).

**Test Scores**

Harris (1974) and Alkin (1974) presented five "metrics" that are directly interpretable in terms of the referenced domains:

1. A rate metric simply refers to the time it takes to complete the specified task.
2. A sign metric indicates the mastery or non- mastery of the task.
3. An accuracy metric gives the proportion of times the examinee is successful/unsuccess- ful.
4. A proportion metric specifies the portion or percentage of the items in a domain on which the student performs accurately.
5. A scaling metric describes the point along a continuum at which the student's perfor- mance occurs.

Ebel (1962) makes a cogent defense of the use of content standard test scores: the "percent of a systematic sample which an individual has performed successfully" (p. 15). Although Ebel has been something of an opponent of criterion-referenced tests, his description of content standard test scores is remarkably similar to current descriptions of criterion-referenced tests and their scoring procedures. For example, he says the word "content" indicated that the score was directly interpretable in terms of the tasks or content of the test. The word "standard" referred to the use of a common scale, the percentage of items the individual has answered correctly. "Administration and scoring are explicit and objective enough so that independent investigators would obtain substantially the same scores for the same persons" (Ebel, 1962, p. 16). The content standard test score is a proportion metric (Harris, 1974) and essentially a raw score. Thorndike and Hagen (1969) argue that a raw score in and of itself is generally meaningless and that only derived scores such as percentiles and standard scores are meaningful. This is a poor argument and suggests a blind spot on their part. In fact, a percentile is meaningless unless you know the test content and the characteristics of the norm group. A raw score or content standard test score, to use Ebel's (1962) phrase, is meaningful if the content domain and test specification are clearly and precisely described.

Nitko (1974), in the same "bit of heresy" proposed by Popham (1978), stated that all the typical norm-referenced test scores we have discussed in this chapter can also be obtained for criterion-referenced tests. He argued as Popham did that "relating acquired levels of performance to chances of being successful in new instructional situations broadens the interpretation of criterion-referenced scores" (p. 77).

In summary, criterion-referenced test scores generally depend on the types of metrics described by Harris (1974) and Alkin (1974). Several of these are basically what has been described in the past as raw scores. Popham (1978) and Nitko (1974) have suggested that the types of scores most often associated with norm-referenced measurement could also be useful in expanding the interpretation of criterion-referenced measures.

## Guidelines for Excellence

Selecting well-constructed, criterion-referenced tests is a major problem for educators. Because the shortcomings of standardized norm-referenced tests are being regularly demonstrated in many journals, many educators are seeking alternative measurement approaches. Tests labeled criterion-referenced are beginning to appear in test catalogs; some seem to be included for the sole purpose of taking advantage of this relatively new concept in testing. Unfortunately, many of these tests fall into Nitko's (1980) category of tests having ill-defined or undefined domains. Popham (1978) has suggested six characteristics of a well-constructed criterion-referenced test that are helpful in evaluation:

1. *Unambiguous descriptive scheme.* As Popham (1978), Nitko (1980), Hively (1973), and Ebel (1962) have repeatedly stated, there must be a clear description of what behavior is and is not included in a criterion-referenced measure. Popham's test specification and Hively's items forms are examples.
2. *Adequate number of items per measured behavior.* The question that always goes with such a statement is, "What is adequate?" The answer that often follows in educational measurement is, "That depends on the kind of decision that is to be made." Obviously if such a test is the final step in the certification of educational diagnosticians, as it is in the state of New Mexico, five questions per behavioral domain would be inadequate. On the other hand, if the test is to measure one subset in a behavioral domain in which there will be other measures administered, five items may well be very adequate. Novick and Lewis (1974) recommended "guidelines which effectively say that it is very desirable to have test lengths of twelve or less, tolerable but undesirable to have test lengths as high

as twenty, and discomforting to have tests that are longer than this" (p. 158). Popham (1978) also indicated that between five and twenty items per measured behavior was a useful rule of thumb. However, in an empirical study, Haladyna and Roid (1983) obtained "satisfactory precision" with twenty to thirty items per test. Obviously the length of the test is directly related to the number of concepts to be measured.

3. *Sufficiently limited focus.* How does one define *sufficiently* and *limited*? Popham (1978) suggested that the main goal here is to avoid tests that obviously have a very broad focus. One way to do this is to ask whether the number of measured behaviors is limited enough that the test user would be able to take "meaningful action based on the test results." In other words, would the test user be able to pinpoint student problems and instructional difficulties well enough to know where to introduce changes in the student's program?

4. *High level of reliability (measurement of test consistency).* If educators are to use criterion-referenced tests to make decisions about instructional programs, the tests must help the educator make appropriate decisions regarding program changes (Popham, 1978). Reliability on a student-by-student basis is only necessary when the test is to be used in the planning of individual student programs.

5. *Adequate validity (what the test says it measures).* Popham (1978) stated that test manuals should supply data on three types of validity. The first of these involves a description of the process by which the specific behaviors in the given domain were selected. Second, evidence of the degree of congruence between the description of the items in the manual and the actual items on the test is required. Third, when specific uses of tests are described in the manual, validity data on each of the uses should be provided.

6. *Sufficient comparative test data.* A precise description of what a student can do only answers some of the questions asked by educators and parents. Generally, they also want to know how this behavior compares with the behavior of other children with similar backgrounds. Popham (1978) admitted that serving this need would result in a test that is both norm-referenced, with one reference point being the norm group, and criterion-referenced, with a domain of content as the other reference point. Although such a test could be possible with some simple content domains, it would be difficult to construct and probably very long.

Hambleton and Eignor (1978) developed a detailed set of guidelines for the evaluation of criterion-referenced tests and test manuals; their guidelines are similar in format to the *Standards for Educational and Psychological Tests and Manuals* (AERA, APS, & NCME, 1985). They developed the guidelines by asking, "What questions would we want to answer before making a decision to use a criterion-referenced test in a particular situation?" (p. 322). They organized their guidelines around ten categories: objectives, test items, administration, test layout, reliability, cutoff scores, validity, norms, reporting of test score information, and test score interpretations. The guidelines were then used to evaluate the eleven commercially available criterion-referenced tests shown in Table 2-3. Most of these tests are referenced to objectives. None of the manuals included test specifications in the way Popham (1978) and Hively (1973) used the term. Hambleton and Eignor also found no rationale offered for levels at which cutoff scores were set and major problems with explanations and procedures used in item analysis.

## CURRICULUM-BASED ASSESSMENT

Curriculum-based assessment is a relatively new term that describes what teachers have been

**Table 2-3**
Tests selected for review.

| Code | Test | Grades | Levels | Forms | Publication date | Publisher |
|------|------|--------|--------|-------|------------------|-----------|
| 1 | 1976 Stanford Diagnostic Mathematics Test | 1–12 | 4 | 2 | 1976 | Harcourt Brace Jovanovich |
| 2 | 1976 Stanford Diagnostic Reading Test | 1–12 | 4 | 2 | 1976 | Harcourt Brace Jovanovich |
| 3 | Skills Monitoring System—Reading | 3–5 | 3 | 5 | 1975 | Harcourt Brace Jovanovich |
| 4 | Individual Pupil Monitoring System—Mathematics | 1–6 | 6 | 2 | 1975 | Houghton Mifflin |
| 5 | Individual Pupil Monitoring System—Mathematics | 1–8 | 8 | 2 | 1975 | Houghton Mifflin |
| 6 | Diagnostic Mathematics Inventory | 1.5–7.5 | 7 | 1 | 1977 | CTB/McGraw-Hill |
| 7 | Prescriptive Reading Inventory | K–6.5 | 6 | 1 | 1977 | CTB/McGraw-Hill |
| 8 | Diagnosis: An Instructional Aid—Mathematics and Reading | 1–6 | 2 | 2 | 1974 | Science Research Associates |
| 9 | Mastery: An Evaluation Tool—SOBAR Reading | K–9 | 10 | 2 | 1975 | Science Research Associates |
| 10 | Mastery: An Evaluation Tool—Mathematics | K–8 | 9 | 2 | 1974 | Science Research Associates |
| 11 | Fountain Valley Support System in Mathematics | K–8 | 9 | 1 | 1974 | Richard L. Zweig Associates |

attempting to do for a very long time. It is a form of criterion-referenced assessment (Neisworth & Bagnato, 1986) in which the criterion being referenced is the school curriculum. As criterion-referenced testing grew out of the belief that standardized tests were not the optimal means for the evaluation of either individual students or instructional programs, curriculum-based assessment was developed because of the perception that criterion (domain)-referenced testing did not produce the most effective database for instructors to use in their making of day-to-day instructional decisions for individual students as they progress or fail to progress through school curriculum.

The need to tie assessment more closely to curriculum appears to have come from the demand for accountability in school programs. These demands were first made on early childhood programs. The federal government provided enormous sums of money for such programs as Head Start, which included an extensive assessment component. Unfortunately, the instructional program and the evaluation program were not closely related, and, as might be expected, the results of the evaluations were in general not supportive of the instructional program. In recent years the discrepancy between curriculum and assessment goals has been reduced; early-childhood educators have declared the need for a close relationship between assessment systems and the early-childhood curriculum (Bailey & Bricker, 1986; Paget & Nagle, 1986). However, the call for a link between assessment and curriculum is not limited to the early-childhood area (Baker & Herman, 1983; Fuchs & Fuchs, 1986a; Linn, 1983).

Another way of looking at the problem of linkage between assessment and curriculum is that the instruments that have been used, whether they are norm-referenced or criterion-referenced, did not have adequate content validity. To some extent this problem is alleviated when the test items are drawn from the content covered in the curriculum. The problem is not entirely solved, however. As Neisworth and Bagnato (1986) noted, "Curriculum based assessment can be no better than the curriculum it employs" (p. 181), and they present guidelines for an optimal curriculum. Thus, an assessment system based on a poor curriculum could show excellent progress in the curriculum, when in fact the students' knowledge and skills in the domain were very limited.

A review of the curriculum-based assessment literature shows that relatively little attention has been given to the evaluation of tests' construction procedures, reliability, and validity. For example, Deno (1985) cited as evidence of the validity of a curriculum-based reading test, the fact that scores on their test were highly correlated with scores on norm-referenced reading tests. Later in the same article he argued that these same norm-referenced tests were not reliable measures of a student's improvement in reading. At best the reasoning is circular. However, he also presented data comparing performance on the reading measure by different types of students: students in special education, in Chapter 1 programs, and in regular education. These data support the criterion validity of

the measure. Fuchs, Fuchs, and Deno (1982) investigated the reliability and validity of procedures used in the selection of passages and the setting of criteria for mastery, for curriculum-based informal reading inventories. They found that the procedure of arbitrarily selecting passages from reading texts did not produce reliable data, because there are great differences in the readability levels of reading texts used in their study, that are purported to be at the same reading level; there are variations even in passages from the same text.

Fuchs, Fuchs, and Deno (1982) also investigated the validity of several criteria used in determining instructional level. Some of these criteria, including the traditional, informal reading-inventory criteria of 95% accuracy, were appropriate and others would lead to erroneous conclusions. Other authors (Idol, Nevin, & Paolucci-Whitcomb, 1986) apparently have assumed that, by basing the test on the curriculum and by collaborating on these tasks with the classroom teacher and the consulting teacher, researchers can solve problems in item construction, item selection, item sequence, test form development, performance criteria, reliability, and validity. On the other hand, these authors describe extensive and time-consuming procedures in which students are administered alternate forms on separate occasions. Various other procedures are also described but no data are presented to support the validity of the procedures. Time required to implement assessment tasks is an important factor for the teacher. Wesson, King, and Deno (1984) found that, without careful training, teachers tend to become inefficient in the use of direct and frequent measurement of student performance, and the common perception that such procedures take too much time could in fact be true.

Another problem with curriculum-based assessment that has not been addressed adequately is the fact that the curriculum on which the assessment is based changes on a regular basis, often in relation to textbook adoption. The extent to which the tests will have to be revised with each major curriculum change has yet to be explored.

Curriculum-based measurement is an important aspect of the instructional program. Its use in diagnosis, classification, and program evaluation has yet to be established. Undoubtedly research will continue on the problems and solutions will be found. On a discouraging note, the most significant problems in curriculum-based assessment are the same ones that have plagued norm-referenced assessment for a long time.

## SUMMARY

The type of test selected should be determined by the purpose of the testing. Norm-referenced tests are the instruments of choice when the task at hand is to diagnose or determine eligibility for placement in special programs. When the need is to plan for instruction, to evaluate the effectiveness of an instructional program, or to determine progress in a school curriculum, criterion-referenced or curriculum-based tests are the most appropriate. However, regardless of the type of educational test data available, a careful analysis of items answered correctly and incorrectly will provide useful information for teaching. Many problems remain in item construction, item selection, test form development, performance criteria, and reliability and validity. Educational personnel must rely on aids in test evaluation such as the *Standards for Educational and Psychological Tests and Manuals*.

# CHAPTER 3

# Measurement

## Reliability and Validity

### OUTLINE

Nonabsolute properties of testing
Reliability
Validity
Summary

**C** hapter 2 reviewed some key issues in the selection of norm-referenced versus criterion-referenced measures. However, an important assumption in an assessment process is that tests are *indirect measurements* of a child's functioning. In other words, not all classroom behavior is directly measurable; therefore, not all of a child's activities can be described as observable phenomena (see Chapter 8 for discussion). Testing a child implies quantifiability, and quantifiability means that some number can be applied to behavior. For instance, silent reading might require that ten questions be answered. A score on a numerical scale of 1 to 10 can be assigned from answers to the comprehensive questions at the end of the passage. Similarly, a specific occurrence of silent reading comprehension might be regarded as *adequate* according to a comprehension rating scale composed of three categories: competent, adequate, deficient. (Specific aspects of this measurement will be introduced later.)

At first thought, it may seem that there is no such thing as unmeasurable activity. If a teacher can test the occurrence or existence of a specific activity, it can be measured, the assumption here being that existence and quantification are the same thing. This assumption might be true for a low level of analysis involving factors such as reading comprehension performance or conduct problems. But the technical aspects of measuring child performance go beyond the simple question of occurrence or existence.

## NONABSOLUTE PROPERTIES OF TESTING

When one takes into account the technical aspects of measurement, one can see that the activities that occur refer to the characteristic of the measurement device, not whether that behavior exists or does not exist. For example, a measuring device must be consistent in the value or number achieved in successive applications (must be reliable) as well as measure what it is supposed to measure (must be valid). Unfortunately, reliability and validity are not absolute properties of measurement. They are only relative in degrees less than 100%. In other words, a teacher cannot assume that a raw score represents an accurate picture of the child's ability or knowledge. The score can be influenced by chance events or inadequacies of the test. Regardless of these difficulties, even if the child's obtained score is a true score, measurement provides only indirect information into childhood thinking or problem solving. Let us illustrate with a child's statement: "I see green martians." It is quite difficult to check the existence or nonexistence of that concept within the child because there is no way an observer can get inside the child's brain and determine whether the child's green martians are green as the observer views green or if the child actually sees martians. Thus there is no way to invalidate the existence or nonexistence of that event's reliability from the child's perspective. The individual's verbal report cannot reliably and validly be used in the quantification of aspects of introspective, conscious experience. The individual's verbal report can be reliably and validly used, however, in the quantification of other indirect aspects of the individual's thinking. A verbal report is essentially speech and can be reliably and validly quantified by an external observer.

Although test scores are at best an indirect measure of thinking, an appropriate test can yield measurements that are meaningful and dependable. The meaningfulness of the score depends on the test's content (appropriateness of material) and the nature of the norm group (see Chapter 2). One aspect of the dependability of tests is their reliability.

## RELIABILITY

A standardized test instrument provides a score that consists of two components: a *true score* and an *error component*. A true score is a child-obtained score uncontaminated by chance events or conditions, and an error component (error of measurement) reflects the extent to which scores are attributable to chance. An *obtained* or *raw score* is the measure the child receives on a test.

The relationship between obtained score, true score, and error component is represented by the formula Obtained score = True score + Error component. For a measuring instrument yielding an obtained score, most of the variability of scores can be attributed to variations in the true score. An obtained score would be unsatisfactory if most of its variability (Chapter 2) were a reflection of chance. The variations in a child's obtained score represent the degree to which the measuring instrument is reliable. The obtained scores of a highly unreliable test reflect many variations that are caused by chance.

Therefore, in a broad sense, the reliability of a child's obtained score is the extent to which it (obtained score) is attributable to "true" score difference and chance errors. Although reliability can be defined as the consistency of a child's obtained scores on the same test or equivalent items tested on different occasions, it more technically relates to the ratio of true to obtained scores. We know that if a test is given twice to an individual, the same score will probably not be obtained on each administration: scores vary from one administration to another. Repeating the measurement permits an estimate of the true score to be made, and the error of measurement of a single score to be noted. Therefore reliability can be defined as (1) the degree to which score variance results from the true score, or (2) the extent of the subject's performance that will remain constant with repeated administration.

No one can completely divide each measurement into a true score and an error component, because the reliability of the instrument has to be determined by indirect means. However, consistency in measurement is necessary for the determination of test stability. As stated by Popham (1980):

> Suppose you were to sit down on a deserted tropical isle, bookless but not brainless, and try to figure out what qualities a good assessment device should possess. It shouldn't take you long to stumble on the attribute of *consistency* of measurement, since unless a test measures whatever it's measuring with a reasonable degree of consistency, we can't put any faith in its results (p. 30).

Therefore two ways to judge the reliability of a test are to judge its stability and consistency.

## Stability

Stability of a test or observation is determined by the use of one individual over time. Repeating an instrument or an observation is called *test-retest reliability*. Test-retest reliability indicates the ability of the testing device or observer to repeat a measurement. In a test-retest situation, the same test is administered repeatedly, with intervening time periods; this method contrasts with other methods in which two forms of a test are given during the same session. If the process being observed during the test-retest sequence changes somewhat over time, the variability of these changes will reflect the test's reliability. One way of describing the stability of scores over time is to derive the correlation coefficient between two sets of scores.

The correlation coefficient is an expression of a degree and direction of relationship. As discussed in Chapter 2, the correlation statistic is an index that has values from $-1.00$ through $+1.00$. Correlation of a test-retest method in its simplest form requires two scores, one from each administration of the test, for each person taking the tests. The index of correlation suggests the degree and the direction of relationship between the two scores. A 0.00 correlation suggests that there is no relationship between the scores obtained on the same test that was taken at different times. Differences in the scores seem to be caused by chance; that is, the scores obtained on two separate occasions are not systematically related. If an individual's scores are in the same rank order on two occasions (that is, the person's highest score on the first occasion is also obtained on the second occasion) and the relative differences between the two scores (errors) are the same on both occasions, the correlation value will be $+1.00$. This reliability coefficient represents a perfect positive relationship between the two tests. Even if a negative correlation is obtained, the reliability coefficient is treated as 0.00, because it is assumed that test reliabilities cannot be negative (Wardrop, 1976).

*Graphic Description of Correlation.* Figure 3-1 is a scatter diagram of correlation. To dem-

onstrate the relationship between form A and form B of a test, form A could be the variable represented on the vertical axis and form B on the horizontal axis. The zero score for both axes is to the left and down; high scores are to the right and up. Either variable can be located on the axis as long as it is properly labeled. In a predictive relationship (discussed later in this chapter), the vertical axis would serve as the predictive variable.

In diagram *A* the correlation would be positive and strong, near $+.60$. In diagram *B* the correlation is about equal in strength to that in diagram *A* but occurs from the lower right-hand corner to the upper left-hand corner. This relationship may be represented perhaps as $-.60$.

**Figure 3-1**
Scatter diagram of
correlation between form A
and form B of a sample test.

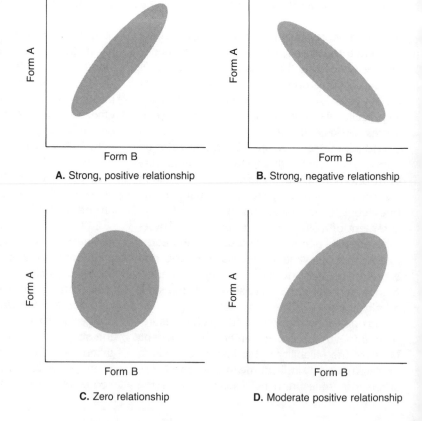

A. Strong, positive relationship

B. Strong, negative relationship

C. Zero relationship

D. Moderate positive relationship

Form A in this diagram could represent a test of academic behaviors and form B a test on self-concept or anxiety. In diagram C, no particular relationship exists between form A and form B. A moderately positive relation is shown in box D; the scores spread out and do not lie directly from the lower left-hand corner to the upper right-hand corner. Procedures for computing the correlation coefficient will now be explained.

*Correlation Coefficient.* If a group of children has two scores on tests, a correlation between the two scores can be calculated. The formula used to compute the correlation coefficient is:

$$r = \frac{\Sigma XY - [(\Sigma X)(\Sigma Y)/N]}{\sqrt{\left[\Sigma X^2 - \frac{(\Sigma X)^2}{N}\right]\left[\Sigma Y^2 - \frac{(\Sigma Y)^2}{N}\right]}}$$

where

$r$ = Correlation coefficient
$\Sigma X$ = Sum of all scores in variable $X$
$\Sigma Y$ = Sum of all scores in variable $Y$
$\Sigma X^2$ = Square each $X$ score and sum the squared scores
$\Sigma Y^2$ = Square each $Y$ score and sum the squared scores
$X$ = Variable of one characteristic
$Y$ = Variable of other characteristic
$N$ = Number of children

The scores for variable $X$ (test A) and variable $Y$ (test B) are as follows:

| Child | Test A (variable X) | Test B (variable Y) | $X^2$ | $Y^2$ | $XY$ |
|---|---|---|---|---|---|
| Jim | 7 | 1 | 49 | 1 | 7 |
| Ray | 5 | 1 | 25 | 1 | 5 |
| Lorie | 5 | 2 | 25 | 4 | 10 |
| Casey | 4 | 4 | 16 | 16 | 16 |
| Louis | 3 | 6 | 9 | 36 | 18 |
| Kathy | 1 | 6 | 1 | 36 | 6 |
| | $\Sigma X = 25$ | $\Sigma Y = 20$ | $\Sigma X^2 = 125$ | $\Sigma Y^2 = 94$ | $\Sigma XY = 62$ |

The square of $\Sigma X$ is 625, $(\Sigma Y)^2 = 400$, and $N = 6$. With these figures the correlation coefficient can be calculated.

$$r = \frac{62 - (25)(20)/6}{\sqrt{\left[125 - \frac{625}{6}\right]\left[94 - \frac{400}{6}\right]}}$$

$$= \frac{62 - 83.3}{\sqrt{(125 - 104.06)(94 - 66.6)}}$$

$$= \frac{-21.3}{\sqrt{(20.84)(27.4)}}$$

$$= \frac{-21.3}{\sqrt{571.02}}$$

$$r = -.89$$

*Correlation Functions.* A correlation coefficient serves three important purposes. First, it provides information on the reliability of the measure. Second, the correlation between two measures can aid in the evaluation of one test score as a prediction of another test or related construct (for example, school success). One way this is done is through a linear regression formula, expressed through the equation $Y = {}^bX + a$. $Y$ represents the test scores on one test, $X$ represents the scores on the other test, $b$ represents the slope or linear (straight line) representation of the test scores, and $a$ is a constant that adjusts the line to differing test scores. In prediction, we are essentially constructing a plot of test variables, called a scatter diagram, and drawing the straight line that best uniformly divides the test scores as shown as follows:

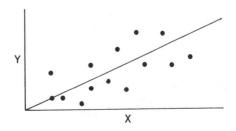

Because test scores might not be represented by a straight line, it can be necessary to use a linear equation to determine how well test scores actually fit on a straight line. The formula to determine (predict) scores for test $X$ from test $Y$ is,

$$^b YX = r\ \frac{\text{standard deviation of } X}{\text{standard deviation of } Y}$$

and "$^a xy$" is $\bar{X} - (\bar{Y})(^b xy)$. The mean and standard deviation of test X are 4.17 and 2.04, and of test Y, 3.33 and 2.38, respectively. From the correlation data discussed earlier, the equation for predicting the score of test X from the score of test Y is:

$$^b xy = -.89\left(\frac{2.04}{2.38}\right), \text{ or } ^b XY = -.76$$

$$^a xy = 4.17 - 3.33(-.89) = 4.17 + 2.96 = 7.13$$

$$X = -.76(Y) + 7.13$$

$$Y = \text{Any test score from test Y}$$

To predict the Y test score from the X test score, the reverse of the same equation requires a somewhat different prediction formula.

The third use for correlation scores is descriptive. Test research is concerned with the relationship between variables. The utilization of correlations requires great care; Sax (1974) lists several cautions:

1. The number of children in the standardization must be considered.
2. Correlations can only be interpreted meaningfully when relationships are expressed in regression lines.
3. Direction or magnitude correlation are suggested, but not causal relationships.
4. Correlations cannot be interpreted as percentages.

*Variations in Stability.* As discussed, the correlation coefficient expresses the stability of test scores. For example, the test-retest reliability coefficient represents the stability of scores over time. In this example, the same test is administered to the same children on two occasions. A variation of this procedure involves retesting with an *alternative* form of the test on another occasion. (Parallel test forms are used.)

Repeated measurements of the same test are influenced by several factors. First, variation in response to the demands of the test can influence reliability. For example, an intelligence test is given once a year while the child is in special education classes. The school assumes that the intelligence score remains stable over a one-year period. However, the stability of this score reflects that very few chance factors enter into the measurement. The score determined the first time the test is given may reflect the student's lack of test-taking sophistication; the score from the second testing could rise because of practice effects that result from the first testing.

Second, the length of time between testing sessions is critical to reliability. Obviously, if it is too short a time, students will remember the questions and the answers they gave on the first test; if the time lapse is too long, the characteristic being measured could change. Because there is no single accepted time interval between the variety of tests, test-retest procedures tend to reflect an excessive amount of measurement error.

**Parallel Forms**

Parallel test forms are the construction of two or more forms of some construct(s) that are administered to the same person during the same testing period. Several authors (among them, Anastasi, 1982) suggest that equivalent or parallel forms are never perfectly correlated or reliable. Errors of measurement occur because the two tests are highly likely to differ on item sampling. The reasons for this difference are apparent. The content of the test can include items from a large array of objectives. These items are pretested with an appropriate norm group in which some objectives are screened out. A cross-sectional sample of test items that represent the same level of difficulty or the same level of importance as the original pool of objectives is modified.

The chance error involved in the equivalent forms is different. While the instrument-centered chance error can exist, so can difficulties arise about the time interval between testings. Different time intervals can cause variations due to differences in test measurement and variations occurring in the child between testings. Thus, test manuals specify such time periods, in instructions such as, "The parallel-form reliability of this test was .89 when the alternate forms were administered eight days apart to 900 third-grade children." Of course, this interpretation assumes that a "stable" construct does not vary over eight days and that a low correlation between both forms represents changes that have occurred in the children.

### Internal-Consistency Method

Another reflection of reliability is the extent to which tests are consistent internally; that is, the extent to which test items measure the same construct. Methods that reflect internal consistency include the split-half method and the analysis of variance procedure.

*Split-Half Method.* In the split-half method, a test is divided into two shorter forms. The division of items provides two tests that have the properties of parallel forms. An odd-even procedure (forming half-tests by placing odd-numbered items in one test and even-numbered items in the other test) provides a parallel form distributing items in different categories over two halves. It should be noted that this method for estimating reliability would be inappropriate if the test were timed or if not all children completed the test.

Because increasing a test's length will ensure greater reliability, it can be necessary to determine the reliability of the half-tests (correlate the internal divisions of the whole test) and the reliability of the whole test. This may be necessary for estimating the reliability from a single

administration of a single test. To estimate the expected coefficient of reliability of a total test (combined halves), one uses a formula known as the Spearman-Brown *prophecy formula*:

$$r_{11} = \frac{2r\frac{1}{2}\frac{1}{2}}{1 + r\frac{1}{2}\frac{1}{2}}$$

where $r_{11}$ is the coefficient of reliability of the total test and $r\frac{1}{2}\frac{1}{2}$ is the coefficient of correlation between the odd-half and the even-half scores. Thus, if the correlation between the two halves of a test is .86, the Spearman-Brown prophecy formula would yield:

$$r_{11} = \frac{2(.86)}{1 + .86} = \frac{1.72}{1.86} = .92$$

Thus the two halves of this test are shown to be equivalent. As the items become less equivalent, the coefficient of reliability for the total test is underestimated. In many cases the subdivided test, because items are inadequate, provides a conservative estimate of the total test's reliability.

Several limitations in the split-half method are apparent. First, split-half reliability methods cannot be used when items are timed; for example, when a test includes a comprehension question but also imposes a 5-minute time limit. Wide differences will occur in the test scores, but the differences will most likely reflect how quickly the child can read. Differences occur because subjects are unable to complete either set of balanced items (odd or even). Second, scores obtained on a single testing are not sensitive to individual's variation from day to day. In other words, the test score is accurate only during a specific testing period. Third, items on the test might not be experimentally independent. If tests are divided on an odd-even basis, items can overlap on content rather than provide an equivalent sample of a construct.

*Analysis of Variance Method.* A procedure for estimating the reliability of pupils' performance from item to item is the *analysis of variance* (ANOVA) method. The ANOVA method is applied to testing information for the purpose of sorting out various factors influencing final scores. Although the method is intricate and beyond the scope of this chapter, using it, one could determine from test scores the extent to which students showed consistency of performance from item to item, or make a sorting out of various factors. The ANOVA method most often utilizes Kuder-Richardson (1927) formulas. A widely used procedure is the formula $KR_{20}$, which takes the form:

$$KR_{20} = \left(\frac{N}{N-1}\right)\left(\frac{SD_t^2 - \Sigma pq}{SD_t^2}\right)$$

where

$KR_{20}$ = Reliability estimate
$SD_t^2$ = Standard deviation of total scores on the test squared
$N^t$ = Number of items within test
$p$ = Percentage or proportion of students passing each item correctly
$q$ = Proportion or percentage of students failing some item, or $1 - p$

The essential assumption of this procedure is that items are homogeneous or represent general factors of ability or personality. The method provides an estimate of reliability without dividing the test, because it is assumed that items have much in common with other items. The $KR_{20}$, as is the split-half technique, is meant to be applied to power not speed tests. The formula is applicable to test items that are scored within an all-or-none system (for example, right or wrong). Some tests have multiple-scored items (for example, most of the time, some of the time, rarely) and therefore need a more generalized formula. Cronbach (1951) has developed a less restrictive formula known as *coefficient alpha*. In this formula, the $\Sigma pq$ is replaced by $\Sigma SD_i$, the sum of variances of item scores. The variance of all individual scores for each item is determined and then added to the variance across all items:

$$r = \left(\frac{N}{N-1}\right)\left(\frac{SD_t^2 - SD_i^2}{SD_t^2}\right)$$

## Correlation Coefficient Significance

In testing, we are usually interested in generalizing beyond the particular sample represented. For example, we might want to know if reading abilities in emotionally disturbed children are correlated with abilities of mentally retarded children of the same age, as revealed by a particular standardized test. Statistical procedures are available for estimating the probability of correlation, although discussion of these procedures is beyond the purpose of this chapter (see Chapter 2). When one is using these procedures, it is necessary to apply a test of probability, because the correlation of a small sample of children is more likely to involve testing error than is a computed correlation of a large sample.

The purpose of looking at significance usually centers around the question, "To what extent is a correlation coefficient greater than .00?" Table 3-1 suggests that, to be considered statistically significant at the 1% (.01) or 5% (.05) level, a correlation coefficient must be of a certain magnitude. When a correlation coefficient is significant at the .01 level, the chance of error is 1 out of 100 that the sample correlation is not greater than a zero correlation. If a correlation is significant at the .05 level, the probability of error is 5 out of 100. Table 3-1 is used to test the coefficients of correlation of various sample sizes.

## Reliability of Difference Scores

Teachers and psychologists are often placed in a position in which they compare differences between tests. For example, it is currently in vogue to make comparisons between discrepancies between intelligence and academic achievement. For the analysis of both test scores, it is important to know how reliable these differences are, because "difference scores" provide a reliability coefficient lower than the single reliability coefficient of each test. Therefore, the reliability of a difference score is related to (1) standardization differences between tests, (2) reliability of each test, and (3) correlation of each

**Table 3-1**
Values of correlation coefficient, by sample size and level of significance.

| Number of samples | Degrees of freedom (df) | 80% | 90% | 95% | 99% | 99.9% |
|---|---|---|---|---|---|---|
| 3 | 1 | .951 | .988 | .997 | 1.000 | 1.000 |
| 4 | 2 | .800 | .900 | .950 | .990 | .999 |
| 5 | 3 | .687 | .805 | .878 | .959 | .991 |
| 6 | 4 | .608 | .729 | .811 | .917 | .974 |
| 7 | 5 | .551 | .669 | .755 | .875 | .951 |
| 8 | 6 | .507 | .621 | .707 | .834 | .925 |
| 9 | 7 | .472 | .582 | .666 | .798 | .898 |
| 10 | 8 | .443 | .549 | .632 | .765 | .872 |
| 11 | 9 | .419 | .521 | .602 | .735 | .847 |
| 12 | 10 | .398 | .497 | .576 | .708 | .823 |
| 13 | 11 | .380 | .476 | .553 | .684 | .801 |
| 14 | 12 | .365 | .457 | .532 | .661 | .780 |
| 15 | 13 | .351 | .441 | .514 | .641 | .760 |
| 16 | 14 | .338 | .426 | .497 | .623 | .742 |
| 17 | 15 | .327 | .412 | .482 | .606 | .725 |
| 18 | 16 | .317 | .400 | .468 | .590 | .708 |
| 19 | 17 | .308 | .389 | .456 | .575 | .693 |
| 20 | 18 | .299 | .378 | .444 | .561 | .679 |
| 21 | 19 | .291 | .369 | .433 | .549 | .665 |
| 22 | 20 | .284 | .360 | .423 | .537 | .652 |
| 23 | 21 | .277 | .352 | .413 | .526 | .640 |
| 24 | 22 | .271 | .344 | .404 | .515 | .629 |
| 25 | 23 | .265 | .337 | .396 | .505 | .618 |
| 26 | 24 | .260 | .330 | .388 | .496 | .607 |
| 27 | 25 | .255 | .323 | .381 | .487 | .597 |
| 28 | 26 | .250 | .317 | .374 | .479 | .588 |
| 29 | 27 | .245 | .311 | .367 | .471 | .579 |
| 30 | 28 | .241 | .306 | .361 | .463 | .570 |
| 31 | 29 | .237 | .301 | .355 | .456 | .562 |
| 32 | 30 | .233 | .296 | .349 | .449 | .554 |
| 42 | 40 | .202 | .257 | .304 | .393 | .490 |
| 62 | 60 | .165 | .211 | .250 | .325 | .408 |
| 122 | 120 | .117 | .150 | .178 | .232 | .294 |

Based on material from Fisher, R. *Statistical method for research workers,* Edinburgh: Oliver & Boyd, 1963.

test. It is assumed that all tests have an expressed standard score (which indicates the number of standard deviation units a score is from the mean; for example, z scores) and that they are somewhat equivalent in reliability. Gulliksen (1950) provides the following formula for calculating reliability of difference scores:

$$r_x = \frac{r_t - r_{a,b}}{1 - r_{a,b}}$$

where

$r_x$ = Reliability of difference scores
$r_t$ = Reliability of two tests
$r_{a,b}$ = Reliability between two tests

If the reliability of the two tests is .70 and they correlate .63 between each other, the reliability of difference scores is:

$$r_x = \frac{.70 - .63}{1 - .63} = \frac{.07}{.37} = .19$$

This formula demonstrates how quickly the difference scores between tests become unreliable as related to the correlation of two tests and their average reliability.

The reliability of difference scores has three implications for educational settings. First, decisions for a child's placement are based on the differences between scores of various tests. Unfortunately, decisions are based not on the reliability of difference scores, but on haphazard interpretation of discrepancy scores. Second, the actual correlation between two tests is usually lower than the scores gained when a simple comparison is made between them. A typical example is the comparison of IQ scores and achievement test scores on learning quotients: when the student's actual performance on tests is compared with classroom expectations, an arbitrary decision is made regarding what is significant about the differences.

One of the most frequently used approaches to the analysis of difference scores is the learning quotient (LQ). Calculations are based on the mental age (MA) of the child (score on intelligence test), chronological age (CA), and grade age (GA), derived from the student's score on an achievement test. These three units of information are used in a two-step calculation. The first step yields the expectancy age (EA):

$$EA = \frac{MA + CA + GA}{3}$$

The learning quotient is then determined by dividing the achievement-test-score age (AA) by the expectancy age:

$$LQ = \frac{AA}{EA}$$

A learning quotient of 89 and below is considered indicative of a significant discrepancy (Myklebust, 1968).

A major problem with this approach is that many times the individual behaviors that need to be measured have not been adequately defined, isolated, and described, and, consequently, satisfactory measuring instruments and techniques are often lacking.

## Standard Error of Measurement

If a student were to take a test and then repeat this process on several other occasions, it would almost be certain that the student's scores would vary from occasion to occasion. This variability of scores reflects the notion that any particular test is not a perfectly reliable instrument. This variability reflects what is called the *standard error of measurement*; that is, the standard error of measurement represents how well an individual's score compares with his or her true score. Because administering the same test to a single child is likely to induce carryover effects (for example, practice, memory), the student's true score can only be estimated. The formula used to compute this estimate is

$$SE_m = s\sqrt{1 - r}$$

where

$r$ = Reliability coefficient for the particular test

$s$ = Standard deviation of test scores for group of examinees

$SE_m$ = Standard error of measurement

The use of a standard error of measurement suggests not only that test scores are inconsistent, but also that a pupil's obtained score is only an approximation of the pupil's true achievement or ability. For example, if a student had a score of 50 on an achievement test, some estimate of the student's true score must be made. The standard deviation of this test was 9 and the reliability was .89. Using the formula for estimating the student's true score, we obtain the following information:

$$SE_m = 9\sqrt{1 - .89} = 9\sqrt{.11}$$
$$= 9 \times .33 = 2.97 = @3$$

The $SE_m$ defines a band or interval that depicts where the child's actual level of ability is likely to lie. Because the $SE_m$ was approximately 3, the child's true score is $50 \pm 3$, or 47 to 53. The distribution of the $SE_m$ is assumed to conform to a normal curve (depicted in Chapter 2), so that 68% of the time the student's score will fall within 1 $SE_m$ of his or her true score. This means that a child's score fluctuates within 3 points on either side of the true score 68 times out of 100. Note that by adopting this procedure, we are going to see that the test underestimates the child's true score in about 15% of the cases and overestimates it in another 15%.

An alternate approach is to use a confidence band or to extend the band to 95% of the cases. The implication of this confidence band is straightforward. Consider a child who has taken an IQ test that has a mean of 100, a standard deviation of 15, and a reliability of .89. The child obtains a score of 75. Using the formula just discussed ($SE_m = 15\sqrt{1 - .89} = 5$), we find that a 68% confidence represents an interval for this child of 70 to 80. A 95% confidence band includes scores of 65 to 85. Thus, even though the student's score was in the mentally retarded range, it is possible that the true intelligence score was in fact in the slow learner category.

## Summary of Sources of Error in Reliability

The different reliability coefficients described in this chapter are summarized in Table 3-2. The table shows which sources of error are possible in each of the procedures for estimating reliability. The summary might not be accurate for unique tests, but the table serves as a reference for most testing manuals. The majority of factors that appreciably influence reliability can be divided into situational factors or test factors.

**Table 3-2**
Reliability coefficients.

| Reliability | Classification | Description | Source of error |
|---|---|---|---|
| Kuder-Richardson | Internal consistency (no time interval between testing) | Correlation estimated from item statistics | Content diversity; item sampling |
| Split-half | Internal consistency | Correlation of entire power test (minimal emphasis on time) to two halves of test | Item sampling; variation in measurement procedure |
| Test-retest | Stability (measurement over specific time period) | Correlation of test with retest given immediately after, or after interval | Variation in measurement procedure; effects of time period; changes in individual child |
| Equivalent forms (parallel or alternate forms) | Stability and/or equivalence (specific time period or no time period) | Correlation between scores on two or more forms of same test given within specific time period or with no interval between testings | Effects of time period; content diversity; child variation |

The environment (for example, use of different test administrators) and the psychological condition of the child (changes in the child from day to day) are situational factors. Test factors may include ambiguity of questions, length of test, level of difficulties, or standardization of subjects within test.

## VALIDITY

Another factor that determines the usefulness of a test is its validity. As Popham (1978) states:

> In addition to measuring with consistency, a test really ought to measure what it claims to be measuring. That's only fair. Measurement folks refer to this concept as *validity* and define it technically as the extent to which a test measures what it purports to measure (p. 31).

Validity is thus the extent to which a test is serving its stated purposes or the extent to which a particular test measures or predicts. Within the Popham tradition, a basic approach to the study of validity includes (1) the reasonable qualities of a test, and (2) the empirical basis of the test.

### Reasonable Qualities

Determining which of several types of validity is important depends on the intended use of a test. Because *validity* is a term denoting the usefulness of a test, a beginning assumption is that a test must adequately represent a particular content area being assessed.

### Content Validity

*Content validity* refers to the extent to which a test samples a particular domain, trait, or characteristic. In establishing the content validity of a particular test, its makers should choose items from a well-defined domain. However, the sampling should be sufficiently representative of the conceptualized area (Messick, 1980). Assessing the content validity involves determining the adequacy with which items reflect (1) the curriculum of instruction, and/or (2) the desired

cognitive and/or affective behaviors. The adequacy with which items reflect curricular activities can be evaluated on the basis of textbooks, teacher objectives, opinions of educators, and the degree to which these items are an adequate sample. A more technical evaluation of content validity may be performed through (1) subjective judgment, (2) homogeneity or interval consistency of items (reliability), or (3) factor analysis (discussed in Chapter 4). Determining generalized student behaviors is less clear (see Messick, 1980, for extensive discussion). Bloom and Gagné offer much direction in this area, however.

*Bloom.* Desired pupil behavior in content items may be classified in two domains—affective and cognitive. This breakdown is similar to the general educational taxonomies of Bloom (Bloom, 1956; Krathwohl, Bloom, & Masia, 1964), which are the core of developmental educational curriculum. The affective domain includes objectives concerned with changes in a child's emotional state or degree of acceptance or rejection of some entity. This domain represents areas of personal-social adjustment. The cognitive domain includes educational objectives related to the recall of knowledge and the development of intellectual abilities and skill (Krathwohl, Bloom, & Massia, 1964).

Bloom's taxonomy of educational objectives provides a format for organization of a curriculum hierarchy. Bloom lists those necessary skills that should be assessed in a curriculum. His emphasis is along the lines of Gagné's work.

*Gagné.* The following is a review of Gagné's *The conditions of learning* (1977), in which he theorized that there are eight types of learning, beginning with the very simple stimulus-response units, which can be built up hierarchically. They are as follows.

*Type 1: signal learning.* A particular stimulus (for example, loud noise) always elicits a particular response (muscle twitch) until eventually the very sight of the person or object making the noise may evoke the response. This is also called *respondent conditioning.*

*Type 2: stimulus-response learning.* A slightly more complex type of learning built out of simple signals, it is normally called *operant conditioning.* A child recalls the word *ball,* the teacher smiles, and the word *ball* is repeated, because it brought a rewarding outcome.

*Type 3: chaining.* Stimulus-response (S-R) units, formed in Type 2 learning, are connected. A child learns to make a verbal response (*chair,* for example) and also learns to discriminate between the *chair* and the *sofa.* The word is then connected to the right object, and a *concept* of *chair* has been formed.

*Type 4: verbal association.* This type is a subvariety of chaining. To discover the meaning of one word, for example, the child recognizes its connection to another word. Thus *duct* (to lead) is chained to *aqua: aqueduct.*

*Type 5: multiple discrimination.* These are stimulus-response chains that work in combination. To discriminate between homonyms, a child might recognize that one word that sounds the same as another word but is spelled differently is connected to one concept, while the second word is connected to another concept.

*Type 6: concept learning.* Tests of multiple discrimination come together under a verbal label. (For example, words that sound alike but are spelled differently are called *homonyms.*)

*Type 7: principle learning.* This is use of a chain of concepts. (For example, the principles of phonetics involve many rules.)

*Type 8: problem solving.* This is the combining of principles into divergent, novel, and higher order principles.

Development of an instructional program for the ordering of numbers proceeds from the final step to the first. The teacher who is developing test items sets the top objective, and then asks, in effect, what children need to know before they can order numbers. The instructional program

is then set up to match each step. Starting at the bottom (S-R connections), the child learns to say the names of the numbers and mark each number with a pencil. As each step is mastered, the child moves to the next. Finally, when the top step is reached, the child generalizes to other types of problems. It should be noted that from the teacher's standpoint this hierarchy is static, because it does not contain a system for maintaining earlier structures.

*Educational Taxonomy.* As stated earlier, Bloom's taxonomy is along the same lines as Gagné's. Bloom incorporates both a cognitive and a behavioral approach to curriculum development, but instead of focusing on a hierarchy of learning as Gagné does, Bloom applies the hierarchy of learning to curriculum objectives. The taxonomies organized for each domain are close representations of the hierarchical structure of Gagné. For the cognitive domain, for example, the main organizing principle is the degree of complexity of the cognitive process involved in the objective. Comparatively simple cognitive behaviors combine with others of a simple nature to yield more complex behaviors.

Bloom's (1956) major categories in the cognitive domain are knowledge (recall of specifics and abstractions), comprehension (translation, interpretation, and extrapolation of what is being communicated), application (use of abstraction in specific or generalized situations), analysis (study of communication or knowledge in terms of relationships or organizational principles), synthesis (putting elements together to form a whole), and evaluation (quantitative and qualitative judgments).

For some purposes, the taxonomies for the development of test items might not be precise on the cognitive level. For example, the cognitive taxonomy deals with mental processes but does not identify either overt behavior performed by the student or the classroom conditions necessary for performance. By combining Bloom's taxonomy and Gagné's learning hierarchy component, one can evaluate tasks that lead to the assessment of pupil performance.

A backward analysis is very useful for pupil placement and for diagnosis and remediation of behavior and learning difficulties. In this regard, criterion-referenced tests play a significant role (see Chapter 2).

*Affective Domain.* Bloom's taxonomy can be more directly applied to children with behavioral difficulties, in the affective domain. A main organizing principle for a taxonomy of the affective domain is the process of internalization. Internalization is a process through which there is, first, a tentative adoption of behavior (overt manifestation) and later a more complete adoption (internal). Five chief categories of objective behavior, related to Bloom's taxonomy, have been identified; each of these has two or three subdivisions. The major categories of Bloom's (Krathwohl, Bloom, & Masia, 1964) affective domain are (1) receiving (willingness to receive or attend to stimuli), (2) responding (willingness and satisfaction in responding), (3) valuing (acceptance that a thing, behavior, or phenomenon has worth), (4) organizing (conceptualizing and organizing a value system), and (5) characterizing by a value or value complex (integration of beliefs and attitudes and control, the behavior of the individual).

The utility of assessing the affective taxonomy is influenced by several factors. In terms of its effect on curriculum development, affective behavior is a precursor of cognitive skills. Willingness to receive stimuli would obviously have to be a mastered skill before recall of specifics is possible. Another factor is the comparatively small amount of research on the affective domain in general. Terms related to a child's learning beliefs, values, and attitudes are often used without being precisely defined. The wide range of definitions from teacher to teacher would affect actual assessment of the affective area.

*Summary of Content Validity.* Content validity is an essential step in the establishment of the other types (for example, construct) of validity discussed. Because content validity is not represented as a correlation coefficient, agreement on the extent of this validity can be obtained through independent judgments of items, to determine whether they do measure what they are supposed to measure. The usual procedure is to allow a group of individuals who did not compose the test to judge each item.

Two procedures in a test's construction can enhance its content validity. First, the test instrument should be based on curriculum items or list of objectives. Second, test items must represent the appropriate vocabulary, style, and ideas embedded within educational instruction.

## Item Analysis

Scrutinizing the strengths and weaknesses of each test item is known as *item analysis.* Examination of each item is done in terms of (1) level of difficulty, (2) discriminating power, and (3) ambiguity. Item analysis also serves as a basis for the development of informal testing instruments for classroom practices (see Chapter 2).

*Difficulty.* Determining an item's level of difficulty focuses on the proportion of students who correctly answer that item. What percentage of students who attempted to answer a test item did so correctly? The formula for determining this percentage is

$$P = \frac{N_c(100)}{N_T}$$

where

$P$ = Percentage of children answering test item correctly

$N_c$ = Number of children answering test item correctly

$N_T$ = Total number of children who answered item

As indicated from this formula, the higher the percentage, the easier the item. By examining items in this manner, testers can identify those items that are (1) more discriminating, (2) more functional, or (3) less ambiguous. Two factors that are not considered by this procedure are the extent to which the time needed to complete an item determines difficulty and the extent to which guessing is a differential power (Findley, 1956).

**Discrimination Index.** The extent to which an item separates test-takers into two extreme groups is called the *discrimination index*. This procedure separates those individuals who score in the upper group from those who score in the unsuccessful or lower group. The purpose of this index is to provide a measure that would place every child into the appropriate upper or lower group; its success depends on the extent to which items discriminate group differences. The discrimination index could be used to (1) improve the quality of items so that there is less discrimination between different children's performances, and (2) analyze teacher-made tests for homogeneous item selection. The formula to compute this index is (Findley, 1956)

$$D_i = \frac{N_u - N_L}{N_T}$$

where

$D_i$ = Discrimination index
$N_u$ = Number of children in upper group (approximately top 27%)
$N_L$ = Number of children in lower group (lower 27%)
$N_T$ = Total number of the two groups

Values range from +1.0 to −1.0. If a test's index is negative, its items are usually considered to be heterogeneous, poorly written, or ambiguous. Sax (1974) suggests that items with an index between 0 and .30 provide minimal information for the separation of individual differences and should be rewritten to reflect similar objectives of the overall test.

**Ambiguity.** Children who perform generally well on the test (upper group) might perform incorrectly as often as they do correctly on a

particular item of the test. Ambiguity reflects the extent to which this phenomenon occurs. Therefore, interpretation of children's performance has to be done on marked discrepancies in item performances.

**Item Analysis and Informal Tests.** While item analysis of standardized tests is useful in discriminating among individuals and controlling the difficulty level of items, a logical analysis of appropriate items would provide teachers with a basis on which they could develop their own informal testing procedures. In such an analysis, items are selected from standardized tests (for sample items) or tied into teaching objectives. The analysis asks, can this item that discriminates among many children be used as a basis for teacher assessment and instruction?

Specific task- or item-oriented tests provide valuable teaching data, whose worth often exceeds that of information obtained through standardized testing procedures. Although informal tests may be given by the teacher in the classroom, test information derived from item analysis must be considered part of the regular classroom curriculum. Instruments included at this level of evaluation include (1) individually administered written assignments, (2) informal teaching lessons assessing various skills, and (3) orally administered exercises. An illustration of an informal test evaluation of a series of classroom sight-word objectives and teaching procedures is given in Figure 3-2.

Alternatives to such an informal testing procedure could include a survey of academic needs. An informal survey is intended to provide a quick estimate of pupils' best starting places. The informal testing survey below is intended for grades three to eight. Potential places for beginning instruction would include the highest level at which the child correctly solves three out of four problems.

**Math survey**

| *Level 3* | 35 | 116 | 42 | 3)‾6‾6‾9‾ |
|---|---|---|---|---|
| | +42 | −81 | ×2 | |

| Level 4 | $6.50<br>+3.25 | 6)762 | 25<br>42<br>37 | 692<br>×6 |
|---|---|---|---|---|

| Level 5 | 421<br>×53 | 62)3560 | 6¼<br>−3 | 4.8<br>5.2<br>6.7<br>4.9 |
|---|---|---|---|---|

Level 6    98.7 + 6.4 + 297.5 + .8 =

|  | 729<br>×405 | 39)874 | 13½<br>72¼<br>6½ |
|---|---|---|---|

Level 7    125)43751          76)4.408

15% of 60 gallons =

Find the area of a rectangle 26.2 inches long and 14.8 inches wide.

This instrument is not intended to be time-consuming for the teacher to administer, but should provide the teacher with data to use in

---

OBJECTIVE:    Sight-word skill—Dolch sight words.

CATEGORY:    A test exercise for a sight-word objective will require the child to associate a written word with its oral speech equivalent.

EXERCISE:    Show the child a card containing one word, such as cat. Ask the child to pronounce the word.

RESPONSE:    The test exercise must be designed so that

1. The child will either respond or indicate that he cannot respond.
2. The teacher will be able to determine which response each child makes.
3. An answer that will be considered adequate is indicated.

ADEQUATE ANSWER:    The child will pronounce the word correctly in 5 seconds or less.

INTERPRETATION:    The child's responses are interpreted in terms of the specific objective for which the test was designed.

---

**Figure 3-2**
Informal test.

the planning for specific needs of individual students. Although the informal instruments have many advantages, they also carry some inherent dangers, such as possible lack of reliability.

**Construct Validity**

The theory underlying the test must be assessed on both logical (reasonable) and empirical grounds. *Construct validity* refers to the constructs (psychological or educational) of a test. To what extent does the test represent the theoretical trait (for example, intelligence, abstract reasoning) under study? How does the measurement instrument fit into an organized body of knowledge? Very few measures used in testing research are applied to the analysis of construct validity. For example, there are no definable content areas called *intelligence*. To determine the construct validity of a test, one must first make a complete and precise definition of the characteristic being studied. On the basis of that definition, predictions are made concerning how or what individuals possess variations of this construct and those who possess lower levels. For some measures (for example, Anxiety-Taylor Manifest Anxiety Scale, Tennessee Self-Concept Scale), a considerable body of information is emerging. This amount of study indicates that these measures are on a threshold of fitting into a developing theoretical framework.

Also made on the basis of definition of the characteristic being studied, some predictions are made to serve as a guide for test development. For example, a relationship or correlation is made between the present test score and scores from other tests derived from a theoretically similar framework. Since it is difficult to empirically prove that a theory or construct is absolutely true (probability provides one frame of reference), a test serves as a primary dimension along which a theory is evaluated. The factors that determine the theoretical value of a test are endless, but five prominent ones are

1. The heuristic value of a test—the test's ability to provide a descriptive analysis of theoretical statements
2. The generality of a test—the amount and extent of descriptive analysis of child behavior that the theory is supposed to generate
3. The compatibility of the test to previously constructed tests of that theoretical orientation—the correlation between that and similar tests
4. The ease with which the test can be subjected to empirical evaluation—the preciseness of the test item(s) of the theory
5. The degree to which the test includes items whose usefulness have already been confirmed through empirical evaluation

Knowing precisely what a test relates to theoretically is of more value than any other method of validation. Also, understanding the social outcome and criticism of testing interacts with the determining of construct validity (as discussed, for example, in Crawford, 1979; Messick, 1980). Messick (1980) considers test validity to be an overall judgment of the adequacy of inferences drawn from the test construct. This evaluation is based on four ideas: (1) the potential of social consequence of the proposed test, (2) the relevance of construct and its utility in practical situations, (3) the implications of interpretation of the test, and (4) evidence drawn from research of the test.

Putting these ideas together, Messick had devised a model linking the source of construct justification to the actual outcome of the test. In other words, the implications of using the test (for example, social consequences, relevance, utility) interact with the proper meaning or construct of the test. In an attempt to show this relationship, Messick provided a flow diagram linking test construct validity and test interpretations as a continuous process (Figure 3-3). The primary concern of this continuous process is the "balancing of the instrumental value of the test in accomplishing its intended purpose with the instrumental value of any negative side effects and positive by-products of the testing" (p. 1025). In the final analysis, the value of the test construct rests on an individual's interpretation of it within a theoretical and value-based framework. The next section discusses three forms of criterion-related validity: congruent, concurrent, and predictive.

## Congruent Validity

The process of validating one test in terms of another earlier test is called *congruent validity*. The validity of the new test is validated against another through a correlational analysis. Difficulties arise when a new measure is correlated with another test of doubtful construct validity; the new measure therefore can be no better than the original measure. One example of congruent validity is the extent to which test $X$ correlates with the Stanford-Binet.

## Concurrent Validity

*Concurrent validity* is defined as the matching of test scores to measures of contemporary criterion performance. Stated another way, concurrent validity refers to statements about the prediction of events that occur at roughly the same time the testing instrument is applied. Contemporary measures may include current school marks, criterion-referenced measures, or counseling interviews. Sax (1974) suggests that the determination of concurrent validity is appropriate when a recently developed measure is to be substituted for a better established, ongoing measure. However, Anastasi (1982) suggests that, because of criterion complexity, validating a test against composite criterions (for example, classroom achievement) might be of questionable value and of limited generality. Success in school or related activities depends not on one trait but on many traits. Hence, classroom criteria are multifaceted. Procedures, however, for developing an accurate estimate of concurrent validity (also called *synthetic validity,* cf. Anastasi, 1982) include (1) detailing

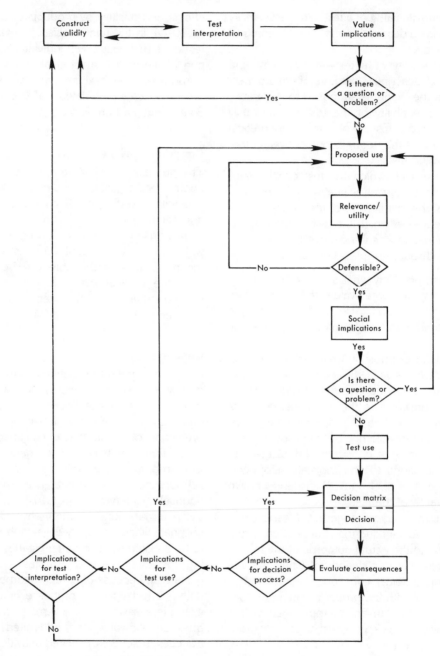

**Figure 3-3**

Feedback model for test validity. (From Messick, S. Test validity and ethics of assessment, *American Psychologist*, 1980, *35*, 1024. Copyright 1980 by the American Psychological Association. Reprinted by permission.)

classroom performance and its relative contribution to predictive success, (2) analyzing the extent to which the test in question measures proficiency in performance of each school task, and (3) finding the validity of each test for a given academic (or related) task.

### Predictive Validity

As the name suggests, predictive validity attempts to forecast some future measurement based on a current test or observation. A typical example in education is the prediction of success (for example, in reading or math) in school. The basic evidence in support of predictive validity is a relationship between two variables. The two variables are criterion (construct of interest) and prediction (construct of test). A test is said to have predictive validity for reading performance, for example, if the scores on a test correlate with grades or other measures that are given at some future time. A test cannot have predictive validity if the construct of concern has not been empirically investigated. The manuals of some tests include statements whose validity has not yet been tested.

The predictive function of a test is important because it is the only way in which the appropriateness of its construct(s) can be empirically assessed. For a theoretical base of a test to be empirically testable, the test must yield predictions that can be directly evaluated by classroom assessment. Why a test needs be tested at all might be puzzling to some because the test might have been previously characterized as having good content or congruent validity. The basic point is that more constructs that will generate specific descriptive levels of classroom functioning must be postulated.

## SUMMARY

Without validity, a test or observational procedure is of little value. Validity and reliability are related in that if a test is demonstrated to have content, construct, congruent, concurrent, or predictive validity, it must have some degree of reliability. However, it is important to remember that tests can be reliable and have little or no validity. Validity is best conceptualized as having both a reasonable and an empirical base. This conceptualization is shown in Figure 3-4. In summary, special emphasis should be given to the theoretical base from which the test is derived, as well as its value in determining classroom functioning. Some of the major points in this chapter are summarized in the following discussion on test selection.

Sternberg (1979) suggests that the selection of tests be based on four criteria of the test: (1) quantifiability, or the assignment of events to rules, (2) reliability, or the extent to which the quantification is externally consistent, (3) empirical validity, or the extent to which the task measures the constructs, and (4) construct validity, or the assurance that the task has a basis in psychological theory. Sternberg's fourth point is important because he believes that a theory must dictate the choice of testing instruments, rather than the test being chosen arbitrarily and this choice "giving rise to a post hoc theory of task performance" (p. 218). Sternberg's concepts are further elaborated in Chapter 4.

| Reasonableness of test | Empirical base of test |
|---|---|
| Content validity | Construct |
|   Curriculum representation |   Heuristic value |
|   Desired behaviors |   Generality |
|     Hierarchical example |   Compatibility |
|     Cognitive objectives |   Precision |
|     Affective objectives |   Confirmation |
| Item analysis | Congruent |
|   Level of difficulty |   Historical bases |
|   Discriminating index | Concurrent |
|   Ambiguity |   Contemporary criterion |
|   Informal assessment | Predictive |
| |   Theoretical base |
| |   Specific descriptive level |

**Figure 3-4**

A conceptualization of validity.

With this overall view in mind, we can review several aspects of developing and using tests. These aspects include

1. Complete description in the text manual of the development of the test (for example, rationale, observational procedures, results of item analysis)
2. Responsibility for making inferences about meaning and legitimate use of the test
3. Revision procedures of the test
4. Stated purposes of the test and user qualifications
5. Direction for administration and scoring
6. Standard for reports of research on reliability and validity
7. Detailed description of norms and scales that should be included (for example, details of sample group with means, standard deviations)
8. Discussion of measure error
9. Standard uses of the test

# PART TWO

# TESTING DOMAIN

# CHAPTER 4

# Intelligence

## An Information Processing View

### OUTLINE

What makes a child intelligent and what constitutes intellectual behavior are questions that have generated much theoretical debate over the last century (Binet & Henri, 1895; Snow, 1980; Sternberg, 1988). To date many questions remain unanswered. Is intelligence a unitary or generalized function, or is it composed of a group of relatively separate abilities (Carew, 1981; Guilford, 1967, 1980; Sternberg, 1988)? How modifiable is intelligence? Is its development determined mostly by genetic factors or is it dependent on learning experiences in environments of varying degrees of stimulation or deprivation (Hunt, 1969; Jensen, 1969; Kagan, 1969; Scarr & Carter-Saltzman, 1982)? More specifically, can intelligence as an underlying construct, trait, ability, or capacity be directly assessed, or should it be defined only in terms of performance on a specific cognitive task (Piaget & Inhelder, 1969)? If the latter position is accepted, a child's ability may be related to his or her score for a particular intelligence test under certain circumstances.

Differing positions on the above issues are reflected in frequently cited definitions. Wechsler (1958) asserts that intelligence cannot be the sum of measured abilities or elements but reflects more the way elements are combined. Factors such as drives and incentives are involved, and one ability contributes little to the effectiveness of behavior as a whole. According to Wechsler, intelligence is the "aggregate of global capacities of the individual to act purposefully, to think rationally, and to deal effectively with his environment" (p. 7). Therefore the only way intelligence can be measured quantitatively is by a measurement of various elements. Similarly, Spearman (1927) and Thurstone (1938a), in their analyses of many individuals acting on a wide variety of test items, concluded that individuals have different strengths and weaknesses in facets of intelligence ranging from verbal fluency to adeptness in seeing spatial relationships. Whereas Thurstone placed emphasis on the specific facets of intellectual behavior, Spearman (1927) maintains that an overall global capacity

or innate intelligence accounts for variations in test scores.

In contrast to Wechsler, Thurstone, and Spearman, Burt (1958) views intelligence as "an innate, general cognitive ability" (p. 162). Differences in intelligence seem to depend on the combined action of numerous genes whose influence accounts for 75% of measured variance in IQ. Burt's work laid the groundwork for Jensen's (1969) thesis that retarded and low-functioning children could not be helped intellectually by earlier intervention.

In contrast to all others mentioned, Wesman (1968) views intelligence "as the summation of learning experiences" (p. 267). Tests with different names (intelligence, achievement, aptitude) are for the most part measuring cumulative learning experience. Different tests merely reflect different criteria that have been selected for investigation. Table 4-1 provides a brief summary of major authors, with their definitions and components of intelligent behavior.

## HISTORICAL VIEW

The view of intelligence as delineated in this chapter is made from an information-processing model. Several recent theorists and reviews have also adapted this perspective (Carroll, 1978; Humphreys & Revelle, 1984; Neisser, 1979; Snow, 1980; Spear & Sternberg, 1987). Even an earlier article of Binet (Binet & Henri, 1895) expressed a conviction that a central problem of intellectual assessment focused on the interrelationship of various subcomponent processes of individual performance. Several generations later, the psychometric movement was motivated partly by a behaviorism (see Chapter 8) that operationalized intellectual performance and provided precise measurement. This psychometric movement succeeded in exorcising the idea of introspective processes of problem solving. Since then, the dominant trend in the study of intelligence, including the components of intelligence, has followed a strict statistical model, which forms the theoretical

**Table 4-1**

Major authors.

| Author | Description of intelligence | Components of intelligence |
|---|---|---|
| Goddard (1908); Binet (1909); Terman (1921) | Proportional ability to carry out abstract thinking | Judgment, practical sense, initiative, and ability to adapt to circumstances |
| Boring (1923) | Intelligence is what the tests test | Depend on construct validity of test |
| Spearman (1927) | General factor to deduce abstract relationships ($g$) plus one specific factor per test | Verbal and numerical abilities |
| Thorndike (1927) | Stimulus-response connections | Completion of sentences, mathematical reasoning, ability to use vocabulary and to follow directions |
| Thurstone (1938) | Primary mental abilities that are independent of each other | Number, facility, verbal meaning, inductive reasoning, perceptual speed, spatial relations, memory, and verbal fluency |
| Vernon (1960) | Complexity and flexibility of person's schemata | General factor ($g$) followed by verbal, educational and practical, mechanical, spatial, and other specific factors |
| Guilford (1967) | Composed of operations, products, and content in a multifaceted structure, with focus on the mental operations performed | 120 cells (see Chapter 1) |
| Wesman (1968) | Bits or modules of information formed either in content or processes | Summation of learning experience |
| Jensen (1969) | IQ is related to socially valued criteria (for example, upward mobility, scholastic success) | Associative ability (level 1—digit-span memory, free recall); cognitive ability (level 2—abstract reasoning tasks) |
| Piaget (1970) | Extension of biological adaptation | Processes of assimilation (processes responsive to inner schema) and accommodation (processes responsive to environmental cues that differ from existing inner schema) |
| Neisser (1979) | Includes abilities that tests do not test | Intelligence does not exist except as a resemblance to a prototype (what an intelligent person does) |
| Snow (1980) | Views as fluid (fluid versus crystallized intelligence) involving the assembly, adaptation, and solving of novel problems in the physical and social world | Synthesis of cognition, affect, and conation (coordination of affect and cognition) |

basis of most intelligence tests (see Sternberg, 1979, for review).

Clear evidence exists to support the information processing theory that models of human cognitive processes can account for a variety of child responses by means of intellectual tests or other psychometric measures (e.g., Snow, 1980; Wagner & Sternberg, 1984). Theories of children's information processing can be implemented at various levels: neural processes, higher mental processes (for example, concept attainment), or basic structural components (for example, attention, short-term memory, long-term memory).

Although this chapter will not present a neurological basis for information processing, it will focus on some of the elementary and complex processes accounting for the methods by which a child adapts to his or her environment. Information processing tends to encourage attention to processes rather than to the stated functional relationships between classroom learning and test performance. Information processing also encourages the building of a theoretical base for a whole range of cognitive tasks in which the child may engage, in various environmental settings. The method by which a child develops strategies, rather than the isolation of a single attribute (for example, vocabulary), is certainly a focus. This chapter will provide a brief overview of information processing theory as related to intellectual functioning and standardized tests. However, before that discussion is begun, a brief review of factor analysis is necessary, because this procedure is perhaps the most popular method used to understand the intellectual abilities of handicapped children.

## FACTOR ANALYTICAL MODELS

Factor analysis is a mathematical procedure used to identify the number of abilities or traits that determine test scores. A test can measure a single factor such as "general knowledge" or a number of factors such as vocabulary, numerical reasoning, spatial orientation. A basic theorem of factor analysis is that the sum of variance (discussed in Chapter 3) of items (common factors) and the specific factors (items unique to a particular test), plus the error variance (essentially any condition that is irrelevant to the purpose of a test), equals the total variance of the test. Factor analysis further subdivides the sources of variance contributing to a child's performance so that what remains is a "true variance." The smaller the contributions of spe-

cific and error factors to the test, the more accurate this "true" estimate would be.

A second theorem of factor analysis is that specific and error factors cannot contribute to the correlation between variables. In other words, correlations between variables occur only on items in which they share. Therefore one of the main questions that factor analysis attempts to answer is whether intelligence is unitary or whether a diversity of intellectual abilities resides within the individual child.

Factor analysis starts with a table of correlations such as that shown in Table 4-2, but ordinarily a much larger set of test variables is involved. By the use of computational procedures, factor analysis attempts to identify a small number of underlying factors that can account for a complete set of relationships among test variables. Each factor of each test has a loading, corresponding to a correlation of that test with the particular factor. The analysis attempts to describe a pattern of factor loading within a theoretical framework. Table 4-2 presents a study in which tests were given to learning-disabled males (eight to eleven years of age) so that related measures to IQ could be determined.

The Children's Embedded Figures Test (CEFT) (Witkin, Oltman, Raskin, & Karp, 1971), discussed later in this chapter, was used as a measure of field dependence. The test requires the subject to locate a specific, two-dimensional figure (for example, tent or house shape) embedded within designs in varying degrees of complexity. This test distinguishes between subjects who experience visual information as discrete from the organized context of which it is a part (field independent) and those for whom perceptual ability is dominated by the overall organization of the field (field dependent). The mean score was 8.0 (standard deviation [SD] = 6.96).

The Locus of Control Scale for Children was administered orally (Nowicki & Strickland, 1973, discussed in Chapter 9). This scale is a forty-item yes-no instrument based on the dimension

Table 4-2

Factor analysis: correlations.

| Dependent measure | Factors being tested | | | |
| --- | --- | --- | --- | --- |
| | 1 | 2 | 3 | 4 |
| Embedded figures | .091 | .088 | .027 | .613 |
| Locus of control | .472 | .033 | .100 | −.030 |
| Slosson intelligence test | −.238 | .827 | −.219 | .263 |
| Mathematics | −.755 | .029 | −.063 | .211 |
| Reading recognition | −.878 | .126 | −.225 | .303 |
| Reading comprehension | −.750 | .323 | −.158 | .051 |
| Spelling | −.822 | .194 | −.243 | .147 |
| General information | −.740 | .221 | .189 | −.025 |
| Motor-free test | −.130 | .428 | .051 | −.110 |
| Chronological age | .098 | .006 | .896 | .210 |

of internal-external control of reinforcement. The mean score was 19.2 (SD = 5.08).

The Slosson Intelligence Test (SIT) is an individually administered test designed to evaluate mental ability (Slosson, 1981). The test includes many items that appear in the Stanford-Binet Intelligence Scale. The mean IQ score was 96.71 (SD = 5.60).

The Peabody Individual Achievement Test (PIAT) is an individually administered test designed to provide a wide-range screening measure of academic achievement in five content areas (Dunn & Markwardt, 1970). Topics of the five subtests include mathematics, reading recognition, reading comprehension, spelling, and general information. Respective mean percentile scores were 38.54 (SD = 27.63), 38.16 (SD = 32.02), 35.76 (SD = 31.16), 36.74 (SD = 28.83), and 42.84 (SD = 30.09).

The Motor-Free Test of Visual Perception (Colarusso & Hammill, 1972) provides a quick, reliable, and motor-free test of visual perception. It contains thirty-six multiple-choice items; the child points to the item of his or her choice. Different perceptual items, such as visual discrimination, closure, figure-ground, and position in space, yield an overall perceptual quotient (PQ) score. The mean PQ score was 93.95 (SD = 23.05).

Ideally each subtest should correlate with one factor but not with any others. If the contents of the tests and subtests that correlate most highly with each factor are examined, it is possible to deduce the nature of each factor. As shown in Table 4-2, Factor 1 is most clearly defined by tests of achievement and locus of control. This relationship corresponds with Nowicki and Strickland's (1973) concept that locus of control affects achievement and that high achievement is associated with internality. Factor 2 is responsible for 23.5% of the variance and yields loadings in intelligence and perceptual performance. Factor 3 is an age-related factor. Factor 4 is a small factor of cognitive style, distinct from intelligence and achievement. Although not all of the subtests are unambiguous measures of a single factor, most of the correlations make sense educationally. In short, it is important to note that while these ability factors are interpreted by an understanding of the theoretical nature of the tests, alternative interpretations are possible.

Some individuals have stated that the usefulness of factor analysis in describing intelligence has diminished, not only in terms of the number of factors, the subjectivity in naming factors, and choice of items serving in the initial pool analysis, but more specifically in its ability to determine the characteristics of the subjects answering the items (McNemar, 1964; Sternberg, 1988; Vernon, 1960). Many considerations—the individual differences of children and of models of structural relations among dimensions, differences in intellectual ability as a function of genetics, the effects of maturational and environmental factors in terms of opportunities of learning, transfer, and the application to problems of assessment—have been sorely lacking. Most of the factors obtained in factor-analysis studies, such as those of Guilford, tend to depend on some degree of correlation with each other. This dependency has led many psychologists (Vernon, 1960) to question both the conceptual and practical utility of such a fractional approach to the study of intelligence. McNemar states that "the structure of the intellect that requires 120 factors may very well lead us . . . to regard . . . fractionalization and fragmentation of ability into more and more factors of less and less importance as indicative of scatterbrainedness" (p. 872).

From an assessment point of view, the notion of general intelligence has not been discarded (Carroll & Maxwell, 1979). However, important questions posed by recent theorists (e.g., Sternberg, 1988) examine whether the factor of intelligence is linked to psychological processes or mental operation. Do factors represent individual differences or capacities in memory, attention, strategies on particular tasks, use of appropriate cues, or generalizability of skills to other tasks? Such questions have led recent theorists to study intelligence within the framework of an information processing model. The question "To what extent do psychometric and information-processing variables measure the same abilities?" has not been answered.

## INTELLIGENCE: A PROTOTYPE

The simplest way to measure intelligence in children (as suggested by factorial models) would be to combine all the relevant dimensions of adapting behavior (for example, classroom

functioning) into an overall test or index. Such a test would be somewhat arbitrary, as discussed earlier, as to the items used, but in principle it might provide some device to separate children according to individual differences. Currently, this ideal is unattainable because many of the relevant dimensions of children's behavior are not standardized or even identified. The characteristics of a "normal" adapting child would include not only vocabulary, analogical reasoning, social judgments, and general information, but also creativity, flexibility in learning, wit, and common sense. As suggested by many authors (for example, Torrance, 1970) these characteristics exhibit themselves only in practical or unique situations; others cannot be evaluated unless the child is observed over an extended period.

Thus there seem to be only two possibilities for assessment: not to measure intelligence at all or to measure it inadequately. In relation to civil rights, subcultural differences, distribution of economic and social benefits of children, and genetic and biological differences in intelligence, much could be said for the first alternative, but for various reasons society has adopted the second. Probably the most relevant argument for the second alternative is that at present IQ tests serve one function extremely well: they predict academic success or failure.

Thus, the basic structure of intelligence tests was designed to fill the pragmatic need of predicting school success (Binet, 1902). Intelligence tests are composed of items representative of the kinds of problems manifested in the mastering of school curricula. Furthermore, the typical intelligence test consists of a large number of problems that a prototypical child would respond to correctly. An individual child's score represents his or her resemblance to the prototypical child (average or smart) who would get all the items correct. If intelligence can be conceptualized as a resemblance and not a quality, how can it be measured in atypical or exceptional learners? A tautology in thinking exists at this point. Perhaps an orientation toward a child's potential is an alternative consideration.

## ASSESSING INTELLECTUAL POTENTIAL

### Potential Zone

Research by Brown and French (1979) and later by Brown, Campione and Palincsar (1987) considers the first problem of diagnosis to focus on the improvement of school performance rather than the mere correlation of test scores with overall classroom adjustment. Utilizing Vygotsky's (1978) zone of potential development, Brown and French make a distinction between the child's potential development and actual developmental level:

> A distinction is made between a child's actual developmental level, i.e. his completed development as might be measured on a standardized test, and his level of potential development, the degree of competence he can achieve with aid. Both measures are seen as essential for the diagnosis of learning disabilities and the concomitant design of remedial programs (p. 210).

Child-standardized intelligence performance provides a quantitative index of developmental status, but does not provide information on those functions that have not developed nor on the route by which the child arrived at his or her current developmental state. Therefore, the zone of proximal development is assessed, so that cognitive potential can be determined. This would include first giving the child an IQ test such as the Binet, WISC-R, or Wechsler Preschool and Primary Scale of Intelligence (WPPSI) in a standardized fashion. If the child fails to determine a problem's solution or concept, the examiner provides progressive cues to facilitate problem solution. The number of cues or promptings needed is considered the *width* of their zone potential. Another similar problem is given to the child, and the examiner makes note if fewer cues are needed. A transfer test is especially important and reflects the child's attempts to implement a strategy. The ability of the child to benefit from cues given by the examiner provides valuable information in terms of the child's starting competence on a variety of cognitive and academic tasks. Children who have a wide zone of potential are those who show a reduction in the number of prompts needed from problem to problem and who show "effective transfer to new solutions across similar problems" (p. 260).

Brown and French suggest that a necessary battery of transfer tests are appropriate to tap underlying rules suitable to task domains. Such tasks have largely been defined as isomorphs—tasks in which the child's strategies can be mapped from one problem to another. For example, number scrabble is an isomorph of the familiar game tic-tac-toe. In number scrabble, nine tiles, numbered 1 to 9, are placed face up between two players. Players draw single tiles alternately and the player who is first able to complete the triad of tiles and whose numbers add up to 15 wins the game. Specific information gathered in the solution of such a task can determine: (1) if the skills gained in solving one form of the problem will transfer to an isomorphic form of the same problem, (2) the extent to which instruction facilitates transfer of problem solving, and (3) the degree to which the problem's difficulties are associated with problem representation and the extent to which the solver assimilates the examiner's instructions.

### Thinking

Ann Brown, among others (Vygotsky, 1978), views the assessment of intelligence or problem solving that occurs in a context outside the traditional testing milieu, such as in mother-child dyads, group problem-solving sessions, or social settings. Special attention is given to the child's ability to mimic a normal process of development. Problem-solving behavior is seen as born of a social context. The assessment of intelligence in a social context represents a further deviation from traditional assessment practices. The primary goal of this assessment is not necessarily to locate the deficiencies in cognitive structures nor to discover generalized abilities across social situations. Rather the focus is to explicate the relation between the social context and the child's potential zone. Socialization practices certainly determine the organizational model from problem solving, and provide a firm understanding of the child's zone of potential. The varieties in cues in the environmental context are used to maximize problem solving.

## Regulation

Focus is now given to a variety of child self-regulation skills (e.g., Meichenbaum, 1987). The internalization process is said to be related to the internalization of language. This process begins with nonverbal mediation and is subsequently replaced by more advanced cognitive activity. Overt behavior becomes regulated through means of verbal mediation. Regulatory role and function are especially useful in mother-child dyads, and determination of them includes assessment of the child's monitoring, reality testing, predicting, and checking skills in a social situation.

In their model for assessment and training of daily problem solving, D'Zurilla and Goldfried (1971) have proposed five components: (1) problem orientation, (2) problem definition and formulation, (3) generation of alternatives, (4) decision making, and (5) verification. The growing efficacy of this approach has been noted in studies of cognitive behavior modification (Meichenbaum, 1977); it is also seen as a means of enhancing academic performance (Douglas & co-workers, 1976). Of course, when components of intelligence are being modified, a number of practical issues arise, such as (1) the cognitive capacity of the child to benefit from instruction, (2) the concomitant use of incentives, and (3) the generalization of the strategies to other tasks.

## Everyday Thinking

In summarizing their suggested diagnostic orientation, Brown and French state that IQ tests are predictive of school achievement, but the general welfare of a student requires a diagnostic approach that does more than predict. For improving diagnosis and remediation of academic problems, the following suggestions are made:

1. Consideration must be given to the limitations of tests in assessing everyday cognitive efficiencies. A contrast should be made between academic intelligence (for example, abstractness, speed of processing, correct solution) and everyday reasoning (for example, speed is irrelevant, abstract is less desirable than concrete solution).
2. Measure competence in relation to the demands of the child's individual environment.
3. What are the minimum demands of everyday life for the child of a blue-collar worker, that provide insight into the child's assimilation?
4. Also needed is a theoretical base that measures functional literacy, minimal competence, and mundane cognition, so that life adaptation and academic success can be predicted.

## INFORMATION PROCESSING

Perhaps no other theoretical base currently adds to our understanding of intellectual behavior more than that of information processing (Snow, 1980; Sternberg, 1985). Although the information processing model is both metaphor and methodology, it is extremely useful in explaining individual differences in intellectual functioning. Some limitations, however, have been noted by Snow (1980). Information processing theory implies that by examining an entire sequence of responses we can only begin to appreciate a child's intellectual activity.

Gradually it has become apparent that the child controls much and in some cases all of what is learned, relatively independently of the teacher. *What has happened is that the child's strategic knowledge has become a focus for assessment.* There has been a growing recognition that understanding a child's awareness of a given task, of what and how to remember or retrieve at a later time, is the most important topic for understanding learning and ability phenomena (e.g., Brown & Campione, 1986). In recalling, for example, a child must elaborate tasks and materials, then transform, recode, encode, reorganize, and give meaning to seemingly nonsense material. To recall the child must search and retrieve appropriate information, decode it into something meaningful, and decide on its accuracy and whether or not to verbalize it as the answer. Admittedly this is a gross simplification of a child's intelligence and an inadequate description of a child's functioning, but it captures the information-processing point of view. This point of view contrasts radically with an applied behavioral orientation (see Chapter 8) as well as factor analytical models of intellectual abilities.

Perhaps one of the most ambitious approaches to intellectual assessment from an information-processing framework is that of Sternberg (1977, 1981, 1985, 1988), to be discussed later. Utilizing six information-processing components, Sternberg has noted that these components account for large proportions of variance in ability testing (particularly reasoning and vocabulary). Furthermore, individual child differences are related to the extent to which strategies are used to identify relevant variables.

Similarly, Whitely (1977), in analyzing analogy reasoning, identified components of short-term and long-term memory, control processes, and response implementation as it contributed to verbal, analogy test performance. Whitely noted that individual differences, apparent in the item-solving strategies and the content of memory scores, seem central to the performance. Relating this analysis to intervention, Holtzman, Glaser, and Pellegrino (1975), utilizing a computer-simulated model, gave children explicit training instructions on component processes. Their results across age groups suggest that hypothesized components are trainable, support the "psychological reality of the identified processes, and suggest the potential of instruction in these processes for improving intellectual

competence" (p. 356). Therefore, intellectual assessment from an information-processing approach must account for the types of problems under study, the individual child's knowledge base, and the strategies that interact with problem solution.

Traditionally, test taking has been viewed as an activity that takes place in an unfamiliar context when an unmotivated child is initially unsuccessful in achieving some goal in the classroom. While this could describe the initial stages of a learning experience, contemporary assessment begins to reflect on a child's response as something distinct from learning. Instead of right or wrong responses, information processing stresses a child's search patterns, discovery, and strategy changes or shifts. Within the field of information processing, perhaps the most influential, as well as most strongly based in history, expositions are those of Bruner (Bruner, Goodnow, & Austin, 1956), Newell and Simon (Newell, Shaw, & Simon, 1958; Newell & Simon, 1972), Atkinson and Shiffren (1968), Craik and Lockhart (1972), and Brown (1977). Each theorist and the implications of his ideas for assessment will be reviewed briefly.

### Bruner, Goodnow, and Austin

An organized sequence of responses that a child makes in an effort to achieve the solution to a problem is called a *strategy*. It is a plan that includes stages of information gathering (what information the child chooses as important) and information processing (how the gathered information is processed). A pioneer work on strategy development is that of Bruner, Goodnow, and Austin (1956). There are many facets to their research; however, a major task included a conjunctive concept (red and square) in which the experimenters discovered that children used several distinct strategies in their problem-solving behavior. Four decision sequences have been identified.

*Conservative Focusing.* By a process of elimination, *focusing* yields relevant pieces of information about a concept. By comparing each successively encountered stimulus with a salient example of the concept, the child begins to eliminate an untenable hypothesis. Conservative focus begins when the child accepts the instance of positive comparison with the concept. Each time the concept is encountered, the child varies his or her idea of the concept by only one attribute. In other words, if the first card—an example of the concept—were red and the next card were green and square, the child in considering the second card would focus on the second attribute—square—because *red* has already been established as part of the conjunctive concept. This approach imposes minimal strain on memory and inferential ability, and ensures that the concept will eventually be obtained.

*Focus Gambling.* Focus gambling involves varying the choices of relevant attributes (shape, color, size) to more than one value at a time. Contingent on the occurrence of negative and positive instances of the attribute of the rule, this method can require fewer or more trials to gather the same evidence as gathered in the conservative focus.

*Simultaneous Scanning.* Instead of adopting a single attribute or two attributes as a basis for the elimination of irrelevant pieces of information, in the search for concept attainment, some children form a simple hypothesis about the solution (for example, all red and square forms are an example of the rule). *Simultaneous scanning* involves the generation of all possible hypotheses on the basis of the first positive instance of the concept, and the use of each following instance to eliminate untenable hypotheses. To scan optimally the child must have considerable use of memory so that he or she can avoid redundant stimulus selection and tests. Bruner noted that children generally have only limited success with the scanning strategy.

*Successive Scanning.* By following a "trial and error" approach (to one hypothesis at a time), *successive scanning* imposes less strain

on a child's memory. Again, the child must remember which hypothesis has been tried so that he or she can avoid redundant stimulus selections.

*Implications.* Bruner's research is multifaceted, and the essential outcome suggests that children's conceptual, problem-solving behavior is highly organized and consciously planned and integrated. Any theory for assessment based on children's problem-solving strategies must account for the fact that there are wide individual differences in behavior on tasks (tests) and that these can fluctuate with relatively small changes in the conditions (instructions, practicing before test taking, motivation) in which the tasks are performed.

Bruner's findings can be applied to assessment models in two ways. First, the strategies that are available to children for their forming of concepts vary. Hunt (1974) has shown that items on the Raven Progressive Matrices Test (to be considered later in this chapter) can be solved by means of two different strategies. One uses perceptual Gestalt-like relations, and the other uses a more analytical or cognitive relation. Although Hunt does not offer empirical evidence that these two distinct procedures are used by different children, a case can be made for such a conclusion. Even if children of different exceptionalities use the same basic strategies for organizing information, their test responses can be quite different if they use dissimilar strategies while taking the test. As shown in Bruner's findings on problem solving, some children's strategies can be more effective than others' and this difference becomes a crucial intervening variable between the task (environment) and the response produced on a test. Second, some strategies might be more effective than others, but effective strategies can be difficult to discover. It cannot be assumed that all children come equipped with the best strategies or will be able to discover the best strategies during test taking or learning conditions.

## Newell and Simon

A computer analogy to human behavior provides a means by which attention is directed to processes taught rather than environmental relations and response outcomes. Unquestionably a major contribution to a general theory of problem-solving behavior is the research of Newell, Shaw, and Simon (1958). Their theory has taken the form of the discovering of proofs for theorems in symbolic logic (Whitehead & Russell, 1925) through a complex computer program. This program, called the Logic Theorist, follows certain patterns of human processing. First, information follows a set in which instructions indicate the order in which various operations are to be performed. Second, insight or solution is based on the logical elimination and selection of alternative hypotheses. Effective learning is not done through simple trial and error but is determined by the extent to which behavior is governed by understanding of a rule. Third, learning is accomplished in a hierarchy (or task analysis of processes), in which a sequence of operations that generate and remember problems is done in an ordered fashion.

From an information-processing perspective, a problem exists when a child is required to choose the correct alternative or problem solution when several are presented. Newell and Simon (1972) studied the means in which a problem-solver making a choice would evaluate the properties of alternative solutions, and the difficulty imposed by this evaluation. They considered the chess player who has the problem of choosing moves, any of which can determine the outcome of the game. The evaluation of alternatives is extremely complex because of the number of alternatives available to the player as well as to the opponent. Alternatives in moves lead to a multitude of possibilities eventually leading to a tie, loss, or win.

In explaining these complexities, Newell and Simon detail the following classes of problems: cryptarithmetic (solving for a code that substitutes letters for numerical equivalents), developing proofs of symbolic logic through the application of rules, and choosing correct alternatives. Each class of problems is subject to a task analysis (discussed in Chapter 1), based on the responses of subjects who are instructed to think aloud while problem solving. The usefulness of a subject's verbalization as data rests on two assumptions. First, thinking aloud does not interfere with the subject's performance on the problem-solving task, and second, verbalization provides a complete record of the basic processes that are being executed. Available evidence supports these assumptions (Ericson, 1975).

Newell and Simon's research indicates that the essence of human problem solving can be understood through a description of three major determinants: (1) the space the solver uses to represent the environment—the task—and to accumulate knowledge about it, (2) task demands, and (3) the environment in which the task takes place. The task environment describes a general class of problems to which a problem belongs (for example, logic). Therefore the task environment is objective and external to the subject's perceived definition of the task. The problem solver, on the other hand, defines the problem-space or constraints (decisions, moves, strategies, logical relationships) incorporated into task solution. Theoretically, the problem solver strives to reduce the problem space so that each decision eliminates a number of available alternatives and solving the task becomes easier. Four propositions determine the relation of the three components:

1. The structure of problem-space (for example, the subjective nature of the task environment—strategies) determines the number of possible alternatives used for problem solving.
2. The task-environment structure (for example, memory, attention) determines the constraints of problem-space.
3. The structural features of the information are few, but do not vary among subjects regardless of task.

4. The structural characteristics are sufficiently strong in subjects so that they can determine problem space, and solution behavior occurs there.

The actual structural features of Newell and Simon's theory are few but represent a sensory register, short-term memory, and long-term memory. A description of each structure will be given when Atkinson and Shiffren's model is reviewed.

*Implications.* Newell and Simon's model has two major implications for the assessment of intelligence. First, protocol analysis of subjects who talk aloud verifies whether actual problem-space (strategies, relationships) is occurring. The usefulness of children's verbalization about answers given during tests allows the diagnostician to identify appropriate or inappropriate strategies. Understanding language instruction may provide successful modeling to precede models of problem-solving processes. Thinking skills and cognitive strategies, for example, have been developed by Covington and co-workers (1973) in an instructional unit called the Productive Thinking Program. Strategies identified in this series include (1) generating unusual or new ideas (divergent thinking), (2) breaking mental set, to look at a problem differently, (3) avoiding premature judgments, (4) clarifying the essentials of a problem, and (5) attending to relevant facts and conditions of the problem.

Second, and of more importance, Newell and Simon's model offers a paradigm in which intellectual behavior is analogous to an information-processing system. Children's knowledge represented in long-term memory consists of networks or strategies used at appropriate solving times. Only a few gross characteristics are invariant (for example, short-term, long-term memory). An important area of assessment becomes the child's problem-space, or the internal problem-representation of task demands. For example, the child is presented a math word problem that offers some initial information, a desired outcome from the child's

perspective, and certain constraints by which the initial teaching conditions can be transformed into the final goal (answer). The activity of the child is seen as a goal-directed search within the problem-space. Individual strategic differences result because there are a number of ways through which a final state can be reached from the same starting condition. At a level of classroom observation, assessment is made of the child's sequence of thought. Observation would include a condition (stimulus) and an action (behavior). A basic rule of interpretation is that whenever the condition of production is satisfied, the action of production will be executed.

## Atkinson and Shiffrin

The general theoretical framework of Atkinson and Shiffrin (1968) proposes a categorization of an information-processing system (memory) along two major dimensions. One dimension distinguishes the permanent structural features (similar to Newell and Simon) of an information-processing system, and other focuses on the control processes that are under the volition of the child or subject. Permanent features of memory include a physical system that is fixed or unvarying from one situation to another. Control processes are constructed and used at the option of the child and can vacillate from task to task. A general observation of a child's control processes in the classroom would further demonstrate that the nature of instruction, meaningfulness of material, and child's organization strategies, affect the child's recall performance. As Newell and Simon used (1972), a computer analogy is used to illustrate the distinction between memory structure and control process. Each component will be reviewed briefly.

*Sensory Register.* Figure 4-1 illustrates three basic structural components of information processing: sensory register, short-term store, and long-term store. Information in the multi-modality is assumed to first enter the appropri-

**Figure 4-1**

Atkinson and Shiffrin model. Three structural components of information processing. (Based on material from Atkinson, R., & Shiffrin, R. Human memory. In K. Spence & J. Spence [Eds.], *The psychology of learning and motivation* [Vol. 2]. New York: Academic Press, 1968, p. 11.)

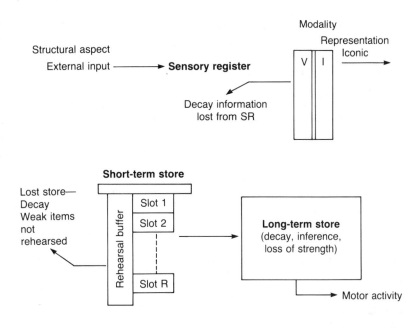

ate sensory register. Information in this initial store is thought to be a relatively complete copy of the physical stimulus that is available for further processing, for a maximum of three to five seconds. An example of sensory registration for the visual modality is an image or icon. For example, in a reading task, if an array of letters is presented tachistoscopically and the child is then asked to write out those letters after a 30-second delay (Sperling, 1967), the child will be able to reproduce about six or seven letters.

As shown in Figure 4-1, incoming information for other modalities (auditory, kinesthetic) receives sensory registration, but less is known about their representation. For example, children who are presented a letter of the alphabet might produce a photographic trace that decays quickly, or they might physically scan the letter and transfer the information into an auditory (for example, echo of sound), visual, or linguistic (meaning) representation. In other words, information presented visually could be recorded into other modalities. The transfer of a visual image to the auditory-visual-linguistic store, is made at the discretion of the child.

In the reading process, each letter or word is scanned against information in long-term memory and the verbal name. Certainly this representation will facilitate the transfer of information from the sensory register to a higher level of information processing. Less understood from the Atkinson and Shiffren model is what happens if information in the sensory register matches a long-term memory representation or needs to be mediated in the short-term store.

*Short-Term Memory.* From the sensory register, information is transferred into the limited capacity, short-term memory. (Its capacity is seven items plus or minus two; Miller, 1956.) The short-term memory represents the subject's working memory, and is in many respects the heart of Atkinson and Shiffren's model. Information lost in this memory is assumed to decay or disappear, but actual time of decay is longer than time available in the sensory register. Furthermore, as just discussed, the information from input (processed through the sensory register) does not have to represent its actual sensory input form. The exact rate of decay of information cannot be estimated, because this component is greatly controlled by the subject. A child can evoke rehearsal and thereby influence the structural characteristic of the decay process.

The short-term memory retains information in terms of auditory-verbal-linguistic representations. Atkinson and Shiffren have found it difficult to separate verbal and linguistic aspects from an auditory representation. When a child recalls letters, for example, the child may subvocally rehearse a letter by voicing the quality of the letter as well as the place of articulation in the mouth. These kinesthetic activities are difficult to separate from the actual linguistic aspects of recall. More recently, Tulving (1986) has differentiated between episodic (memory for order of events) and semantic (meaning) memory components that include a number of separate properties.

The exact nature of the capacity of short-term memory is somewhat obscure for atypical populations of children (Torgesen & Houck, 1980; Swanson, 1986). Research has been unclear as to whether the limitation is one of processing capacity, storage capacity, or some interaction between the two. Capacity measures usually include between five and nine items, depending on whether the items are letters, words, pictures, or digits. Variation in capacity is explained again by variations in the control processes (to be discussed in the following section) and in the meaningfulness of the material. The crucial factor in capacity is the child's ability to encode units or sequence the items so that they can be recoded into smaller units (Miller, 1956). Other factors that affect capacity include (1) information load, (2) similarity of items, (3) number of items processed during subsequent activities, and (4) passage of time (Atkinson & Shiffrin, 1968).

Analogous with the Atkinson and Shiffrin model, Ellis' (1970) view is that a pathology in the central nervous system is an underlying factor in short-term memory deficits of retarded children. Recent research suggests that deficits in these children's capacity can be attributed to a lack of separation between control processes (for example, retrieval strategies and actual short-term memory capacity). Unfortunately some studies have shown that short-term memory is not related to IQ (Belmont & Butterfield, 1971). Recent studies have produced data that suggest short-term memory deficits in atypical learners that represent structural as well as control process deficits (Swanson, 1986).

*Long-Term Memory.* The amount of information, as well as the form of information, transferred to long-term memory is primarily a function of control processes (for example, rehearsal). A permanent storage of information, long-term memory has unlimited capacity. The means by which information is stored is determined by the use of links, associations, and general organizational plans. Information stored in long-term memory is primarily semantic. Forgetting is caused by item decay (loss of information) or interference.

*Control Processes.* The term *control processes,* those processes that work within and between structural components, refers to schemes, coding techniques, or mneumonics used by subjects attempting to remember information. The variety is unlimited, and classification is rather difficult. In the sensory register, control processes include the child's decision to attend to information as well as the ability to determine when to scan information by matching input in the sensory register against long-term memory and thereby identifying input. Sample strategies may include scanning information and generating names for information, matching features or differences among stimuli, or focusing on one distinct feature.

Control processes inherent in short-term memory include a choice as to which information to scan and a choice of what and how to rehearse. Rehearsal refers to the conscious repetition of information, either subvocally or orally, to aid in the recall of information at a later time. Learning a telephone number or street address illustrates the primary use of rehearsal. Rehearsal also follows some individual systems in which a subject obtains an organizational form from the information being presented or imposes organization on that information. Two processes are involved: organization (ordering, classifying, or tagging information to facilitate retrieval) and mediation (comparing new items with items already in memory). Organizational schemes can include

1. Chunking: Grouping items so that each one brings to mind a complete series of items (for example, grouping words into a sentence)
2. Clustering: Organizing items into categories (for example, animal, furniture)
3. Mneumonics: Idiosyncratic methods for organizing materials
4. Coding: Varying the qualitative form of information (for example, using images rather than verbal labels or substituting pictures for words)

Mediation may be facilitated by use of these methods:

1. Making use of preexisting associations, eliminating the necessity for new ones
2. Utilizing instructions, either verbal or asking the child to imagine, to aid in retrieval and organization
3. Cuing at recall by using verbal and imaginary information to facilitate mediation

Short-term memory also uses a rehearsal buffer (as shown in Figure 4-1), which gives the subject some control over which items should be eliminated from rehearsal and which items should be included.

Control processes in long-term memory are involved in determining the mediational links or general plans. The search of long-term memory varies in degrees of order, such as a letter-by-letter search, conceptual categories, and temporal events.

***Summary and Implications.*** The Atkinson and Shiffrin model views information as flowing through component stores in a well-regulated fashion: the information progresses from sensory registers to short-term memory, and finally to long-term memory. To differentiate these stores in terms of children's functioning, one should realize that:

1. Short-term memory has a limited capacity and thus makes effective use of rehearsal and organizational mechanisms.
2. Storage in long-term memory is mostly semantic.
3. Two critical determinants of forgetting from long-term memory are displacement and interference as a result of a lack of retrieval strategy.

Therefore, assessment of intelligence must differentiate between the structural features of a memory system and the child's control processes. Focus on control processes can provide the information necessary to facilitate the flow of information to long-term memory.

### Levels of Processing Approach

Craik and Lockhart (1972) suggest that multistore models of information processing are inadequate in explaining the various characteristics of memory stores. For example, they cite literature (Cermack & Craik, 1979) suggesting that information in short-term store is both visual and semantic rather than being coded in an auditory-verbal-linguistic manner. They provide a description of various structural features of multistore models (Table 4-3). The Craik and Lockhart model deemphasizes the component structures of a memory system and proposes that control processes are a central focus of information processing. Processing depth is thought to be a product of the level at which incoming information is processed.

The memory system of Craik and Lockhart focuses on the processing or interpretation of incoming information in the content (for example, cognitive structures of the memory system).

**Table 4-3**
Multistore models.

| Feature | Sensory registers | Short-term memory | Long-term memory |
|---|---|---|---|
| Entry of information | Preattentive; before awareness | Requires attention | Rehearsal |
| Maintenance of information | Not possible | Continued attention; rehearsal | Repetition; organization |
| Format of information | Literal copy of input | Auditory-semantic; visual | Semantic; auditory and visual |
| Capacity | Large | Small (7 $\pm$2) | No known limit |
| Information loss | Decay | Displacement; possible decay | Possibly no loss; loss of accessibility |
| Trace duration | One-fourth to 2 seconds | Up to 30 seconds | Minutes to years |
| Retrieval | Readout | Automatic chunking; conscious awareness | Retrieval cues; search process; executive function |

Based on material from Craik, F., & Lockhart, R. Level of processing: A framework for memory research. *Journal of Verbal Learning and Verbal Behavior,* 1972, *11,* 671–684.

Processing is considered to occur in a series of analyses. For example, a child is presented with several words. The child could remember the words very shallowly or in terms of the orthographic features, and thus give rise to a short-lived memory trace; the child could process the words into phonological features represented by the printed word, and thus produce a somewhat more stable memory trace; or the child could process the word into semantic terms, and thus form a much more durable memory trace. A shallow analysis is concerned with perceptual or sensory features of information (for example, angles, brightness). The child merely matches the input against past learning. A deeper analysis is concerned with stimulus enrichment and elaboration through a semantic analysis. The child may put words into a sentence, free-associate other comparable words, or make a story with the word. The focus at this level is on the extraction of meaning.

Perhaps a major distinction of this model is the differentiation it makes between two deliberate control processes or rehearsal mechanisms. The first type of rehearsal refers to recycling of items in memory while the depth of encoding (for example, phonemic) remains unchanged. The second type of rehearsal refers to processes that increase the depth of encoding. In these terms, simple repetition of words represents the first type of rehearsal, whereas a word-elaboration technique is an example of the second type. Implicit in this distinction is the assumption that the simple repetitions of items to be remembered serve to maintain information in consciousness, whereas stimulus enrichment and elaborations are required for deeper encoding.

For assessment purposes, a diagnostician might give a list of words to be recalled. After the child has recalled the words, the diagnostician asks the child how he or she remembered the words. The child who responds by focusing on organization of words (for example, "I made them into a sentence," "they reminded me of..." is considered to be processing at an automatic level, rather than focusing on rehearsal activity. The child who responds both by focusing on the words (for example, "I made them into a sentence" ) and by rehearsal activity (for example, "I said the words over to myself," "I said the sentence I made up over again") is considered to be showing the second type of rehearsal. The child who makes reference only to the number of times he or she said the words ("I said the word each time you said it") is demonstrating the first type of rehearsal. The child who does not report having gone through the words systematically by elaboration, association, or rehearsal activity, is considered to have no apparent strategy.

*Implications.* Although this model is plagued with recent criticism in terms of its being tautological (e.g., Baddeley, 1978) and ignoring iconic memory processes and independent variables in its measure of depth of processing (Nelson, Walling, & Evoy, 1979), it can be applied in several ways to help in the understanding of children's information processing. First, focus is placed on the type of control processes used by subjects rather than on structural differences in information processing (for example, recall). Second, the model implies a continuum of depth rather than a series of stores (for example, short-term memory) or domains of processing. Third, what a child does with material to be processed is more important than what is recalled. Mere repetition of material enhances recall and recognition, but factors such as the child's imposing meaningfulness give greater coherence and integration of information. Therefore, assessment procedures could categorize control processes into a continuum of operations running from minimal processing (repeat a word in a reading lesson) to various types of elaborate processing, involved in either further enrichment of one item or associative linkage of several items.

## Neisser: The "Executive" Function

Neisser (1967) focuses on how information is retrieved from long-term memory. The storage of information is viewed from the individual's own concept of the event. Memory is made up not only of a verbal synthesis but also of visual images and reconstructions of events. As stated by Neisser:

> We store traces of earlier cognitive acts, not the product of those acts. The traces are not simply "revived" or "reactivated" in recall; instead, the stored fragments are used as information to support a new construction. It is as if the bone fragments used by the paleontologist did not appear in the model he builds at all—as indeed they need not, if it is to represent a fully fleshed-out, skin-covered dinosaur. The bones can be thought of somewhat loosely, as remnants of the structure which created and supported the original dinosaur, and thus as sources of information about how to reconstruct it (p. 285).

The fragments of information recalled are based on key pieces of information that have been salvaged. Relying on Bartlett's earlier work (1932), Neisser considers that subjects rely only on cues or fragments of information, and the reconstruction of information for retrieval becomes information of the processed cues. For example, if a child thought that a letter of the alphabet looked something like a human figure and then tried to remember that item according to its encoding, the recall might not include an actual representation of the letter. In Neisser's model, an item can be partially retrieved and be only half correct.

To explain the reconstruction processes that lead to retrieval of information, an *executive* routine is performed. The executive routine is a program that determines the order in which subprograms will be performed. In other words, it is the organization directive for various retrieval strategies. The executive function does not perform the searching task, organize, nor sort out material, but programs the various routines. Simply, it is the *how-to* search mechanism. Whereas a computer system has the executive function built in, humans have the ability to modify and develop an overall routine of information retrieval that can direct search procedures.

Neisser sums up his model in six points that reflect the retrieval process:

1. Information stored in memory does not have a 1:1 relationship to what subjects originally perceived. Information exists as fragments of overt and covert activity.
2. The retrieval of information consists of many programmed searches conducted simultaneously and independently (parallel search or multiple search).
3. A search strategy, separate from the executive function, seeks actively to organize and reconstruct retrieval information step by step (sequential analysis). The search strategy lays out all information to be organized and sorted.
4. The control of parallel and sequential processes is directed by the executive routine.
5. Executive routine and search processes are learned and based on earlier processing, the implications being that
   a. Subjects learn to organize and retrieve.
   b. There are individual styles of organization.
6. Failure to recall is failure to perceive, the implication being that
   a. Subjects are attending to the wrong stimulus.
   b. Executive routine is attending to the wrong traces.
   c. There is a misguided search strategy.

*Implications.* Neisser's model, based on extensive research and computer analogies, provides a format with which the retrieval processes of stored information can be understood. The implications of this model to the assessment of intelligence are obvious. First, the retrieval of information represents a reconstruction of the input or original stimulus. This reconstruction includes not only verbal information, but also visual information. Second, the *how-to* of a search or executive function can be learned and modified. Third, the child can be seen as having his or her unique executive routine.

In assessment, focus should be placed on the child's ability to select a retrieval strategy initially,

abandon it when it is no longer effective or required, and reinstate it when its use is again required. Working within this tradition, Butterfield and Belmont (1979) have trained mentally retarded persons in the role of executive control, by which they learn to select, evaluate, and revise or abandon control process operations. Their data suggests that executive control is an instructional variable and is developmentally based. Their data also suggests that retarded persons do not use executive control spontaneously, but that they can be taught.

### Brown: Knowing, Knowing About Knowing, and Knowing How to Know

Brown (1975) views memory development as being integrated with cognitive development; it includes such skills as language, problem solving, and comprehension. Because memory is complex, Brown proposes that it be broken down into three knowledge systems: (1) knowing—development of a knowledge system, especially semantic memory (Tulving, 1983), (2) knowing about knowing—introspective knowledge of a child's memory system (Flavell, 1970), and (3) knowing how to know—utilizing those strategies and skills a child possesses for deliberate memorization.

In Brown's model, a distinction or separation is made between semantic and episodic memory. *Semantic memory* refers to the storage of information about concepts and words; such a memory is embedded within the structure of language. *Episodic memory,* on the other hand, refers to remembered biographical events ("you visited me") or repetitive experiences or events.

Another distinction is made in Brown's model between the concepts of production and mediation deficiencies. Based on the work of Flavell (1970), the term *mediational deficiencies* refers to the fact that children are unable to utilize a mediator or strategy efficiently. For example, young children might not spontaneously produce a potential mediator to process task requirements, but even if they did, they would fail to direct their overt responses. Theories of production deficiencies suggest that children can be taught efficient strategies that they fail to produce spontaneously, and that these taught strategies will direct and improve the children's overt behaviors.

A third distinction made in Brown's model is that the more strategic information is needed for effective performance, the more likely it is that the task will be affected by growth and change in the child. Therefore Brown recognizes that (1) tasks have semantic or episodic require-

ments, (2) failure to use a strategy is related to mediation and production deficiencies, and (3) tasks that require strategies are sensitive to developmental changes in the child. Brown's development model is represented in Figure 4-2.

Perhaps the unique focus of Brown's model (as opposed to other models reviewed) is on child's metamemorial functioning. As might be expected, metamemory, or knowledge and awareness of memory operations, changes with age (Campione & Brown, 1986). Metavariables

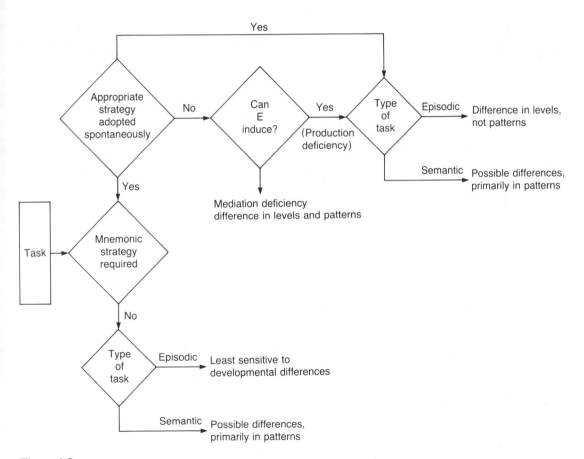

**Figure 4-2**
Brown's developmental model. (Based on material from Brown, A. L. The development of memory: Knowing, knowing about knowing, and knowing how to know. In H. W. Reese [Ed.], *Advances in child development and behavior* [Vol. 10]. New York: Academic Press, 1975, p. 139.)

refer to the child's concept of the requirements of particular tasks, the concept of mneumonic behavior, and the relation of these variables to actual memory performance.

*Implications.* Because memory, as suggested by Brown, is applied cognition, special attention should be given to the knowing, knowing about knowing, and knowing about how to know the ability of children. Such an assessment should be sensitive enough to (1) differentiate strategic from nonstrategic qualities, (2) differentiate semantic from episodic sequences, and (3) identify those tasks most susceptible to developmental changes.

## The Piagetian Model

Most information models that focus on cognitive structures and control processes have been concerned with the performance of tasks rather than the methods of learning how to perform them or with the cognitive abilities developmentally necessary to perform them. Once the structures and control processes of information processing are fairly well understood, it seems feasible to undertake understanding the specific developmental processes that create intelligent performance. Developing a model of children's performance on Piagetian tasks constitutes another step in building an assessment model of intelligence.

In Piaget's theory of intellectual development (1952), focus is placed on the means by which children adapt to and interpret objects and events in their environment. Therefore Piaget's concept of intelligence differs markedly from the traditional approach, which is concerned with measurement on a theoretical basis. Intelligence from a Piagetian perspective can be understood in terms of a complete process of adaptation. Adaptation depends on the two processes of assimilation and accommodation. It is the cognitive striving of human beings to find equilibrium between themselves and their environment through the processes of assimilation and accommodation.

In a simple view of Piaget's model, the child is seen as an active organism in which knowledge or reality must be discovered and constructed by the activity of the child (Flavell, 1963). Therefore knowledge involves a biological interaction between the child and the environment. The principal structure and functions of intelligent behavior, and the sequential stages of development are identified by Piaget as two areas of concern related to this interaction. These areas are only different facets of the same totality.

Heredity, one of the variables related to the child's interaction with the environment, determines the structure of intelligence and is related to the child's automatic behavior reactions (for example, reflexes) and physical structures (for example, eyes). The principle of functioning involves two invariant processes of organization and adaptation. The child systematically organizes interactions with the environment into a coherent system, either physically or psychologically. Physical interactions relate to the functioning and coordination of limbs. Psychological organization includes the coordination that must occur between grasping an object (physical) and then viewing it (psychological).

Maturation, experience, and social environment are, according to Piaget, not sufficient to explain intellectual development, because these factors alone cannot account for the sequential nature of development. Biological development is self-regulatory. The equilibration factor is the fundamental factor of development and is necessary for the coordination of the three other factors (maturation, experience, and social environment). The work of equilibration is the establishment or construction of structures not by balance of opposing forces but by self-regulation. Equilibration is a set of active reactions of the subject to external demands.

*Invariant Functions.* Adaptation is the need for the learning organism to achieve a state of dynamic equilibrium; behaviors seek a higher level of equilibrium according to the child's structure and organizational functions (physical and psychological) (Piaget, 1970). This optimal level is best understood as the state of learning in which the child is comfortable and operating at peak efficiency.

Two invariant functions involved in the process of adaptation are assimilation and accommodation (Piaget, 1970). Piaget states that *assimilation* is the integration of external elements into evolving or completed structures of an organism. He explains this by using the illustration of a biochemical reaction: food is digested (assimilated) in the body to form the basic substance of the organism. This process can be represented by the following reaction: $T + I = AT + E$, where T is a structure, I is substance or energies, E is eliminated substance or energies, and A is a coefficient $\geq 1$.

Assimilation strengthens or increases an already existing structure. It is the process whereby the organism adapts the environment to biological systems already in existence. The individual uses the environment as he or she conceives of it; the individual assimilates only as much as he or she can "digest" at the present time. In other words, the child acts on environmental stimuli as long as there exists a continuous or unified relationship of familiarity between the child and the object.

*Accommodation* is any modification of the existing psychological representation that forces some type of change. It is a modification of an assimilatory scheme or structure by the elements it assimilates. It is the process that involves the adaptation of the organism to the environment. Piaget illustrates this with an example of embryological development: "A phenotype assimilates the substances necessary to the conservation of its structure as specified by its genotype. But, depending on whether these substances are plentiful or rare or whether the usual substances are replaced by other slightly different ones, nonhereditary variations such as changes in shape or height may occur" (p. 105).

The psychological representation of information in assimilation and accommodation processes is called a *schema*—the pattern of a meaningful psychological event, which is repeatable. In a sense, the schema is a behavioral event that can be repeated and coordinated with the behavioral events of accommodation and assimilation. Mental assimilation involves the incorporation of the sensory data into the existing response patterns, and accommodation involves adjustment of the patterns.

***Stages of Development.*** The other variable related to the child's interaction with the environment is the stage of development. Characteristics of the stages are illustrated by the terms *hierarchization, integration, consolidation,* and *structuring.* A brief description of each term follows.

1. *Hierarchization:* It is necessary to have a fixed order of succession of the different levels that constitute a developmental sequence. This is not saying that the phases must adhere to specific age levels, but that there is an orderly succession to each level. The sequence cannot be altered.
2. *Integration:* In essence, this states that a given state (such as *preoperational*) incorporates or integrates the development of the preceding stage (*sensorimotor*). A stage is not merely a developmental entity.
3. *Consolidation:* A stage always involves an aspect of achievement of the recently acquired behavior as well as an aspect of behavior from the next level.
4. *Structuring:* The actual organization of the intellectual behavior characteristic of a particular level of functioning is called structuring. The operations of a given stage are not simply juxtaposed with another in an additive fashion but are interconnected by the ties of behavior that group them into total structures.

Piaget believes there are four major stages of intellectual development: sensorimotor (zero to eighteen months of age), preoperational (eighteen months to seven years of age), concrete operations (seven to twelve years of age), and formal operation (twelve years of age and upward). These stages are continuous, and each is built on and is a derivative of the earlier one. The sensorimotor period is perceived as a time of general development, in which reflexes move from one point of behavior to a type of discovery learning that does not use language. Figure 4-3 provides an overview of the stages of intellectual development.

The child's interactions with the environment are based on sensations, imagery, and manipulation. Before the appearance of language, the child can perform motor actions but not thought processes that depend on symbolic language;

---

**SENSORIMOTOR STAGE (0 to 2 months)**

Before the appearance of language, a child can perform only motor actions and not thought processes that depend on symbolic language. Because intelligence is adaptation, there is intelligence before the development of symbolic operations. Subphase descriptions include:

A. Reflexes (0 to 1 month)—innate (thumb sucking).
B. Primary circular reactions (1 to 4 months)—repeated act for sake, and first acquired adaptations (for example, repetitive opening of fists, fingering of blanket).
C. Secondary circular reactions (4 to 6 months)—produces stimulus effects (for example, kicks object and waits for results, shakes rattle to hear it).
D. Coordination of secondary reactions (7 to 10 months)—applies skills to new situations (for example, begins problem solving—knocks down object (pillow) to retrieve hidden object; object permanence obtained).
E. Tertiary circular reactions (11 to 18 months)—acts with trial and error or experimentation; varies overt response to same object (for example, knocks down pillow with rattle instead of feet); varies movement—accommodates.
F. Innovation of new means through internal mental combinations—a form of representation (18 to 24 months) (for example, solves a detour problem by going around barrier).

**PREOPERATIONAL STAGE (1½ to 7 years)**

Increased use of verbal representation, but speech is egocentric. The beginnings of symbolic rather than simple motor play. Transductive reasoning. Subphase descriptions include:

A. Preconceptual phase (2 to 4 years)—transition period of egocentric to socialized behavior.

1. Not concerned with communicating with others. Discovers new symbols for language. Symbols have personal reference. The child knows the world only as he or she sees it.
2. Assimilation of new experiences takes place through active exploring of environment.
3. Play occupies most of child's waking hours. Imaginary or symbolic play has all the elements of reality, while to the uninitiated bystander, this play is fantasy, for example, a wooden block "horse" "eats" a block "apple."
4. The child repeats words and connects these words with visual objects or perceived actions. Proper phonation and approximate correct use of words (2 to 3 years); symbolic imitation (mostly spontaneous).
5. Thought and reason are egocentric (a predominant language of self-reference).
6. Causal relationships deal with proximity (for example, young child interprets the act of walking past a stool and tripping on the leg as the cause: the stool is to blame for tripping [animism]). The child cannot do reversal conceptualizations.
7. Events are reasoned and judged by their outward appearance regardless of their objective logic (for example, a child will select a filled glass of water [to the brim] in preference to a glass three-fourths full but twice as large [based on child's idea of fullness]).
8. Takes orders from others literally (for example, "be good" confuses the child—does not know what to do in the absence of a demand of a specific behavior).

B. Phase of intuitive thought (4 to 7 years).

1. Gradual awareness of conservation of mass, weight, and volume (amount remains the same if transferred to a different size or shape).
2. Child does not have a set of categories when sorting; quantities judged by more or less.

---

**Figure 4-3**

Piaget's developmental stages.

because intelligence is adaptation, there is intelligence before the development of symbolic operations. This level of development of intelligent behavior has only limited application to the assessment of an exceptional child. However, the notion that development is a continual process not linked to time means that some children (for example, autistic children) might be arrested at one stage.

Intellectual behavior (formal operations) is characterized as the child's ability to deal efficiently with verbal propositions and a "hypothetic-deductive" method of inquiry and problem solution. A typical experiment utilized

---

3. Unilateral authority for adults (rules have always existed).
4. Limited to actual, not potential. Incapable of thinking in terms of whole; still deals in parts.
5. Outside clues still define a situation (for example, if a child's bed is moved to another room, the bed becomes a new and different bed).
6. Uses appropriate language without fully understanding it (knows right arm from left but no idea of right and left).
7. In reasoning, outcome justifies logic (for example, car that finishes first in race is the fastest even if it covered only a short distance).
8. Speech is a means to excitation instead of a means of exchange of ideas or messages.
9. Lacks mental representation of series of actions (can walk but cannot draw action on paper).
10. Quantity is not conserved, not aware of degrees (darker, lighter, larger); interprets darker as very dark (absolute) rather than darker than another. (Young children do conserve as long as facts presented to them are within their expectations.)
11. A child will select those parts of sensory impressions that are most salient. Example: Present a photograph of a picnic scene. A 4-year-old will describe the scene as boys and girls playing. An older child (differentiating more aspects of stimulus) will call it a happy school picnic. With increasing age and practice (learning), the child tends to make more differentiations among stimuli in the environment.

### CONCRETE OPERATIONAL STAGE (7 to 11 years)

Evidence for organized, logical thought. Thinking becomes less transductive and less egocentric. The child is capable of concrete problem solving.

A. Socialized speech—more likely to consider the point of view of others.
B. Mental representations—has a sequential mental representation of a series of actions. Can tell how to get from one place to another or draw it on paper. Knows that liquids or solids are not transformed without changing their mass or volume.
C. Reversibility—capable of reversible operations (can state correctly the constancy of a piece of clay).
D. Class inclusion—sees object with common features and is able to form a class of objects with similar characteristics.
E. Serialization—understands relationships (for example, dark, darker, darkest; has the ability to arrange objects according to some quantified dimension (such as weight, size) on an ordinal scale).
F. Mode of thinking—returning mentally to starting point to overcome perceptual contradictions.

### FORMAL OPERATIONS (12 years and upward)

Comprehension of abstract concepts (for example, ability to form "ideals" and reason about the future), ability to handle contrary-to-fact propositions and to develop and test hypotheses.

A. Can deal with many possible ways of solving problems.
B. Can deal in hypothetical propositions (ideas don't have to fit reality—concrete reality oriented).
C. Organizes problems into high order operations using abstract rules.
D. Groping with hypothesis about the possible (11 years).
E. Naive idealism—change the world by thought (12 years).
F. Ability to use hypothetical reasoning based on a logic of all possible components.
G. Undertakes and performs controlled experimentation.
H. Integrated group lattice of total structure.

**Figure 4-3**

*continued*

by Piaget to assess concrete and formal operations is the assessment of the conservation of mass, weight, and volume. Following are some assessment procedures from Swanson, Minifie, and Minifie (1979). Materials used for testing the child's concept of the conservation of mass, weight, and volume include two clay balls that are identical in size, shape, and weight. Each child was tested individually three times on each conservation task. Conservation or nonconservation responses to prediction, judgment, and explanation questions were evaluated. For example, on the conservation of mass task the child was asked, "Do both balls have the same amount of clay? Is there as much clay in this ball as in this one?" Further questions were then asked.

1. Prediction: "Suppose I roll one of the balls out into a hot dog. Will there be as much clay in the hot dog as in the ball? Will both have the same amount of clay?"
2. Judgment: "Is there as much clay in the ball as in the hot dog? Do they both have the same amount of clay?"
3. Explanation: "Why is that?"

The same procedure can be used to test for conservation of weight and volume. Children's responses on prediction, judgment, and explanation questions can be used in the derivation of a conservation score. For example, each conservation response can be given a score of 1 and each nonconservation response a score of 0. Criteria of conservation or nonconservation for explanation responses are based on Piaget and Inhelder's (1969) categorizations. Other tests and references from a Piagetian perspective are provided in Table 4-4.

*Implications.* The implication of Piaget's theory is that there is a constant sequence in cognitive development. Stages do not necessarily adhere to specific age levels, but there is orderly succession to each level. Diagnosticians need to recognize and understand the following implications of Piaget's work:

1. The development of cognitive behavior is a continuous process, not limited by time.
2. Each child progresses along his or her unique continuum, and progress is noted by behavioral manifestations (for example, conservation).
3. Cognitive structures are built on past stages and should not contradict the purposes of the lower act.
4. Assessment's focus is on the controlled equilibrium of the learning environment (assessing of the accommodation process).

### Sternberg's Model: Componential Analysis

Sternberg's theory of mental ability (1978, 1979, 1988; Sternberg & Suben, 1986) is organized into four levels: composite tasks, subtasks, information-processing components, and metacomponents. According to Sternberg, a theory of each of the four levels of analysis tells something about the structure and content of mental abilities responsible for intelligent performance.

*Composite Tasks.* Because many tasks or tests of mental ability lack a theoretical point or perspective, Sternberg proposes that the selection of tasks (composite tasks) be based on four criteria. First, the concept under study must be quantifiable—the unit to be assessed can be assigned a numerical value. Second, the concept under study must be reliable—the quantification obtained must be internally consistent. Third, the task chosen must have a basis in psychological theory—construct validity (see Chapter 3). The task is not chosen because the task is well used (for example, utilizing the Wechsler Test for its own sake), but because it serves as a vehicle for the testing of one or more psychological theories. As stated by Sternberg (1979), "the theory thus dictates the choice of task(s) rather than the task(s) being chosen more or less arbitrarily and then giving rise to a post hoc theory of task performance" (p. 218). Fourth, the task chosen must measure to some extent the construct(s) of the supposed theory of intelligence—must have empirical validity.

**Table 4-4**
Tests and references from a Piagetian perspective.

| Task name | Description and purpose* | Cognitive ability—assessment stage |
|---|---|---|
| Rotation of beads | To assess child's ability to predict when a colored bead enters a tube (regardless of how rotated) that it will exit the bottom first | Maintain imagery—preoperational |
| Euclidean space | Ability to recognize Euclidean shapes and represent them motorically (drawing) | Spatial reasoning—preoperational |
| One-for-one exchange | Using equal number of pennies and packages, child is asked who has the most or do both examiner and child have the same | Comprehension of corresponding sets—begin concrete operational |
| Term-to-term correspondence | Place blocks into two rows of one-to-one correspondence, then collapse one row of blocks so one is longer and the other is shorter; child is asked if both rows have the same number of blocks | Comprehension of correspondence and number—begin concrete operational |
| Conservation of length | After child establishes equivalence of two rods, they are placed parallel to one another; child is asked if rods are the same length or if one is longer | Reasoning on object changes as result of displacement—begin concrete operational |
| Conservation of liquids | Equivalence is established with two beakers of water, then water is displaced into four other beakers of various sizes; child is asked if there is more water in one or if they have the same amount of water | Comprehension on quantities of liquid in various container shapes—concrete operational |
| Conservation of mass, weight, and volume | Discussed in chapter | First two are concrete operational; last one is formal operational |
| Class inclusion | Child is shown various objects (e.g., beads, animals) and asked to classify and to use two classifications (one that encompasses all and another pertaining to one attribute) at the same time | Comprehension of subcategories—concrete operational |
| Relationships | Identify right and left placement of three objects or comprehension of brother/sister relations | Relational sense—concrete operational |
| Probability | Judgment based on the number of objects (e.g., blocks) of each category (e.g., color) that remain after a displacement procedure | Make predictions—formal operational |

*Total task description can be found in Piaget, J., & Inhelder, B. *The psychology of the child.* New York: Basic Books, 1969.

Applying these four criteria suggests that a number of composite tasks representing complex mental abilities could be used.

1. *Analogies:* An analogy demonstrates a relationship among four or more items. A political science item could measure the student's understanding of the relationship among four terms designated by the letters a, b, c, and d:

   Fourscore and seven years ago (a) is to Lincoln (b) as I'm not a crook (c) is to:
   a. Reagan
   b. Carter
   c. Kennedy
   d. Nixon

2. *Classifications:* A classification consists of the determining of a series of objective items based on a common set of data. The data may be in the form of written materials, tables, charts, graphs/maps, or pictures. Sternberg suggests that a classification be utilized to identify relationships of data; for example:

   Shangri-la, Eden, El Dorado. Which of the following terms best fits with these three:
   a. Denver, Colorado
   b. Utopia

3. *Series completion:* Completion tasks require the student to complete a series of logically related terms with an appropriate word; for example:

   Sit, stand, walk, _____ . Choose from the following terms to fill in the blank:
   a. lie
   b. run

4. *Metaphorical completions and ratings:* Metaphorical tasks require the student to supply concrete examples of an abstract notion. In the completion task, children may be presented with an incomplete sentence followed by a blank in which a "goodness of fit" is to be determined. For example:

   Grasshoppers in the crops are like bears in the:
   a. cave
   b. honey

   In the rating task, children rate the appropriateness of metaphors such as, "the digestive system is like thinking."

5. *Syllogisms:* Syllogisms require that a deduction or conclusion be made from two or more premises. Sternberg suggests using three types of syllogisms:
   a. *Linear syllogisms*—subject receives two premises. For example,

      Jane is kinder than Dracula, Dracula is kinder than my teacher, who is the kindest?

   b. *Categorical syllogisms*—student receives two premises and an analysis of a logical conclusion. For example,

      Some teachers like McDonald's hamburgers, some students like McDonald's hamburgers, therefore, some students are teachers.

   c. *Conditional syllogisms*—student receives two premises and an analysis of an if-then conclusion. For example,

      If the day is gloomy, it must be Monday; the day is not gloomy; then it must not be Monday.

*Level of Subtask.* A mere listing of children's scores on mental-abilities tasks is at present theoretically barren because it gives no understanding of the determinants of a child's performance. Although items correlate across subject and task manipulations (for example, subjects who perform well on categorical syllogisms perform well on conditional syllogisms), a decomposition of the composite task is necessary if strategies and processes that specify task performance are to be determined. Sternberg suggests that tasks that appear quite different on the surface can require similar processes or strategies for their solution. Therefore, so that the proliferation of possible tasks is controlled, a subset of information-processing components must be identified. Such an analysis of subtask levels allows the assessor to more closely specify the relationship between task structure and the components that act on that structure. This intermediate step in the analysis of the nature of mental abilities "guards against the spurious good fit between model (intelligence) and data that can result when the number of parameters to be estimated becomes large relative to the number of data points predicted" (Sternberg, 1979, p. 220).

Although the decomposition of composite tasks can be done in a variety of ways (Sternberg, 1985), two groupings can be inductive tasks (for example, analogies, classifications, series completions, metaphorical completions) and deductive tasks (for example, syllogisms). An inductive analysis is fairly explicit. Faced with a series of tasks, the child induces the appropriate number of the statement and/or constructs that generate (summarize) them. In contrast to deductive tasks in which the child starts at the top and works down, an inductive analysis begins at the bottom and works up. Inductive tasks involve a precuing phase (for example, analysis of the given information). This phase requires a breakdown of each subtask into a series of trials, in which successively less information is presented. For example, in an analogy problem, precuing may include zero to five terms. Consider the following analogy: teacher:classroom :: doctor: (a) hospital, (b) courtroom. The child might receive no precuing terms (a blank field), one term (teacher), two terms (teacher:classroom), three terms (teacher:classroom :: doctor), four terms (teacher:classroom :: doctor: [a] hospital), or five terms (teacher:classroom :: doctor: [a] hospital, [b] courtroom). The purpose of this breakdown into information-processing units is to select only those conditions of precuing that (1) do not alter the strategy by which a child can solve a problem, and (2) more closely isolate information-processing components. Child difficulty may

involve encoding (knowledge of each term of the analogy), inference (relationship of the first two terms), mapping (relationship of the first and third terms), application (relationship of the third term to the answer options), and/or response (correct answer or justification process).

A second method, deductive tasks, involves the analysis of similar subtasks, such as series completion and metaphorical completion. This method involves analysis of the full problem. Explanations of difficulties in problem solution are facilitated by an analysis of precues. The application of precues and the analysis of problem solution without precues (full task) is easily transferable to deductive tasks. For example, two components of syllogistic reasoning may include encoding (given syllogistic premise) and combination (set relations encoded for two syllogistic premises). Errors in the syllogistic reasoning of atypical learners may originate in the combination rather than encoding stage.

To summarize, a decomposition of composite tasks (for example, analogies, syllogisms) into subtasks (inductive, deductive) is useful in the isolation of information-processing components. The next step in the breakdown of child task-performance is the isolation of component processes.

*Componential Analysis.* A componential analysis consists of a series of intensive task analyses of elementary information processes. Components are of three kinds: general (performance required on all tasks), class (skill required for various tasks), and specific components (skill required for a single task). In many respects this classification of components is similar to Guilford's factorial model (discussed in Chapter 1). The purpose of analyzing these components is to seek out a theoretical base that is practically sound (for example, applies to classroom learning). This theoretical base would include

1. Identification of task components and the types of information on which they act
2. Comparison of components to those in a standard test of mental abilities

3. Estimation of child difficulty and probability of execution of each component
4. Comparison of the amounts of consistency with which various strategies are employed within and between components

Sternberg suggests that a successful, detailed specification of task performance provides information that gives the best account of the child's responses (time, response-choice, error data) and also relates those responses to standard ability tests. Component analysis provides insight into the child's abilities; however, further analysis must take into consideration the "control" the child has over his or her own cognitive processes.

*Metacomponents.* The child's awareness of or control of his or her own cognitive processes is called *metacognition.* Solving problems, remembering words, and comprehending what is read are deliberate actions that require self-invoked plans and cognitive skills. To accomplish these activities, the child must coordinate a variety of information regarding the material to be learned. The child's general knowledge guides the effective selection and implementation of task-relevant skills (Palincsar & Brown, 1987). Sternberg regards metacognition as a level of thinking higher than task-specific strategies, because metacognition constitutes information about learning parameters. Metacognition serves as an executive function, directing and coordinating the learner's thinking and behavior.

Drawing on developmental literature (Flavell & Wellman, 1977), Sternberg discusses three important categories of metacognition that might be related to the theory of componential level. First, an assessment must be made of the child's knowledge of enduring characteristics and transient conditions that apply to such things as syllogisms and analogies. To engage component skills commensurate with their ability, learners need to appraise their potential realistically. Second, an assessment of the child's knowledge of the purposes, scope, and requirements of the task must be made before

problems can be efficiently executed. Third, an assessment must be made of the child's awareness of existing strategies and the recognition of the need to apply them. A child must be able to form plans, generate hypotheses, check on progress, evaluate responses, and apply learned behavior to similar problem-solving tasks. Because the development of children's metacognition is associated with efficient learning, remembering, and problem solving, it could provide, according to Sternberg (1979), processes responsible for the solution of problems in an intelligent way.

*Implications.* To conceptualize intellectual behavior, one needs a pretheoretical framework. Sternberg views intelligence as being based on an information-processing framework; intelligence is seen as the child's ability to adapt to the environment. Adaptation, of course, takes many forms and can include social competence, effective motivation, and a basic knowledge of the real world (Sternberg, 1988). In Sternberg's model, intellectual behavior is understood in part by a focus on components; this approach is similar in analogy to that of Newell and Simon (1972), in which information processing is concerned with the internal representation of objects and symbols. These components form an information-processing concept that translates input into conceptual representations of physical movement. Some aspects of Sternberg's model are

1. *Performance components:* processes used in a problem-solving strategy; for example, encoding, short-term memory, inferring relations, justifying the best solution over other alternatives, responding to a problem situation
2. *Acquisition components:* skills used in learning new information
3. *Retention components:* skills used in remembering previous information that has been learned
4. *Transfer components:* representation of information in another context or variety of contexts

According to Sternberg, these components, which are closely integrated, represent an intellectual system. Metacomponents are higher-order control processes that determine the means by which a problem can be solved. Examples include the selection of low-order components, deciding on an appropriate strategy and the point at which to switch to another decision or solution, and allocating the time necessary to complete a problem so an accurate response can occur.

*Remediation.* Some support for the modifiability of intellectual performance within Sternberg's conceptualization comes from the earlier work of Butterfield and Belmont (Butterfield & Belmont, 1979; Butterfield, Wambold, & Belmont, 1973) and Feurstein (1979). Butterfield and Belmont, from their decade of research with mentally retarded persons, have concluded that deficiencies in recall are largely a result of a person's failure to rehearse information actively. When instructed to rehearse, some people can make significant gains in recall performance. Although some caution is needed in the interpretation of their results, favorable performances have been found when (1) information speed has been controlled (Butterfield, Wambold, & Belmont, 1973), (2) an appropriate strategy can be generated (Butterfield & Belmont, 1977), and (3) the child can execute functions (Butterfield & Belmont, in press).

Consistent with Butterfield and Belmont, Brown (1978) has outlined a series of steps by which a successful intervention of problem-solving strategies can be planned.

1. It might be necessary to train persons in motivation as well as cognition.
2. All cognitive components must be analyzed in relation to task and capacity requirements.
3. Assessment must be made of spontaneous strategy efficiencies and deficiencies, and the deliberate training of them.
4. Assessment must be made of the transfer of strategies to a variety of tasks.
5. Techniques should be developed that teach retarded children monitoring and realistic

evaluation of strategy production, as related to their capacity and array of skills (pp. 101–102).

Feurstein's (1979) views of retardation and its assessment focus on the processes of thinking, not the products of thinking (for example, vocabulary, general information). The evaluation of retarded children, who lack control processes (inadequate definition of problem, inability to select relevant cues, lack of hypothesis testing), must go beyond psychometric evaluation and assess the modifiability of strategies and conditions. While data are still pending, Feurstein has utilized several metacomponential exercises to facilitate mediation (learning how to learn). One exercise influences the identification of similarities and differences of words by function, another by categorization exercises that develop systematic exploration, discrimination, and summative behavior.

## STANDARDIZED INSTRUMENTS TO ASSESS INTELLECTUAL COMPONENTS

The purpose of this section is to review the major test instruments available to psychologists and educators. Although many of these tests were not developed from an information-processing framework, they may all be adapted as such. Each test is reviewed according to its purpose, sample items, standardization, reliability, and validity. The tests are divided into (1) individually administered intelligence tests of general abilities, (2) group administered intelligence tests of general abilities, and (3) individually administered tests of specific abilities.

### INDIVIDUALLY ADMINISTERED INTELLIGENCE TESTS OF GENERAL ABILITIES

#### Wechsler Test Series

Four different Wechsler Intelligence Scales are widely used in the public schools by certified psychologists.* The main difference among the scales is the age group for which each is intended. The Wechsler Preschool and Primary Scale of Intelligence (WPPSI; 1967) is used with children between 4 and 6½ years of age. One of the most widely used tests of general intelligence for children 5 to 15 years of age is the Wechsler Intelligence Scale for Children (WISC; 1949). A revision of the Wechsler Intelligence Scale for Children (WISC-R; 1974) is used with students who are between 6 and 16 years, 11 months of age. The Wechsler Adult Intelligence Scale (WAIS-R; 1981) is used for older persons.

Because the WISC-R test is used most often, special attention will be given to it. The verbal scale and the performance scale contain five subtests and one alternate test each. The full scale score is the total of the verbal and performance scales. Scores on the subtests are converted to standard scores, which can be summed and converted to deviation IQ scores for each of the scales. The distribution of deviation IQ scores has a mean of 100 and a standard deviation of 15, so results for all ages are comparable. A scaled score of 10 indicates average ability for age in a particular subtest. The following is a list of skills measured by each subtest of the WISC and WISC-R.

**Verbal scale subtests**

**Information** Information gained from experience and education; alertness to world around child; statement of learned facts

**Comprehension** Practical knowledge and social judgment; anticipation and judging consequences of behavioral situations

**Arithmetic** Concentration and arithmetic reasoning; specific school learning; mental alertness; ability to manipulate numerical concepts

---

*Because the purpose of this chapter is to provide a conceptualization of information-processing research as applied to the construct of intelligence, idiosyncratic research for each test as it applied to atypical learners was not included. A good reference for the Wechsler Scales is Kaufman (1980).

**Similarities** Ability to recognize and describe essential relations between objects or ideas; verbal concept formation; concrete versus abstract kinds of thinking; ability to see relationships between facts and ideas

**Vocabulary** Cultural environment reflected; potentiality for dealing with symbols; quality and character of thought process; provides information about the quality of language used

**Digit span** Attention, and auditory memory and sequencing; measures ability to attend to rather simple situations

**Performance scale subtests**

**Picture completion** Visual alertness and organization; ability to recognize essential details; contact with reality; measures ability to identify and discriminate between essential and nonessential details in pictures

**Picture arrangement** Nonverbal judgment, anticipation, and planning (through use of essential picture clues); responsiveness to interpersonal relations; indication of social alertness and common sense

**Block design** Analysis and reproduction of abstract designs; logical insight into space relationships; visual-motor perception and coordination

**Object assembly** Seeing relationship of parts to whole in a familiar configuration; critical appraisal of small details; visual-motor coordination; concentration and simple assembly skills

**Coding** Speed of visual-motor reaction and association of symbols; ability to learn unfamiliar tasks; ability to learn symbols and shapes and to recreate them

**Mazes** Visual-motor planning and following of a visual pattern

The interpretive rationale for the subtests and suggestions for administering, scoring, and interpreting performance are given in a training manual by Glasser and Zimmerman (1967).

*Reliability and Validity.* Few discussions of validity occur within the Wechsler Scale manuals. The scales have been repeatedly correlated with the Stanford-Binet and other tests of intelligence. A correlation of .75 was found between the WPPSI and the Stanford-Binet. Investigators have found concurrent validity coefficients between the WISC and achievement tests to be between .50 and .60.

Reliability coefficients of the WAIS were computed within the 18–19-year-old, 24–34-year-old, and 45–54-year-old samples. For all three age groups, full-scale IQs yielded reliability coefficients of .97, verbal IQs .96, and performance IQs .93 and .94. On the WISC-R, average split-half reliability coefficients for verbal, performance, and full-scale IQs were .94, .90, and .96, respectively. Retest coefficients were .93, .90, and .95. On the WPPSI the reliability of full-scale IQs varied between .92 and .94, verbal IQs between .87 and .90, and performance IQs between .84 and .91. Retest reliability, after an interval of eleven weeks, averaged .89.

*Standardization.* The size and representativeness of the standardization samples of the Wechsler Scales are impressive. On the WAIS, 1700 cases were used as normative data. An equal number of men and women in seven age levels was used. They were proportionately chosen to match the 1950 census, in regard to geographical region, urban-rural, race, occupational level, and education. At each age level, one man and one woman from an institution for mentally retarded persons were also used. An "old age" sample of aged sixty and over was also taken.

The standardization sample for the WISC-R included 100 boys and 100 girls, ranging from 6½ to 16½ years of age. The sample was stratified on the basis of the 1970 census, with respect to geographical region, urban-rural, occupation of head of household, and race. Testing was conducted in thirty-two states.

The WPPSI was standardized on 1200 children, 100 boys and 100 girls in each of six half-year age groups from 4 to 6½ years. The sample was stratified according to the 1960 census, with reference to geographical region, urban-rural, proportion of white and nonwhite, and father's occupational level. The Wechsler

Scales as applied to minority assessment are discussed in Chapter 13.

### STANFORD-BINET INTELLIGENCE SCALE

(Terman, L., & Merrill, M., 1960 revision, Houghton Mifflin; Third Revision, 1973, Riverside Publishing Company)

The Stanford-Binet Intelligence Scale is recommended for use with subjects from two years of age through adulthood. (For a more extensive review of the test, see Anastasi, 1982.) Practically speaking, the test is seldom used in school systems for children over ten or twelve years of age because of its length and the time required for administration (Sattler, 1974). In such cases, the WISC-R or the WAIS is normally used. The Stanford-Binet contains a series of items, increasing in difficulty and grouped by age level, starting at two years of age and progressing to adulthood. There are six test items and an alternate item for each age level, with the exception of the average adult level, which has eight items and an alternate item. Tests items for each age level are shown in Table 4-5, and the table suggests the number of months given toward the subject's mental age (MA). To determine MA, add to the basal age the month of credit earned above the basal age. Deviation IQs are determined from standard scores on an assumed mean of 100 and standard deviation of 16. As an illustration of the content of various subtests, a description is provided for items in year six.

1. *Vocabulary:* Child gives the meanings or definitions of words of varying difficulty.
2. *Differences:* Child states a difference between certain animals or objects (such as a bird and a dog).
3. *Mutilated pictures:* Child looks at a card on which there are objects with parts missing, and child is asked to tell what parts are missing.
4. *Number concepts:* Child is asked to count out a specified number of blocks.
5. *Opposite analogies:* Child completes statements that express analogies.

**Table 4-5**
Age levels for Stanford-Binet test items.

| Age level | | Number of items plus alternate (A) | Months added to MA for each item passed |
|---|---|---|---|
| **Years** | **Months** | | |
| 2 | 0 | 6 plus A | Subject must pass all items for the test to be valid |
| 2 | 6 | 6 plus A | 1 month |
| 3 | 0 | 6 plus A | 1 month |
| 3 | 6 | 6 plus A | 1 month |
| 4 | 0 | 6 plus A | 1 month |
| 4 | 6 | 6 plus A | 1 month |
| 5 | | 6 plus A | 2 months |
| 6 | | 6 plus A | 2 months |
| 7 | | 6 plus A | 2 months |
| 8 | | 6 plus A | 2 months |
| 9 | | 6 plus A | 2 months |
| 10 | | 6 plus A | 2 months |
| 11 | | 6 plus A | 2 months |
| 12 | | 6 plus A | 2 months |
| 13 | | 6 plus A | 2 months |
| 14 | | 6 plus A | 2 months |
| Average Adult | | 8 plus A | 2 months |
| Superior Adult I | | 6 plus A | 4 months |
| Superior Adult II | | 6 plus A | 5 months |
| Superior Adult III | | 6 plus A | 6 months |

6. *Maze tracing:* Child is shown a picture of a schoolhouse and a little boy, and is then asked to draw the shortest path between the boy and the schoolhouse.

   *Alternate: response to pictures, level II:* Child is asked to look at pictures and describe them.

Terman and Merrill stated (1960) that intelligence is regarded as general mental adaptability, and thus an inspection of their scale reveals a variety of subtests measuring a considerable range of mental abilities. Sattler (1982) has analyzed the functions of the scale according to item-content categories. The schema includes seven major groupings.

1. *Language:* Includes vocabulary items at the prekindergarten level (vocabulary referring to the number of words the child can define) and quality of vocabulary (measured by such tests as abstract words, rhymes, word naming, definitions, and comprehension of verbal relations)

2. *Memory:* Subclassified into meaningful, non-meaningful, and visual memory; some other designations for this category include rote auditory memory, ideational memory, and attention span

3. *Conceptual thinking:* Primarily concerned with abstract thinking

4. *Reasoning:* Subclassified into verbal and nonverbal reasoning; verbal absurdity items are examples of this category; pictorial and orientational problems are examples of nonverbal reasoning items; reasoning refers to the perception of logical relations, discrimination ability, and analysis and synthesis

5. *Numerical reasoning:* Includes arithmetical problems; content is closely related to school learning
6. *Visual motor:* Contains items of manual dexterity, eye-hand coordination, and perception of spatial relations; constructive visual imagery can include such items as paper folding
7. *Social intelligence:* Closely related to the reasoning category; social intelligence includes social maturity and social judgment; comprehension and finding reason items reflect social judgment; items concerning obeyance of simple commands, response to pictures, and comparison illustrate social maturity

The revised scale reflects the validity of the two forms of the 1937 scale. A .82 correlation between the revised scale and the 1937 scale suggests a high level of agreement. A biserial correlation of the revised scale is .66, with a .61 for all tests in the two forms of the 1937 scale. Standardization was originally done on 3184 persons, with approximately 100 boys and 100 girls at each age. Age scales are postulated on the assumption of fairly regular and progressive increases in mental growth.

### KAUFMAN ASSESSMENT BATTERY FOR CHILDREN
(See Chapter 11)

### NEBRASKA TEST OF LEARNING APTITUDE (NTLA)
(Hiskey, M., 1966, Psychological Corporation)

The NTLA is designed to assess the learning aptitude of hearing and deaf individuals. The age range is three to sixteen years. The test includes twelve subtests, with pantomime instructions for administration to deaf persons and verbal instructions for administration to hearing children. Administration of the test requires much experience. The twelve subtests are bead patterns, memory for color, picture identification, picture association, paper folding (patterns), visual attention span, block patterns, completion of drawings, memory for digits, puzzle blocks, picture analogies, and spatial reason-

ing. Each subtest is scored separately and plotted on the appropriate table of norms (that is, deaf norms if deaf persons are being tested) on the back of the record sheet. All items were chosen with special reference to the limitations of deaf children, and the final item selection was based chiefly on the criterion of age differentiation.

Subtest learning ages and median learning ages for the total test range from .55 to .89 for deaf children three to ten years of age, from .59 to .67 for deaf children eleven to seventeen years of age, from .51 to .77 for hearing children three to ten years of age, and from .54 to .67 for hearing children eleven to seventeen years of age. Concurrent validity scores are .86 between the NTLA and the Stanford-Binet administered to ninety-nine hearing children between three and ten years of age, .78 between the NTLA and Stanford-Binet for fifty hearing children between eleven and seventeen years of age, and .82 between the NTLA and WISC for fifty-two hearing children between five and eleven years of age.

Split-half reliabilities for the NTLAs standardization groups are .95 for deaf children three to ten years of age, .92 for deaf children eleven to seventeen years of age, .93 for hearing children three to ten years of age, and .90 for hearing children eleven to seventeen years of age. The standardization sample of the revised NTLA included 1107 deaf children and 1101 hearing children between 2 years, 6 months and 17 years, 5 months of age from ten states. The hearing children were grouped according to their parents' occupational levels as used in the 1960 census. The deaf children were from state schools for the deaf.

### DETROIT TEST OF LEARNING APTITUDE, SECOND EDITION (DTLA-2)
(Hammill, D., 1985, Pro-Ed.)

The DTLA is a comprehensive instrument for persons aged six to eighteen years. The test includes eleven subtests measuring a wide range of psychological abilities; these subtests include word opposites, symbolic relations, conceptual matching, and object sequences. Nine composite scores can cover verbal, nonverbal, conceptual structure, attention enhanced, attention reduced, motor enhanced, motor reduced, and overall aptitude skills. The DTLA is individually administered and the test kit includes student response and examiner forms, manual summary, and profile sheets. Administering the test takes approximately 50–120 minutes, and a software scoring system is available.

The test provides a score for each subtest, which can be converted to an MA for each subtest. A general MA is derived from the median ages of subjects who have taken whatever subtests have been administered. To provide a readily visible pattern for diagnostic interpretations, the manual contains a table of the subtests that has been cross-matched with the eight psychological functions assessed by the test. The manual also provides a comprehensive explanation of the eight psychological functions and their relationship to the subtests.

The test items have concurrent validity, which was determined by a comparison of a sampling of the IQ distribution of subjects tested with the DTLA with a similar number who had been tested with another instrument. Overall test reliability is high (.95), as shown by the test-retest method with a lapse of five months between testings. Correlations between subjects ranged from 20 to 67.

The earlier edition of the DTLA was standardized on a representative sample of students from the Detroit public schools. Testing for development of the norms involved 150 pupils at each age level whose IQs ranged from 90 to 110 and who were considered to be at their normal grade for their age. Caution should be exercised when age norms are interpreted for adults, because the norms only apply up to eighteen years of age.

### TEST OF CONCEPT UTILIZATION (TCU)

(Crager, P., & Spriggs, A., 1972, Western Psychological Services)

The TCU is a fifty-item instrument; each item consists of two pictures of everyday objects. One picture is made up of ten standard objects; the second picture consists of fifty other objects. The subject must tell the examiner ways in which the two pictures are related. The standard items have outstanding characteristics in one of five categories: (1) color, (2) shape, (3) relational function, (4) homogeneous function, and (5) abstract function, principle, or noun class. The kit consists of a manual, a set of spiral-bound plates, and a scoring booklet. The scoring booklet is designed to provide a variety of information, including item analysis and positive and negative correlations with grade point averages. Validity scores are not provided. Test-retest reliability is .89. Scores were normed for five to eighteen years of age and yield a $T$ score and percentile rank. The normative sample consisted of 700 urban and metropolitan children in Denver schools and preschools. The children were selected randomly from stratified socioeconomic groups according to the 1960 census. Approximately 1% of the children were from minority groups.

### BASIC CONCEPT INVENTORY (BCI)

(Engelman, S., 1975, Follett Publishing Company)

The purpose of the BCI is to evaluate the instruction in certain beginning, academically related concepts. The test can be given either to a group of children or to an individual child. The emphasis is on specific concepts to be taught. It is intended mostly for culturally disadvantaged preschool and kindergarten children, slow learners, emotionally disturbed children, and mentally retarded children. It may be given to children as old as ten years of age. Scores on the BCI are reported as the number of items missed in four areas: basic concepts, statement repetition, comprehension, and pattern awareness. This test is recommended for deaf or hard of hearing and physically impaired persons.

The BCI is a criterion-referenced measure, and the scores are not ranked or spread over a distribution. Emphasis is placed on the child's individual score, so that the instruction received by the child on specific skills can be evaluated. The process of item construction and selection was informal and subjective. Many concept problems were identified from the inadequacies of children in the Bereiter-Engelmann preschool and kindergarten classes.

The content and criterion validity of the BCI were built-in, and predictive and construct validity for the BCI have not been established. No numerical coefficients were given. It is published as a field research edition. Many items were tested for reliability, but data are insufficient and not reported.

The individually administered BCI is read aloud to the child, and the four scores on the subtests are tallied to give one total for the number of errors. The lower the score, the more adequate the child's performance. A child who misses forty or more tasks is considered to be a child who might experience difficulties in new learning situations. The test is a research edition, and no age or grade norms are given. The test manual offers three reasons for these omissions: applying a single norm to subgroups obscures natural development, a child's age is irrelevant to the learning of certain concepts, and age norms are achievement norms that hide the basis of knowledge acquisition and potential remedy.

### LEITER INTERNATIONAL PERFORMANCE SCALE
(Leiter, R., & Arthur, G., 1969, Stoelting Company)

The Leiter Scale is a nonverbal performance scale used for measuring intelligence. It consists of sixty-eight standardized items and can be used with persons from two to eighteen years of age. The test consists of wooden blocks that fit into a frame. The subject matches the blocks to a printed strip that fits into the top of the frame. Matching for younger children involves simple pairing and matching advances to complex relationships for older children. The entire test is given without verbal instructions; instead the examiner uses pantomime or gestures. There are no time limits except for subtests on block design. The first test in the examination is one at an age level that is two years below the subject's estimated mental age. Because there are no verbal instructions, tasks for early age levels must be simple so that what is expected is obvious. The age level at which all tests are performed correctly is determined to be the basal level. Testing is continued until all tests at two consecutive year levels are failed.

Because the Leiter Scale is completely nonverbal, its assessment validity with those individuals who have verbal difficulties is more valid. The hypothesis is that general intelligence is the ability to solve problems with which an individual has had no previous experience. Overall, this test appears to be valuable in the assessment of those individuals who have one or more of various handicaps (for example, deaf, ESL, multiple handicaps).

Concurrent validity was determined with the Stanford-Binet and the WISC. The correlations between the Leiter Scale and the Stanford-Binet on children four, five, six, seven, or eight years of age ranged from .63 to .93. The performance scale of the WISC showed a correlation of .79 to .80. This was higher than that of the verbal scale, which showed a correlation of .40 to .78. No study has been done on predictive validity. Split-half reliabilities of .91 to .94 are reported from several studies. The samples were quite heterogeneous in age as well as in other characteristics. The norms were established on a sample of 289 children of middle-class status from the metropolitan midwest. This sample should be expanded to include different types of children from a more varied area.

Sample descriptions of test items for the two-, nine-, and eighteen-year-old levels are as follows.

### Two-year-olds' test
*Test 1: Matching colors (black, red, green, blue, yellow)*

DESCRIPTION: The five colored blocks are matched to a sheet containing pictures of the five colors.

PROCEDURE: The examiner places the black block in the first stall and tries to get the subject to put the red block in place by placing it on the table, then in the appropriate stall, then on the table again, nodding to the subject to do it and at the same time pointing to the second or red stall.

SCORING: Accurately places four colors without assistance during any one trial.

### Nine-year-olds' test

*Test 1: Dot estimation*

DESCRIPTION: Fifteen dots are on the left end of the strip and eighty-five on the right end. The blocks have varying numbers of dots on them, between fifteen and eighty-five.

PROCEDURE: Place the blocks in random order before the subject. Give no help.

SCORING: All blocks must be properly placed to match the strip.

### Eighteen-year-olds' tests

*Test 4: Concealed cubes test*

DESCRIPTION: The strip contains pictures of blocks divided into numerous cubes. Not all cubes are showing. The blocks have numbers from fifty-six to eighty-two on them.

PROCEDURE: Place test material before the subject, with blocks in random order. No help is given. There will be three blocks left over when the test is finished.

SCORING: All blocks must be correctly placed to match the strip, for credit to be given.

*Test 5: Spatial relations test*

DESCRIPTION: The strip contains hands in various positions. The blocks contain feet in various positions. Analogies are made.

PROCEDURE: Place test material before the subject in random order. Give no clues.

SCORING: All blocks must be placed correctly for credit.

#### COLUMBIA MENTAL MATURITY SCALE (CMMS)

(Burgemeister, L., & Lorge, I., 1972, Harcourt Brace Jovanovich)

The CMMS provides an estimate of the general reasoning ability of children three years, six months through nine years, eleven months of age. It is a 92-item, pictorial classification test; each item consists of three, four, or five drawings on a large card. No verbal response and minimal motor response are required from the child, thus it is especially suitable for children with cerebral palsy, mental retardation, and visual, speech, and hearing impairments. It does not rely on language or reading skills, thus it is also appropriate for children who do not speak English.

Scores are expressed as age deviation scores, which are normalized standard scores within age groups, with a mean of 100 and a standard deviation of 16. Percentile and stanine equivalents are also provided. The manual includes a maturity index, indicating the age group in the standardized sample in which test performance is most similar to that of the child.

A correlation of .67 with the Stanford-Binet was found in a group of fifty-two preschool and first-grade children. Correlations with achievement test scores of first- and second-graders were between the high .40s and low .60s. High reliability, ranging from .85 to .91, was found by the split-half method. A test-retest of three age groups, after intervals of seven to ten days, yielded a high reliability, of .84 to .86.

Administration includes teaching the child the task, using three sample items, presenting the test items included in the level appropriate for the child's chronological age, and recording each item on the individual record form. There are no specific examiner qualifications.

Norms were derived from testing a selected sample of 2600 children at sixty-seven test centers in twenty-five states. The norming was controlled so that a representative national sample of 200 children was tested at each age level. Controls were used so that the sample met proportional quotas in terms of parental occupation, race, and urban-rural.

#### SLOSSON INTELLIGENCE TEST (SIT)

(Slosson, R., 1981, Slosson Educational Publications)

The SIT is useful as an individual screening instrument, because it allows an evaluation of the individual's mental ability to be made in a brief period of time. The SIT is based upon the constructs of the Stanford-Binet Intelligence Test and the Gesell Development Scales. The subjects' age range is from two weeks to twenty-seven years; the majority of the 194 items are designed to test the lower age range. After the test is completed, a mental age is calculated in the normal way and IQ is determined; or a deviation IQ can be calculated through the use of the 1981 norm tables.

The norm group consisted of 1109 persons from New England; they ranged in age from two to eighteen years. Demographic information on the norm group is not included. The SIT mean is .97, and the standard deviation is 20. Test-retest reliability is reported at .97 and a standard error of measurement at 4.3. Validity for the SIT is stated in its relationship to the Stanford-Binet Intelligence Test and is discussed as such. The SIT should not be used to estimate the IQs of mentally retarded or gifted children and its use with persons having visual acuity or auditory problems should be avoided.

Test items were chosen from other IQ tests and have "face" validity. Published validity studies show a confusing picture, with validity ranging from .54 to .93. The manual states .90 and .98 correlations with the Stanford-Binet. Test-retest within a period of two months revealed a .97 reliability coefficient. A sample of 139 individuals from four to fifty years of age was used in the initial standardization process. Since then many other studies of various sample sizes have been done. The IQ scale is one of ratio rather than deviation.

### MINNESOTA PRE-SCHOOL SCALE

(Goodenough, F., Maurer, K., & Wagenen, M., 1971, American Guidance Service)

Designed for children $1\frac{1}{2}$ to 6 years of age, this scale tests verbal and nonverbal intelligence. Three scores (verbal, nonverbal, total) yield an intelligence quotient equivalent. The test consists of twenty-six subtests, equally divided into verbal and nonverbal items in the areas of response to pictures, comprehension, absurdities, vocabulary, speech, and opposites. Some actions the child must perform during the test are point, follow directions, name things, draw, trace, and build with blocks.

There is no validity report. Reliability ranged from .68 to .94 for the verbal scale, and from .67

to .92 for the nonverbal scale. Combined scores ranged from .80 to .94. The norms are based on the results of testing 100 children (50 boys and 50 girls) at each of nine half-year age levels, or 900 children in all. Within each age level, children were selected to represent a cross-section of the population. Test items eliminated during selection included those that had little interest to children and those that produced emotional reactions.

### MCCARTHY SCALES OF CHILDREN'S ABILITIES

(McCarthy, D., 1972, Psychological Corporation)

This test for children between $2\frac{1}{2}$ and $8\frac{1}{2}$ years of age has eighteen subtests grouped into six overlapping scales. The scales are verbal, perceptual-performance, quantitative, general cognitive, memory, and motor. The general cognitive score comes closest to the traditional global measure of intellectual development. The behaviors sampled by the subtests include block building, puzzle solving, right-left orientation, leg coordination, arm coordination, imitative action, drawing a design, drawing a child, numerical memory, verbal fluency, counting and sorting, opposite analogies, and conceptual grouping.

The manual cites suggestive data on predictive validity of this test compared against an educational achievement battery administered at the end of the first grade. The McCarthy Scales were used to test thirty-one children, who were then tested four months later with the Metropolitan Achievement Test. Correlations were high for the perceptual-performance and quantitative scales, moderate for the general cognitive scale, and weak for the verbal, memory, and motor scales. Split-half reliability for the general cognitive index averaged .93 within age levels; average coefficients for the other five scales ranged from .79 to .88. Retest reliabilities over a one-month interval for 125 children classified into three age groups averaged .90 for the general cognitive index and from .69 to .89 for the separate scales. The scales were standardized on 1032 children, approximately 100 children at each of the ten age levels between

$2\frac{1}{2}$ and $8\frac{1}{2}$ years of age. The sample contained an equal number of boys and girls and was stratified by geographic region, father's occupational level, urban-rural, and "color." Bilingual children were tested only if they could speak and understand English.

### WOODCOCK-JOHNSON PSYCHO-EDUCATIONAL BATTERY

(Woodcock, R., & Johnson, M., 1977, American Guidance Service and DLM Teaching Resources)

This test is a comprehensive set of twenty-seven subtests, measuring cognitive abilities, scholastic aptitudes, achievement, and interests at preschool through adult levels. Tests are administered orally and individually. All required materials, including tests, scoring tables, response booklets, and a cassette, are included in the kit.

A number of options are provided for the conversion of raw scores into more meaningful information. In addition to grade scores, age scores, standard scores, and percentile ranks, performance evaluation may be based on the extended age scale, the extended grade scale, or the suggested instructional range. Profiles provide a graphic representation of the information derived from a subject's test scores. As suggested by Salvia and Ysseldyke (1985), this test is very suitable for use with special education populations.

The entire battery may be administered in one two-hour session or in separate sessions. Single tests or a cluster of tests may be used to meet specific needs. A summary and interpretation of test results can be completed in approximately one hour. If only certain assessment information is needed, the examiner can eliminate those parts of the battery that are not applicable and thereby save considerable time.

A high degree of correlation with other commonly used tests is demonstrated. In terms of reliability, with few exceptions, cluster scores are above .90; many are above .95. Norming population was based on 4732 subjects ranging from three to over eighty years of age and representing forty-nine communities across the United States. The following variables were considered: sex, race, occupational status, geographic region, and type of community.

### BAYLEY SCALES OF INFANT DEVELOPMENT

(Bayley, N., 1969, 1984, Psychological Corporation)

This test is designed to yield a three-part evaluation of a child's developmental status during the first $2\frac{1}{2}$ years of life. According to Bayley, "The primary value of the development index is to provide the basis for establishing a child's current status, and thus the extent of any deviation from normal expectancy" (1969, p. 4). The 1984 revision provides a manual supplement that clarifies the administration and scoring directions.

Functions of the Bayley Scale include:

1. The Mental Scale assesses sensory-perceptual acuities and discrimination; the early acquisition of "object permanency" and memory, learning and problem-solving ability; vocalization and early evidence of the ability to form generalizations and classifications, which are the basis of abstract thinking. Results are expressed as a standard score, the MDI, or Mental Development Index.
2. The Motor Scale provides a measure of body control, coordination of the large muscles, and finger manipulative skills. Results are expressed as a standard score, the PDI, or Psychomotor Development Index.
3. The Infant Behavior Record assesses the child's social and objective orientations toward his environment, as expressed in attitudes, interests, emotions, energy, activity, and tendencies to approach or withdraw from stimulation (pp. 3–4).

Split-half reliability coefficients for the mental scale range from .81 to .93, with a median value of .88. Split-half coefficients for the motor scale range from .68 to .92, with a median of .84. Bayley attributes the lower coefficients for the motor scale to the fact that it has about half as many items as the mental scale (Bayley, 1969).

Evidence for the validity of the tests is limited, the primary evidence being an increase in performance with an increase in age. Bayley also reports correlation between the MDIs and the Stanford-Binet IQs for groups of children twenty-four, twenty-seven, or thirty months of age. The correlations range between .47 for children who are thirty months of age to .57 for the total group. The scales were standardized on a sample of 1262 children selected to reflect the proportions of children from two through thirty months of age in various subgroups (sex, race, socioeconomic status, rural-urban, geographic region), as described in the 1960 census.

### CATTELL INFANT INTELLIGENCE SCALE
(Cattell, P., 1940, Psychological Corporation)

Cattell's purpose in developing this scale was to construct a downward extension of the Stanford-Binet. The scale is arranged so that there are five test items at each age by month, through twelve months, then at two-month intervals to thirty months. At the lower age levels, the items are composed of such tasks as attending to voice, using the eyes to follow a dangling ring or person, and head lifting. At higher age levels, the scale requires more complex behavior, such as manipulating blocks, spoons, cups, pegboards, and form boards. There is also an increasing use of verbal functions and oral instructions. At the upper age levels, Stanford-Binet items are mingled with other items in the scale. If the child passes an item at the thirty-month level, the examiner proceeds to the Stanford-Binet, beginning at the three-year level. Scores are expressed in terms of MAs and IQs.

Reliability was determined by use of the split-half technique. The reported reliability coefficients vary from .56 at the three-month level to .90 at the eighteen-month level. Most of the coefficients are in the .80s (Cattell, 1940). Cattell attributes the relatively low reliability coefficients to the heterogeneity of the item content.

Validity of the scale is expressed in terms of the increase in percentage of persons passing each item at successive age levels, and in terms of correlations with scores on the Stanford-Binet administered to children at thirty-six months of age. The validity coefficients range from .10

(three-month level of Cattell Scale) to .83 (thirty-month level of the Cattell Scale). Tests administered to infants less than nine months of age are of little value in predicting later measured status. "The standardization is based on 1346 examinations made on 274 children at the ages of three, six, nine, twelve, eighteen, twenty-four, thirty and thirty-six months" (Cattell, 1940, p. 25). The children represented a rather restricted sample from the "lower middle classes."

## GROUP INTELLIGENCE TESTS OF GENERAL ABILITIES

### BOEHM TEST OF BASIC CONCEPTS
(Boehm, A., 1970, Psychological Corporation)

This test measures abstract concepts that frequently occur in the curriculum at the primary levels. Age range on the test is from kindergarten through eight years. The test is available in two forms, A and B. Each form contains two levels of twenty-five concepts each. The concepts can be categorized into four groups: space, quantity, time, and miscellaneous. When the test is administered, the child is shown a set of pictures while the teacher reads a set of statements. The child marks the picture that is most closely related to the statement that the teacher read. There are two booklets for each form, and the items in booklet one should be given first. A raw score is obtained and then interpreted for grade level and socioeconomic status.

The manual presents only face validity, but it is believed that this is strong. Boehm claims that content validity has been established, in that items were selected from currently used curriculum materials. Reliability was established by use of the split-half method with correction; the Spearman-Brown formula was used for grade levels and socioeconomic levels for both forms. Form A was found to be more reliable than Form B. Reliabilities from both forms had a median coefficient of .81; the standard error of measurement in raw score points ranged from 0.9 to 3.4 and had a median of 2.15.

Boehm intended for this test to be a criterion-referenced measure. The standardization procedure was done on a group of children who were in mixed grades—kindergarten through third grade. The sample was tested at the beginning, middle, and end of the year. The sample was also divided into different socioeconomic groups, although the studies show only marginal reliabilities for the three socioeconomic levels. Form B was designed to be equivalent to Form A, but the correlations between the two forms are too low for the forms to be actually equivalent.

### COGNITIVE ABILITIES TEST (1979) (CAT)

(Thorndike, R., & Hagen, E., Riverside Publishing Co.)

The CAT is an integrated test series designed to assess the development of cognitive abilities in children in grades ranging from kindergarten through the first year of college. The series consists of Primary I, Primary II, and CAT-Multilevel (based on the Lorge-Thorndike tests). The complete series yields comparable scores in cognitive development for the same individual at different times. Instructions and questions are given orally; students' responses are represented by pictures. Hand scoring is done by use of a pictorial strip key with the correct answers for each page. The number of correct answers for each subtest is totaled and computed with the chronological age; this computation and use of a normative table yields a deviation IQ. The CAT yields three scores: verbal, quantitative, and nonverbal. Skills measured by the CAT are in part learned skills. A low score is a sign that the individual might need more intensive, more varied, and more directed experience to help in the improvement of such skills. Therefore scores should be used by the classroom teacher and others to structure the learning environment and to plan learning experiences.

Reliability coefficients range from .76 to .94, for retesting at a six-month interval. When construct validity was determined, the CAT multilevel batteries were correlated with the Stanford-Binet for 550 individuals. Reported correlations were .65 to .75. Concurrent correlations were highest (.70 to .80) between the verbal battery and the Iowa Test of Basic Skills; the Tests of Achievement and Proficiency subtest Norms for the CAT were done concurrently with the ITBS and the TAP in 1977 and 1978. Efforts were made to insure racial-ethnic composition and other major variables, such as size of enrollment of school district, geographic region, and the community's socioeconomic status, were considered in the selection of the sample. Both 1978 and 1979 norms are available for the primary and multilevel batteries.

### PRIMARY MENTAL ABILITIES TEST (PMA)

(Thurstone, L., & Thurstone, T., 1962, Science Research Associates)

The PMA is a group test with five levels for children according to grade: kindergarten to first, second to fourth, fourth to sixth, sixth to ninth, and ninth to twelfth. An adult level is also included. Each level has six scores: verbal meaning, perceptual speed, number facility, spatial relations, reasoning, and a total score. The profile of five primary mental abilities helps teachers evaluate and interpret individual differences in behavior and performance among children who appear to be of comparable intelligence.

The manual claims that the verbal meaning score is related to all academic courses, and that the reasoning score is related to achievement and is useful in predictions of how well children will score in arithmetic. The score in perceptual speed is important to predictions of how well younger children will learn symbols. Deviation IQs are used in levels after the fourth grade, but ratio IQs are used before the fourth grade.

Validity was established by correlations of the PMA scores with grade point average (GPA), grades in individual subjects, Kuhlman-Anderson Intelligence Test scores, and scores on the Iowa Test of Basic Skills. Test-retest reliability was .83 to .95. The standardization sample was made up of 32,393 children, four to twenty years of age. Subjects were from public schools in five different regions of the United States. Economic status, race, and sex were not reported.

### LORGE-THORNDIKE INTELLIGENCE TEST

(Lorge, I., & Thorndike, R., 1966, Riverside Publishing Co.)

This test can be given to children from kindergarten to grade 13. The test has five levels. Suggestions are given as to what level is appropriate for children with varying socioeconomic status. Most of the materials test "abstract intelligence," which is defined as the "ability to work with ideas and relationships among ideas." The tests are based on the premise that most of the abstract ideas with which the school child or working adult deals are expressed in verbal symbols. There are two series in the test: verbal and nonverbal. The subtests in the verbal series include word knowledge, sentence completion, verbal classification, verbal analogies, and arithmetic reasoning. The subtests in the nonverbal series are oral vocabulary, cross-out, and pairing (lower level) and figure analogies, figure classification, and number series (higher levels). The test manual states that scores on the nonverbal series will not predict success in school as well as the verbal series will. It is suggested that both series be given together to reveal significant facts about reading achievement, school progress, or vocational prospects.

This test correlates moderately (.60 to .70) with achievement tests. One study reported that the test was given at the beginning of the ninth grade and correlated .67 with average achievement at the end of the ninth grade. Construct validity intercorrelations of the subtests range from .30 to .70. Correlation between the verbal and nonverbal series ranges from .54 to .70. Individual items correlated .43 to .70 with the subtests of which they are a part. Correlations with four "other group tests," the Stanford-Binet, and the WISC, were for the most part .60 or higher. Alternate forms of the test have reported correlations of .76 to .90 in one study and .79 to .87 in another. Odd-even correlations are very high, ranging from .88 to .94. The test was standardized on 136,000 children in forty-four communities in twenty-two states. Some bias in the norms was assumed because participation was voluntary. Norms were given as grade percentiles, grade equivalents, age equivalents, and IQ equivalents (mean = 100, standard deviation = 16).

### CALIFORNIA SHORT FORM TEST OF MENTAL MATURITY (CTMM)

(Sullivan, E., Clark, W., & Tiegs, E., 1963, California Test Bureau)

There are two forms of the CTMM: the long form and the short form. The seven subtests of the short form contribute to five factor scores: logical reasoning, numerical reasoning, spatial relationships, verbal concepts, and memory. From these subtests, scores in language, nonlanguage, total MAs and IQs are derived. It is possible to obtain a separate mental age and IQ for each subtest as well as for the total battery. Some levels of tests range from preprimary (level 0) to adult (level 5). The test contains two individual profiles: a percentile rank that has a standard score scale that delineates factor, section, and total scores; and a profile for plotting the language, nonlanguage, and total short-form IQs. The examiner can compare performance across areas tested by both inter- and intraindividual responses. Step-by-step instructions for obtaining and plotting IQs, mental age, percentile, standard scores, and stanines are given.

Validity correlation (.70 to .80) is noted with other group tests and with the California Achievement Tests. Total score reliability was high (.93 to .96). Normative data were based on chronological age groups derived from 253 schools (total of 38,793 cases) representing seven geographic regions and forty-nine states. The test was compared with other intelligence and mental ability tests, including the Stanford-Binet. The test was scaled to Stanford-Binet so that total IQ and corresponding total mental age were obtained (derived from a relationship of IQ and chronological age in the same manner as the MA for the Stanford-Binet).

### CULTURE FAIR INTELLIGENCE TESTS (CFIT)
(Cattell, R., & Cattell, A., 1973, Institute for Personality and Ability Testing)

Based on Cattell's theory of fluid general ability (adaptive mental behavior in unfamiliar situations) rather than on traditional concepts of crystallized intelligence, this test includes mostly nonsense material that is universally unfamiliar. The CFIT has three different scales: (1) four to eight years of age and mentally retarded adults; takes about 22 to 60 minutes to administer; (2) eight to fourteen years of age and average adults; takes about 30 minutes to administer; and (3) nine to sixteen years of age and superior adults; takes about 30 minutes to administer. In their measures of intelligence, the two forms of the test (A and B) reduce the influence of verbal fluency, educational level, and culture climate. There are eight subtests: substitutions, classification, mazes, selecting named objects, following directions, wrong pictures, riddles, and similarities. All of the subtests, except tests five and seven, can be given in a small group setting.

Validity rests with the series of factor analytical studies that were conducted by Cattell; he correlated a general ability factor ($g$) with the performance on each of the subtests containing that factor. The correlations of the subtests with the $g$ ranged from .53 to .99. The test was also correlated with the Stanford-Binet (.62 for underprivileged children) and the Goodenough-Harris (.46 for 72 unspecified children). Other correlations ranged from .49 with the Otis Beta to .72 with the full scale WISC. Test-retest reliability on fifty-seven Head Start children was .80 for the total test and ranged from .57 to .71 for the subtests. Internal consistency and equivalent form, and test-retest reliabilities were reported for scale 2. Internal consistency ranged from .77 to .81 for Form A and from .71 to .76 for Form B. Split-half reliability ranged from .95 to .97. Equivalent-form reliability ranged from .58 to .72. Test-retest reliability ranged from .82 to .85. Reliability for scale 3

included internal consistency—.51 to .68, and equivalent-form—.32 to .68. Scale 1 was standardized on only 117 children, with 20 being the largest number for any year. Age variation makes a difference in the IQ. The reliability and validity for this particular scale is not very high. Scale 2 was standardized on 713 pupils in two midwestern towns. The SD was 24, which is high in comparison with the Revised Stanford-Binet Scale, which has an SD of 16 (ranges from 12 to 20). Scale 3 was standardized on 886 high school students and 600 college/university students. IQs of some distance from the mean will be much higher or much lower than those usually obtained.

### ANALYSIS OF LEARNING POTENTIAL (ALP)
(Durost, W., Gardner, E., & Madden, R., 1970, Harcourt Brace Jovanovich)

This test (Primary I—Grade 1, Primary II—Grades 2 to 3, Elementary—Grades 4 to 6, Advanced I—Grades 7 to 9, Advanced II—Grades 10 to 12) was developed to assess the school learning ability of pupils typically found in grades 1 to 12. The test has two forms, A and B. The Advanced II portion of the ALP contains nine subtests: word meaning, number relations, word categories, spatial reasoning, number fluency, number operations reasoning, word clues, syntactic clues, and evidence evaluation. The tests may be given in the form of a complete battery (all nine subtests given in two separate sessions; first session, tests 1 to 5; second session, tests 6 to 9), a reading prognostic cluster (tests 1, 3, 8, 9 in one session), or a mathematics prognostic cluster (tests 2, 5, 6 in one session). Each subtest has a time limit, and students are expected to stop working on a particular subtest when the time has elapsed. The examiner has a copy of the Manual for Administration, which contains the specific instructions for procedures in each subtest. The examiner reads instructions word for word to the students. Students are given a test booklet and an answer sheet, and are instructed to mark all responses on the answer sheet and to leave the test booklet without any marks.

Concurrent validity correlation with the Metropolitan and Stanford Achievement batteries is in the .70s. The Kuder-Richardson formula for the total battery for age ranged from .96 to .97. The Kuder-Richardson formula for the total battery for grade ranged from .95 to .96. Norms are based on testing of 165,000 pupils in approximately seventy-five school districts from forty-four states. Testing was conducted during the fall and winter of 1967–1968 with students in grades 1 to 12.

### KUHLMANN-ANDERSON INTELLIGENCE TESTS, 8TH EDITION

(Kuhlmann, F., & Anderson, R., 1982, Scholastic Testing Service)

This test is designed to assess the learning aptitude of students in kindergarten through grade twelve. Each test battery consists of twelve subtests. The results of over 150 concurrent validity studies are reported in the manual. Most were correlated with deviation IQs earned on achievement and other intelligence tests. Correlations were moderate at the various levels. K, D, EF, G, and H batteries are reported to have adequate predictive validity. A, B, and CD batteries are either lacking in evidence of predictive validity or are not reported in the manual. Machine-scorable booklets are available for grades K–3.

Internal consistency coefficients for Forms K, A, B, and CD range from .93 to .95. Subtest scores range from .51 to .69 for B battery, from .51 to .86 for CD, from .48 to .80 for D, and from .71 to .81 for EF. Test-retest reliability data are reported for all batteries. For levels K through EF, test-retest coefficients over two- to four-month intervals are reported for deviation IQs: coefficients range from .83 to .90. For levels G and H, test-retest reliabilities for deviation IQs over periods from one to two years range from .83 to .92. Raw scores can be transformed to mental ages, deviation IQs, and percentile ranks. Scores are obtained for the total test, not for the subtests. The test was standardized on 27,853 students, selected according to community size, geographical location, and socioeconomic level.

The normative sample consisted of at least 3000 students per grade level and between 700 and 800 students per three-month interval. No information on standardization for the 8th edition is available.

## INDIVIDUAL TESTS OF SPECIFIC AREAS*

### RAVEN PROGRESSIVE MATRICES TEST

(Raven, J., 1938, 1951, 1958, Los Angeles: Western Psychological Service)

This test measures a person's capacity to "apprehend meaningless figures, see the relations between them, conceive the nature of the figure completing each system of relations presented, and . . . develop a logical method of reasoning." The Coloured Progressive Matrices (CPM) (1949), which was constructed for children from five to eleven years of age and mentally subnormal or impaired individuals, is designed to be used before the person's ability to reason by analogy has developed. The original Standard Progressive Matrices consists of five sets of twelve designs each that require completion: completion of a pattern, completion of an analogy, systematic alteration of a pattern, introduction of systematic permutation, and systematic resolution of figures into parts. The CPM consists of three sets, A, AB, and B (AB being transitional problems), of twelve designs each. The designs of the CPM are brightly colored so that they attract the attention of a young child.

The CPM is available in either board form or book form. With the board form, the child actually manipulates the blocks, and places his or her choices into the blank space. The examiner can thus demonstrate nonverbally what the child is to do. The book form requires more guidance because the child can only point to his

---

*These tests might or might not be correlates of intelligence; research at present is conflicting. Because intellectual functioning is broadly conceptualized in this text from an information-processing orientation, a brief review of these unique tests is included.

or her choice. Standard instructions allow the examiner to demonstrate the first design completion as many times as is necessary for the child's comprehension; during the first five designs of each set, the examiner may encourage the child to make an alternate choice without penalty. Responses are recorded by the examiner; the test is hand scored. Scores (correct responses) of the three sets are compared with norms of children of the same age, and a grade of 1 to 5 is assigned on the basis of percentile rank. Length of test varies with the individual but generally does not exceed one hour.

Raven states that differences between bright, average, and dull children from 10 years of age on become increasingly significant on the CPM. Because the CPM is easy to administer and score, and because significant relations exist between the CPM and other IQ measures, the CPM might be a valuable screening device of intellectual ability. It is not of much value as a diagnostic tool for purposes of remediation, because the perceptual processes involved in the problem solving are not analyzed. The board form of the test is valuable for estimations of the capacity for rational judgment of persons who are partially paralyzed or deaf, those who do not speak or do not speak English, and those who have speech handicaps. The board form, however, is not readily available for use, whereas other nonverbal tests are.

None of the three manuals provides standardization and validity data. The only mention of reliability is in the Advanced Progressive Matrices Level I, in which a reliability coefficient of .76 to .91 is given. Although there is no mention of normative data, other authors mention a correlation of .91 with full-scale WISC IQs.

### GOODENOUGH-HARRIS DRAWING TEST

(Harris, D., & Goodenough, L., 1963, Harcourt Brace Jovanovich)

Designed to evaluate intelligence in children (five to fifteen years of age), this test has the children draw a man and a woman. The test can be used for such purposes as screening; as a rapid, nonthreatening means of gaining an impression of a child's general ability level; and of estimating the mental ability of children for whom the usual verbal tests of ability are inappropriate. The test provides three spaces in which the child can produce the drawings—one for the drawing of a man, one for the drawing of a woman, and one for a "self" drawing. Beside each space, 73 blanks are provided for scoring purposes. The child is asked to draw the very best picture he or she can of a man, woman, and himself or herself. The child is cautioned to make a whole person, not simply a head-and-shoulders view. There is no time limit for the test, but according to the authors, young children rarely take more than ten to fifteen minutes. The test can be administered either as a group test or as an individual test. The authors recommend children under eight or nine years of age take a short rest period between the second and third drawings. The examiner should avoid making any suggestion except to remind the child to draw a whole person.

Over the years the Draw-A-Man has been subject to a considerable amount of research. Most of the data collected are applicable to the Harris revision (at least on the man scale). Interscore reliability coefficients around the .90s have been reported. A number of studies have reported retest reliability coefficients ranging from .94 for a one-day interval between testings, to a .65 for a three-year interval between testings. Most of the retest coefficients are in the .60s and .70s.

To demonstrate the validity of the Draw-A-Man, researchers have correlated the Draw-A-Man scores to those of other tests. Correlations with the Stanford-Binet range from .43 to .74. Correlations with other tests are about the same range and magnitude. Research has found a correlation of .43 with the WISC and .51 to .72 with the California Test of Mental Maturity.

The scoring of this test is not based on the subject's artistic skill but on the presence of essential details and their relationship to each other. Credit is given for the inclusion of such things as individual body parts, clothing details, proportion, and perspective. Scorable items were selected according to age differentiation, relation to the total score on the test, and the relation to scores on group intelligence tests. There are seventy-three scorable items on the man scale and seventy-one scorable items on the woman scale.

Norms for the man and woman scales were established on samples of 300 children at each age level from five to fifteen years. They were selected to be representative of the population of the United States with regard to father's occupation and geographic region. The manual provides standard score norms that have a mean of 100 and a standard deviation of 15. There are also percentile equivalents for the standard scores.

### TORRANCE TESTS OF CREATIVE THINKING (TTCT)

(Torrance, E. P., 1984, Scholastic Testing Service)

This test measures four aspects of "creative thinking": fluency, flexibility, originality, and elaboration. Provided are two scores for each aspect: verbal and figural. The author and publisher of the TTCT recommend that it be used in research studies of cognitive functions, individualized instruction, remedial programs, and new educational programs, as well as for the assessment of an individual student's potential.

The test can be administered individually or in a group. One form, Thinking Creatively with Pictures, can be administered to anyone from kindergarten up and takes a total of thirty minutes. There are three subtests: picture construction, picture completion, and lines. Each represents a different aspect of creativity or a different creative tendency. For example, the picture-construction activity sets in motion the tendency toward finding a purpose for something that has no definite purpose and to elaborate in such a way that that purpose is achieved.

A second form of the test, Thinking Creatively with Words, is administered to those in fourth-grade through college-graduate level. The total

test takes forty-five minutes and is timed according to specific subtests. There are several subtests, each requiring a written response from the subject. The ask-guess category was created to give subjects an opportunity to express their curiosity and to give a picture of their ability to develop hypotheses and think in terms of possibilities. The product-improvement activity enables the subject to play with ideas and manipulate an object. The unusual-uses activity offers the subject the opportunity to free himself or herself of well-established sets and create new ones. The unusual questions activity measures "divergent power," and the just-suppose activity, a variation of the guess consequences aspect of the ask and guess activity, is designed to elicit a high degree of fantasy; the subject must play with possibilities and imagine events that might occur as a consequence of an improbable situation.

These are not intelligence tests but are designed to help teachers "sift out the more- from the less-talented students." However, they do correlate with intelligence tests. Creativity is defined as a problem-solving ability in a general sense. The following definitions may clarify this:

*Fluency:* Number of relevant responses given.

*Flexibility:* Number of different categories of response.

*Originality:* Sum of credits, in which routine responses count zero, less common responses get a unit score, and infrequent responses get a credit of 2.

*Elaboration:* Count of the additional details used in each response totaled over responses.

Studies concerned with construct validity are studies of the personalities of high and low scorers. Studies suggest that the test does measure behaviors consistent with the literature on creative behavior. In a section on concurrent validity, the TTCT seems to have low relations to teacher nominations but seems to be related to both academic intelligence and educational achievement test scores.

Creative thinking can be influenced by personality and situational variables, so, as the manual points out, "it is to be expected that motivational conditions affect test-retest reliability and that motivational aspects are probably controlled more adequately in research studies than in normative studies." Thus test-retest reliabilities range from .35 to .73 over three-year periods. Although the reliability studies of the TTCT are well summarized in the manual, many of the studies are not fully reported, and so it is difficult to assess them. However, the diversity of studies and samples suggests that the scales have adequate reliability.

Means and standard deviations are provided for a number of samples. The basic groups used for the two main score conversion tables are 118 fifth-graders in St. Croix, Wisconsin, and 108 seventh-graders. No other conversion tables are provided, and the scores are converted into $T$ scores, but not to percentile ranks or other scores.

### MEMORY FOR DESIGNS

(Graham, F., & Kendall, B., 1960, Psychological Test Specialists)

This simple test of drawing is designed to assess immediate memory and perceptual motor coordination. The subject sees a design for 5 seconds, then attempts to draw it from memory. This procedure is repeated for each of the fifteen designs. To assign a score from 0 to 3 points, the tester compares each drawing with carefully chosen sample drawings, representative of the productions of psychiatric controls and persons with varying degrees of brain injury. A raw score is the sum of the points for all fifteen drawings. This total is corrected for age and intelligence by reference to a table.

The validity coefficient is .67, and scorer agreement on the Memory for Designs test is significantly higher than on the Bender-Gestalt. Test and immediate retest reliability was .89. Norms are based on the performance of 825 individuals (including normal persons, psychotic persons, and persons with brain disorders or

idiopathic epilepsy) ranging in age from $8\frac{1}{2}$ to 60 years. Groups were matched for sex, age, race, education, and occupational status.

### SPATIAL ORIENTATION MEMORY TEST

(Wepman, J., & Turaids, D., 1975, Language Research Associates)

This test is designed to assess the development of a child's ability to remember the direction of forms that are presented visually. The test includes twenty designs and twenty arrays of four to five of the same design in different orientations. The test is administered individually to children five to nine years of age. Each design is presented to the child for 5 seconds. The child is then asked to point to the same design that is turned in the same direction on a separate card. The raw score can be converted into a rating that ranges from $-2$ to 2.

The test correlates .42 with a reading readiness test given to six-year-old children. It also correlates .51 with a reading test in an achievement battery given to seven-year-old children. Reliability coefficients of Form I versus Form II range from .60 to .74; the median is .62. These reliabilities are reported on children from five to eight years of age. This test was standardized on 100 children from five through ten years of age.

### AMMONS QUICK TEST

(Ammons, R., & Ammons, C., 1962, Psychological Test Specialists)

This is an intelligence test (a derivative of the Full-Range Picture Vocabulary Test) based on language concepts; the subject hears a word and points to the appropriate picture. Age range for the test is two to eighteen years. There are three 50-word forms, each form having as its basis a single plate of four complex drawings. Clear information about percentiles and quotients is provided (mean quotient is about 101 and standard deviation about 15) in the manual.

Reported validities concern correlations of this test with the Full-Range Picture Vocabulary Test. These correlations are high, from .60 to .96. The congruent validity of the Full-Range is satisfactory; such measures as the SB, WISC, WAIS, and various achievement measures were used. Correlations usually are in the .70s and .80s, although with the WISC they are in the .60s and .70s. Correlations are in the .40s with college samples, which suggests that the Full-Range is more efficient for the screening of individuals in the average (or below) range of intelligence than those of superior intelligence. Alternate-form reliabilities in a variety of child and adult samples are in the .90s. The standardization sample was 458 cases ranging from two years of age to adulthood; these were controlled for age, grade, placement, own (or husband's or father's) occupation, and sex.

### PEABODY PICTURE VOCABULARY TEST

This test is discussed in Chapter 5.

### OHWAKI-KOHS TACTILE BLOCK DESIGN INTELLIGENCE TEST FOR THE BLIND

(Ohwaki, Y., 1965, Western Psychological Services)

The Ohwaki-Kohs test is used to measure intelligence in totally blind persons, six years of age to adulthood. It is made up of eighteen designs and sixteen tactile blocks. The subject combines four or more blocks and attempts to reproduce the designs presented to him or her. The subject's mental age and IQ are measured by the duration and number of successful subtests. The test includes one practice trial and eighteen subtests, arranged in order of difficulty. The examiner allows the subject to explore the block many times; fingers of both hands can be used so that the subject becomes acquainted with the tactile differences of the surfaces. The examiner turns the block to all six surfaces so they can be tactilely examined, over and over until the subject appears to understand the tactile differences of each surface. The examiner then places the practice design card on the table in front of the subject; the four blocks are placed to the right of the card, readily available to the right hand of the subject. The examiner takes the subject's hand and places it on the design to show that the surfaces on the card are the same

as found on the blocks. The examiner tells the subject to take the four blocks and put them together so the tops of the four blocks make the same design as that on the design card. The examiner makes the first design for demonstration purposes.

In terms of validity, moderately predictive correlations (.55) were found for arithmetic, drawing, and reading Braille. In a group of thirty-three blind subjects, ranging from eight to twenty years of age, a test-retest study made within $3\frac{1}{2}$ months resulted in a coefficient of .846. The standardization of the test does not show a normal curve when the distribution was made on the 345 subjects. The distribution of IQ extends to the lower part in general, and the higher part is distinct from the lower. The children in the normal zone of IQ were relatively few. More children need to be tested to determine if this was a result of the few subjects tested, the intelligence distribution of the blind, or the characteristics of the test.

### EMBEDDED FIGURES TEST (EFT)

(Witkin, A., Oltman, K., Raskin, E., & Karp, S., 1971, Palo Alto, CA: Consulting Psychologists Press)

The EFT is not an intelligence test but a test assessing cognitive style in intellectual functioning; it is appropriate for use on subjects ten years of age and up. The subject's task on the EFT is to locate a previously seen simple figure within a larger complex figure that has been organized to obscure or embed the simple figure. Scores on the EFT reflect ability at perceptual disembedding, which has been interpreted as determining the cognitive style of the subject. Cognitive styles have been divided into field dependence and field independence; characteristics peculiar to each are outlined in the manual. The test kit consists of two sets of twelve cards with complex figures, a set of eight cards with simple forms, a stylus, a stopwatch, and data sheets. The examiner first shows a complex figure, then the simple figure, then the complex figure again, each for a specified time. The student's score is determined by the amount of time he or she takes to find and trace the simple figure within the complex figure. The EFT provides a score that is a mean-solution-time per item, which can be compared with the mean number of seconds per item for subjects ten years of age to adulthood. These scores can also be compared on the basis of sex differences. A high score on the EFT indicates a high degree of field-independent cognitive functioning. A detailed explanation on the interpretation of the relationship between field dependence or independence and the three main IQ factors on the WAIS has been provided.

The EFT presents two types of validity: construct validity and congruent validity. Construct validity has been used to determine that the EFT is indeed a test of field dependence and independence in perception and that items of the EFT are assessing cognitive style in intellectual functioning. Several factor analytical studies were conducted. Congruent validity was determined by comparisons with several earlier established measures: the WAIS, the Rod and Frame Test, and the Body Adjustment Test.

Reliability is high—.90 for split-half method and .89 for test-retest methods.

The test was standardized on 880 students between ten years of age and adulthood. A different number of students was tested at each age level, and not all age levels were actually tested. Use of the EFT is appropriate in certain situations in which specific knowledge of cognitive style is desired. Although field independence on the EFT has correlated highly with certain intelligence-related factors on other tests, it is not recommended as a test for general intelligence.

## SUMMARY

The purpose of this chapter is to provide a basic understanding of information-processing theory. The works of Brown, Bruner, Newell and Simon, Atkinson and Shiffrin, Neisser, Craik and Lockhart, Piaget, and Sternberg were discussed. Standardized tests believed to cover some basic components of intelligence were reviewed.

# CHAPTER 5

# Assessment of Language

PATRICIA TOMLIN
H. LEE SWANSON

## OUTLINE

**L**anguage is one of the most complex systems of rules a child ever learns. Experiences with the outside world and a capacity from within the child must mesh, for language to develop (deVilliers & deVilliers, 1979). Theories as to the development and nature of language vary. Each school of thought has developed its interpretation, with its own slightly different slant to terminology. Yet professionals interested in our unique communication system have taken a sensible approach. Acceptance of any single point of view about language is believed to force artificial, restrictive boundaries on assessment and therapy (Carrow-Woolfolk & Lynch, 1982). Each attempt to analyze and describe, integrate and synthesize language components has been accepted as an expansion of knowledge. The profession is characterized by its propensity to integrate the old with the new and allow for the evaluation of ideas; the field thus resists the temptation to "throw the baby out with the bath." Thus, the study of the processes of language, its development and its interface with cognition, is perhaps the most exciting, alive, growing professional arena in education today.

*Language* in this chapter will be viewed as a method by which humans communicate. Although it is not possible to make a comprehensive review of all theories related to language processes, a representative overview of current constructs will be presented. Perhaps Clark and Clark (1977) best expressed the integral role of language in human functioning:

> Language stands at the center of human affairs, from the most prosaic to the most profound. It is used for haggling with store clerks, telling off umpires and gossiping.... Indeed, it is a basic ingredient in virtually every social situation. The thread that runs through all these activities is communication, people trying to put their ideas over to others. As the main vehicle of human communication, language is indispensable. (p. 3)

Early in the field's history, language was primarily defined in terms of its auditory-vocal-linguistic code or its structural and semantic rules (Carrow-Woolfolk & Lynch, 1982). The assessment of language was often equated with the assessment of speech and on the human anatomy necessary for central auditory processing. Yet speech is not necessarily language, and language is not always speech. The domains of speech, phonology and audiology have gained recognition as separate disciplines in their own right. Contemporary views of language processes are more representative of psycholinguistic and cognitive perspectives. Thus, the communicative options within language range from private, self-regulatory speech, through verbalization, to nonverbal gestures.

This chapter is designed as an overview of past practices, current developments in assessment, and future directions. In an attempt to provide a framework for assessment and evaluation, it will mainly address language acquisition, development, and disorders. It describes the development and assessment of speech, its articulation and phonological characteristics, but shies away from the more medical orientation of central auditory processing. A section on language disorders primarily addresses the largest population of school-aged children in need of assistance, the language-learning disabled. This chapter concludes with a listing of representative assessment instruments published since 1960.

## THEORETICAL CONSIDERATIONS

Early language theories were based primarily upon behavioral theory. Behavioral theories describe a passive language learner, who is taught to speak through stimulus-response conditioning and reinforcement. Thus, correct sentence form is learned through a person's interaction with and imitation of others in the environment. Skinner's (1957) interpretation specified that verbal units result from a child's being rewarded for saying wordlike sounds. Language application was transferred from one stimulus to another according to the similarity between stimuli. Rewarding a word's use increases the probability of that word's future occurrence. Thus, undifferentiated verbal responses are shaped by appropriate stimulus reinforcement, reinforcement provided by the child's experience, social interaction, or the situational context.

Language acquisition theory presents a hypothesis based upon uniquely human, innate capacities. Using their innate capacity for linguistic knowledge, children develop language naturally, automatically, effortlessly, and quickly. Nativists refer to human language as the product of evolutionary specialization, a process that has given the human species the internal construct that they need to take in linguistic knowledge and transform this knowledge. Chomsky (1965) refers to this theoretical construct as a language acquisition device (LAD), a device that determines the general form of language's structure. Thus, the acquisition of the structure of language depends upon use of an intact knowledge that the child is born with. The regularities in language behavior discovered through cross-cultural (Slobin, 1979) and longitudinal research (Brown, 1973), plus the observed universal syntactic features across languages, have provided support for this position.

Interactionist theory takes the nativists' predisposition for language into account, but sees that predisposition takes on a sociohistorical nature as children learn language through interaction with their speech communities. In refining the nativist notion of language acquisition, Bruner (1983) has thus described a language acquisition support system, the LASS. His theory recognizes the predisposition of humans toward linguistic knowledge, yet he emphasizes the communicative interactions between child and primary caretaker within a specific cultural context. These interactions shape the linguistic development of the child. Bruner (1983) writes:

> While the capacity for intelligent action has deep biological roots and a discernible evolutionary history, the exercise of that capacity depends upon man appropriating to himself modes of acting and

thinking that exist not in his genes but in his culture. (p. 23)

## COGNITION AND LANGUAGE

Presently, there are two major viewpoints from which the development of cognition and language in children are regarded. The old adage, "Which came first, the chicken or the egg?" aptly describes these conflicting views. Some professionals accept that concepts are first introduced to children by means of language, while others believe that when children come to the task of language learning, they are already equipped with the basic concepts that they have built up through their interactions with the world. Much of speech/language assessment and intervention has been based upon the developmental framework proposed by Piaget. Piaget (Piaget & Inhelder, 1969) suggested that children develop language by means of complementary cognitive capacities and maturation (see Chapter 4). Language and thought thus develop simultaneously as the child passes through a series of fixed developmental stages, requiring progressive, increasingly complex strategies of cognitive organization. Piagetian theory predicts that children's thinking is qualitatively different at different levels of development, and that therefore, assessment is best conducted through the use of sequential, ordinal scales (e.g., see Finch-Williams, 1984). All mental development (in language) is an extension of biological organization and adaptation. He postulates that what is inherited is a set of functional invariants—processes that are basic to all biological adaptation and that reflect sensitivities to internal as well as external function.

The pacesetter for language development, according to Piaget, is the child's cognitive development. Thus, the emergence of symbolic function occurs when the child makes something stand for or represent an object or event that might not be perceptually present. This symbolic function, in the form of drawing, mental imagery, gestures, or deferred imitation, is an early manifestation of language. Many investigations have studied the relationship between Piagetian milestones and linguistic structures. Although there appears to be correspondence between sensorimotor stages and characteristics of language production, the inconsistency of research's findings preclude a decision that one emerges prior to the other (Ingram, 1976a; Dihoff & Chapman, 1977; Miller, Chapman, Branson & Reichle, 1980).

In contrast to Piaget, Vygotsky (1962) hypothesized that mature concept-formation is a function of social and cultural growth, and that language becomes the means by which children and adults systematize their diverse perceptions. Mature functioning thus utilizes *the word* as a means of concept formation:

> Learning to direct one's own mental processes with the aid of words or signs is an integral part of the process of concept formation (p. 59). . . . This operation is guided by the use of words as a means of actively centering attention, of abstracting certain traits, synthesizing them and symbolizing them. (p. 81)

According to Vygotsky, conceptual thinking begins with the child's construction of *heaps,* i.e., unorganized groupings of thoughts without apparent basis, an undirected extension of categories created by chance. At this level, items are brought together and given a label solely by subjective impression. The next level of concept development, *thinking in complexes,* allows for the learning of basic rules of categorization and grouping, as the child manipulates various attributes of stimuli. Items are grouped and labeled according to both subjective impressions and similarities that actually exist; related "families" of items are thus created. At the complex level,

> word meanings as perceived by the child refer to the same objects the adult has in mind, which ensures understanding between child and adult, but . . . the child thinks the same thing in a different way, by means of different mental operations (p. 69). . . . The coincidence, in practice, of many word meanings for the adult and the three year old

child, the possibility of mutual understanding, and the apparent similarity of their thought processes have led to the false assumption that all the forms of adult intellectual activity are already present in embryo in child thinking and that no drastic change occurs at the age of puberty. (p. 68)

As development progresses, the adolescent will form and use a concept correctly in a concrete situation, but will find it difficult to express that concept in words. Thus, at the adolescent level, there is a marked discrepancy between the ability to process and the ability to express that process. Only when the individual has attained the ability to decontextualize, examine, deduce, and apply generalizations to unique situations, has mature concept-formation been achieved.

The interest in theorizing on the relationship between language and cognition has not abated with time. In fact, with the recent psycholinguistic influence on language assessment and intervention, discussions occur more often and with less resolution than before. Many of today's thinkers view Vygotskian thought as an extension of, perhaps a refinement of, Piagetian theory. In terms of assessment, practice-language use becomes the evaluator's window to the mind. The analysis of children's production of language yields inferences about their cognitive ability. Yet, in many respects, language is the catalyst for cognition. Children must organize the ideas they have acquired. Children also must acquire the linguistic rules with which they can verbalize those ideas. As stated by Carrow-Woolfolk and Lynch (1982):

> Although it is possible to develop concepts without language, the presence of language influences the further development of concepts, particularly abstract concepts that have no sensory referent and those that are conveyed by the grammatical structure itself. Words point to distinctions that have meaning; e.g., a small glass with a handle is a cup. If a child does not understand cup as a concept separate from glass until the label of word is used in his environment, it might be said that the word preceded the concept. The child perceives the difference, but does not consider it significant until

it is labeled. [Thus] language of some kind (spoken, written or signed) is essential to the acquisition, elaboration, and oral refinement of certain abstract concepts. (p. 123)

Given this brief introduction to the relationship between language and cognition, we now turn our attention to speech acquisition.

## SPEECH ACQUISITION

The acquisition of speech is orderly and at times appears to be operating in accordance with a developmental scale. Speech is closely associated with chronological age and with normal physical and intellectual maturation. Numerous measures have been used to describe speech development, and the information in Table 5-1 was compiled from the works of Blair (1980), Carrow (1968), Gesell and Amatruda (1941), Hauserman (1958), Templin (1957), and Terman and Merrill (1960).

The first sound an infant makes is purely reflexive—sounds are caused by air passing through the vocal cords. The infant engages in undifferentiated crying with random vocalizations and cooing. At about four to six months of age, the infant enters the lallation stage—the imitation of sounds purely for pleasure. The infant engages in babbling, verbalization in response to speech of others, and immediate responses that approximate human interactional patterns. At seven to eleven months of age, the echolalic stage, the child automatically repeats words and phrases. The child's tongue, of course, moves with vocalizations (*lalling*).

At 1 year of age, a child says his or her first word. At approximately 18 months of age, the child is at the one-word sentence stage in which nouns are primarily used. At 2 years of age, the child uses two-word sentences. Sentences are functionally complete, and pronouns and verbs are used most frequently. At approximately 2½ years of age, the child uses three-word sentences. Speech is presented in a telegraphic manner (the child systematically omits all but the most important words). By 3

years of age, the child can use a complete, simple, active sentence. The child can use sentences to tell stories that are understood by others. At 3½ years of age, the child can express concepts with words and sentence length is four or five words. At 5 years of age, the child has excessive verbalization and engages in imaginary speech. Articulation errors, however, are still common and may include omission (only portions of words pronounced), substitutions (substituting phonemes in words), additions (extra sound to words), and distortions (alterations in sounds). By 5 years of age, the child also uses negation and inflexional forms of verbs. Sentences are well developed and include complex syntax. By 6 to 8 years of age, the child has fairly sophisticated speech and acceptable articulation.

In describing an informal assessment of speech acquisition (as well as production), Gaffner and co-workers (1978) developed a five-point rating scale designed to assess language production, speech reception, and speech intelligibility (Table 5-2). While the element of subjectivity is apparent in these items, Gaffner and co-workers note that these measures provide an estimate of linguistic ability. The classroom teacher can develop other items by which to compare a child's performance with those of the peers.

A more detailed informal assessment has been described by Oslerger and co-workers (1978); in it speech is assessed on three tasks. Task one requires the child to produce sounds of various patterns from auditory cues only. Production of syllables and strings of syllables is done in one breath. These syllables include four different durations, intensities, and pitches. Thus, the child is assessed on imitative skills. The second task assesses the child's ability to spontaneously produce different syllables and strings of syllables. To elicit specific patterns, visual cues are used. The third task requires the child to discriminate the syllables or strings of syllables produced by the teacher. Each of these tasks incorporates a training scheme.

**Table 5-1**    Speech development.

| Approximate age | Language behavior | |
|---|---|---|
| | Receptive | Expressive |
| 6 mo. | Responds to sound that is out of sight (car drives up, bell); Hears sound and plays with noise-making toys; Turns to speaking voice | Laughs or squeals aloud, babbles several sounds in one breath; Vocalizes dadda or mamma, but is not specific |
| 7–9 mo. | Recognizes name; Listens and locates sound; Recognizes mamma; Waves bye-bye or plays patty-cake at verbal request | Front vowels, babbles, or lalling—intonation; Imitates sounds such as cough or tongue click |
| 10–12 mo. | Identifies picture on card (show me the car, house, cup ...); Comes when called; Smiles and pats mirror; Understands gesture; Repeats performance when someone laughs | Spontaneous repetition of sound made by others; Imitates /m/, /n/, /p/, /b/; Points to object while babbling; First words appear |
| 13–15 mo. | Responds to words and phrases (no, come); Generalized use of vocabulary (e.g., "dadda" might mean Where's Daddy; Daddy is coming) | Sentence length—1 word; Vocabulary—1–15 words; Recognizes several objects by name |
| 14–18 mo. | Follows simple instructions (e.g., Put the ball on the table.); Identifies picture on card (e.g., Show me the kitty.) | Speaking vocabulary—5–10 words; Uses two-word sentences |
| 19–21 mo. | Identifies picture when named (e.g., book, basket, star); Points to doll parts (e.g., head, eyes, hair) | Vocabulary of 20 words, combines words to express different ideas (e.g., Mamma go bye-bye.) |
| 20–24 mo. | Follows simple directions (e.g., Show me a dog, Show me a man, Show me a hat.) | Has approximately 300-word vocabulary, 25% use of consonants (e.g., initial and final) |
| 2–3 yr. | Can follow preposition directions (e.g., Put the ball on the chair, under the chair, in front of ...); Identifies action in pictures (e.g., Show me the girl jumping, sitting); Understands "many" and "few" | Repeats two or three digits after presentation (e.g., 2–4, 6–4–1); Can tell how simple objects are used; Vocabulary of 500–1000 words; uses pronouns, adverbs, adjectives, and prepositions; Sentence length of three to four words; Correct articulation of consonants: /m/, /n/, /p/, /f/, /h/, /w/ |

# LANGUAGE PROCESSES: FORM-CONTENT-USE

In order to best organize the information to be presented, we'll begin with the broad categorization of language processes that Bloom and Lahey (1978) provide within their descriptive-linguistic *form-content-use* paradigm. This model describes language in terms of linguistic representations, and introduces the components of language most often subject to assessment.

**Table 5-1** *continued*

| Approximate age | Language behavior | |
|---|---|---|
| | Receptive | Expressive |
| 3–4 yr. | Interpretation of pictures (e.g., Which one tells you it is night time?); Object identification through function (e.g., Show the one that gives us milk.); Number concept of 2; Opposite analysis (e.g., In daytime it is light, at night it is ___ ; Father is a man, Mother is a ___); Follows a two-stage command | Sentence length of four to eight words; Vocabulary in excess of 1500 words; Identifies two to three colors by name; Articulates consonant blends (e.g., /gr/, /mp/, /br/, /rt/), single phonemes /k/, /b/, /d/, /g/, /r/, and beginning articulation of /y/; Past tense appears and simple active-declarative sentences |
| 4–5 yr. | Follows a three-stage command; Has number concept of 3 or 4; Can repeat four digits; Definitions of familiar objects (e.g., What is a hat?); Memory for sentence of 10 words in length | Correct articulation of /s/, /sch/, /ch/, /sh/; Counts 10 objects; Vocabulary in excess of 2000 words; Correct use of all parts of speech; How and why questions; Can tell a story by pointing to pictures and describing action in multiword sentences |
| 5–6 yr. | Knows right and left; Number concept to 10; Understands words of quantity (e.g., more or less; bigger; many, few); Simple analogies (e.g., A lemon is sour, sugar is ___.) | Articulation of /t/, /th/, /v/, /l/; Vocabulary in excess of 2500 words; Can count to 30 by ones; Asks meanings of words; Syntactical development essentially complete |
| 6–7 yr. | Reads on pre-primer level; Can use picture dictionary; Defines and explains words | Correct articulation of /y/, /th/, /z/, /zh/, /s/; Experimentation with larger words |
| 7+ yr. | Comprehends cause-and-effect relationships; Compares and contrasts relationships (e.g., How is a submarine different from a fish?) | Fluent use of language; Correct articulation of sounds /kt/, /tr/, /sp/ |

## Form

The features and characteristics of the words used for communication are referred to as the *form* of language. The most basic elements of a word's form include phonology, morphology and syntax. Because these components provide a foundation for language assessment and research, these forms of language will be reviewed.

*Phonology.* Phonology is the term applied to knowledge of the sounds and sound sequences required by one's language. The phonemic system also encompasses the knowledge of the means in which stress, intonation, and pitch affect oral communication. The elementary sounds of the English language, *phonemes,* (for the most part vowels and consonants), correspond roughly to the letters of our alphabetic writing system. For example, the word *cat* consists of an ordered set of three phonemes: /c/, /a/, /t/. The three letters used to spell *cat* in English orthography are often referred to as *graphemes.* Although there is a rough correspondence in English between graphemes and phonemes, the relationship is definitely not one-to-one (see Panagos, 1978, for review).

Whereas words stand for concepts that have meanings, phonemes stand for structural components of words and generally have no mean-

**Table 5-2**
Five-point rating scale.

| Nonsubstantial | | | | Substantial |
|---|---|---|---|---|
| **1** | **2** | **3** | **4** | **5** |
| **Language production** | | | | |
| Language not measurable | Isolated words, holophrastic utterance, one-word utterance | Use of phrases, two- to three-word utterances, including nouns and verbs | Simple sentence structure | Substantial output |
| **Speech reception** | | | | |
| Not understood | Understands a few spoken words | Understands two- to three-word utterances | Understands simple sentences | Complete understanding |
| **Speech expression** | | | | |
| Cannot be understood | Isolated phrases or words are intelligible | Gist of content can be understood | Speech intelligible with exception of a few phrases or words | Speech completely intelligible |

Based on material from Gaffner, D., et al. Speech and language assessment scale of deaf children. *Journal of Communication Disorders,* 1978, *11,* 215–226.

ing at all. Communicating concepts to other individuals requires that words be represented by a succession of phonemic segments. The number of unique, hearable positions of the vocal sounds is many orders of magnitude fewer than the number of different concepts that individuals possess (deVilliers & deVilliers, 1974). Because a child's vocal system is essentially a one-word-at-a-time system, it is necessary to represent all of the concepts that children possess; the difficulty of achieving this puts the process of assessment in perspective.

Several authors (Jakobson, 1968; Jakobson, Fant, & Halle, 1963) have devised an economical set of contrasts so that every phoneme of every language can be featured. There are usually considered to be approximately forty consonant and vowel phonemes in the English language. There is some disagreement regarding the exact number of phonemes characteristic of English (McNeill, 1970), particularly concerning whether complex vowels should be considered

phonemes. There is little disagreement, however, concerning the methods with which children phonetically spell a particular word.

Of course, phonemes may differ in the number of features they share. Consider the words *pit* and *spit,* in which we focus on the phoneme /p/. Phonetically the /p/ in the two words has different sounds; the /p/ that occurs in *pit* is an aspirated sound, while the /p/ that occurs after /s/ in all words is an unaspirated sound. A segment of a sound is phonemic in the language of a child if it differs from all other sounds in the location and means by which it is articulated (Fromkin & Rodman, 1974; Jakobson, 1968; Jakobson, Fant, & Halle, 1963).

Articulation in English involves seven major mouth formations:

1. The two lips together (bilabial)
2. The bottom lip against the upper front teeth (labiodental)
3. The tongue against the teeth (dental)

4. The tongue against the alveolar ridge of the gums just behind the upper front teeth (alveolar)
5. The tongue against the hard palate in the roof of the mouth just behind the alveolar ridge (palatal)
6. The tongue against the soft palate, or velum, in the rear roof of the mouth (velar)
7. The glottis in the throat (glottal)

These formations divide the consonants into seven places of articulation:

1. *Bilabial:* p, b, m, w
2. *Labiodental:* f, v
3. *Dental:* θ, ð
4. *Alveolar:* t, d, s, z, n, l, r
5. *Palatal:* š, ž, č, ǰ, y
6. *Velar:* k, g
7. *Glottal:* h

The sounds of consonants also differ in the manner or the mechanical means by which they are produced. The eight features representing the manner of articulation include:

1. *Nasals:* m, n, ŋ (walking)—sound is directly through the nasal cavities.
2. *Stops:* p, b, t, d, k, g—airflow is abruptly interrupted.
3. *Affricates:* c (chew), j—sound is made by forcing air through a narrow constriction.
4. *Fricatives:* f, v, θ (voiceless, ether), ð (voiced, either), s, z, š (shoes), ž (delusion), h— produced by constriction at the point of articulation.
5. *Liquid:* l, r—some obstruction in the airflow but not enough to cause friction.
6. *Voiced:* b, m, g, v, z, y—presence of a laryngeal tone.
7. *Glide:* w, ʍ (whistle), y, h, ʔ (Hugo)—sound is determined by movement to or from the vowel with no obstruction of the airflow.
8. *Sibilant:* s, z, š, ž, č, ǰ—friction between two articulators produces a hissing noise.

Vowels, according to Clark and Clark (1977), are classified by the position of the tongue in the

mouth during articulation (*front*—pit; *center*— putt; *back*—put). The height of the tongue is also used for classification in terms of *high* (pit), *mid* (pet), or *low* (pat). The two-way classification is illustrated in Table 5-3.

In general, phonemes that share many features are more confusing to children than sounds that have few features in common. The relationship between phonemes' features might be considered analogous to the relationship between a chord and the individual notes that constitute the chord. Errors of mispronunciation result from a failure to differentiate the features, or the notes constituting the chord. Errors of mispronunciation and speech recognition involve difficulty with sound segments (phonemes) that are relatively complex in their distinctive-feature description; there are few errors in sounds with which children have no difficulties. The late-developing aspects of phonology are potentially significant to the assessment of children who have language deficits (Ingram, 1976a).

There is agreement in some reviews that stops (/b/, /d/, /g/, /p/, /t/, /k/), nasals (/m/, /n/), and glides (/w/, /y/, /h/) are mastered early (Menyuk, 1971; Moore, 1973). Shvachkin (cited in Moore, 1973) and Jakobson (1968) hypothesized from observations of children that phonemic speech perception develops concomitantly with word meaning during the second year of life, and that the development follows an

**Table 5-3**

Two-way classification of English vowels.

| Height of tongue | Part of tongue involved | | |
|---|---|---|---|
| | Front | Central | Back |
| High | i beet | — | u boot |
| | ɪ bit | ɨ marry | ʊ put |
| Mid | e bait | | o boat |
| | | ə sofa | |
| | ɛ bet | | ɔ bought |
| Low | æ bat | ʌ but | a pot |

ontogenetic sequence. Table 5-4 shows the stages in the development of phonemic speech as suggested by Shvachkin and Jakobson.

Menyuk (1971) suggests that use of voiced consonants is a distinction acquired by four years of age. Later acquisitions, stages eleven and twelve, are mainly continuants (/s/, /z/, /š/, /ž/) or sounds that have a gradual release (/č/, /ǰ/). It is difficult to relate such generalizations, on the maturation of standard English phonemes, to traditional developmental stages. Inconsistency in development can include the acquisition of stops (with the exception of /t/) before the development of other sounds. Conversely, continuants (with the exception of /f/ and /h/) are acquired relatively late and voiced is mastered initially (/d/ before /t/), while in other instances devoiced is acquired first (for example, /s/ before /z/).

Summary data on phonological acquisition are presented in more detail by Brown (1973)

and Clark and Clark (1977). Some agreed-upon conclusions include the following:

1. Phoneme production increases with age; vowels are more common than consonants in the first years of life after vowel-consonant patterns are reached.
2. At onset, front-mouth vowels (for example, /i/, /e/) are most frequently uttered; the use of back vowels (for example, /u/) increases with age. Adult vowel approximations are achieved around 2½ to 3 years of age.
3. Uses of postdentals, labials, and labiodentals increase with age, while glottal consonant stops (for example, /g/) and fricatives (for example, /h/) are characteristic of younger ages. The use of velars and dentals remains unaffected by age.

Some common observational assessments that may be used to informally assess children's phonological developments may focus on the

**Table 5-4**
Stages in the development of phonemic speech perception.

| Stage | Phonemic distribution | Approximate age |
|-------|----------------------|-----------------|
| 1 | Vowels | 1–2 yr. |
|   | a. *a* versus other vowels | |
|   | b. Front versus back; i-u, e-o, i-o, e-u | |
|   | c. High versus low: i-e, u-o | |
| 2 | Presence versus absence of consonant: CVC-VC | |
| 3 | Sonorant versus articulated obstruent: m-b, r-d, n-g, y-v | 3 yr. |
| 4 | Palatalized versus nonpalatalized: ń-n, ḿ-m, b́-b, v́-v, ź-z, ĺ-l, ŕ-r | |
| 5 | Sonorants | |
|   | a. Nasal versus liquid or glide: m-l, m-r, n-l, n-r, n-y, m-y | |
|   | b. Nasal versus nasal: m-n | |
|   | c. Liquid versus liquid: l-r | |
| 6 | Sonorant versus nonarticulated obstruent: m-z, l-x, n-ž | |
| 7 | Labial versus nonlabial: b-d, b-g, v-z, f-x | |
| 8 | Stop versus fricative: b-v, d-z, k-x, d-ž | |
| 9 | Velar versus dental or palatal: g-d, x-s, x-š | |
| 10 | Voiced versus voiceless: b-p, d-t, g-k, v-f, z-s, ž-š | 4 yr. |
| 11 | "Hushing" versus "hissing" sibilants: ž-z, š-s | 5 yr. |
| 12 | Liquid versus glide: r-y, l-y | |

syllabic structure and assimilatory and substitution processes (Ingram, 1976a). A reference for informal phonological assessment is provided in the following outline.

## Common errors in the phonological process of children of all ages*

A. Substitution processes
  1. Stopping—fricatives and occasionally other sounds are replaced with a stop consonant: seat (tit), soup (dup).
  2. Fronting of velars—velar consonants tend to be replaced with alveolar ones: book (but), coat (towt).
  3. Fronting of palatals—similar to above; shoe (su), juice (dzus).
  4. Denasalization—the replacement of a nasal consonant with an oral one; no (dow), home (hub)
  5. Gliding—the substitution of a glide (w) or (y) for a liquid sound; rock (wak), lap (yæp).
  6. Vocalization—the replacement of a syllabic consonant with a vowel: apple (æpo), flower (fawo).
  7. Vowel neutralization—the reduction of vowels to a central /a/ or /ə/: bath (bat), book (ba).
B. Assimilatory processes
  1. Prevocalic voicing of consonants—consonants tend to be voiced when preceding a vowel: pen (bɛn), tea (di).
  2. Devoicing of final consonants: bed (bɛt), big (bɪk).
  3. Nasalization of vowels—vowels tend to take on the nasality of a following nasal consonant: friend (frẽ).
  4. Velar assimilation—apical consonants tend to assimilate to a following velar consonant: duck (gək), tongue (gəŋ).
  5. Labial assimilation: top (bap).

---

*Adapted from Ingram, D. Current issues in child phonology. In D. Morehead & A. Morehead (Eds.), *Normal and deficient child language.* Baltimore: University Park Press, 1976, p.15.

  6. Progressive vowel assimilation—an unstressed vowel will assimilate to a preceding stressed vowel: apple (ʔaba).
C. Syllabic structure processes
  1. Deletion of final consonant: out (æw), bike (bay).
  2. Reduction of clusters—the reduction of a consonant cluster to a single consonant: floor (fər), step (dɛp).
  3. Deletion of unstressed syllables: banana (næna).
  4. Reduplication: noodle (nunu).

## Common phonological errors for children up to six or seven years of age (Compton, 1976)

1. Alveolar stops are substituted for velar ones.
2. Affricatives are usually substituted by /t/ or /d/.
3. Initial consonants are rarely omitted; the final consonants have a higher chance of being omitted.
4. Errors of omission for final stops occur more often than the omission of final fricative consonants.
5. The omission of the final alveolar consonant is much more common than any other articulation error.

In summary, most work in standardized assessment has concentrated on phonological acquisition that occurs before five or six years of age; it is uncertain how aspects such as articulation of sound interact on the child's comprehension of word meanings. However, articulation errors are common and can include omissions (only portions of words being pronounced), substitutes (substituting phonemes in words), additions (extra sound added to words), and distortions (alterations in sounds).

*Morphology.* Morphology refers to the study of the smallest meaningful unit of language. Phonemes in combination, morphemes are important components of basic word structure; this category includes prefixes, suffixes, and word endings used to indicate number, gender, or tense. For example, *cats* contains two morphemes, *cat* and *s*. The phrase *unhappy boy* contains three morphological units: *un* (meaning *not*), *happy* and *boy*. A phonemic sequence can be used as a morpheme in one word (*un* in *unkind*) and not in another (the *un* in *under*). As more morphemes are added to the child's repertoire, the child's language structures become more complex. The main classifications of morphemes are as follows:

1. *Bound versus free:* Bound morphemes cannot stand alone in meaning (for example, prefixes such as *pre, un, anti*) while free morphemes can (for example, *car, an, black*).
2. *Affix versus root:* Affix is what is added to a word (for example, prefix, suffix) while a *root* is the core of full morphemes.

Characteristics of morphemes are:

1. Different morphemes can be spelled differently but pronounced alike (for example, *blue* and *blew*).
2. Different morphemes may be spelled alike but sound different (for example, *read* and *read*).
3. A phonemic sequence can be a morpheme in one word but not in another (for example, *un* in *unkind* is a morpheme while *un* in *under* is not).
4. A phoneme can change a morpheme (for example, *s*).
5. Some ostensibly meaningless morphemes do exist (for example, *to*).

At approximately one year of age, children first acquire free morphemes. As they learn phonemes and sequences of phonemes that form meaningful units, their morphological development expands. Berko (1958), in a classic study, found that use of nonsense words made no differences in preschoolers' and first-graders' knowledge of inflectional morphology (for example, *s, ed,* and variations of each). Each child was shown cartoon-like drawings while the examiner read the following statements:

This is a wug.
Now there is another one.
There are two of them.
There are two _____.

Berko's results suggest that children learn general rules for plural inflection at a relatively young age. Because general rules can be applied to new material, those rules can form the core of generative grammar.

One of the interesting achievements of the early phases of grammar acquisition is the way in which children learn to qualify the meanings of their simple sentences. Brown (1973) has provided the most complete description of the course of grammar development in children. Based on a longitudinal study, his findings suggest that children acquire morphemes (modifiers, *ing, s, ed*) in a somewhat regular order. Table 5-5 lists fourteen morphemes that Brown studied and the order in which they occur in development of the English language. In terms of complexity, simple morphemes (such as /s/) are acquired earlier than the copula *be*. And of course the development from simple to complex is characteristic of children's cognitive development. Morphemes are important components of basic word structure, and the determination of a model of their appropriate use by children is vital to the development of an appropriate assessment procedure.

The rate of children's language development varies greatly, so chronological age is a poor index of linguistic level. According to Brown (1973), the best index of language level during the early period is *mean length of utterance* (MLU) in morphemes (the average number of morphemes used in utterances). For example, a child who says, "Baby walk" (2 morphemes), "Ball" (1 morpheme), "See Mama" (2 morphemes), and "Baby ball" (2 morphemes), has an average MLU of 1.75 morphemes.

Informal language analysis in terms of MLUs is useful but time consuming. Furthermore, there is doubt about the reliability and validity of MLU as an index of language development. Yet teachers need a means of evaluating a child's

**Table 5-5**

Suffixes and function words.

| Form | Meaning | Example |
| --- | --- | --- |
| Present progressive; -ing | Ongoing process | He is *riding.* |
| Preposition: in | Containment | The cat is *in* the house. |
| Preposition: on | Support | The box is *on* the chair. |
| Plural: -s | Number | The *dogs* ran away. |
| Past irregular: went, saw | Earlier in time relative to time of speaking | They all *went* to the playground. |
| Possessive: -'s | Possession | *Mother's* hat is big. |
| Uncontractible copula be: are, was | Number; earlier in time | *Are* they boys or girls? *Was* that a dog? |
| Articles: the, a | Definite/indefinite | He has *the* toy. |
| Past regular: -ed | Earlier in time | He *wanted* the book. |
| Third person regular: -s | Number; earlier in time | She *goes* fast. |
| Third person irregular: has, does | Number; earlier in time | *Does* the dog bark? |
| Uncontractible auxiliary be: is, were | Number; earlier in time; ongoing process | *Is* he running? *Were* they at home? |
| Contractible copula be: -'s, -'re | Number; earlier in time | *That's* what happened. |
| Contractible auxiliary be: -'s, -'re | Number; earlier in time; ongoing process | *They're* running very slowly. |

Adapted from material by R. Brown (1973). Cited in Clark, H. H., & Clark, E. V. *Psychology and language: An introduction to psycholinguistics.* New York: Harcourt Brace Jovanovich, 1977.

linguistic development. Brown (1973) recommends using 100 utterances to determine MLUs. Spontaneous language can be developed from story pictures or other visual stimuli. The teacher can use open-ended imperatives or interrogatives (for example, tell me about this, tell me more). Language samples can then be tape-recorded. The calculation of the mean number of morphological units can follow a procedure outlined by Brown (1973), and Chapman and Miller (1975):

1. Only fully transcribable utterances are used.
2. Utterance repetition is counted if it serves a purpose in the story such as for emphasis (for example, *no, no, no*).
3. Filler-type utterances are not counted (for example, *mm* or *ok*).

4. All compound words, proper names, and ritualized reduplications are counted as single words (for example, *choo-choo, night-night, see-saw, pocketbook*).
5. Auxiliaries are counted as separate morphemes (for example, *is, have*).
6. Diminutive forms are counted as one morpheme (for example, *mommy, doggy*).
7. Contractions are counted as two morphemes (for example, *won't*).
8. Utterances that are imitations of preceding adult speeches are counted if they do not comprise more than 20% of the child's utterances.

*Syntax.* Words are composed of morphemes, and sentences are composed according to syntactic rules. Syntax, a part of grammar, refers to the set of rules whereby sentences are ordered from words; that is, with syntax, phrases and sentences can be generated. Syntax is a set of rules that allows the production of grammatically correct word strings. Syntax identifies the relationships of the various parts of the sentences, such as the relationships among the subject, the object, and the verb.

Through use of relationships determined by the syntax of language, children can convey their meaning or intentions. An initial phase of syntactical behavior occurs when a child joins two words that have an underlying relationship; the child subsequently begins to acquire new response units.

Although both the length and the number of sentences in language are theoretically infinite, sentences are generated from a finite set of symbols or rules. These symbols may be formally written as a set of phrase-structure rules, as shown in Figure 5-1.

These rules are not complete but are representative of rules discussed by Chomsky (1968). The symbols are abbreviations for classes of grammatical elements or constituents: S = sentence, NP = noun phrase, VP = verb phrase, Det = determiner, N = noun, V = verb, Aux = auxiliary, and Past = past tense.

The earliest stages of a person's syntactical development are relatively well studied (Limber, 1973; McNeill, 1970; Wood, 1976).

A striking feature of early language is that one word means several different things. One-word sentences, "holophrases," mean what older persons would express in a complete sentence. McNeill (1970) suggests that holophrastic speech is relational or grammatical speech. Between approximately six and twelve months of age, an infant relates one-word utterances to various events and objects.

As the child learns, he or she begins to form two-word sentences, which follow a distinct pattern. This small sentence contains a pivot (most frequently used word) and an open class (more words but infrequently used). A small group of morphemes in the pivot class occurs with many morphemes in the open class. Thus, young

| Symbol | Rewritten as |
|--------|--------------|
| S | S and/or $*S^n$ |
| S | NP + Aux + VP or Pre S + NP + Aux + VP or NP + Aux + VP + Adv or Pre S + NP + Aux + VP + Adv |
| Pre S | Q or Imp or Neg or Emp or any combination of the above except Q + Imp |
| NP | Det + N or NP (+S)* (for example, The boy, who go sub) |
| VP | V + Part or V + NP or V + PP or V + NP (+S)* or be + Adj (+S)* or be + PP or be + NP (+S)* |
| Adv | PP |
| PP | P + NP |
| Aux | Tense or Mod or Perf or Prog or Pass |
| Perf | have + en (participle) |
| Prog | be + ing (participle) |
| Pass | be + en (participle) |
| Det | Article, quantifier, demonstrative |
| N | Count, mass |

**Figure 5-1**
Common rules of syntax. (Based on material from McNeill, D. *The acquisition of language: The study of developmental psycholinguistics.* New York: Harper & Row, 1970.)

children utter such phrases as "See shoe," "See horsie," "See daddy," with "see" belonging to the pivot class.

This concept of pivoted language development was supported by the findings of others, such as Slobin (1975), so that pivot and open class structures are generally regarded as universal features of early language development. However, other investigators have discarded this idea (Bloom, 1970; Bowerman, 1973; Braine, 1976). Regardless, the earliest intelligible words are simple names or predicates (for example, *milk, Ma*). These first words, spoken at approximately one year of age, begin to stand for an entire sentence. Thus, the single word "ball" may mean "This is a ball," "Catch the ball," or "Give me the ball." Children begin to combine words at eighteen to twenty-four months of age, beginning with such simple sentences as "All gone" or "All done" (meaning "I'm through sitting in my high chair").

McNeill (1970) suggests that most children acquire the syntax of their own language by about 3½ to 5½ years of age. By 3 years of age, children can generate syntactically complex names and descriptions (Limber, 1973). They can (1) generate common simple sentences (for example, N-V-N), (2) form complements (for example, expand an N-V-N sequence for noun phrases), and (3) join sentences (using, for example, a conjunction—and; an adverb—where, how, when; or a relative—that).

By 5 years of age, children begin matching the sentence structure of an utterance to structures in their grammar (Wood, 1976). Children search for underlying relationships such as those between subject and verb, or subject, verb, and object, and apply those operations within their grammar to match those in the sentence. Menyuk (1971) suggests that the usage of syntactical operation appropriately follows logically in terms of (1) addition (introducing an element in sentence formation), (2) deletion (omitting elements in a sentence), (3) substitution (replacing an element or phrase in a sentence), (4) permutation (changing sequence of phrases in a sentence), (5) embedding (placing a clause within a sentence), and (6) nesting (embedding two or more phrases within a sentence). In summary, the formulation of a sentence, in order of development, is as follows:

1. Joining words to make a sentence
2. Subject-plus-predicate sentence
3. Verb phrase expanded to include auxiliary verb and copula (form of verb to be or equivalent)
4. Embedding and permutations within a sentence

In studies of exceptional children, Morehead and Ingram (1976) found that normal and linguistically deficient children differed in the amount of time they needed for learning basic syntax structures, rather than in the organization or occurrence of specific subcomponents of the basic structure. In other words, linguistically deficient children do not develop linguistic systems that are quantitatively different from those of normal children; the acquisition of the linguistic system is merely delayed.

Syntactical problems can be related to disorders in other structures of language. Several developmental studies (for example, Menyuk & Looney, 1972; Panagos, 1978) offer evidence of the interrelationships between syntactical and phonological deficits; that is, children who make syntactical errors in the formulation of utterances also make phonological (articulation) errors. For example, Lenneberg, Nichols, and Rosenberger (1966) observed that mentally retarded subjects misarticulated more consonants in connected speech and in phonetically complex words than they did in simple, isolated words taken from articulation tests.

Several authors (Carrow, 1974; Schwartz & Daly, 1978) describe a procedure known as "elicited imitation," which is used to examine a child's syntactical or morphological competence. These authors assumed that when a sentence is given to a child, the child, in repeating the sentence, will use productive rules commensurate with but not exceeding his or her level of linguistic development. If a sentence is beyond the child's linguistic competence, the child is most likely to recode the model sentence into a more simplified version. To evaluate linguistic performance, the examiner analyzes discrepancies between the model and the child's version. Children's acquisition of various syntactical structures is examined in some of the following ways:

1. Repetition of sentence containing various structures
2. Sentence completion, given as example of the structure desired (for example, *The boy*

*hit the girl, The teacher thanked the boy,*
_____—passive structure)
3. Adding correct inflection when given either real words or nonsense items (see Berko discussed earlier)
4. Manipulate object to portray meaning of utterance (for example, Give the boy the ball—indirect object structure)
5. Identification of a set of pictures representing an orally presented model sentence (for example, Show the picture in which the boy is not listening—negation structure)

## Content: Semantics

The syntactic construction of "Horses talk sadly about their homelands" is appropriate (Wiig & Semel, 1984). The noun, verb, and modifiers are aligned as the rules of English usage would dictate. Yet the sentence is not semantically correct; its meaning registers in our minds as nonsensical. The verb *talk* requires a human, animate noun. Unless this sentence were to be presented within the context of a children's book, we would instinctively judge it inappropriate. Bloom and Lahey's *content* paradigm incorporates those "meaning" components of language, the various aspects of semantics. *Semantics* involves word knowledge (vocabulary), knowledge of word relationships, and the understanding of time-and-event relationships. Thus, meaning comes through consideration of both the arrangement and the relationships among different words in a sentence.

Not all theorists agree about the nature of semantic development in children. Research has shown that English-speaking children initially express a limited range of meanings (Brown, 1973). Word meanings, whether deployed in holophrases or two-word utterances, depend upon the child's understanding of his world (deVilliers & deVilliers, 1979). Children's use of language allows them to talk about actions ("Me fall"), recurrence ("More milk"), labeling ("That Teddy"), and nonexistence ("All gone"). Each language draws attention to alternative ways by which information can be presented, to enhance the similarities of some relationships and contrast others. Young children's word relationships are characterized by synonomy (mother/mom), antonymy (mom /dad) and taxonomy (dog/animal). In learning each new word, the child accumulates more knowledge about his world, knowledge that the child then absorbs into a developing hierarchical system of concepts (Wiig & Semel, 1984).

An assumption made in theories of semantic development is that word association is a consequence of linguistic competence and that the ability to produce language is therefore evidence of meaning acquisition. The meaning of a sentence is derived from the meaning of its constituent phrases, which are in turn derived from the meanings of words that compose them. Therefore, the meaning of each of the words is a compositional function of primitive semantic features. Semantic features can be thought of as similar to speech segments, whose patterns distinguish sound segments or phonemes.

Clark's (1973) semantic-feature hypothesis states that children first begin to use word meanings that only partially represent those of an adult lexicon. As speech improves, the word's meaning develops from a general to a specific feature fashion. Simply, a word's meaning has two parts. The sense of a word is the concept it denotes (*chair* denotes the concept of chair), and the reference of a word is the set of things to which it applies (*chair* applies to all real and imaginary entities that belong to the concept *chair*). Semantics is then both cognitive and perceptual. There are abstract relations, for example, that define logical propositions paired with underlying sentences or phrases. At the same time, perceptual modes also define certain kinds of semantic relations. Piaget's concept of images in the sensorimotor period testifies to this relationship.

A common form of assessment of children's language focuses on the sense of a word. A child's ability to gain meaning for words would most logically include these elements:

1. The ability to analyze or segment material into manageable "words" (also included are grammatical phrases)
2. The ability to generate associations for each word that are mutually compatible with the environment
3. The ability to choose from these associations those that are mutually compatible for development of a sentence

But the purpose of assessment is to distinguish what children know about words from what they know about their environment. Therefore, by building plausible interpretations for words and utterances from what they know and from cues in their environmental context, children play an active role in the acquisition of meaning. In doing this, they start with two assumptions about the function of language and the content of language (Clark, 1975). The first assumption is that speech develops out of a reliance on cues from adult speech (for example, features). The logical step for children is to infer that language is for communication. The second assumption is that children make a logical connection between what speakers say within a particular context and the language that is being used. Children develop skills to determine precisely what these connections are—the child's mapping between concepts and language.

Common errors resulting from these two assumptions include, according to Bowerman (1976), strategies that overextend, underextend, or do not replicate adult meaning. Overextension includes using words that might be appropriate in only one use, in another; for example, the child says bow-wow when he sees a dog but later extends the word to include cows or horses. An example of underextension would be using the word *dog* only for the family pet. At other times, the child's meaning does not overlap at all with the meaning required for the environmental context. Therefore, no one knows for sure the number of words a child will comprehend or be able to say when he or she begins school. Certainly, individual cultural experiences

will influence production (Panagos, 1978). Regardless of individual differences, the child knows more words than he or she can say; that is, the size of the child's receptive vocabulary is greater than his or her expressive vocabulary.

If the opposite is true—a child can say more than the words that he or she understands—we might have reason for concern, because this suggests that the child has difficulty in either receiving or processing auditory stimuli (Wiig & Semel, 1984). Largely because of such considerations, most investigations of vocabulary growth have focused on changes in the child's expressive vocabulary. Studies of vocabulary growth (Lenneberg, 1975; Smith, 1926) place the average vocabulary size for one year of age at 3 words, two years of age at 272 words, three years of age at 896 words, four years of age at 1540 words, five years of age at 2072 words, and six years of age at 2562 words. Developing frequent word usage, however, is not necessarily a cumulative process. Bloom (1975) found that children might use several different words for a few days but not say them again for several months. These words are still understood; children simply do not say them during some periods.

## Use

The *use* of language involves the *pragmatic* functions of language in varying contexts; *use* involves the ways in which different social situations affect the linguistic forms one uses in communicative attempts. Pragmatics, the study of language in context, regards the *speech act* rather than the sentence as the basic unit of communication. An assessment model considers word selections and combinations to be contextually based uses of language, which reflect the intentions and beliefs of the speaker and the intended impact of utterances on listeners. *Speech acts* are described in terms of their intended impact on the listener. A pragmatics assessment model of children's communication is therefore more expansive than simply phonemic or morphological development. The model attempts to describe the child as a communicator.

A crucial limitation of the study of a child's syntax is that it focuses on the child's linguistic competency or knowledge of language structure, not the child's communicative competence and the appropriate and effective use of structure in context. The lack of information regarding the effective communicative structures of children has critically limited assessment procedures. An informal assessment of pragmatics might include these questions:

1. When a teacher indicates that he or she does not understand the child's utterances, are there changes in the frequency of the child's repetition of that utterance, is the utterance revised, or is there no response?
2. Are the differences in these utterances across Piagetian stages?
3. Are the children sensitive to the conversational demands inherent in peer communicative failure and do they respond to those demands? Semantically? Syntactically?
4. Is the child's strategy in restructuring conversation unsystematic or systematic?

Further examination of these qualities in children within their speech environment is necessary for complete language assessment.

The study of use also incorporates the *function* of language. Halliday (1975) has suggested the following seven functions of language:

1. *Informative function:* Children communicate new information by means of language, the "let me tell you about this" function.
2. *Imaginative function:* Language permits an escape from realities into a universe of the child's own thinking, the poetic and/or "let's pretend" function.
3. *Heuristic function:* Language is used to discover or explore the environment, the "tell me why" function.
4. *Personal function:* Child expresses unique views, the "what I feel" or "what I think" function.
5. *Interpersonal function:* Children interact for socialization purposes, the "me and you" function.
6. *Regulatory function:* The child is able to control own behavior as well as that of others, through self-vocalization and instructions, the "do that" function.
7. *Instrumental function:* Language permits the child to satisfy needs and express concerns, the "I want" function.

As this list suggests, language serves a wide range of purposes for the developing child. Although these functions have been known to most teachers, research has only recently begun to understand some of the processes underlying language development. For example, what is the relationship between children's "awareness" of their language and their actual production of language?

### Related Processes of Language

*Metalinguistics, Competence, and Performance.* Several authors (deVilliers & deVilliers, 1974; Luria, 1975; Valian & Caplan, 1979) assume that there is a distinction between the language user's knowledge of the language and observed linguistic activities. This ability to know language, not merely the ability to speak or write, is called "metalinguistic awareness." It does not emerge until the child is about five years of age (deVilliers & deVilliers, 1974) and is generally evaluated by the use of questions asking children to judge between acceptable and unacceptable word order. DeVilliers and deVilliers found a clear relationship between the child's level of language development and metalinguistic awareness: as production in sentences increases, awareness increases; but insight lags behind production. Although it is known that metalinguistic awareness can lag production, the main focus in assessment has been on what a child knows or knows how to do, *competence,* and what a child actually does, *performance. Competence* means that a child knows language but still makes errors when the child engages in certain performances. Assessment is an attempt to describe what children know that allows them to perform in a variety of ways. Such a system divides a child's production into correct and incorrect instances of a sentence, for example. In other words, an assumption is made that the child knows appropriate sentence structure but that competence alone does not fully explain the child's performance. Competence and performance are interdependent but separate parameters of behavior.

***Language and Behavior Regulation.*** Luria (1961) has described language as a regulator of overt behavior. The verbal regulation of behavior is initiated externally and then is internalized within the child. Luria differentiates the truly meaningful use of language (semantic) from language that functions merely as sound stimulus (impulsive), and describes the developmental progression of verbal regulation of behavior as follows:

1. *Other-external:* At first, speech is an initiatory function for children from one to three years of age. Language originates outside the child, from other people (for example, someone says, "Clap your hands," and the child's action follows).
2. *Inhibitory-external:* An inhibitory function of speech begins to develop from 3 to 4½ years of age. The child can stop a behavioral action once it has started (for example, "Take off your sock," and the child's correct action follows even though the child was in the process of putting on a sock).
3. *Self-external:* A regulatory function also occurs at 3 to 4½ years of age when the child responds to a set of instructions (for example, "When you see the light, squeeze the button").
4. *Self-internal:* Self-regulation occurs at 4½ years of age. The child uses verbal symbols to organize and arrange behavior (for example, the child saying internally, "I am going to listen to mommy this time").

Self-regulation is most likely to relate to the social context as well as to the development of inner language. The child's ability to recognize semantic properties within the language experience would provide a basis for self-regulation.

Verbal control becomes more frequently and more generally semantic than impulsive. Children's behavior can be increasingly controlled by what is said to them (semantic aspect) rather than by the purely physical-stimulus effect when something is said to them at that particular moment (impulsive speech). Given this fundamental information, let us now direct our attention to the assessment process.

## ASSESSMENT OF LANGUAGE

A typical speech and language evaluation involves administering standardized tests as well as obtaining and later analyzing a spontaneous (spoken or written) language sample. In attempts to judge the appropriateness of a child's language, the areas of imitation, comprehension, and production are often examined. Because language-impaired children might not exhibit a uniform depression of abilities across linguistic, cognitive, or pragmatic functions, assessment of individual strengths and weaknesses is required.

Wiig and Semel (1984) propose that the process of language evaluation should be hierarchical. Thus, evaluation consists of several steps or levels, each of which depends upon the outcome of the previous level. Diagnosis of an individual's language problem requires the same problem-solving skills that research requires—formulating, testing, confirming, confirming the accuracies and inaccuracies of the hypothesis, and reformulating the hypothesis (Kamhi, 1984). The type of approach used during the assessment will depend in large part upon the diagnostician's theoretical views as to the nature of language disabilities and appropriate intervention approaches and strategies. Unfortunately, many professionals possess limited knowledge of the biologic, cognitive, psychologic, social, and environmental forces involved in normal language development (Kamhi, 1984). Without adequate understanding of the many factors that affect normal functioning, evaluators of abnormal functioning walk on thin ice. Recent publications on early language development (deVilliers & deVilliers, 1979) or child language disorders (Carrow-Woolfolk & Lynch, 1982) contain excellent discussions and models of the factors that interact to affect language-disordered children.

Wiig and Semel (1984) also describe four approaches to language assessment with which the testor should be familiar, as he or she examines testing instruments. The first, the diagnostic-prescriptive approach, focuses on the linguistic characteristics of either the child's performance or the task at hand. Instruments designed from this perspective attempt to identify an individual's strengths and weaknesses, and thus lead the diagnostician to make correct decisions for remediation/intervention. Within this approach, the process or ability model coexists with the task-analysis model (see Chapter 1).

The second approach to assessment, the behavior-learning approach, attempts to identify the stimulus-response-reinforcement relations in the student's language and communication behaviors. This construct seeks to determine the relative frequencies and probabilities of occurrence of specific language behaviors. To obtain some of these behavioral measures (i.e., a count of syllables or words spoken, duration of pauses, etc.), electronic equipment is often utilized.

The third approach, the interactive-interpersonal, assesses aspects of the student's ability to communicate effectively in interpersonal-social contexts. Effectiveness in communication across contexts and with varying goals and audiences is evaluated through the use of role-playing or story-telling formats. The final and fourth approach is referred to as the total environmental approach. This form of language evaluation combines process and task analysis, behavior learning, and interpersonal-interactive approaches, with an academic orientation. Thus, language skills inherent to reading, spelling, writing, and the gaining of information from the classroom and the textbook, are evaluated. This approach requires a multidisciplinary evaluation of all facets of students' language performance.

A comprehensive assessment of student language should include (1.) observations of the student's phonological, morphological, syntactic, semantic, and pragmatic abilities across language modes (listening, speaking, reading, writing), (2.) observations across a variety of contexts (from highly structured tasks to peer-group interactions), and (3.) observations of a student's cognitive skills, from the ability to focus and maintain attention to the organization of information for recall (Nelson, 1986). Table 5-6 provides an assessment overview. A number of formats are used in the evaluation of language performance; the choice of a particular one depends on the age of the child and the area(s) of concern. Clinical analysis involves both formal and informal measures. An evaluation of a very young child can include role-playing and symbolic play activities as well as analyses of two-word utterances and the use of auxiliaries and common grammatical structures (Bliss, 1985). Older students are commonly evaluated with sentence repetition formats, which provide evidence of the interaction between short-term memory and syntactic abilities, when highly familiar vocabulary and typical contexts are avoided (Wiig & Semel, 1984).

Current assessment procedures include oral storytelling and narratives from which judgments can be made about children's organization, attention to detail, sense of cause-and-effect relationships, sequencing skills, and goal directiveness. Written expository text is also becoming an eval-

**Table 5-6**

Summary of assessment components.

| Components of Assessment | | |
|---|---|---|
| *Rule Systems* | *Modes* | *Levels* |
| Phonological | Listening | Sound |
| Morphological | Reading | Syllable |
| Syntactic | Speaking | Word |
| Semantic | Writing | Sentence |
| Pragmatic | Thinking | Text |

Adapted from N. W. Nelson, 1986.

uative tool, to measure metalinguistic awareness, cognitive organization, abilities to decenter (audience consideration), and the child's capacity to handle the multiple, simultaneous processes that writing requires (Tomlan, 1986).

## PRACTICAL CONCERNS IN ASSESSMENT

A discussion of speech and language assessment should include a number of practical concerns. Particularly high levels of attention should be given to these factors:

1. The relevance of the assessment process to the identification, description, and analysis of language in the instructional setting. "The language of the classroom" includes the conceptual and linguistic abilities of the child, the content and concepts involved in the task, and the teacher's language of instruction (speaking mode, grammatical complexity, etc.). The relationship between the student's ability and the teacher/curricular expectations can not be discounted. "Many students referred for testing may not have a specific disability; rather, the language interaction in the environment may be disabling" (Gruenewald & Pollak, 1984, p. 7).

2. Consideration that standardized diagnostic tests are generally insensitive to the subtleties of ongoing functional communication. Short, fragmented responses to predetermined test items are not thoroughly indicative of the language skills required for successful interactions with others. To supplement standardized assessment procedures, checklists or observational recording systems should be employed. Figure 5-2 provides a sample check list for observation of classroom communication, adapted from the work of Sanger, Keith and Maher (1987).

3. The contextual factors influencing test administration and performance. What is your purpose in testing? Can you define your goal and choose an appropriate instrument accordingly? Is your purpose to screen, to determine eligibility, to plan an intervention program, to measure progress? To measure individual gain or group gain? (Schery, 1981). Does the test measure what its title proclaims it should? The skill or skills that a specific test evaluates might or might not be reflected in the name of the test. How broad or narrow is the instrument's scope? The competence of test administration goes beyond the recording of pluses and minuses in response to items that are often artificial and irrelevant (Stark, 1981). Again, a background in the nature and disorders of language is a necessity.

4. The need for nonbiased assessment. Nonbiased assessment differs from traditional assessment in one fundamental way: a traditional assessment often depends upon the cultural/linguistic orientation of the service provider, whereas a nonbiased assessment is based primarily upon the cultural/linguistic orientation of the child himself. Evaluators must be in touch with their own attitudes and stereotypical opinions regarding a child's ethnic identity and values, language style, gender, socioeconomic class, and appearance. The development of dialect-sensitive or culture-fair language instruments has not kept pace with the development of testing materials for standard English speakers (Terrell & Terrell, 1983). When they reviewed a number of tests, Adler and Birdsong (1983) found the Daily Language Facility Test, the Denver Articulation Screening Exam (1973), and the Sentence Repetition Task, to be culture-fair.

When nonstandard English usage must be assessed, informal assessment procedures (Leonard & Weiss, 1983), such as the collection of spontaneous speech samples across contexts, might be used. To uncover a student's particular competencies, the evaluator may choose to use purposeful probes, materials, and content appropriate to the child's culture. For an overview of cultural-bias issues in language assessment, the reader is referred to *Topics in Language Disorders* (1983).

| Student behavior | Yes | No |
|---|---|---|
| 1. Inattentive or distracted, especially when background noise is present | — | — |
| 2. Learns better in one-to-one situations | — | — |
| 3. Learning seems to be affected by where the child is seated in relation to the teacher | — | — |
| 4. Has more difficulty learning when two or more speakers participate in conversation | — | — |
| 5. Obvious difficulty learning when there are several distractions | — | — |
| 6. Has trouble picking up new information and may require several repetitions | — | — |
| 7. Has difficulty following multistage commands | — | — |
| 8. Requires additional cues to understand information presented in class (i.e., visual cues to accompany oral information) | — | — |
| 9. Misunderstands what is said, especially if presented at a fast rate | — | — |
| 10. More difficulty understanding teachers when they move around the room than when they are stationary | — | — |
| 11. Frequently requires redundancy such as asking for questions to be repeated | — | — |
| 12. Seems to hold eye contact with the teacher's face/mouth more so than other students | — | — |
| 13. Rarely rehearses information as a strategy for remembering it | — | — |
| 14. Generally unaware of errors and does not seek clarification of information | — | — |
| 15. Does not paraphrase information when having difficulty with understanding | — | — |
| 16. Often gives inappropriate, immediate, or delayed responses | — | — |
| 17. Has difficulty providing complex explanations to questions | — | — |
| 18. Has difficulty recalling sequences of information such as telling a story or talking about an event | — | — |
| 19. Produces intermittent or inconsistent responses to questions or commands | — | — |
| 20. Has difficulty formulating or generating oral expressive language | — | — |
| 21. Has difficulty formulating or generating written expressive language | — | — |

**Figure 5-2**
Checklist for observation of classroom communication. (Adapted from
Sanger, D., Keith, R., and Maher, B. (1987). An assessment technique for
children with auditory-language processing problems. *Journal of
Communication Disorders, 5,* pp. 265–280.)

5. Administering a test according to established criteria does not necessarily result in the surfacing of critical information. To understand a child's language behavior, one must understand the child's method of arriving at an answer. Thus, through analysis of error patterns and open discussion with the student as to how he/she arrived at a given response, we gain valuable diagnostic information.

6. Once assessment has been completed, professional interpretations of a child's performance can require a high degree of interprofessional communication and flexibility. Differing theoretical models across education-related disciplines emphasize different performance components and/or describe similar performances with unique vocabulary. Hopefully, a mechanism is in place that allows the practitioner to become more than casually familiar with the assessment instruments.

## EARLY SCREENING AND IDENTIFICATION

The profession has placed priority on the early identification of language-related deficits. The gap between the language-impaired child and the normal child widens with age. Research indicates that the early language disability is often the seed of later learning and behavioral problems. Thus, assessment issues relative to predictive validity are of paramount importance.

Preschool and kindergarten screening programs incorporate single tests or test batteries as well as teacher rating scales. The aim of any screening device is to produce results such that the total number of impaired children who are not identified is at a minimum. Although it has been estimated that an elementary teacher's observations can predict children who will experience academic failure with 80% accuracy, screening tools add objective data to good pedagogical practice. Among the most familiar screening tools used for language and/or articulation assessment are the Northwestern Syntax Screening Test (1970), the Predictive Screening Test of Articulation (1968), and the Denver Developmental Screening Test (1970).

A number of assessment instruments have been scrutinized for their reliability and validity. One way of evaluating the predictive validity and reliability of any screening test is to inspect the correlation coefficients between select screening tools, and between each screening tool and a diagnostic criterion measure. Perhaps the instrument that enjoys widespread popularity due to financial and time constraints is not the most reliable measure available. A number of recent studies have addressed these issues.

Schetz (1985) evaluated the discriminating potential of the Fluharty Preschool Speech and Language Test (1976) and the Compton Speech and Language Screening Evaluation (1979). The Fluharty is designed to screen youngsters from ages two through six years. It purports to sample vocabulary, articulation, and language (both receptive and expressive) performance. The Compton is designed for children between the ages of three and six years. This instrument addresses areas of articulation and vocabulary, color naming, shape recognition, auditory-visual memory and language; it includes a spontaneous language sample. The accuracy of these two tests was compared in four areas: vocabulary, articulation, language comprehension, and language expression. Of the total number of kindergarten subjects (N = 107), 23 were identified by the Fluharty as being in need of further evaluation, while 29 were identified by the Compton. Both tests identified the same children in only seven instances: two students were similarly identified as being at risk on vocabulary, four students on articulation, and one student for language expression. No subject was identified by both tests as being deficient in language comprehension. When screening was validated through the administration of diagnostic instruments [the Peabody Picture Vocabulary

Test-Revised (1981) and the Goldman-Fristoe Test of Articulation (1969)], scores for the majority of those tested were not low enough to indicate a real problem. Schetz (1985) concluded that the Fluharty overestimated difficulties in language comprehension, while the Compton overestimated difficulties in vocabulary.

Illerbrun, Haines, and Greenough (1985) included five screening instruments and three diagnostic criterion measures in their study with 136 Canadian kindergarten children. The Kindergarten Language Screening Test (1978), the Bankson Language Screening Test—38-Item Short Form (1977), the Fluharty Preschool Speech and Language Screening Test (1978), the Clinical Evaluation of Language Functions—Elementary Screening Test (1980), and the Language Identification Screening Test for Kindergarten (1984) were correlated with collapsed values for the criterion measures, which were the Test of Language Development (1977), the Test for Auditory Comprehension of Language (1973) and the Carrow Elicited Language Inventory (1974). To determine which screening tool provided the most reliable prediction, an intercorrelation analysis showed that the Language Identification Screening Test for Kindergarten, at .85, was the winner. The poorest predictor was the Kindergarten Language Screening Test (.68), and the three remaining tests achieved correlations in the mid- to high-70s. Illerbrun, Haines, and Greenough suggested that test users work toward developing local norms, because published screening test norms are often not directly applicable to either community or regional variations.

## TOOLS FOR ASSESSMENT

The following section reviews selected tools that represent the Bloom and Lahey paradigm of *form-content-use*. These tests were selected according to their degree of current popularity, and offer the reader information as to purpose, administration, and norms. Table 5-7 provides an overview of other tests and subtests that can be used to test various language processes.

**Table 5-7**
Tests of language structures (pp. 158–167).

| Test | Assessment purpose | Age/grade range | Reference |
|---|---|---|---|
| **Tests of language development or general ability** | | | |
| Developmental Potential of Preschool Children | For children with cerebral palsy—focus on receptive and expressive language | 2–4½ yr. | Haeussermann (1958). New York: Grune & Stratton |
| Rating Scale for Evaluation of Expressive, Receptive, and Phonetic Language Development in Young Child | Phonological, receptive, and expressive language development | 4 wk.–6 yr. | D'Asaro & Johns (1961). *Cerebral Palsy Review*, 1961, 22, 3–4 |
| Sequenced Inventory of Communication Developments | Response (includes imitating, initiating, and responding), expressive (includes length, grammatical, and syntactical), and articulation | 9 mo.–4 yr. | (1975). Seattle: University of Washington Press |
| Preschool Language Scale | Auditory comprehension, verbal ability, and articulation | 2–6 yr. | Zimmerman, Steiner, & Evatt (1969). Columbus, Ohio: Merrill |
| Language and Learning Disorders of the Pre-Academic Child | Comprehension of single words, connected discourse, expression of connected discourse, auditory memory for sentences, and various perceptual motor skills | Birth–6 yr. | (1968). Los Angeles. Western Psychological Services |
| Early Childhood Education for Handicapped Children | Language reception, language expression, problem solving, social motor | Birth–3 yr. | Houston Speech & Hearing Center (1972). Houston: University of Texas at Houston |
| Houston Test for Language Development | Accent, melody of speech, gesture, vocabulary, sound articulation, content, grammatical usage, and vocabulary | 6 mo.–6 yr. | Crabtree (1963). Houston: Houston Test Company |
| Cirus | Contains subtest on receptive vocabulary (what words mean) and productive language (say and tell) | Nursery–kindergarten | (1974). Princeton, N.J.: Educational Testing Services |
| Utah Test of Language Development | Repetitions of digits, naming colors and pictures, length of sentences, vocabulary, responding to commands and reading | 1–15 yr. | Mecham, Jex, & Jones (1967). Salt Lake City: Communication Research Associates |
| Illinois Test of Psycholinguistic Abilities | Auditory reception, visual reception, auditory association, visual association, verbal expression, manual expression, grammatical closure, visual closure, auditory sequential memory, visual sequential memory, auditory closure, sound blending | 2 yr. 4 mo.–10 yr. 3 mo. | Kirk, McCarthy, & Kirk (1968). Urbana: University of Illinois Press |

| Test | Description | Age range | Reference |
|---|---|---|---|
| Vane Evaluation of Language Scale | Receptive and expressive language, handedness and attention/memory | 2½–6 yr. | Vane (1975). Clinical Psychology Publishing Co. |
| Test of Language Development | Primary and intermediate levels, assesses understanding and meaningful use of spoken words, including optional articulation subtests. Includes Picture vocabulary, oral vocabulary, grammatical understanding, sentence imitation, and grammatical completion | 4 yr.–8 yr., 11 mo. 8½–12 yr., 11 mo. | Newcomer & Hammill (1988) PRO-ED |
| Detroit Tests of Learning Aptitudes - 2 Word Opposites Sentence Imitation Word Sequences Oral Directions Story Construction | Word-finding, vocabulary grammar usage, memory auditory discrimination, memory simultaneous linguistic/perceptual processing dependent upon memory capacities text organization | 6 yrs.–17 yr. 11 mo. | Hammill (1985) PRO-ED |
| Children's Language Processes Inventory | Cognitive, auditory, speech, visual-motor and language | 3–12 yr. | Hutchinson (1977) Conlyn, Inc. |
| Slingerland Screening Tests for Identifying Children with Specific Language Disabilities | Oral sentence completion, retelling a brief story, word repetition; other more general subtests include visual discrimination, auditory memory | Not standardized | Slingerland, (1970). Cambridge, Mass.: Educators Publishing Service |

### Tests of language form

| Test | Description | Age range | Reference |
|---|---|---|---|
| Goldman- Fristoe-Woodcock Test of Auditory Discrimination | Speech-sound discrimination for consonant-vowel (CV) and CVC combinations; test includes (1) vocabulary, (2) auditory discrimination-quiet (word presented with no background noise, audio-taped items in isolation), and (3) auditory discrimination-noise (audio-taped items in isolation) | 3 yr.–adult | Goldman, Fristoe, & Woodcock (1970). Circle Pines, Minn.: American Guidance Service |
| Fruit Distraction Test | Reading time distractibility score, reading error distractibility score, and number of distractors recalled | 6–13 yr. | Santostefano (1964). *Journal of Clinical Psychology, 20,* 213–218. |
| Wepman Auditory Discrimination Test | Discrimination of pairs of words that are same or different; child must understand *same* and *different* to perform task; phonemes vary among initial, medial, and final positions | 5–8 yr. | Wepman (1958). Chicago: Language Research Associates |

**Table 5-7** *continued*

| Test | Assessment purpose | Age/grade range | Reference |
|---|---|---|---|
| **Tests of language form** *continued* | | | |
| Goldman-Fristoe-Woodcock Auditory Skills Test Battery | Auditory selective attention (listen in presence of noise), auditory discrimination (discriminate between speech sounds), auditory memory (recall sequences of auditory stimuli and content of oral story), and sound-symbol (analyze, blend, read, and spell auditory and visual stimuli) | 3 yr.–adult | Goldman, Fristoe, & Woodcock (1976). Circle Pines, Minn.: American Guidance Service |
| Flowers-Costello Test of Central Auditory Abilities | Auditory discrimination of distorted or deleted words at end of sentence or discrimination of words against semantically competing background (competing messages subtest) | Kindergarten–grade 6 | Flowers, Costello, & Small (1970). Dearborn, Mich.: Perceptual Learning Systems |
| Lindamood Auditory Conceptualization Test-Revised | Auditory processing of aurally presented speech sounds | Preschool + | Lindamood (1979). DLM Teaching Resources |
| Carrow Elicited Language Inventory | Basic sentence construction types and specific grammatical morphemes; based on sentence imitation and error analysis | 3–7 yr., 11 mo. | Carrow (1974). Austin, Tex.: Learning Concepts |
| Developmental Sentence Analysis | Classify presentence phrases (predicate and subject) and grammatical structure found in complete sentences; developmental sentence types & developmental sentence scoring | 2 yr.–6 yr. 11 mo. | Lee (1974). Evanston, Ill.: Northwestern University Press |
| Northwestern Syntax Screening Test | Process, recall syntactical structures of increasing complexity; two subtests, receptive and expressive, each contains 20 semantically and syntactically paired sentences | 3 yr.–7 yr. | Lee (1971). Evanston, Ill.: Northwestern University Press |
| Test for Auditory Comprehension of Language | Oral comprehension with pointing response; assesses vocabulary, morphology and syntax | 3 yr.–6 yr. 11 mo. | Carrow-Woolfolk (1973). Austin, Tex.: Learning Concepts |
| Meeting Street School Screening Test: Follow Directions I and II | Direction I contains prepositions (e.g., behind, between) for child action; Direction II contains more difficult prepositions (e.g. from, to, behind, around) | 5 yr.–7 yr. 5 mo. | Hainsworth & Sigueland (1969). Crippled Children and Adults of Rhode Island, Inc. |

| Test | Description | Ages/Grades | Reference |
|---|---|---|---|
| Picture Story Language Test | Syntax, productivity, abstract-concrete; expressed in terms of total words, total sentences, and words per sentence | 7 yr.–17 yr. | Mykelbust (1965). New York: Grune & Stratton |
| Developmental Sentence Types | Four levels of utterances (from one word to subject-predicate model) | Not standardized | Lee (1966). *Journal of Speech and Hearing Disorders, 31,* 311–330 |
| Test of Early Language Development | Screen form and content of expressive and receptive language | 3 yr.–7 yr. 11 mo. | Hresko, Reid, Hammill (1981) PRO-ED |
| Stanford Diagnostic Reading subtests | | | Karlsen, Madden, & Gardner (1966). New York: Harcourt Brace Jovanovich |
| Auditory Discrimination | Identification of identical sounds in initial, medial, and final position (phoneme identification) | Grades 1–12 | |
| Beginning and Ending Sounds | Mark letters or letter matched with pictorial stimuli | Grades 1–12 | |
| Blending | Sound blending within an auditory visual format | Grades 1–12 | |
| Syllabication | Identify first syllables in visual one-, two-, three-syllable words | Grades 1–12 | |
| Clymer-Barrett Prereading Battery Beginning Sound Subtest | Auditory discrimination of beginning sounds | Kindergarten–grade 1 | Clymer & Barrett (1967). Princeton, N.J.: Personnel Press |
| Ending Sounds in Words Subtest | Auditory discrimination of ending sounds | Grades 1–4 | |
| Roswell-Chall Auditory Blending Test | Auditory blending of sounds into words | Grades 1–4 | Roswell & Chall (1963). New York: Essay Press |
| Illinois Test of Psycholinguistic Abilities Sound Blending Subtest | Synthesize phoneme sequences | 2 yr. 4 mo.–10 yr. 3 mo. | Kirk, McCarthy, & Kirk (1968). Urbana: University of Illinois Press |
| Auditory Closure Subtest | Reconstruct oral words with deleted phonemes (e.g., _aseball) | 2 yr. 4 mo.–10 yr. 3 mo. | |
| Structured Photographic Language Test | Formulation of critical morphophonemic and syntactic structures | 4–8 yr. 11 mo. | Werner & Krescheck (1977). Janelle Publications |
| System Fore: Developmental Language Program | Phonology, morphology, syntax and semantics, Spanish translation for ages 3 to 7 yr. Domain referenced | Birth–10 yr. | Division of Special Education Los Angeles Unified Schools (1972) |
| Berko Experimental Test of Morphology | Use of nonsense words for noun plurals, past tense, singular possessives, plural possessives, derivation, singular of verbs, adjectival inflection, progressive tense, and compounding (e.g., This is a wug. Now there are two _____.) | Not standardized | Berko (1958). *Word, 14,* 150–177. |

161

**Table 5-7** *continued*

| Test | Assessment purpose | Age/grade range | Reference |
|---|---|---|---|
| **Tests of language form** *continued* | | | |
| Grammatic Closure Subtest of the Illinois Test of Psycholinguistic Abilities | Knowledge of regular and irregular noun plurals, noun possessive singular, noun derivation, progressive tense, regular and irregular past tense, past participle, comparative and superlative, adverbs, preposition, and pronouns | 2 yr.–10 yr. 3 mo. | Kirk, McCarthy, & Kirk (1968). Urbana: University of Illinois Press |
| Bankson Language Screening Test | Semantic knowledge, morphological and syntactical rules, perception | 4–7 yr. | Bankson (1977). University Park Press |
| **Tests of language content** | | | |
| Test for Auditory Comprehension of Language | Oral language comprehension without language expression; represents categories by form classes, function words, morphological construction, grammatical categories, oral syntactical structures; syntactical structures of predictive, modification, and comprehension | 3 yr. 11 mo.–6 yr. 11 mo. | Carrow (1973). Austin, Tex.: Learning Concepts |
| Meeting Street School Screening Test: Follow Directions I and II | Direction I contains prepositions (e.g., behind, between) for child action; Direction II contains more difficult prepositions (e.g., from, to, behind, around) | 5 yr.–7 yr. 5 mo. | Hainsworth & Sigueland (1969). Crippled Children and Adults of Rhode Island, Inc. |
| Vocabulary Comprehension Scale | Vocabulary appropriate for school entry; pronouns, words of position, size, quality and quantity | 2–6 yr. | Bangs (1972). Learning Concepts |
| Boehm Test of Basic Concepts | Comprehension of labels for concepts of quantity, number, space, etc. | Kindergarten–grade 2 | Boehm (1970). New York: Psychological Corporation |
| Assessment of Children's Language Comprehension | Vocabulary comprehension and comprehension of critical elements in sequences (e.g., monkey sitting on the fence) | 3 yr.–6 yr. 5 mo. | Foster, Gidden, & Stark (1972). Palo Alto, Calif.: Consulting Psychologists Press |
| Peabody Picture Vocabulary Subtest-Revised | Receptive vocabulary (comprehension of words) | 2 yr.–adult | Dunn (1981). Circle Pines, Minn.: American Guidance Service |

| Test | Age Range | Description | Reference |
|---|---|---|---|
| Irwin-Hammill Abstraction Test | 6–17 yr. | Identify missing item in sequence (e.g., numeral between 3 and 5); identify words that do not belong in category (e.g., cat, dog, horse, house) | Hammill & Irwin (1966). *American Journal of Mental Deficiency, 70,* 866–872 |
| Assessment of Children's Language Comprehension | 3 yr.–6 yr. 11 mo. | Vocabulary comprehension; comprehension of 2-, 3-, and 4-element sentences; pictures with pointing response | Foster, Giddan & Stark (1972). Consulting Psychologists Press |
| Reynell Developmental Language Scales | 1–7 yr. | Verbal comprehension (specifically designed for limited response repertoires) and expressive language | Reynell (1977). Western Psychological Services |
| Auditory Comprehension Test for Sentences | 7–12 yr. | Auditory comprehension across three parameters (length, vocabulary and syntax) using picture stimulus and pointing response. | Shewan (1979). Biolinguistics Clinical Institutes |
| McCarthy Scale of Children's Abilities Conceptual Grouping/Subtest | 2 yr. 6 mo.–8 yr. 6 mo. | Ability to understand verbal instruction on categorizing blocks (instructions on dimensions such as size, form, and color) | McCarthy (1970). New York: Psychological Corporation |
| Stanford-Binet Intelligence Scale Opposite Analogies/Subtest | 2 yr.–adult | Formation of specific verbal opposites to complete analogy (e.g., A debt is a liability; an income is ____) | Terman & Merrill (1960). Boston: Houghton Mifflin |
| Illinois Test of Psycholinguistic Abilities Auditory Association Subtest | 2 yr. 4 mo.–10 yr. 3 mo. | Formation of verbal analogies (e.g., A rabbit is fast; a turtle is ____.) | Kirk, McCarthy, & Kirk (1960). Urbana; University of Illinois Press |
| Wiig-Semel Test of Linguistic Concepts | Grades 1–8 | Comprehension of linguistic relationship (e.g., comparative, passive, temporal, spatial—comparative relationship: Are watermelons bigger than apples?) | Wiig & Semel (1973). *Journal of Speech and Hearing Research, 16,* 627–636 |
| Boston Diagnostic Aphasia Examination | No normative data | Inferred or implied cause-effect relationship from stories | Goodglass & Kaplan (1972). Philadelphia: Lea & Febiger |
| Proverbs Test | Not standardized | Verbal abstraction ability | Gorham (1956). *Psychological Reports, 2,* 1–12 |
| WISC-R Similarities/Subtest of | 6–16 yr. | Verbal identification of likeness between objects, substances, facts, or ideas | Wechsler (1975). New York: Psychological Corporation |
| Botel Reading Inventory Word Opposites/Subtest of | Grade 1–high school | Knowledge of word opposites | Botel (1970). Chicago: Follett |

**Table 5-7** *continued*

| Test | Assessment purpose | Age/grade range | Reference |
|---|---|---|---|
| **Tests of language content** *continued* | | | |
| Gates-McKillop Reading Diagnostic Test Oral Vocabulary/Subtest of | Vocabulary meaning in a sentence-completion task (e.g., A turbine is part of a ____. Choices: stomach, machine) | Grades 2—12 | Gates & McKillop (1962). New York: Teachers College Press |
| Stanford-Binet | | | |
| Proverbs | Describe abstract, generalized meaning | 2 yr.–adult | |
| Differences, Similarities | Similarities and/or differences between two or three things or abstract words | 2 yr.–adult | |
| Verbal Absurdities | Perception and verbal identification of illogical cause-effect relationships | 2 yr.–adult | |
| Finding Reasons | Implied cause-effect relationship | 2 yr.–adult | |
| Opposite Analogies | Formulation of specific verbal opposite to complete analogy (e.g., A debt is a liability; an income is ____.) | 2 yr.–adult | |
| **Tests of language use** | | | |
| Communication Evaluation Chart | Capacity to use receptive and expressive language, motor coordination, visual-motor perceptual skills | Infancy–5 yr. | Anderson, Miles, & Matheny (1963). Cambridge, Mass.: Educators Publishing Service |
| Language and Learning Disorders of the Pre-Academic Child | Comprehension of single words, connected discourse, expression of connected discourse, auditory memory for sentences, and various perceptual motor skills | Birth–6 yr. | (1968). Los Angeles: Western Psychological Services |
| Environmental Language Inventory | Mean length of utterances in play, conversation, and imitation | 2–6 yr. | (1974). Columbus: Nisonger Center, Ohio State University |
| Adaptive Behavior Scale | Contains items on language development | Child–adult | American Association on Mental Deficiency (1975). Washington, D.C. |
| Porch Index of Communicative Ability in Children | Overall, gestural, verbal, graphic, general communication, visual & auditory abilities | 3–10 yr. | Porch (1977). Consulting Psychologists Press |
| Test of Language Competence | Understanding ambiguous sentences, making inferences, recreating sentences and understanding metaphoric expressions | 9 yr.–18 yr. 11 mo. | Wiig & Secord (1985). The Psychological Corp. |

| Test | Age range | Description | Reference |
|---|---|---|---|
| Verbal Language Development Scale | Preschool–15 yr. | Speaking, listening, reading, and writing extension of Vineland Social Maturity Scale | (1971). Circle Pines, Minn.: American Guidance Service |
| Test of Written Language | 7 yr.–18 yr. 11 mo. | Word usage, spelling, style, handwriting, vocabulary and thematic maturity | Hammill & Larsen (1983). PRO-ED |
| Test of Adolescent Language-2 | 12 yr.–18 yr. 5 mo. | Contrasts vocabulary & grammatical abilities across listening, reading, writing and speaking modes | Hammill, Brown, Larsen & Weiderholt (1987). PRO-ED |

**Bilingual/bicultural tests**

| Test | Age range | Description | Reference |
|---|---|---|---|
| Dailey Language Facility Test | 3 yr.–grade 12 | Expressive language (tests consist of a series of pictures that the child describes or tells story about); scores child's ability to conceptualize and communicate in native language (e.g., Spanish) or codes errors from standard English pronunciation | Dailey (1966). Alexandria, Va.: Allington Corporation |
| Bilingual Syntax Measure | 3 yr.–12 yr. | Language dominates with respect to syntactical structure in terms of English as a second language or Spanish as a second language; conversation-type tests | Burt, Dulay, & Chavez (1978). The Psychological Corp. |
| Dos Amigos Verbal Language Scale | 6–10 yr. | English-Spanish dominance measure to assess production of lexical items (words and their opposites) | Cirtchlow (1974). Academic Therapy Publications |
| Basic Inventory of Natural Language | Not standardized | Which language (English or Spanish) child possesses in terms of dominance and dialect; measures include fluency score, level of complexity score, average sentence length | Herbert, Moesser, & Sancho (1974). San Bernardino, Calif.: Chess and Associates |
| Basic Language Competency Battery | Kindergarten–grade 9 | Measure basic language competency for a child learning second language (Spanish & English version); subtests include oral vocabulary, sound perception, sentence structure. | Cervenka (1972). Edward Cervenka, 617 W. 3rd Avenue, New York |
| Home Bilingual Usage Estimate | All ages | Classify child as monolingual, English dominant, apparent bilingual, Spanish dominant, or Spanish monolingual through use of home interview schedule | Skoczylas (1971). Gilroy, Calif.: author |

**Table 5-7** *continued*

| Test | Assessment purpose | Age/grade range | Reference |
|---|---|---|---|
| **Bilingual/bicultural tests** *continued* | | | |
| James Language Dominance Test | Determine language dominance in Mexican-American children | Kindergarten–grade 1 | James (1974). Austin, Tex.: Learning Concepts |
| Language Dominance Index Form | Index to evaluate children's English proficiency (items include listening and reading comprehension, speaking, writing) | Not standardized | Wilson Riles (not copyrighted). Superintendent of Public Instruction, State of California |
| Linguistic Capacity Index | Measure English readiness of children for English language instruction (measure of receptive English language) | Primary grades when natural language is Spanish | Brengelman (1964). Austin, Tex.: Southwest Educational Development Laboratory |
| Mat-Sea-Cal | Oral test to determine ability to (1) produce and understand distinctive characteristics of English, (2) express known cognitive concepts, and (3) perform learning task in English | Kindergarten–grade 4 | Matluck & Matluck (1974). Seattle: Center for Applied Linguistics |
| Oral Language Evaluation | Identify child who needs second language training | Not standardized | Silvaroli & Maynes (1975). Los Angeles: D. A. Lewis Associates |
| Bilingual Oral Language Test | Oral language in Spanish or English | 7–12 yr. | (1978). Bilingual Media Productions, Inc. |
| **Other tests of auditory processing/articulation** | | | |
| Goldman-Fristoe Test of Articulation | Production of all consonant sounds, with the exception of /zh/ for sounds in a word, sounds in sentences, and correct articulation of sounds when provided stimulation. Articulation of consonant sounds | 6–16 yr. | Goldman & Fristoe (1972). American Guidance Service |
| Templin-Darley Tests of Articulation | Articulation of first grade vocabulary using cloze procedures; ability to produce vowels, diphthongs, single consonants (medial, initial, final position), and consonant blends in varying combinations | 3–8 yr. | Templin & Darley (1969). Univ. of Iowa, Educational Research & Service |
| Arizona Articulation Profile | Determination of misarticulation and total articulatory proficiency | 6 yr.–11 yr. 11 mo. | Fudola (1970). Los Angeles: Western Psychological Services |

| Test | Description | Age/Grade | Reference |
|---|---|---|---|
| Dailey Language Facility Test | Ability to use oral language independently of pronunciation (also vocabulary, information, and grammar) | 3 yr.–grade 12 | Dailey (1966). Alexandria, Va.: Allington Corporation |
| Deep Test of Articulation | Assessment of nine frequently misarticulated consonant sounds: /s/, /l/, /b/, /t/, /c/, /s/, /k/, /f/, and /t/ | Not standardized | McDonald (1964). Pittsburgh: Stonery House |
| Edinburgh Articulation Test | Naming of well-known objects to assess consonants and consonant clusters | 3–6 yr. | Ingram, Anthony, Bogle, & McIsaac (1971). Edinburgh, Scotland: Livingstone |
| Predictive Screening Test of Articulation | Separates children who have articulation disorders into two categories: (1) children who will correct their misarticulations and (2) those who require speech therapy | Kindergarten–grade 3 | Van Riper & Erickson (1969). J. Speech Hear. Disord. 34:214–219 |
| Picture Articulation and Language Screening | Elicits sentence responses for picture stimulation for language and articulation performance (e.g., sounds in initial and final positions) | Not standardized; appropriate for grade 1 | Rogers (1970). Salt Lake City: Word Making Productions |
| Fisher-Logemann Test of Articulation Competency | Phonological rules that govern selection of distinctive features in misarticulations | Not standardized | Fisher & Logemann (1971). Boston: Houghton Mifflin |
| English and Spanish Phonemic Unit Production Test | Ability to reproduce English and Spanish phonemic units through sentence repetition | Kindergarten–college | Skoczylas (1972). 2649 Santa Ynez, Gilroy, Calif. |
| Michigan Oral Language Test | Ability to produce standard phonological and grammatical features | Not standardized; focus from kindergarten–grade 3 | Robinett & Benjamin (not copyrighted). Michigan Department of Education |
| Test of Non-Verbal Auditory Discrimination | Tonal patterns assessing discrimination of pitch, loudness, rhythm, duration, and timbre | 6–8 yr. | Buktenica (1968). Nashville, Tenn. |

# SCREENING INSTRUMENTS

### SCREENING TESTS FOR IDENTIFYING CHILDREN WITH SPECIFIC LANGUAGE DISABILITY
(Slingerland, B. H., 1970, Educators Publishing Service, Inc.)

The Slingerland tests presume that failure to achieve adequate progress in acquisition of basic school skills can be the result of learning difficulties characterized by poor use of language, including poor writing and poor spelling, and inadequate performance in certain kinds of perceptual, motor, and visual-motor patterning activities. Therefore, this test is not a test of language as such. Consistent with the underlying educational treatment theory, the tests are intended to provide early identification of potential learning difficulties and to help the teacher determine which sensory channels or modalities are responsible for depressed performance in areas presumed essential to skill acquisition. No data are available on reliability and validity.

### NORTHWESTERN SYNTAX SCREENING TEST (NSST)
(Lee, L., 1971, Northwestern University Press)

The NSST is a screening test for syntactical development but is not an in-depth study of syntax. The NSST tests receptive and expressive grammatical competence. The test consists of two parts, each containing twenty pairs of sentences; each pair uses four pictures. In the first part, the child points to the picture that corresponds to the sentences read by the examiner. In the second part, the child repeats the sentences that indicate the correct pictures. It takes 20 minutes to administer the test.

Interpretation guidelines are available in the manual, but traditionally a child whose score is more than 2 standard deviations below the mean on either the receptive or expressive level is considered in need of further assessment. A perfect raw score would be 40 on each of the two parts of the test. Scores on each part of the test are converted to percentile ranges (90th, 75th, 50th, 25th, and 10th). A score below the 10th percentile is specified for follow-up.

No data on reliability accompany the test, although the NSST claims content validity. Scores have been collected on 344 children between 3 years and 7 years, 11 months of age—164 boys and 180 girls. The subjects represented middle- to upper-middle income families. All families spoke standard American English.

A short version of the NSST has been developed by Ratusnik, Klee, and Ratusnik (1980) in an effort to address the need for adequate norms. This screening version was specifically designed to discriminate normal from linguistically different children. Ratusnik, Klee, and Ratusnik (1980) reported that, when the short form was used, the screening decisions made in 99% of the cases were the same as those made with the original NSST instrument.

### UTAH TEST OF LANGUAGE DEVELOPMENT, REVISED EDITION
(Mecham, M. J., Jex, J. L., and Jones, J. D., 1967, Communications Research Associates, Inc.)

The Utah Test of Language Development is a 51-item instrument for measuring the expressive and receptive language skills of children, 1½ to 4½ years of age. The test takes 30 to 45 minutes to administer. A number of sequencing tasks, such as repeating digits, repeating sentences, and indicating the days of the week, are included, as well as visual-motor tasks in which the cross, square, and diamond are produced. The test provides a score that can be converted to the child's language age. As an attempt to survey childhood expressive and receptive language skills, it does provide a screening device that is as well-suited to this purpose as any test currently available for the preschool level. Test items have "face" validity because they were selected from previously standardized sources. Their age-equivalent scores correlate .98 with age levels in the original tests. Reliability as determined by split-half correlation is high (.94). This edition was standardized on "273 normal white children in Utah"; of this number, only 30 served as the normative population for the 12½- to 14½-year-old group. Language ages have been computed by the plotting of raw scores against age in 2-year intervals. The test is not yet ready for unrestricted use as a diagnostic test.

### AUDITORY CONCEPTUALIZATION TEST (ACT)

(Lindamood, C. H., and Lindamood, P. C., 1971, Teaching Resources Corporation)

This test measures a student's ability to discriminate one speech sound from another and to perceive the number and order of sounds in sequences. Prerequisite concepts for the test are same/different, first / last, numbers 1 to 4, and left to right. Alternate forms are given, and the test is individually administered. Completing the 28 items requires about 10 to 30 minutes, but there is no time limit. The manual states that the ACT is valuable in identifying children who will experience difficulty in reading and spelling, yet it does not support this claim. The authors of the test claim that it is able to predict 55% of the variance among the combined reading and spelling scores at each grade. Correlations with the Wide-Range Achievement Test (WRAT), which was administered at the same time to the norm population, was .73. An alternate forms reliability of .96 was based on a sample of 52 students, kindergarten to grade 12. The test can be administered by any professional, but a background in the international phonetic alphabet or training in phonetic skills is recommended. A training tape provides some standardization of examiner performance. The test was normed on 660 students, kindergarten to grade 12, in the Monterey, California, public schools. A full range of socioeconomic-ethnic groups was represented; teachers selected students that would supply a range of "upper" and "lower" performances.

### GOLDMAN-FRISTOE-WOODCOCK TEST OF AUDITORY DISCRIMINATION (GFW)

(Goldman, R., Fristoe, M., and Woodcock, R. W., 1970, American Guidance Services, Inc.)

The GFW is intended to assess the listener's ability to distinguish speech sounds under conditions of noisy and quiet backgrounds; it is used on children four years of age and up.

Pretraining picture cards are available. A tape recorder is needed for the 7½-minute tape for the two subtests, and earphones are recommended. The test takes 20 to 30 minutes to administer. The GFW is one special-education instrument with reasonably adequate development and research. The manual contains clear directions for administering, scoring, and interpreting the results of the test, as well as a discussion of some problems associated with discrimination testing. Research in analyzing errors can indicate the techniques to be used, as well as the skills needed by the child in auditory training for those with speech and hearing defects. Test-retest reliability was .87 on the quiet subtest and .81 on the noise subtest. Tables of percentiles show how a listener compares with the standard population of a comparable age. Data are given for nine clinical samples, including those with speech and language problems, hearing defects, mental retardation, and learning problems. The test was standardized on a general population sample numbering 745 and ranging from three to eighty-four years of age.

Baran and Gengel (1984) speak to an issue that applies to the GFW series: small differences in raw scores can be reflected as large shifts in percentile rank and age equivalent.

### CARROW ELICITED LANGUAGE INVENTORY (CELI)

(Carrow, E., 1974, Learning Concepts)

The CELI is a set of fifty-two sentences that subjects are asked to imitate. Some sentences are longer than the child's memory, so the child must recode the information in a manner more like that used to code spontaneous speech. The types of errors include substitutions, omissions, additions, transpositions, and reversals. Because complex sentences are excluded, the test is limited to use with children from three to eight years of age. It is not suitable for children with severe misarticulations, severe jargon speech, or echolalia. Subjects are tested individually; their responses are recorded on cassette tape. Instructions are modified for different ages. The test includes a manual, verb protocol sheet, and tapes for administration. The administration time is 45 minutes. The test assigns a numerical error score that quantifies language status. The product-moment correlation coefficient between age and total *error* score was $-0.62$, suggesting that the CELI has concurrent validity. (Performance decreases with chronological age.) The CELI also has congruent validity because the correlation with the Developmental Sentence Scoring (DSS) was $-0.79$. Test-retest reliability (2-week interval) was high, at .98. Interexaminer reliability was also high, at .99. The test was standardized on 475 white children from church and day-care centers of middle socioeconomic level homes in which standard American English was the only language spoken. Children with apparent language disorders were eliminated. The subjects ranged from 3 years to 7 years, 11 months of age. There was no apparent scoring difference between the sexes. Mean scores for total error scores and subcategory scores are presented, as are percentile ranks and standard scores (stanines).

## GENERAL LANGUAGE ABILITY TESTS

### BOEHM TEST OF BASIC CONCEPTS (BTBC)

(Boehm, A. E., 1971 edition, Forms A and B, The Psychological Corporation)

The BTBC measures children's mastery of concepts considered necessary for achievement in the first years of school. The test is read aloud by the teacher and is appropriate for children in kindergarten to grade 2. It takes 15 to 20 minutes to administer the test. The testing materials consist of a manual and a demonstration copy of both test booklets for the teacher, and two test booklets plus a pencil for the child.

This test is intended both as a detector and as an instructional device for use by the classroom teacher. It identifies individual children whose overall level of concept mastery is low and who therefore might need special attention; it also identifies individual concepts with which large numbers of children in a class are not familiar.

Both forms are administered in the same manner. Each of the forms consists of 50 pictorial items arranged in approximate order of increasing difficulty and divided evenly between two booklets; each booklet contains three sample questions followed by twenty-five test questions. The second level (booklet 2) is more difficult than the first level. Each item consists of a set of pictures; the teacher reads a statement aloud that illustrates one of the pictures. The child marks the picture that best illustrates the statement. Test items were selected from relevant curriculum materials and represent concepts basic to the understanding of directions and other oral communications from teachers at the preschool and primary grade level (content validity).

The split-half reliability coefficients for the total score on Form A range from .68 to .90; the corresponding coefficients for the total score on Form B range from .12 to .94. The coefficient of .12 is, of course, quite low. It was obtained for the grade 2, high-socioeconomic-level sample. The BTBC has been presumed applicable for such a group. Tests were standardized on 2647 children in grades from kindergarten to grade 2. Children's socioeconomic status ranged from low to high; the middle socioeconomic status having the highest number of middle-level children were in California, District of Columbia, Florida, Kansas, Missouri, New York, and New Jersey. Raw scores can be converted to percentiles, but this test is more a screening device than a diagnostic test.

### PEABODY PICTURE VOCABULARY TEST-R (PPVT-R)

(Dunn, L. M., 1981, American Guidance Services, Inc.)

The PPVT-R is an untimed individual test of receptive vocabulary that usually takes 10 to 15 minutes to administer; it consists of a booklet with three practice and 175 test plates, each with four numbered pictures. The same booklet is used for form L and form M. The forms differ only in the stimulus words. The answer sheet provides the stimulus word for each item, the correct response number, and space for recording the subject's response; the reverse side contains space for identifying information and recording behavioral observations.

The total score achieved on the test can be converted to any of four types of derived scores: a percentile rank, stanines, an age equivalent (mental age), or a standard deviation score IQ with a mean of 100 and a standard deviation of 15. Percentile ranks and stanines can also be computed by grade level, K through 12. The original form of the test, the PPVT, had been criticized primarily for its inadequate standardization. The PPVT-R's sampling method employed the 1970 U.S. Census information to locate its subjects from different sized communities of varying socioeconomic status and ethnic classification. Norms for ages 2 years, 6 months through 40 years of age are based on a total of 5028 subjects (4200 children and adolescents, 828 adults).

To administer the test, the examiner reads the stimulus word and the subject responds by pointing to, giving the number of, or otherwise indicating the picture best illustrating the word. The examiner, according to the manual, must not spell, define, or even show the word to the subject. Items are arranged in ascending order of difficulty, and subjects respond only to the items between their basal (eight consecutive correct responses) and ceiling (six failures out of eight consecutive responses) scores. Appropriate starting points for different ages are suggested in the manual.

Choong and McMahon (1983) compared age-equivalent scores across the two test versions, for 80 children from 3½ years to 4½ years. Results of a two-tailed t-test analysis established that the mean PPVT age equivalent was higher than the mean PPVT-R beyond the .001 level of statistical significance. The PPVT-R's age equivalents were one to three months higher than students' chronological age; the PPVT's equivalencies were ten to twelve months higher than students' chronological age. Choong and McMahon concluded that confidence in the PPVT-R would be well placed.

## THE FULLERTON LANGUAGE TEST FOR ADOLESCENTS
(Thorum, A. R., 1986, Consulting Psychologists, Inc.)

The purpose of the test is to discriminate between adolescent language-impaired and normal populations. Based on the premise that grammatical skills are largely developed by the age of twelve, this test was standardized on normal students from ages eleven to eighteen. It consists of eight subtests, the majority of which are adaptations of well-recognized language assessment instruments. The subtests provide the means for indepth clinical evaluation; the quality and quantity of information to be gathered is dependent upon the expertise of the examiner. Subtest topics include auditory synthesis, morphological competency, oral commands, convergent production and divergent production (word-finding/retrieval abilities), syllabication, grammatic competence, and idioms. The test requires 35 minutes to administer in toto, and the examiner needs a stop watch and tape recorder for some of the subtests. The number of correct responses is converted to standard deviations from the mean of average students. Items on the subtests were selected for their ability to discriminate between those youngsters who were language-impaired and those who were not. As such, items are presented randomly and do not reflect a developmental or hierarchical ordering. The manual offers an adequate description of interpretation, including suggestions for remediation. The manual reports that test-retest reliability coefficients range from .84 to .96, and internal consistency coefficients from .70 to .85.

## TEST OF ADOLESCENT LANGUAGE (TOAL-2)
(Hammill, D., Brown, V., Larsen, S. and Wiederholt, J., 1987, Pro-Ed)

A revision of the original TOAL, the TOAL-2 provides more items and revised standardization for assessment of students from ages 12 through 18½. As with all Pro-Ed manuals developed within the last 5 years, the TOAL-2 manual fully describes all aspects of rationale, standardization, administration, and scoring. This norm-referenced test contrasts student performance across eight subtests: listening vocabulary and listening grammar, speaking vocabulary and speaking grammar, reading vocabulary and reading grammar, and writing vocabulary and writing grammar. The test allows for comparisons across composite scores (i.e., listening, speaking, vocabulary, grammar, receptive abilities, expressive abilities, etc.), and provides the means by which TOAL-2 standard scores (mean of 10, standard deviation 3) can be converted to NCE scores, T-scores, z-scores, stanines, and an 'adolescent language quotient'. Administration time for the entire battery to language impaired students is usually 2 to 2½ hours. The instrument was standardized on 2628 students, predominantly urban and white. The majority of research on reliability and validity issues has used the original version of the TOAL. The manual reports findings that the TOAL correlated well with the PPVT, the CTBS, the TWS, and the TLC, among others.

### ILLINOIS TEST OF PSYCHOLINGUISTIC ABILITIES (ITPA), REVISED EDITION

(Kirk, S. A., McCarthy, J., and Kirk, W., 1961, 1968, University of Illinois Press)

The ITPA is designed to provide intraindividual assessment and testing for educational purposes through analysis of individual discrepancy in subtest scores. The test can be used with children between 2½ and 10 years of age. The ITPA may be of value for both highly intelligent 9- and 10-year-olds who score off the top in several tests but relatively low in one or two subtests (suggesting the need for remediation in the weak areas), and for educable retarded children of 11 or 12 years of age, for whom it can provide a guide for remedial efforts. Because the emphasis of the ITPA is on differences within the child, the major thrust of the test is the determination of discrepancies in scores for the various psycholinguistic functions. The ITPA is a diagnostic instrument that can be utilized as a major tool on which to base remediation. Time for administration is 45 to 60 minutes.

The ITPA consists of twelve subtests that evaluate the abilities of children in the two major channels of communication—visual-motor and auditory-vocal; in the three types of psycholinguistic processes—receptive, organizing, and expressive; and in the two levels of organization— representational or symbolic and automatic or nonsymbolic. Thus it is possible to determine a child's strength or weakness within a specific channel or process or as a pattern on a particular level.

Scores on the twelve subtests are recorded on the profile of abilities and the summary sheet of the ITPA record form. The raw scores and the table of norms are used to obtain a psycholinguistic age (PLA) and a scaled score (SS) for each subtest. The composite psycholinguistic age, which is from the composite raw score on the ten basic subtests, is a global score indicating an overall index of psycholinguistic abilities and disabilities. Scaled scores of each subtest allow comparisons of a child's performance from test to test to be made; scaled scores can be plotted on a profile of abilities. This profile is helpful in the determination of discrepancies in scores for the various psycholinguistic functions measured, (that is, those items in which the student is particularly strong or weak) and in the development of remedial programs. A psycholinguistic quotient or ratio IQ is also found. Remediation of disabilities indicated by subtests of the ITPA is discussed by Kirk and Kirk (1971).

Hallahan and Cruickshank (1973) have reviewed research on the ITPA, and their conclusions can be summarized by the following two points:

1. Abilities assessed might not correspond with the subtest named; for example, attention and distractibility can account for low subtest performance.
2. Subtests do not test completely distinct areas of ability. Similar psycholinguistic abilities may be tapped over subtests. (The reader is referred to Hammill and Larsen [1974a] and Newcomer and Hammill [1976] for an extensive review.)

Retest reliabilities conducted after a 5- to 6-month interval for three age groups yielded a range from .12 to .86, median .50; the corrected-for-range estimates range from .28 to .90, median .71. Retest correlations for the composite score of the three age groups yielded .83, .70, and .70, respectively. Median reliabilities of the differences among all subtest pairs range from .57 and .88, median .74; the corrected-for-range reliabilities range from .67 to .91, median .81. The ITPA is a difficult battery to administer. The norm group consisted of 962 children of "average" intelligence, from schools with achievements in the "middle range," in middle-class communities, and free from physical handicaps and emotional disturbances. The standardization group, therefore, has a "middle America" bias with minority groups underrepresented.

## TESTS OF SPEECH: ARTICULATION

### GOLDMAN-FRISTOE TEST OF ARTICULATION

(Goldman, R., and Fristoe, M., 1972, American Guidance Services, Inc.)

The Goldman-Fristoe Test of Articulation evaluates the consonant sounds in English at three levels of complexity: sounds in words, sounds in sentences, and stimulability. These subtests enable the tester to observe speech sound production under three conditions: picture naming; imitation of sounds in syllables, words, and sentences; and story repetition. The test kit includes picture cards, fifty response forms, and a manual. The scoring relies on the judgment of the tester. Normative data are based on children three to eight years of age. It takes 10 to 15 minutes to administer the test.

### THE RILEY ARTICULATION AND LANGUAGE TEST (RALT), REVISED

(Riley, G. D., 1966 and 1971, Western Psychological Services)

The RALT is used for rapid screening of children most in need of speech therapy. It is designed for kindergarten through second-grade children. It measures four areas: language

proficiency, intelligibility, articulation function, and language function. Imitation and repetition of words are stressed. The test consists of record booklets, manual, and forms. It takes 3 to 5 minutes to administer.

Raw score credit is given for each response on the articulation subtest, which requires the child to imitate eight words, each of which attempts to elicit one of four phonemes. The language subtest consists of six progressively longer sentence repetition items. A correct response on each of these items requires that "syllables must have stress and intonation resembling the examiner's model." A final portion of the test requires the examiner to rate the child's intelligibility and to identify selected oral communication problems during an unspecified type of conversational sample. This information is from a revision of the original test (1966).

Test-retest method was used for reliability measures, but no figures are given for either edition. Standardization data are based on the original edition and were obtained on 436 kindergarten through second-grade children from middle and low socioeconomic levels. However, the age, geographical, and ethnic data of the standardization groups are unspecified.

### ARIZONA ARTICULATION PROFICIENCY SCALE (AAPS), REVISED

(Fudala, J. B., 1970, Western Psychological Services)

The AAPS is a 154-item scale that measures the child's ability to articulate consonants, consonant clusters, vowels, and diphthongs in single words; it uses picture naming and sentences that are read orally. Fifty-one items test initial and final consonants, 20 items test vowels. The AAPS is to be used only as a screening instrument. The test is easy and takes 10 to 15 minutes to administer. Six scores can be obtained: three regular picture test scores and three optional sentence test scores. The scores represent a percentage of the child's intelligibility. A weighted score is assigned to each phoneme. The weighted value for each error is subtracted from 100% intelligibility, to determine the percentage of the child's intelligibility. Validity is high—.92 when AAPS scores were compared with ratings given by judges as to the intelligibility of speech samples. Test-retest reliability over a one-week interval is .96. Interexaminer reliability of the scale is .99. The test was standardized on 702 children, 3 years to 11 years, 11 months of age, from the Seattle public schools. The socioeconomic status and ethnicity of the population were not specified. The manual contains ranges of test scores associated with various degrees of intelligibility and recommends cutoff ages for the normal acquisition of the phonemes.

## MODELS OF LANGUAGE PROCESSING USED WITH DISORDERED LANGUAGE: WIIG AND SEMEL

Perhaps one of the most comprehensive and practical texts on language assessment and intervention is by Wiig and Semel (1984). Their analysis of the sensory, perceptual, linguistic, and cognitive components necessary to expressive and receptive processes has served to clarify and provide a framework for diagnostic purposes.

Wiig and Semel propose that language evaluation function as a link between language comprehension and language formulation/production. This model attempts to delineate the relationships between the sensory processing, perceptual and linguistic units, and semantic interpretation made during receptive and expressive processes. Their model of task analysis places emphasis upon those cognitive processes involved in the manipulation of information, its storage, and retrieval. Thus, task analysis of test items should consider these aspects:

1. The modality of input
2. The response modality
3. The level of processing required (sensation, syntactic, cognitive-semantic, etc.)
4. The type of sensory integration required (intersensory versus intrasensory)
5. The item formats
6. The item contents

Figures 5-3 and 5-4 demonstrate the expressive and receptive model advanced by these authors.

Within this framework, assessment should be dependent upon the critical evaluation of student performance against criteria based upon logical comparison and previously mastered information. The constructs of identity, similarity, and consistency play a fundamental role in the diagnostic process. Thus, a youngster might be considered at risk should he not understand the inconsistency and lack of logic in the meaning of the prepositional phrase in "Jack placed the large box in the table." Another youngster might not have the ability to critically judge the syntactic inconsistencies of "The mens goes home." Wiig and Semel provide information to the tester on the type of questions to pursue in the investigation of a number of language components. Thus, evaluative exploration into morphological and syntactic abilities can include tasks relative to inflectional and derivational word endings, pronouns (personal, demonstrative, etc.), phrase structure rules, use of negation, interrogatives (Yes/No and Wh- questions), passive constructions, conjoined sentences and relative clauses, and embedding. The evaluation of areas related to semantics can include investigations of a student's abilities to appropriately utilize word meanings, the meaning of components for classification, antonymy, synonymy, spatial relationships, time relationships and figurative language.

### Carrow-Woolfolk and Lynch

The integrative model developed by Carrow-Woolfolk and Lynch (1982) has provided a broad, multidimensional approach. This view of language places equal emphasis across four dimensions: the cognitive, the linguistic, the performance, and the communicative environment. Figure 5-5 demonstrates the various components within each dimension. The two-way arrows indicate reciprocal relationships. The dimension of linguistic knowledge incorporates the code and the rules that make up the task that children must learn so that they can use

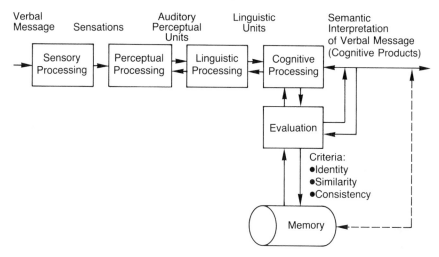

**Figure 5-3**

Relationships between perceptual, linguistic, and cognitive processing in language comprehension. Adapted from Wiig, E., and Semel, E. (1984) *Language assessment and intervention for the learning disabled.* Columbus: Merrill.

language. These invariant rules govern the systematic and structural aspects of the code: the phonological, morphological, syntactic, semantic, and pragmatic components. Each member of a given community learns the same code. The cognitive dimension is the system by which language is learned, the abilities humans must possess so that they can acquire the rules that govern the code and its meaning. This model places particular emphasis on the interactions between perception, memory, concept formation, and representation within the cognitive system, as well as the temporal overlap in their deployment.

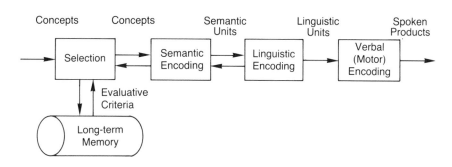

**Figure 5-4**

Relationships between cognitive, linguistic, and expressive aspects in language production. Adapted from Wiig, E., and Semel, E. (1984) *Language assessment and intervention for the learning disabled.* Columbus: Merrill.

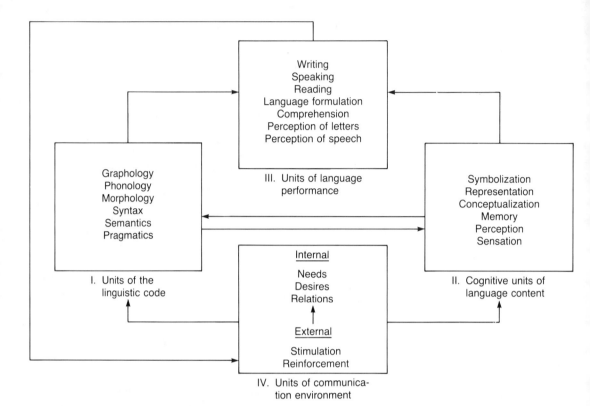

**Figure 5-5**

The four-dimensional model of Carrow-Woolfolk and Lynch.
Carrow-Woolfolk, E., & Lynch, J. (1982) *An integrative approach to language disorders in children.* New York: Grune & Stratton, p. 322.

Cognition is defined as the process by which the world is internalized so that objects and events are grouped, classified, and organized in a manner conducive to efficient memory storage. In turn, this internalization process must allow for ease of access and utilization of stored information, for thinking, acting, communicating and relating. Thus, the development of meaning and the development of language performance are considered to be two separate dimensions of language by Carrow-Woolfolk and Lynch.

The dimension of language performance relates to the behavioral processes that humans learn and use so that they can utilize the code. The integration of performance across systems requires the actualization of processes in sequence. Although we have no direct measure of internal cognitive activity, we do describe and discriminate between the processing stages involved in reading, writing, auditory comprehension, and speaking. These stages are commonly related to neurological processes. Although these are described as discrete, sequential units used for ease of understanding and examination, the performance dimension recognizes their reciprocal, simultaneous nature. The dimension of communicative environment includes both the internal motivations, desires, and needs of the communicative partners and the environmental factors that stimulate language as it emerges. Thus, this dimension respects both the needs for interpersonal communication and the external forces created by the social context, the effects of the child on his/her environment, the effects of the family, and the effects of the culture at large.

A melding of both the Wiig and Semel, and the Carrow-Woolfolk and Lynch approaches, gives the evaluator a complete philosophical framework from which to choose assessment tools, both formal and informal. The former approach provides specific language components for investigation, while the latter provides the awareness of the gestalt—the sociolinguistic considerations inherent to language as communication. An assessment of the quality of language requires equal measure of all domains.

## DISORDERS OF LANGUAGE PROCESSES

The initial diagnosis of a language disorder might be made by a psychologist who has based the diagnosis on a child's IQ test score. The pediatrician might have referred the child for language assessment because of known birth trauma, defects, or developmental delays. The teacher might speak of this child who cannot follow directions, doesn't speak clearly, or doesn't seem to be paying attention in class. Often, parents are concerned because of the lack of school progress, lack of friends, and an instinctive sense that their youngster is growing more frustrated and angry with academics as each year passes. If we're lucky, the child is identified and provided the necessary and appropriate support during elementary school years.

### Prevalence

Speech and language disorders are of multiple types and degrees of severity. Childhood disorders include different forms of speech impediments as well as dysfunctions related to central language abilities. The term *language disorders* umbrellas a number of deficits, from those associated with mental retardation, autism, cerebral palsy, and traumatic aphasia, to disorders associated with cleft palate and hearing impairments. Such disorders are estimated to affect 1.5%–2% of all school-aged children (Wiig & Semel, 1984). Recent work by Beitchman, Nair, Glegg, and Patel (1986) investigated the prevalence of speech/language disorders in Canadian kindergarten children, and found substantially higher percentages.

Beitchman, Nair, Glegg, and Patel (1986) suggest that their study is the first to take a random sample of five-year-old children (N = 1,655), employ a methodologically rigorous approach, and assess both speech production and expressive and receptive language processes. Data were taken from English-speaking, middle-class, predominantly dual-parent kindergarteners living in Ottawa-Carleton. Beitchman, Nair, Glegg, and Patel used a three-stage screening procedure; each stage consisted of a combination of individually administered, standardized tests for language processes (Stage I: Bankson Language Screening, the Screening Test for Auditory Comprehension of Language, the Photo Articulation Test; Stage II: the TOLD, PPVT-R, G-F-W Memory for Content, and Memory for Sequence) and checklists for voice disorders, stuttering, and dysarthria. According to their criteria for identification, the original pool of 1655 children was narrowed to an identified group of 315 youngsters. These 19% (±2.8%) of the original pool were identified as having speech and language disorders; 6.4% were found to have speech disorders in isolation. Of the remaining children, 4.5% had both speech and language disorders, while 8.04% had language disorders only. Thus, the percentage in the "Speech Only" category is a small proportion of the total; those with some type of language problem are the majority of the identified.

### Approaches to Disordered Language

Most theorists and clinicians would agree with Van Kleeck (1984) in her decision to separate approaches to language disorders into three major categories: the medical model, the processing model, and the behavioral-product model. Medical models include all attempts to identify children's disorders with causal and maintaining factors based on anatomical structure or neurological function. Thus, those youngsters determined to have damage to the cleft palate or lip; those with conductive hearing losses; and those with diffuse, global central nervous system damage resulting in mental retardation, would fall under the purview of medical models. For all its value in determining cause, the medical model, in its determination of language intervention goals, does not emphasize the actual language and communication behaviors of the child.

The processing models identify the mental processes that may be causing or contributing to language disorders. There are processing models that relate language disorders to auditory/linguistic processing deficits (e.g., deficits in auditory memory, auditory sequencing, auditory discrimination, etc.), and processing models that relate such disorders to general cognitive deficits (e.g., deficits in information gathering, general symbolic functioning, etc.). The third type, the behavioral product model, emphasizes actual communicative behavior and compares this description with knowledge of normal developmental sequences. The contrast between what is normal and the level of deviance provides information as to what is to be taught.

## The Language-Learning Disabled

Recent research has verified that language difficulties are prevalent among those designated as learning disabled, and that language-learning disabled students may well constitute the largest group of language impaired (Hessler & Kitchen, 1980; Liberman, Moore, & Hutchinson, 1984; Wallach & Leibergott, 1984; Wiig & Semel, 1984). Children with language disorders, reading disabilities, or learning disabilities are not necessarily members of distinct populations (Wallach & Leibergott, 1984). Kamhi and Catts (1986) suggest that these children are best viewed on a continuum or as subgroups of the general category *learning disabled*. "The use of a continuum to differentiate among these chil-

dren seems attractive, but there is some question about which factor should underlie it. The most obvious choice is some measure(s) of language performance" (p. 345).

Parents often are the first to recognize that their child is at risk. Their infant doesn't babble, imitate adult speech, or acquire first words during the expected developmental periods. Their toddler remains at one-word and two-word utterance levels longer than expected. A specific skill or behavior develops that sets this young child apart, and seems to make him or her somehow different from other children of the same age. Early school years bring teachers' comments about this youngster's inability to count in sequence, name the days of the week, or tell the names of items in the same semantic category. This young student is slow to respond and confused, or inattentive and impulsive. The child's speech may be characterized by "cluttering," rapid, jerky spurts of speech, or he or she might seem unnecessarily slow to find the words to say what he means. Certain morphological structures, outside the realm of cultural diversity, are consistently omitted or abused. This youngster develops his own vocabulary: "binglejells" for jinglebells, "buzgetti" for spaghetti, "thumbtoe" for big toe. These words, interpreted in context and reinforced with smiles and chuckles during younger years, linger on, as do other words that indicate reversal difficulties, semantic substitutions, or difficulties in sound discrimination. This youngster doesn't easily adapt to a phonetic approach to reading, or this child might be the student who can decode well but comprehends little of what he or she has read.

As the demands of the classroom become more complex, the language-disordered child becomes easier to identify. Spoken vocabulary is limited. Spoken sentences are not spoken in true sentence form but bear more resemblance to "idea units" or phrases. Ideas are related so as to communicate in context, but there are not the words necessary to allow the message to stand alone. The young adolescent sits quietly at his or her desk, unaware that the temporal and spatial concepts central to prepositions such as *before* and *after* are beyond his or her reach. This teenager finds doing mathematical work the equivalent of learning a foreign language, and words such as *few, many, all except* and *some* represent abstractions that he or she is at a loss to discern. The tasks inherent to writing are overwhelming. The inability to listen, synthesize, and write at the same time affects notetaking. His or her inability to simultaneously generate concepts, recall words, manipulate language, formulate sentences, spell words, and monitor writing processes restricts written performance. This adolescent has difficulty with socialization in high school. One, perhaps two, select friends are preferred to peer group interaction; this child often seeks isolation.

Language-learning disabled persons experience word retrieval problems (Wiig, Lapointe & Semel, 1977), spelling and punctuation difficulties (Gregg, 1982), and syntactic and semantic difficulties (Idol-Maestas, 1980; Kirchner & Skarakis-Doyle, 1983; Wiig, Becker-Redding, & Semel, 1986). These people also have problems in determining appropriate goals and strategies (Strand, 1982; Torgeson, 1979; Wong, 1982; Zakreski, 1982), have memory deficits (Bauer, 1982; Ceci, Ringstrom & Lea, 1981; Kirchner & Klatzky, 1985; Newman & Hagen, 1981) and have difficulty performing mental operations (Maier, 1980). At one time, the assumption was made that mildly handicapped children "outgrew" such "academic" difficulties. Research has shown that the problems of the child become problems of greater or lesser magnitude for the adult. Thus, the adult may experience significant difficulty on the job in which the criteria for employment include the abilities to listen closely, follow directions accurately, and satisfactorily coexist with co-workers. This same adult may experience personal difficulties within his relationships at home—with his wife, his family, and his friends.

## JACKI—A CASE STUDY

This description, of the assessment process utilized with a language-learning–disabled ado-

lescent, is designed to afford the reader a glimpse, from a psycholinguistic/cognitive perspective, of the hierarchical nature of language assessment. The assessment process is described in part; presentation of the whole is not possible within the constraints of this text.

Jacki is of medium build and has blond hair and blue eyes. She is currently a freshman at an in-state, four-year college. Jacki began school in Kansas City, Kansas. Her family relocated to Denver, Colorado, as she was about to attend second grade. Some concerns were shared with her parents as early as grades one and two: the teachers felt that Jacki wasn't developing the necessary word-recognition skills as rapidly as she should be. During the third grade, testing for a reading problem was undertaken. Jacki was placed in a special reading class, and continued to receive support for the next four years, until sixth grade. Her summers were now occupied with math and reading tutorial sessions.

Middle-school years (grades six, seven, and eight) brought some behavioral problems: Jacki began having periodic outbursts and tantrums. This behavior prompted her parents to seek psychological support. Her parents were told that she suffered from an "anger syndrome," a type of biochemical reaction to anger, which resulted in loss of control. She attended behavioral-management therapy (individual, family, and small group) for six months.

Jacki then enrolled in a suburban, parochial high school. Freshman testing showed eighth-grade achievement scores. During her sophomore year, she returned to the psychologist for another two to three months of behavioral therapy, again as a result of behavioral-discipline difficulties at home. Throughout high school she was among the most active students—she was involved in soccer, the campus student association (as an officer), and then acted as representative for her class during her senior year. She was well respected among teachers and peers at school and consistently was voted in or put herself in leadership positions. Throughout her senior year of high school, Jacki also worked part time at a local supermarket.

Jacki's mother and father are professional people; her mother stayed home with Jacki during the early school years. Jacki has two older sisters, one now in college and the other working in management. Until recently, Jacki did not feel close to her parents, but felt very close to her father's mother, an older woman living in another state, who is affectionately referred to as "JoJo." Jacki's parents can recall particulars about her early language development. She seemed to invent words as often as she inverted them: "I gotforit" for *I forgot;* "thumb-toe" for *big toe,* "the day before tomorrow" for *yesterday.* They recall family discussions that became progressively more heated when Jacki seemed to hear only what she wanted to hear. Her father expresses concern about her fragmented lifestyle, her need to be continuously active, her need to be alone, and her vacillating moods, her levels of stress.

Language assessment was initiated at the request of Jacki's English teacher during the first semester of her senior year in high school. The English course was a writing course; entitled "Term Paper," it required that students read various works by a single author and synthesize information as to the author's style across novels. Although Jacki said that she enjoyed writing and considered this course as being pivotal to her education, she had walked out of the class twice in two weeks in tears. When she made the referral, the teacher brought the following sample of Jacki's writing:

> **Loser Takes All** portray a character (Bertram) who endeavors pity from the reader. The reader feels for the character through this characters own pity. Bertram goes to the casinos as his only form of answers in life or source. After having his wife give up on their marriage and his boss ignore him, he dwells on the desperation of some sort of excitement. The portrayal of Bertram's 'hung head' expresses pity from the writer thus the reader. The description of Bertram's hung head is expressed by the writer and interpreted from the reader. The reader reads of a pitiful character, one that indulges in independence but is a failure even at

that. Bertram's failure of independence is seen because he had a desperation for attention, hence pity.

Jacki's writing assignments over the years had always been graded as borderline satisfactory; teachers had added numerous comments on the abuse of sentence fragments. This English teacher believed that Jacki's difficulties warranted special attention.

Jacki's first language assessment was conducted when she had just turned eighteen years of age. Using a diagnostic-prescriptive approach to assessment, the examiner used a number of instruments in the attempt to ascertain her unique profile of strengths and weaknesses. Because the English course required extensive reading, and because Jacki's perception was that her slowness in reading prevented her from performing the tasks required for this course, the evaluation began with a reading test. The Woodcock Reading Mastery Tests (Woodcock, 1973) provided reading achievement scores in grade equivalents: word identification, 12.9; word attack, 6.7; word comprehension, 11.6; passage comprehension, 12.9.

The Test of Adolescent Language-2 (TOAL, 1987) and the Detroit Tests of Learning Aptitude-2 (DTLA-2, 1985) were then administered. The TOAL-2 provides a contrast between vocabulary and grammar skills, across the four academically related skills of listening, speaking, reading, and writing. The DTLA-2 allows the examiner to gather information as to the student's proficiencies across a number of dimensions: language, memory, visual processing, auditory processing, integration, and problem-solving. Each of these tests offers standard score equivalents (mean 10, standard deviation 3) from 1 to 20; scores between 8 and 12 are considered to be within the normal range. The TOAL-2 manual states that "standard scores provide the examiner with an intraindividual comparison of the student's measured abilities, and such scores are the best means of evaluating specific strengths and weaknesses across areas measured" (Hammill, Brown, Larsen & Weiderholt,

1987, p. 34). Jacki's scores on selected subtests ranged from a low of 7 to a high of 15, as shown in Figure 5-6.

With this information, the evaluator could conclude from the TOAL-2 test that Jacki's expressive skills (speaking and writing) are lower than her receptive skills (listening and reading). The examiner could also conclude that the subtest of visual memory and sequencing, the *Letter Sequences* subtest of the DTLA-2, revealed an area for concern. Another area of concern, based on her *Word Opposites* performance, could involve word finding and vocabulary skills.

The problem-solving approach to language assessment requires a higher commitment to the analysis of student responses than simply the accumulation of test scores. Once a particular pattern is discerned, the evaluator pursues indepth analyses of that area of difficulty—its degree of severity and its sphere of influence. The analysis to be shared here is based upon a psycholinguistic orientation; there are different interpretations and approaches to be made of any given set of data.

The subtest items of the DTLA-2 provide many instances for data gathering on language processes. Jacki's subtest scores are shown in Figure 5-7. One subtest was particularly interesting. The *Word Sequences* subtest of the DTLA-2 provides the examiner with a series of unrelated words to be read aloud to the examinee. Jacki had successfully repeated four words in a series. The following sequence then occurred:

*Examiner:*
tub-ball-flag-clock-bird
*Jacki:*
tub-ball-flag-clock-bird

*Examiner:*
pipe-west-fence-coat-mule
*Jacki:*
pipe-fence-bird

*Examiner:*
fish-clock-sun-box-frog
*Jacki:*
fish-clock-sun-box-clog

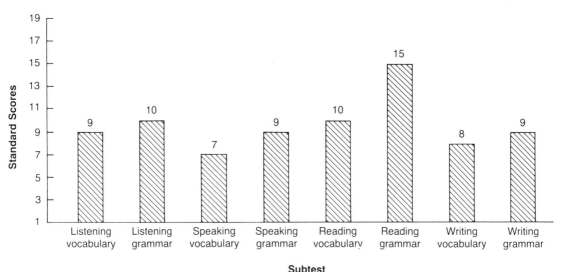

**Figure 5-6**
Jacki's results: Test of Adolescent Language.

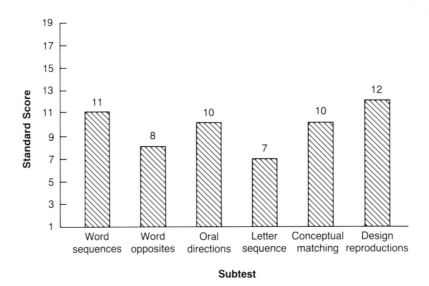

**Figure 5-7**
Jacki's results: Detroit Test of Learning Aptitude.

As the test continued, Jacki made numerous, similar types of errors. The examiner was in a position to make some assumptions as to Jacki's auditory-memory abilities and her propensity to perseverate.

At the conclusion of this particular task, further information was gathered through Jacki's answers of appropriate meta-questions: How did you try to remember these words? Did you listen for the sounds of the words only, or did you try to picture items in your mind? Did you repeat the words to yourself? Which came easier, the words at the beginning of a series or the words at the end? Did you try to create relationships between words to help you remember more of them? Information gathered with administration of the TOAL-2 indicated evidence of vocabulary deficits and a reduced capacity to manipulate language.

On the *Speaking Vocabulary* subtest, Jacki was asked to use each word presented in her own spoken sentence. Her responses are typified by this:

*Excavate:* "They had to excavate the school due to a firedrill."

On the *Writing Vocabulary* subtest, in which Jacki was asked to write each word into a sentence, her incorrect responses included:

*Illustration:* "The illustration I read was about teenage sports."
*Consequences:* "Under the consequences, you will not go out this weekend."
*Solitary:* "The old man loved the solitary of his cabin in the mountains."
*Gaunt:* "People didn't like her because she always would gaunt her riches."

Another subtest within the TOAL-2 is *Written Grammar.* This test requires students to synthesize information into a syntactically correct gestalt. Individual sentences are presented, and the student is asked to formulate one sentence that carries all the propositions of the original. Jacki's responses were typified by:

*Stimulus:* We saw a movie. The one we saw was about a disaster. The earth was dying. It was the earth as we know it.
*Jacki's Written Response:* "We saw a movie, it was about the earth as we know it dying, it was a disaster."

On a superficial level, the response could be corrected for comma overuse, but Jacki's performance demonstrates her difficulties with synthesis of information, syntactic construction, working memory, and self-monitoring of writing processes.

Informal tasks were then employed, to glean further insight and confirm data as to the degree and severity of this student's difficulties. First, the hypothesis of word-finding and vocabulary difficulties required further confirmation. Specific exercises from a workbook on critical thinking, designed for junior-high-school students, were used to assess the nature of Jacki's difficulties. A worksheet requiring the student to recall multiple synonyms for various words resulted in these three responses:

*Workbook Stimulus:* Jacki's Response
*Retain:* step back, hesitate, withdrawal, held back
*Pursue:* attack, initiative, approach, forceful
*Sole:* bottom, surface, one major ("sole purpose")

The semantic associations that Jacki has attached to the stimulus words are clear. Her interpretation of the language she reads and hears, as well as her own use of vocabulary in speaking and writing, reflect an underlying inadequacy to ferret through semantic associations, and to choose the correct word to reflect the exact interpretation she requires. Hence, her access to words representing shades of meaning (comparatives, superlatives, antonyms, and synonyms) is weak.

Again, the description of this evaluation is not complete. It is designed to demonstrate the hierarchical process specific to language assessment, and to offer the reader a sense of the responses typical of a language-learning disabled student. Based upon the information accumulated both formally and informally, an individualized language program was developed for Jacki. This student expected to continue her formal education in college, and this expectation was shared by her family, friends, and her boyfriend. Thus, the goal of intervention was to provide Jacki with explicitly presented metalinquistic skills to improve her written performance. The rationale for using writing as the medium of instruction/intervention included the following tenets: 1. Adequate abilities in written expression are fundamental to post-secondary endeavors, 2. Working with writing as a language expression provides a medium of instruction that bypasses the dependency on working memory and the temporal nature of aural/oral skills; 3. Writing assists the student in decontextualizing and thus readily adapts to use in the development of metalinquistic awareness.

Weekly intervention continued for six months. Jacki did not possess the capacity to self-analyze her language; she talked in phrases and did not use intrinsic self-correction to aid in listener comprehension and clarity, and her writing reflected many of the same characteristics. Thus, information was shared that written sentences are constructed from propositions and that differences exist between deep and surface structure. Using her own written text, we explored the discrepancies between her thought patterns and her written message. To work toward bridging the gap between intent and expression, we tried to achieve better sentence construction and refinement of vocabulary, and explicitly imposed limitations on the number of ideas expressed per sentence. To work on thought organization, we used cognitive webbing techniques as preparations for writing, and showed Jacki how to visually depict her ideas during brainstorm periods. We presented explicit meta-questions that provided her with models from which to formulate her own questions in the future.

Jacki went off to college in August. She carried 15 credits her first semester, lived in a dorm, and experienced much frustration with the curriculum and the environment as she worked toward moderately satisfactory grades. The language demands of a college curriculum far surpassed the demands of high school. The difficulty of the curriculum was aggravated by the distraction of a roommate who believed in continuous noise from TV or stereo.

Jacki was armed with enough information about her particular language difficulties, however, that she was capable of maintaining her own form of problem-solving. She could keep her emotional response to the confusion of the linguistic environment around her under control. She could identify specific words that required difficult or different interpretation as she read assignments. She was able to synthesize information and write her ideas more clearly.

Thus, because she had a framework from which to judge her product, she was able to ask herself those metalinquistic questions so imperative to written text. Her grades for this first semester, all B's except one C, give her a GPA of 2.7. The college she is attending is a college of good reputation and standing, in the community and the state. Jacki's grades are the products of long hours of work and a great deal of determination.

# CHAPTER 6

# Perceptual-Motor Assessment

## OUTLINE

**R**esearch interest in the perceptual-motor assessment of school-aged children has waned somewhat in recent years in education, but not in fields such as neuropsychology. This general waning of interest might be due to the fact that a group of researchers was trained in the 1970s, after the publication of a series of reviews (Hammill, 1972; Hammill & Larson, 1974a, 1974b) that indicated that no educationally significant relationship existed between visual-perceptual or auditory-perceptual skills and reading skills. They also questioned the efficacy of various perceptual training programs in improving reading performance. Kavale's (1981, 1982) meta-analyses of much of the same literature suggest that in fact there is a significant relationship between visual- and auditory-perceptual skills and reading achievement, and between perceptual training programs and improvement in reading for some children. Apparently this publication came after these researchers' "impressionable years," however. At any rate the number of studies of perceptual functioning and its relationship to educational tasks has decreased. A discussion of these studies and others will follow in a separate section.

Despite this sparsity of literature, the literature for studies of infants and young children has increased enormously in recent years. These studies have resulted in major revisions in theories of perceptual development. This chapter will focus on theoretical considerations, the development of perceptual processes, and the assessment of various aspects of visual and auditory perceptual-motor skills.

## THEORETICAL CONSIDERATIONS

### Nativism Versus Empiricism

The study of visual perception has been dominated by two theoretical positions. The nativists viewed perception as entirely genetically determined (Mueller, 1838 [1948], Wertheimer, 1958). The visual process was considered to be a largely passive process in which external stimulation was imposed on the retina; the retinal image was then transmitted to the brain for identification and interpretation. Little attention was given to perceptual development because the nativists maintained that infants perceive their environment in essentially the same way as adults do. However, this hypothesis was inadequate to explain such phenomena as depth perception, because there are no receptors that specifically receive and relay depth perception. Consequently, visual perception cannot be viewed entirely as a passive process.

In contrast, the empiricists considered perception an acquired ability. They viewed the perceptual world of infants as an unpredictable, two-dimensional world of ever-changing patterns; through learning this world becomes increasingly ordered. Operating from an empirical position, Bruner (1957) proposed that perception was unconscious problem solving. However, data from studies of infants indicate that infants do possess perceptual skills that they could not have learned in the traditional sense. Consequently, the empiricist position is also inadequate to explain perception.

Piaget (1967) formulated a hypothesis that draws from both theoretical perspectives. He proposed an innate mechanism that infants use to define basic characteristics of visual stimuli. Through learning and experience, these characteristics are ordered to form basic visual-perceptual concepts.

Also borrowing from both the nativists and the empiricists, Gibson (1966) suggested that there are both passive perceptual organs that receive the form of energy to which they are sensitive, and "active perceptual organs, better called systems, that search out the information in stimulus energy" (p. 20). Perceptual information, then, is obtained from both imposed stimulation and obtained stimulation. *Imposed stimulation* refers to visual inputs that are produced by immediate events that are external to the individual; this is usually referred to as sensation.

*Obtained stimulation* results from the actions of and characteristics of the individual's perceptual system.

## Perceptual-Motor Learning

*Perceptual-motor learning* refers to improvements within the process by which the learner obtains more precise information from stimulation over time. Gibson (1966) stated that "if one considers the senses as perceptual systems, the emphasis on perceptual learning is on the discovery of new stimulus invariants, new properties of the world to which the child's repertory of responses can be applied" (p. 6). *Stimulus invariants* are those relationships between the characteristics of an object or an array, that are constant and critical to object identification or object location in the array (Gibson, 1969; Hochberg, 1964).

Furthermore, Gibson (1969) spoke of three trends in perceptual development. The first was an "increasing specificity of discrimination" (p. 450), which is demonstrated by a decrease in stimulus generalization, reduction of variability, and reduction in discrimination time. The second trend is called "optimization of attention" (p. 456). *Attention* refers specifically to the selective aspects of perception. Gibson cited numerous studies to support the contention that attention becomes "more exploratory and less captive" and that this exploration becomes more systematic with age. She also concluded that as they age, children are increasingly able to focus on information relevant to a task and to actively ignore irrelevant data. The third trend that Gibson suggested as progressing with age and experience is an increasing "economy in the extraction of information from the stimulus" (p. 463) array. Gibson believed that this trend is the result of detection of the distinctive features "by extraction of invariants over time" and by "the processing of larger units of structure" (p. 463). Structure as defined by Gibson referred to the invariant relationships between distinctive features in a stimulus flux, that when considered together constituted a higher-order distinctive feature.

## Perceptual-Motor Disabilities

Conversely, perceptual-motor disabilities are difficulties that occur at some or all points in the processing of stimuli; these disabilities prevent or make more difficult the discovery of constant relationships in the stimulus pattern. The term refers to a wide range of types of difficulties as well as a single difficulty or a plurality of difficulties. Experience suggests that in most problems of educational significance a plurality of difficulties exists.

The disability can be in discrimination. Persons with difficulty in this area may overgeneralize from one stimulus to another; that is, a *b* is said to be a *d* and vice versa. Obviously, the distinctive features of the letters have not been detected. Or a child may discriminate *b* and *d* and be able to attach appropriate labels, but be unable to produce graphically the symbol seen or named.

These are only a few of a virtually infinite combination of difficulties that can be appropriately labeled perceptual-motor disabilities.

In summary, the perceptual-motor process is an active process by which human beings extract information from the environment. Perceptual-motor learning is the means by which the information obtained is made more precise and useful in related situations. If maximum and accurate information from the environment is to be obtained, certain basic abilities must be present and the information-processing mechanism must be functioning efficiently. Disabilities that interfere in this process are referred to as perceptual-motor disabilities.

# PERCEPTUAL-MOTOR DEVELOPMENT

The study of perceptual-motor development in infants has been conducted along lines suggested by the nativistic and empirical theories. However, until the early 1960s study of this problem was limited because the methodology necessary to investigate the perceptual world of infants had not been developed. Even today most scales of infant development contain few basic perceptual items. Instead, they rely heavily on measures of motor accomplishments. The application of classical and operant techniques to the study of infant behavior has resulted in a significant increase in our knowledge of the early development of perception. This information will be presented first in terms of changes in visual preference that occur with age, and then in terms of the perceptual and processing abilities of infants and young children.

## Perceptual-Motor Preferences

In their first months of life, the length of time that infants attend to complex patterns is relatively longer than the time they will attend to stimuli with less complex patterns. They also will attend more to moving objects than to stationary ones. Fantz and Nevis (1967) found pattern to be more compelling than size, color, or reflectance. They concluded that the amount of time that an infant spent in looking at various targets was primarily determined by the characteristics of the stimulus. In contrast, the infant's previous visual experience and similarity of the target to familiar objects were less significant. However, Fantz and Miranda (1975) studied newborn preferences for curved versus straight lines and found that when the patterns formed the outer contour of the stimuli, infants looked longer at curved lines than at straight lines; but when the same stimuli were placed within larger white squares, the infants did not demonstrate a consistent preference. By the time the infant is six months of age, this interest in flat patterns begins to decrease and interest in solid, brightly colored objects increases. Bower (1971) found that even before this time, infants begin to associate such qualities as solidity with the objects they see.

Bower also found that infants 100 days old and younger, in their identification of objects

seen previously, tended to identify objects by their movement rather than by their features. Fantz (1970) also reported an increase in these young infants' attention to moving objects. Lipsitt (1970) and Rovee and Rovee (1969) found that two-month-old infants would not only attend to a mobile but would maintain its movement over 20-minute periods, when the infants controlled the action of the mobile by movement of their arms or legs. When they no longer controlled the movement of the mobile, the infants showed less interest in it and also less movement. These results are consistent with those found by Gibson and Yonas (1968) for a different task with older children (fifteen to thirty-eight months). When these youngsters were given a regular marking pen, they would scribble spontaneously for a time; however, when they were given a marking pen that left no mark, scribbling time was significantly reduced.

Before 1960, theorists in intellectual development generally regarded limb movements as the basic behavior. Visual attention was seen as a secondary result of arm and leg movements. These data from Gibson and Yonas suggested quite the opposite. The visual stimulation was more strongly reinforcing to infants aged to twenty months than was the proprioceptive stimulation that resulted from the motor behavior. Furthermore, the infant's change in interest from flat patterns to moving targets and solid objects is an adaptation made necessary by the child's increasing mobility. Aspects of the environment, such as solid objects, are rich in information important to coping with this new personal characteristic. Although there is something of a gap in the data on perceptual preferences of two- and three-year-old children, the general trend is probably toward stimuli that serve an adaptive function and that include not only highly salient features but also less distinctive characteristics.

More evidence for the importance of visual-perceptual ability, specifically visual-recognition memory, to intellectual functioning is found in a study by Rose and Wallace (1985). They studied the relationship of scores obtained from testing of thirty-five premature infants as they aged. In that sequence of tests, visual-recognition, memory scores were obtained at age six months; scores on the Bayley Scales of Infant Development were taken at ages six, twelve, and twenty-four months; scores on the Stanford-Binet Intelligence Scales were taken at thirty-four and forty months; and scores on the WISC-R were made at six years. Significant relationships were found to begin at twenty-four months. At ages twenty-four months and six years, visual-recognition memory scores made a stronger contribution to intellectual function than did parental education, which was the second best predictor.

## Visual-Perceptual Processing

Visual-perceptual processing abilities develop rapidly in the early years. Infants four to sixty-nine days of age were found to be capable of brightness discrimination (Doris & Cooper, 1966). The threshold level for the discrimination response dropped sharply from four to twenty days of age. Maximum discrimination ability seemed to be reached by about sixty days of age.

Infants' ability to detect the shapes of stationary stimuli has been established for some time (Gibson, Owsley, Walker, & Megaw-Nyce, 1979). Byrne and Horowitz (1984) found that three-month-old infants can discriminate between two geometric shapes moving laterally.

Infants only a few days old have also been found to make adaptive responses, based on visual information, to the approach of objects (Bower, 1971; Bower, Broughton, & Moore, 1970). Ball and Tronick (1971) found that infants two to eleven weeks of age will respond appropriately to symmetrically expanding shadows that visually signify an approaching object. The use of real objects rather than shadows did not modify the response. Further evidence of these infants' ability to discriminate was their lack of response to asymmetrically expanding shadows, which indicated an object that would miss the infant, and to a contracting shadow, which signified an object moving away from the viewer.

Yonas and Pick (1975) and Yonas and co-workers (1977) maintained that, in children less than four months of age, the observed behavior was of a tracking rather than a defensive nature. Bower (1977) indicated that Yonas' results were the result of the mothers' holding the babies; Bower also submitted additional data supporting the theory that the infants' response was a defensive posture in response to an approaching stimulus.

In an ingenious experiment, Aronson and Rosenbloom (1971) found that infants thirty to fifty-five days of age expect a person's voice (auditory stimulus) to emanate from the position in space at which they are seen (visual stimulus). When the person was seen in front and the voice came from the side, the infants expressed consistent and distinct distress.

To determine whether infants up to sixty days of age responded to the characteristics of the real object or to the characteristics of the retinal image, Bower (1966) investigated their perceptions. In the first set of experiments, he found that the infants responded to the actual size of the objects and their actual distance, rather than to the retinal size and retinal distance cues. In the experiments, pictorial cues such as shading and perspective were of little or no value in depth perception. It is important to note that the infants used the actual distance cues long before they were able to "learn" about space from their own motor movements, as empiricists have indicated was necessary.

Instead the data indicated that motion parallax was the major cue to depth and that binocular parallax was the next most important cue to the detection of depth. *Motion parallax* refers to the fact that when the head moves, nearer objects appear to move farther and faster than do distant objects. *Binocular parallax* occurs because a human being's eyes are set apart, and consequently, each eye obtains a slightly different view of the same object. This discrepancy is a cue to depth perception in adults and to some degree in children.

In a second set of experiments, Bower (1966) found that the infants also responded to the true shape of the object rather than to the retinal image, and that although they could discriminate objects' orientations when the task involved both shape and orientation, they focused their attention on shape rather than orientation.

The studies cited in this section indicate that infants and very young children are capable of making fine visual discriminations on a variety of dimensions. The ability to discriminate variations in size, shape, depth, and orientation appeared to be functional and not dependent entirely on a momentary retinal image. The ability to discriminate on these various dimensions continues to improve until about seven years of age (Kubzansky, Rebelsky, & Dorman, 1971; Maslow, Frostig, Lefever, & Whittlesey, 1964).

A child's visual perception undoubtedly improves not only in accuracy of discrimination, but also in the perception of increasingly complex relationships between the basic elements of perception, such as size, shape, depth, and orientation (Ruff, 1980). This conclusion is supported by Bower's (1966) finding that when infants had the opportunity to respond to a stimulus incorporating both shape and orientation, they consistently responded to the shape and ignored the orientation of the object, despite the fact that, as further experimentation indicated, they could discriminate the orientation of the objects. These infants seemed unable to perceive both shape and orientation at the same time even though they could discriminate each component separately. Perhaps the infants were simply unable to process two stimulus characteristics at the same time or they were unable to inhibit their attending response to the dominant cue. Both attention and inhibition undoubtedly play a role in the solution of more complex

perceptual problems such as distinguishing figure from ground.

In a more complex study of three- to-five-year-olds' ability to simultaneously perceive part-whole aspects of a picture, Prather and Bacon (1986) found that the children often named both part and whole features of simple pictures, but were significantly less likely to name both aspects of difficult pictures. They concluded that studies that do not require subjects to identify both parts and wholes (Carey & Diamond, 1977; Smith, 1979) and report that the children named only the whole figure, are methodologically flawed. The results of these studies might reflect the children's deficits in language skills rather than in their ability to perceive both part and whole aspects in the same picture.

There is considerable evidence that the ability to process complex graphic symbols is present at three years of age and continues to develop until approximately nine years of age. For example, normative data (Maslow, Frostig, Lefever, & Whittlesey, 1964) from a 1963 standardization sample of the Marianne Frostig Developmental Test of Visual Perception (Frostig, Lefever, & Whittlesey, 1966) indicated that visual-motor processing of geometric shapes improves rapidly from three to seven years of age. Keogh (1969) studied the copying errors made by British children five to nine years of age who were reproducing the figures on the Bender Visual-Motor Gestalt Test (Bender, 1938). She found rotation errors in more than 85% of the drawings of five-year-olds; the percentage dropped to 30% for nine-year-olds (see Figure 6-1). Integration errors (improper location of subparts of the design) decreased from approximately 70% at five years of age to 10% at nine years of age. Errors of truncation (reduction in number of units in the design) did not occur in the drawings of children older than seven years of age. Workovers and erasures increased with age. These behaviors are probably not seen as corrections of errors by the child but rather are attempts to reduce the apparent discrepancy

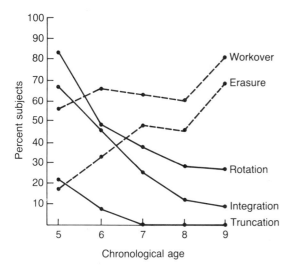

**Figure 6-1**
Developmental copying errors on the Bender Visual-Motor Gestalt Test. (Based on material from Keogh, B. K. The Bender Gestalt with children: Research implications. *Journal of Special Education,* 1969, 3(1), 17.)

between the standard designs and the copied designs.

Gibson, Gibson, Pick, and Osser (1962) studied the development of discrimination of letter-like forms, in a task that did not require graphic production. The real letters and their letter-like transformations are shown in Figure 6-2. Children four to eight years of age were required to select, among twelve letter-like designs, the one that exactly matched a standard design. Errors were classified according to type of transformation. Regardless of the type of transformation, there was a decrease in the number of errors across the age span (Figure 6-3). However, the rate of decrease was considerably different. Relatively few break and close errors were made even at four years of age, and the number of errors decreased over time. This transformation, which is critical to the discrimination of designs, develops very early. Errors in discrimination of line and curve transformations, which are im-

portant to letter differentiation, were quite high at four years of age and very low at eight years of age. Rotational and reversal transformational errors were also high at four years of age but declined to almost zero by eight years of age. However, this transformation is not critical to the identification of all letters. Indeed, some letters are rotations or reversals of other letters. For example, *b* is a 180-degree horizontal rotation of *d* and a 180-degree vertical rotation of *p*. Rotational errors in reading and writing are perhaps the characteristics most often cited by teachers and psychologists as indicative of a problem in visual perception.

However, the data in Figure 6-3 indicate that the age at which these errors occur makes the difference between an age-appropriate performance and a visual-motor perceptual problem. For example, errors in discrimination of line and curve transformations would be expected in a kindergarten youngster, but if a child in grade three consistently made such errors, a perceptual-motor problem would be suspected.

In a longitudinal study designed to assess a set of tasks' effectiveness in predicting achievement in reading and arithmetic, Stevenson, Parker, Wilkinson, Hegion, and Fish (1976) found that a modification of the transformations of Gibson and co-workers (1962), given before kindergarten, was one of the better predictive measures of arithmetic achievement in grade three. Stevenson and co-workers concluded that the measure's predictability lay in the fact that the task required the student to engage in analysis and abstraction. This provides an example of the ways in which a diagnostician can use a developmental task as an aid in assessment. What would not be expected is that a task involving letter transformations would predict arithmetic achievement three years hence.

In summary, developmental data indicate that infants prefer patterned to nonpatterned stimuli and that they are able to respond to the actual size, shape, and orientation of objects (even when they are moving) rather than to the retinal

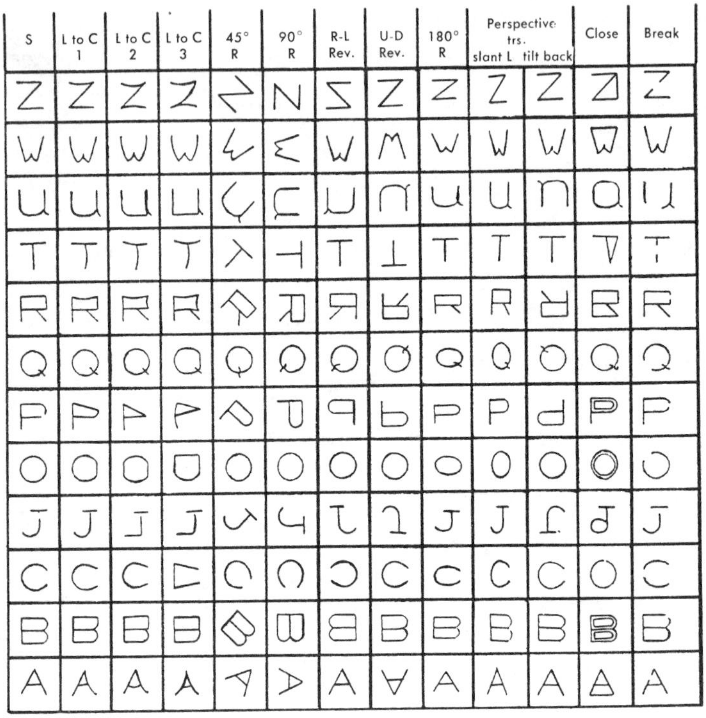

**Figure 6-2**

Real letter standards and their transformations. (From Gibson, E. J., Gibson, J. J., Pick, A. D., and Osser, H. A developmental study of letter-like forms. *Journal of Comparative and Physiological Psychology,* 1962, *55,* 897–906. Copyright 1962 by the American Psychological Association. Reprinted by permission.)

| S | L to C 1 | L to C 2 | L to C 3 | 45° R | 90° R | R-L Rev. | U-D Rev. | 180° R | Perspective trs. slant L / tilt back | Close | Break |
|---|---|---|---|---|---|---|---|---|---|---|---|

image of such objects. Furthermore, they are able to make fine discriminations along these dimensions and are aware of the positions of objects in space. However, infants are probably not able to simultaneously process the multiple, visual characteristics of objects or to perceive the relationships among the basic features of objects. Despite considerable gaps in research data, the development of visual preferences and processing capability is seen to tend generally toward increasingly complex stimuli that have adaptive significance for the child. At about three years of age, children become interested in pictures, drawing, scribbling, and activities related to reading readiness. Their ability to attend to and discriminate between graphic symbols according to their multiple characteristics probably reaches a broad plateau between seven and nine years of age.

A further problem in the assessment of visual-motor perception is that few of the formal tests in this area were designed to measure the process. In the most commonly used tests, the outcome that is scored is the final product of the total process. For example, when an error is made on the Bender Visual-Motor Gestalt Test, the diagnostician does not know whether the problem is a result of poor discrimination, lack of or inability to use mediators, motor difficulty in producing a copy of the design, or any number of other possibilities.

Another consideration in the use of data from perceptual-motor tests is the determination of the amount of the particular ability or skill being measured that is necessary for competence in reading, spelling, arithmetic, and other academic areas. All the reviewed tests determine the presence of deficit or no deficit on a psychometric basis; that is, persons with academic problems who perform below a given point are said to have a deficit in comparison with their age or educational peers, and it is assumed that

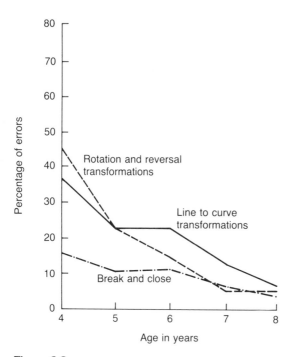

**Figure 6-3**

Developmental error curves for the discrimination of four types of transformation. (From Gibson, E. J., Gibson, J. J., Pick, A. D., and Osser, H. A developmental study of letter-like forms. *Journal of Comparative and Physiological Psychology,* 1962, 55, 897–906. Copyright 1962 by the American Psychological Association. Reprinted by permission.)

the academic problem and the visual-motor deficit are related. The issue is not whether these persons are different from their peers in the assessed area, but whether or not they have the ability or skill needed for them to learn the related academic task. An eleven-year-old boy with word-naming difficulties might score three years below his age on several visual-motor tasks. It seems unlikely that this difficulty is the primary reason that the child is not learning to read, because the great majority of children learn to read with even lower level skills. Unfortunately, research has not addressed the problem of identifying the levels of the various perceptual-motor abilities that are necessary to the satisfactory performance of academic tasks.

## ASSESSMENT OF VISUAL-MOTOR PERCEPTION

Several studies (Bryan 1964; Goins, 1958; Kavale, 1982; Keogh & Smith, 1967; Koppitz, 1964; Watson, 1972) have demonstrated a significant relationship between measures of visual perception and achievement in reading, arithmetic, and spelling. Consequently, the evaluation of visual processing is an important part of the instructional procedure. Some general considerations of assessment will be given in this section. Behaviors that parents and teachers can observe and that are indicative of problems in visual-motor perception will be described. A sample of formal tests will be presented, and research involving the use of the tests will be discussed. However, the diagnostician must realize that visual perception and indeed all aspects of perception are but one component of academic tasks. Numerous studies (de Hirsch, Jansky, & Langford, 1966; Jansky & de Hirsch, 1972; Stevenson, Parker, Wilkinson, Hegion, & Fish, 1976; Stevenson & Newman, 1986) have demonstrated clearly that the prediction of a child's performance in school depends not only on the entire complex of variables that the child brings to the setting, but also on the current parental relationships, the family's socioeconomic status, and school variables.

Before beginning an assessment of visual-motor perception, the diagnostician must determine that the youngster's visual acuity is adequate. If it is not, any visual-perceptual testing should be delayed until the acuity problem is corrected and the child is comfortable with the lens. Following is a brief description of some of the most common screening instruments for visual acuity.

The *Snellen Wall Chart* is the most commonly used and least expensive screening test for visual acuity. The chart evaluates only central visual acuity at a distance of 20 feet. The chart was developed to test preschool children and those who are unable to read. Because of the limited information provided by this test, the diagnostician should be alert to any evidence of visual difficulty during the evaluation. Studies described in the United States Public Health Service Bulletin #2043 (U.S. Department of Health, Education, and Welfare, 1971) indicate that the Snellen chart is a reasonably effective screening test for visual acuity.

The *Keystone Telebinocular,* also a screening instrument, is not designed to give diagnostic data. "Usable binocular vision" is tested at both near and far points. The manual for the test clearly describes the conditions under which referral is made to an optometrist or opthalmologist. A separate set of materials is available for use with preschool children. No statistical data on the reliability or validity of the test are given in the manual. Included is a brief glossary that might be helpful in interpreting the reports of professionals in the area of eye care.

The *Titmus Vision Tester* is used to screen for visual acuity difficulties at near and far points and for phorias—any tendency of the visual axis to deviate from the normal. Like the Telebinocular, special materials are available for use with preschool children.

Data obtained from the assessment of visual perception have two major uses. The first is in achievement of the most efficacious match between the traits of the learner and the methods and materials used in teaching (Ensminger, 1970; Neville, 1970). Unfortunately, most measures of visual processing use geometric shapes rather than alphabetical or numerical symbols, so it is difficult to extrapolate directly from test results to academic programs. The second major use of assessment is in differential diagnosis. When a child is not learning at an appropriate rate, a test of visual perception may be part of the battery administered to determine the area or areas of dysfunction. If a deficit is determined, additional testing can be necessary to obtain all the information necessary for the planning of an educational program.

No single procedure or instrument currently available can be considered to sample all the facets of the visual-motor perceptual process.

Frostig (Maslow, Frostig, Lefever, & Whittlesey, 1964) stated that "it was never believed that these five visual-perceptual abilities were the only ones involved in the total process of visual perception, but they were conceived to be important parts of the process, seemed to have particular relevance to school performance, and were, therefore, studied" (p. 464). Koppitz (1970) has also noted the inadequacy of the Visual-Motor Gestalt Test *alone* to evaluate the whole of visual-motor perceptual functioning.

## Research Studies

This section will review several general studies in perceptual assessment. There are several issues that these researchers address: the existence of meaningful relationships between measures of perceptual factors and school learning (Larsen & Hammill, 1975); the ability of perceptual tests to differentiate between normal and learning-disabled children (Larsen, Rogers, & Sowell, 1976); and the efficacy of perceptual training programs (Hammill, 1972; Hammill & Larsen, 1974a, 1974b).

Larsen and Hammill review several concurrent correlational studies of the relationship between various visual-perceptual factors and reading, arithmetic, and spelling. They reported *median* coefficients ranging from .20 to .30. In studies in which selected tests of visual perception were used as predictors of academic ability, median coefficients ranged from .16 (Visual Sequential Memory—ITPA and Spelling) to .51 (Total Development Test of Visual Perception and Arithmetic). Most of these median coefficients fall within the range of what Guilford (1956) referred to as small but definite relationships, but below the .35 criterion set for significance by Larsen and Hammill.

Larsen, Rogers, and Sowell (1976) concluded that "there seems to be little support for the continued use of these measures as a means of labeling or diagnosing children" (p. 89). However, the Bender Visual-Motor Gestalt Test scores that they reported did significantly ($p < .01$) differentiate between learning-disabled and normal subjects. However, four other measures did not distinguish between the groups.

In his review of several studies, Hammill (1972) concluded that visual-perceptual training did not enhance school learning and questioned whether visual-perceptual processes were trainable. This study has been criticized because of the selection of studies reviewed, the quality of the studies reviewed, and the procedures the reviewers used.

Included in Hammill's review is one study that typifies some of the shortcomings of these studies and suggests why the findings in this area are so variable; it is by Rosen (1966). Of 703 first-grade pupils, one group was randomly assigned to experimental classes in which they received a 29-day adaptation of the Frostig visual-perceptual training programs; the rest of the pupils were in control classes in which they received additional reading instruction. As would be expected for a group of normal children who typically have no need for perceptual training, the scores for the experimental classes were not different from those of the control classes, but the experimental group did show gains in perceptual skills, and the Frostig pre-Perceptual Quotients demonstrated "high predictive validity for reading scores" (p. 985). However, in a post hoc comparison, "50 experimental boys in the low category of pre-perceptual level consistently excelled over a group of 60 comparable perceptual level boys in the control group on mean scores" (pp. 984–985), on the four criterion reading measures. Rosen noted that the differences between scores were small and could represent chance events, but the scores also indicated a reversal of the predominant trend in the rest of the study. One possible explanation for this result is that the critical variable is whether the subjects possess the perceptual skills necessary to learn to read and not whether their perceptual skills are at the level of their age peers. For those pupils who do not possess the prerequisite perceptual skills, perhaps perceptual training is useful as a part of academic instruction.

Kavale (1982) also investigated the role of visual perception and reading achievement. (For a review of these and other studies using meta-analysis and learning-disabled subjects, see Kavale and Forness [1985]). Among the visual-perceptual skills examined in the studies were visual discrimination, visual memory, visual closure, visual spatial relationships, visual-motor integration, visual association, figure-ground discrimination and visual-auditory integration. Reading skills included general reading, reading readiness, word recognition, reading comprehension, vocabulary, and spelling. Kavale found that each perceptual skill was significantly related to reading achievement; however, there were significant differences among the average correlations for the eight visual-perceptual skills. Visual memory and visual discrimination appeared to have a more significant relationship with reading than did the other visual-perceptual skills. Kavale also found that the relationship between visual perceptual skills and reading was independent of IQ.

A recent study (Wade & Kass, 1987) evaluated reading gains in two groups of learning-disabled subjects: Group 1 received three weeks of remediation of component deficits (psychological processes) and then six weeks of academic-deficit remediation; Group 2 received nine weeks of academic-deficit remediation. Using an effect-size analysis (Glass, 1977), the researchers found that scores on the Stanford Diagnostic Reading Test improved after component-deficit remediation only, and that Group 1, who received both types of remediation, gained more than did Group 2, who received only academic-deficit instruction. An important difference between this and the Rosen study is that the component-deficit instruction in this study used academic content, not geometric shapes and drawings of common objects.

Overall, the results of these research studies are clear. First, the relationship of perceptual skills to academic learning is significant, but relatively small. Consequently, programs focused on this one component are unlikely to produce large academic gains. Second, not all handicapped subjects have perceptual-motor problems, and, within the small group that does, there is variety in the aspect of the perceptual-motor process that is involved. Third, perceptual-training programs do not produce academic gains in subjects who have no perceptual difficulties. Subjects with significant perceptual problems will gain only from instructional programs that use academic content and that also deal with the other aspects of their academic difficulties.

Following is a discussion of several standardized tests of visual-motor perception. Unfortunately some of these tests do not meet the primary criteria of the *Standards for Educational and Psychological Testing* (AERA, APA, NCME, 1985). However, we have included in our discussion a number of research studies that should aid diagnosticians in determining the appropriateness of a particular test for their purposes.

### BENDER VISUAL-MOTOR GESTALT TEST (BVMGT)

(Bender, A. L., 1938, American Orthopsychiatric Association Research Monograph)

Bender (1938) developed this test as a means of investigating the applicability of the concepts of Gestalt psychology to the studies of personality and brain injury. The designs used in the test are among those used by Wertheimer (1923) in his studies of perception. Bender (1938) stated that the quality of the reproduction of the designs varies according to the motivational level of the individual and his or her "pathological states either functionally or organically induced" (p. 5). Especially when interpreting the results, the diagnostician must always keep in mind the importance of motivation on performance on the BMVGT.

In the first twenty-five years after its publication, the test was primarily used as a clinical and research instrument with adults. Koppitz (1964) noted that most of the literature concerned exclusively with children was published after 1955. For children, Koppitz (1975) regarded the

BVMGT as a measure of visual-motor integration, with the emphasis on integration.

The BVMGT consists of nine designs. The designs are presented one at a time, and the subject is directed to copy the design as he or she is looking at it. The test is usually administered individually, although Keogh and Smith (1961) have developed a technique for administration to small groups. Siebel, Faust, and Faust (1971) have used similar techniques in grades 1 to 4 with groups of twenty-five to thirty-five children. Individual administration requires approximately 10 minutes; group administration requires about 10 to 35 minutes.

Keogh and Smith have also developed a five-category rating scale for evaluating children's reproductions of the designs on the BVMGT. Other scoring systems include one for adults (Pascal & Suttell, 1964) and one for personality assessment (Hutt, 1977). Watkins developed a scoring system for ages five to fourteen years. However, the scoring system developed by Koppitz (1964, 1975) is the system most widely used at the present time. This system yields age equivalents and percentile scores. Taylor, Kauffman, and Partenio (1984) have questioned whether the Koppitz developmental-scoring system is indeed developmental. In their analyses, the number of errors decreased rapidly between ages five and eight years, and leveled off at ages nine through eleven years. In this latter age group, age accounted for only 3% of the variance in raw scores. Although Koppitz (1975) suggested that the test be considered not developmental for subjects beyond age ten, Taylor, Kauffman, and Partenio's data indicated that the test was not developmental for subjects beyond age eight. Because of these data, users of the Koppitz system and those concerned with research on the test must consider the age of the subjects involved.

*Normative Data.* Using a more representative sample than was used in the 1964 norming study, Koppitz collected new normative data in

1974. Whereas the 1964 sample included only 2% nonwhites, the 1974 norm group included 8.5% black, 1% Oriental, and 4.5% Mexican-American and Puerto Rican. The groups are said to reflect a socioeconomic cross section. The norms for the two sets of data are remarkably similar, except at five years of age; there the mean number of errors is fractionally higher in the 1974 norms. From ten years of age upward, the standard deviations are identical with the means.

Koppitz (1975) reviewed several studies on the clinical validity of the emotional indicators and concluded that the data were supportive. Two new emotional indicators were added in the new volume (Koppitz, 1975). Koppitz cautioned that emotional indicators are only clinical signs from which hypotheses can be developed. The indicators must be evaluated individually against other data. In her first volume, Koppitz identified several neurological indicators. However, in accordance with her review of research, she concluded in the latest volume that a low total score is a better detector of neurological dysfunction than are the neurological indicators identified previously.

*Reliability.* Koppitz (1975) reported studies involving thirty-one interscorer correlations, of which twenty-five were at .89 or better. The lowest was .79. Even though the total interscorer reliability is acceptable, the scoring of rotations has caused difficulty. Consequently, additional instructions were added in the 1975 volume. Test-retest reliability coefficients reported in nine studies (Koppitz, 1975) ranged from .50 to .90 over periods of from one day to eight months. Although these coefficients range from moderate to high, caution must be exercised in the interpretation of individual protocols, as Koppitz urges.

*Validity.* The BVMGT has face validity as a measure of visual-motor integration. In addition, Becker and Sabatino (1973) performed a factor analysis of a number of tests: an IQ test; the Frostig Developmental Test of Visual Perception

(DTVP); a word discrimination test; and the BVMGT. They found that the BVMGT score was heavily weighted on the same factor as that in several parts of the DTVP: subtest 1, Eye-motor Coordination; subtest 5, Spatial Relations; and the Word Discrimination Test.

Testing a sample of ages six through eleven years (with a median age of eight years, eleven months), Wright and DeMers (1982) also found significant relationships between the BVMGT and the Verbal, Performance, and Full Scale IQ scores on the WISC-R. In fact this study revealed that if IQ is a controlled factor, the relationship between the BVMGT and reading and spelling remain significant but low. The correlation with arithmetic was not significant. This finding suggests that the Koppitz developmental scoring system does not account for a significant amount of unique variance in the achievement test scores. Whether this finding is also true of a younger sample, in which the scores are developmental (Taylor, Kauffman, & Partenio, 1984), awaits further research.

Koppitz (1964, 1975) also found statistically significant relationships between BVMGT scores and achievement in reading and arithmetic in grades one through three. The pattern of relationships for both reading and arithmetic was similar. However, the total BVMGT score is more closely related to arithmetic than to reading performance. Becker (1970) found that kindergarten students who perform well on the BVMGT tended to do better on a word discrimination test than those with poor BVMGT performance. Stevenson, Parker, Wilkinson, Hegion, and Fish (1976) did not find significant relationships with reading performances in a prekindergarten sample, but they used only five of the nine figures. However, Smith and Keogh (1962) found significant relationships between BVMGT scores obtained in kindergarten and first-grade reading achievement. A follow-up (Keogh, 1965) of the same group of children at grade three revealed lower and generally nonsignificant relationships between the BVMGT scores and reading and spelling achievement. However, at grade six (Keogh & Smith, 1967), the relationships between the kindergarten BVMGT scores and the achievement scores in reading, spelling, and arithmetic were significantly stronger than the relationships between those achievement scores and BVMGT scores obtained at either grade 3 or grade 6. This study also found that good BVMGT performance was a consistently good predictor of educational achievement but that poor performance was not. In other words, a pupil with a high score would often do well in school, whereas one with a low score might do poor, average, or even excellent work.

Zuelzer and Stedman (1976) studied the relationship of the BVMGT to ethnocultural—Hispanic, black, and white, socioeconomic status, and sex—variables and found significant main effects for ethnicity, sex, and socioeconomic status in a first-grade sample, but this effect disappeared when IQ was added as a covariate.

Several studies have shown moderate (Aylward & Schmidt, 1986; Wright & DeMers, 1982) to high correlations (Breen, Carlson, & Lehman, 1985; Siewert & Breen, 1983) among the BVMGT, Developmental Visual-Motor Integration Test (VMI) (Beery, 1967), and Developmental Visual-Motor Integration Test-Revised (Beery, 1982) (VMI—R). However, both teams of Breen, Carlson and Lehman (1985), and Siewert and Breen (1983), found significant differences in the mean levels of performance of these tests. Although the two tests share some common variance, they are not equivalent.

Using an analysis suggested by Clawson (1962), Schneider and Spivack (1979) found that specific BVMGT signs differentiated between a group of primary and secondary reading-disabled (Rabinovitch, 1959) eight- to ten-year-old children, whereas the developmental scores did not. This is one of very few studies that have attempted such a microanalysis of BVMGT signs, and its results indicate that this approach is worthy of further investigation.

The BVMGT is a valid test of visual-motor integration that can be scored reliably. However,

the score only signals a difficulty; it does not indicate the step in the process at which the difficulty occurred. Unfortunately, test-retest reliability coefficients are marginal, and consequently, interpretations of individual test protocols must be made cautiously. Generally, significant correlations with reading, arithmetic, and IQ scores are obtained.

Watkins (1976) developed the Watkins Bender-Gestalt Scoring System for children from age five to fourteen years. The Watkins system scores forty-two items. Twenty-two of these items are taken from Koppitz (1964, 1975). The other items were developed by the author or drawn from the Pascal and Suttell (1964) scoring system for adults. Standardization was done in forty-two school districts in seven states and included 3355 normal children and 1046 children with learning disabilities. Forty percent of the subjects were from Texas. There were approximately 300 subjects at each age level, 50% boys and 50% girls. Approximately 86% of the subjects were from urban and suburban areas, and 14% were rural. To control socioeconomic status, the researchers' selections of schools were based on the status of the school's neighborhood. Approximately 50% of the group came from low-, 40% from middle-, and 10% from high-level socioeconomic neighborhoods. Anglos made up 80% of the sample, blacks 10%, Mexican-Americans 3%, and other, 2%. Because whole classrooms were used, approximately 1% of the normative sample was mentally retarded. Undoubtedly other handicaps were also included. Although considerable effort was made to obtain a representative sample, the sample cannot be considered truly representative.

*Reliability.* Test-retest reliability was assessed from the normal sample at four different age levels: five, six, eight, and twelve years. The intertest period was approximately one month. For all testing except that at age five, the coefficients were acceptable. A similar study was conducted with the learning-disabled sample.

The reliability coefficients except those at age twelve were lower than the coefficients for the normal group. At ages five and six the coefficients were .66 and .75, respectively. Interrater reliability coefficients were all above .91 for testing at ages six, eight, and twelve. They were considerably lower for the children aged five, because about 10% of the subjects' drawings were unrecognizable.

*Validity.* In a validity study, Watkins (1976) compared the mean number of errors at each age level, of the normal and learning-disabled normative samples. The differences at each age level were significant. The correlation between IQ and the number of errors made by the learning-disabled subjects ranged from $-.11$ to $+.09$; nothing within that range is significant.

Johnston and Lanak (1985) scored the Bender protocols with both the Koppitz and the Watkins scoring systems. Subjects were twenty-five consecutive clients, aged seven through eleven, referred to a neuropsychology service. The scores obtained by the two scoring systems were significantly different; the Watkins system gave the higher scores. The authors concluded that this difference appears "to reflect primarily a difference in terms of level as an artifact of the normative populations, not quality of performance according to the scoring criteria" (p. 378).

### FROSTIG DEVELOPMENTAL TEST OF VISUAL PERCEPTION (DTVP)

(Frostig, M., and others, 1966, Consulting Psychologist Press, Inc.)

The stimulus to develop the DTVP arose from the observation that many children referred to the Marianne Frostig School of Education Therapy had difficulty in processing the visual stimuli necessary for success in school tasks (Maslow, Frostig, Lefever, & Whittlesey, 1964). Analysis of the observations suggested five major areas of difficulty. Frostig's hypothesis was "that each of the five abilities developed relatively independently of the others, and that there should be specific relationships between them and a child's ability to learn and adjust" (p. 464). Each of the five subtests purportedly measures one of these five abilities in children between four and eight years of age. Listed below are the five subtests and the tasks involved in each:

1. *Eye-motor coordination:* The drawing of continuous, straight, curved, or angled lines between boundaries of increasingly narrow width or from point to point
2. *Figure-ground:* The outlining of specific forms against increasingly complex intersecting shapes, and hidden figures
3. *Form constancy:* The recognition and discrimination of certain geometric figures, presented in a variety of sizes, shadings, textures, and positions in space, from other shapes on the page
4. *Position in space:* The discrimination of reversals and rotations of figures presented in a series
5. *Spatial relationships:* The analysis of forms and patterns involving the copying of patterns by linking dots (Frostig, Lefever, and Whittlesey, 1966)

The DTVP can be administered individually or in small groups. Individual administration requires 30 to 40 minutes, and group administration can usually be completed in less than 1 hour.

*Scores.* Three scores can be obtained from the DTVP. A perceptual age score is available for each subtest and for the total test. This score is defined in terms of the performance of the average child in each age group. A scaled score is also available for each subtest. This score is not a standard score, at least not in the traditional sense as those obtained on the WISC-R. Neither Frostig, Lefever, and Whittlesey (1966) nor Maslow, Frostig, Lefever, and Whittlesey, (1964) explained the rationale for their derivation. The rationale is not apparent. Consequently, use of the scale score is not recommended. A perceptual quotient is a deviation score based on the sum of subtest scale scores that have been corrected for age variation. Because the quotient is based on questionable scale scores, it too becomes questionable.

With the exception of the age score, all other derived scores are highly suspect. The test-retest reliability data are undoubtedly affected by the procedures used to derive the scale scores and the perceptual quotient.

Normative data from group administration are available on children between 4 and 8 years of age from California. Approximately 93% of the 1963 standardization sample is assumed to come from middle-class homes, with the remaining 7% from very high- and low-socioeconomic levels. No black children and only a few Mexican-American and Oriental children were included in the sample. Such a limited standardization sample makes interpretation of test results difficult.

*Reliability.* Maslow, Frostig, Lefever, and Whittlesey (1964) report three test-retest reliability studies. Two studies in which the examiners were trained psychologists yielded total test product-moment correlation coefficients ranging from .80 to .98. Subtest coefficients ranged from .42 to .80. In the third study, the persons administering the test were trained in giving the DTVP but were not psychologists or psychometrists. Coefficients for the total test were identical ($r = .69$) for children in kindergarten and grade one. Subtest coefficients ranged from .29 to .74. Because the test-retest interval in these studies was a maximum of three weeks, the total test score reliability would have to be regarded as questionable. Split-half reliabilities for the total test (Maslow, Frostig, Lefever, & Whittlesey, 1964) ranged from .89 at five and six years of age to .78 at eight and nine years of age. Overall, the subtest scores are somewhat lower. Although the total test reliabilities are moderately high at the lower ages, the subtest coefficients are much too low to be used alone for differential diagnosis.

*Validity.* Unfortunately, the only studies provided by Maslow, Frostig, Lefever, and Whittlesey

(1964) deal with construct and predictive validity. They do not provide data that indicate the test is what it claims to be—a test of visual perception. The major source of data on congruent validity is factor analysis.

Many factor analytical studies of the DTVP (Boyd & Randle, 1970; Corach & Powell, 1963; Olson, 1968) have obtained only a single factor rather than the five Frostig hypothesized. These studies have all shared the weakness that no measures other than the DTVP were included in the analysis.

Becker and Sabatino (1973) included, in addition to DTVP, an IQ score, a word discrimination test, and the BVMGT in their factor analysis of test data from children five and six years of age. They obtained three principal components. Factor 1, which accounted for about 65% of the variance, was labeled "visual-motor." The highest loadings were DTVP subtest 1, Eye-motor Coordination; DTVP subtest 5, Spatial Relations; the Word Discrimination Test; and the BVMGT. DTVP subtest 2, Figure-ground Discrimination, and DTVP subtest 3, Form Constancy, constituted the major weightings on Factor 2. This factor accounted for 21% of the total variance. Factor 3 isolated the IQ score, and DTVP subtest 4, Position in Space, accounted for 14% of the total variance. These results indicate that DTVP subtests 1 and 5 measure one factor, subtests 2 and 3 a second, and subtest 4 a third factor. Costello (1976) investigated the factor structure of the DTVP, the Beery Visual-Motor Integration Test, and the BVMGT. Two factors emerged for children in kindergarten and grade one; these were labeled *motor coordination* and *spatial orientation*. At grade two an additional factor, discrimination skills, was obtained. This factor was contributed almost exclusively by the DTVP.

The standardization of the DTVP must be considered inadequate. Except for perceptual age, the other scores are derived in ways that make their use questionable. Total test-retest reliability is marginal, and individual subtest reliabilities are so low as to prohibit their use on an individual basis. Factor analytical studies suggest that the test does measure more than one component of visual perception but does not test the five components that the authors of the test maintain it does.

## DEVELOPMENTAL TEST OF VISUAL-MOTOR INTEGRATION (VMI)

(Beery, K. E., 1982, Follett)

The VMI was the result of an effort, begun in 1961, to develop a test of geometric-form reproduction that (1) included designs appropriate for young children, (2) was well standardized, (3) provided developmental information for individual designs, and (4) was suitable for group administration. The test was first published in 1967 from norms collected in 1964. It was renormed in 1981.

Taking the VMI, children aged two years, nine months through nineteen years, eight months are required to copy geometric figures such as a square, horizontal and vertical diamonds, and a cube, into spaces directly below the standard figures. In the test booklet, the twenty-four figures are placed three per page, in order of increasing difficulty. Testing is terminated when the subject fails to reproduce satisfactorily three consecutive drawings.

The most recent norms provide age-equivalent scores, percentiles, and standard scores, with a mean of 10 and standard deviation of 3. Subjects in the standardization sample included 3090 females and males from urban, suburban, and rural areas. The total sample included 48.7% females and 51.33% males; however breakdowns by sex are not given for each age group. Also, the distribution of subjects across the age groups is very uneven: there are as few as 28 subjects for ages twelve years, nine months through twelve years, eleven months and as many as 116 at six years through six years, two months.

The sample was stratified by net family income and ethnicity; however, no indication of the geographic distribution is given. The author makes no claim that the stratification matches U. S. Census figures. No sex differences were found in the 1981 norming. Consequently, only one set of norms is given for each design.

*Reliability and Validity.* The revised manual for the VMI does not include a single study of reliability or validity study using the new norms. However, Siewert and Breen (1983) compared the VMI, VMI-R and Bender Visual-Motor Gestalt Test: Koppitz (1975) scoring system. Subjects ($n = 111$) were randomly selected from regular education classes, kindergarten through grade three. The researchers found that both the VMI and VMI-R scores were significantly lower than those yielded by the Bender, although the correlations with the Bender were .72 and .70, respectively. VMI and VMI-R scores were highly and significantly correlated ($r = .99$); this correlation indicates that the normative data are very similar. When chronological age was compared with the age-equivalent scores, the Bender score was significantly higher; the VMI and VMI-R scores were not significantly higher.

In a study of forty-four learning-disabled subjects aged seven years through eleven years, nine months, Breen, Carlson, and Lehman (1985) examined the relationships between the VMI-R and VMI, WISC-R, and Bender. Despite the fact that correlations between the three visual-perceptual measures (.75 to .99) are high and significant (especially between the VMI and VMI-R, where $r = .99$), the VMI and VMI-R age-equivalent scores are significantly lower than the Bender age equivalents. All visual-perceptual age equivalents were significantly related to the Performance IQ of the WISC-R.

Aylward and Schmidt (1986) examined the relationships between the VMI-R, the Bender (scored by the Koppitz [1964] system) and the Geometric Design subtest of the WPPSI, in a sample of 103 five-year-olds. Interscorer reliabilities for all three tests by three scorers ranged from .80 to .94. Correlations between the VMI-R and WPPSI Geometric Design scores were highest, although all correlations were significant. The scores of all three tests were significantly related to WPPSI IQs. Subjects were divided into two groups, those with IQs above 120 and those with IQs below 120. The VMI-R correlation with the average-IQ group was significant, but the correlation with the superior group was not. Aylward and Schmidt did not find any significant sex differences.

These data suggest that the VMI-R is equivalent to the VMI. Interrater reliability appears to be satisfactory. No studies evaluating test-retest reliability were located by a review of the literature and none were included in the manual for the revised norms. Although the VMI-R is significantly related to other tests of visual-motor perception, age-equivalent scores for the VMI-R tend to be lower than those of other tests. Consequently, these tests should not be considered equivalent.

### MOTOR-FREE VISUAL PERCEPTION TEST (MVPT)
(Colarusso, R., and Hammill, D. D., 1972, Academic Therapy Publications)

This test is based on the premise that perception is not a unitary process. Bortner and Birch (1960) and Birch and Walker (1966) believe that perception has at least two components. They regard perceptual ability as the input component (that is, the ability to see a design as it really is) and perceptual-motor ability as the integration and execution component. Friedrich, Fuller, and Hawkins (1969) also investigated the concept of perception as a unitary process and concluded from their data that it was not. Interestingly, none of these references, which occurred at least three years before publication of the MVPT, is included in the reference list for that test manual. Similarly, Zach and Kaufman (1972) questioned the adequacy of the perceptual-deficit hypothesis. In regard to BVMGT performance they asked, "Does the child who fails the task do so because he lacks the motor development for copying it, because he cannot discriminate the form or because he

is unable to integrate these two responses?" (p. 352).

The MVPT was designed to measure five types of visual perceptual ability that Colarusso and Hammill (1972) contended were "the most prominent theoretical constructs of visual perception reported in the current literature" (p. 8). The five types are spatial relationships, visual discrimination, figure-ground, visual closure, and visual memory.

The MVPT contains thirty-six items distributed across the hypothesized five types of visual perception. The authors stated that the test is useful for "screening, diagnostic and research purposes." The test takes about ten minutes to administer. The test uses two types of item formats. One requires the subject to match a given stimulus with one of four alternatives; and in the other, the task is to select the one of four alternatives that is different.

Friedrich, Fuller, and Hawkins (1969) questioned the use of a multiple-choice format as a means of investigating an input problem. They argued that the fact that a subject successfully selected the standard figure was not adequate evidence that no perceptual difficulty existed. "If a subject with a perceptual input problem perceives the stimulus design to be rotated $X$ degrees in a certain direction, the exact duplicate of the stimulus design will be perceived likewise" (p. 932).

The test was standardized on an unselected sample of 881 normal children from four through eight years of age, from thirty-two states. Subjects came from all nine geographical divisions used by the United States Census Bureau (1967), except the Mountain Division 8. Heaviest representation was in the East North Central Division 4; all five states were represented. According to the test manual (Colarusso & Hammill, 1972), the sample included children from "all races, economic levels, and residential areas (urban, suburban, rural)" (p. 13). However, no specific data or definition of these terms, numbers included in each group, or the representativeness of these numbers is provided.

*Reliability.* Three types of reliability are reported for each age group and for the total sample. Test-retest reliabilities ranged from .77 at four years of age to .83 at six years of age; the time interval was twenty days. Sample sizes at the various ages ranged from 20 to 45; the total sample was 162.

Split-half and Kuder-Richardson formula 20 reliabilities were calculated for the entire standardization group. All split-half coefficients were in excess of .80, the criterion regarded as evidence of adequate reliability. Kuder-Richardson reliabilities ranged from .71 for subjects four years of age to .86 for the total sample. Because two of the three measures of reliability for four-year-olds were below .80 and because the sample for this age group was comparatively small ($N = 53$ in the norm group), their scores should be interpreted with considerable caution.

*Validity.* Studies of content validity are based entirely on the fact that the items represent five areas of visual perception. No data are presented that indicate whether these factors do actually exist as separate factors.

Three types of construct validity are given by the manual. Age differentiation was determined by use of an analysis of variance procedure on the scores of forty randomly selected subjects, from five through seven years of age. Although the analysis yielded a significant F ratio, no trend analysis or even means and standard deviations were provided to indicate the points at which the differences occurred.

Correlations with other tests of visual perception, intelligence, readiness, and achievement were given as further evidence of construct validity (Table 6-1). All correlations with the DTVP exceed .38. However, this lowest correlation involves the subtest with the least amount of motor involvement, and the subtest with the highest correlation (.60) requires the outlining of forms. This finding must be interpreted in light of the DTVP's exceedingly low subtest reliabilities.

Another finding of interest, consistent with data from other visual perceptual tests, is that the highest correlations with the Metropolitan Readiness Test and the Stanford Achievement Tests (Primary) are with the Numbers and Arithmetic subtests. Correlations of reading are variable across tests, but correlations with all subtests of the Durrell Analysis of Reading Difficulties exceed .33 and are significant ($p = .01$). Relationships with measures of intelligence are relatively low but significant ($p = .05$).

Several studies contribute to an understanding of the test. Newcomer and Hammill (1973) studied the performances of motor-impaired children on the DTVP, BVMGT, and MVPT. They found, as expected, that perceptual ages from tests involving motor components were considerably below the children's chronological ages, whereas the MVPT's perceptual ages were overall within two or three months of chronological age.

In an attempt to sort out the components of a visual-motor integration deficit, Hudgins (1977) administered the MVPT, to assess perception, and the Southern California Motor Accuracy Test (Ayres, 1964), to assess motor difficulties. The tests were administered to 104 children, six and seven years of age, who had scored more than one standard deviation below the mean on the BVMGT. She found that 15.4% of the subjects did not demonstrate difficulties in either visual perception or motor accuracy, 16.5% showed a motor disability only, 26.9% demonstrated a visual perception difficulty only, and 41.3% demonstrated disabilities in both visual perception and motor performance. Hudgins concluded that the results support the hypothesis that the visual, motor, and integrative components in a visual-motor integration task are semiautonomous.

Harber (1979) investigated the relationship of the visual-closure items of the MVPT and the Visual Closure subtest of the ITPA (Kirk, McCarthy, & Kirk, 1968). Normal second graders and learning-disabled students of comparable age were tested. There are several differences between the items on the two tests. The MVPT items are untimed, multiple-choice items; the

**Table 6-1**

Correlations between the MVPT and other tests.

| Test | Ss Description | Ss Location | N | r | Level of Significance |
|------|----------------|-------------|---|---|----------------------|
| Frostig Test (DTVP) | Biracial, urban-suburban, | Chester, Pa. | 107 | | |
| Eye-Motor Coordination | low to middle class | Coatesville, Pa. | | 0.57 | 0.01 |
| Figure-Ground | | | | 0.49 | 0.01 |
| Form Constancy | | | | 0.60 | 0.01 |
| Position in Space | | | | 0.38 | 0.01 |
| Spatial Relationships | | | | 0.59 | 0.01 |
| Total score | | | | 0.73 | 0.01 |
| Stanford Achievement Tests (Primary) | Same as above | Chester, Pa. | 42 | | |
| Word Reading | | | | 0.20 | NS* |
| Word Study Skills | | | | 0.37 | 0.05 |
| Vocabulary | | | | 0.23 | NS |
| Paragraph Meaning | | | | 0.03 | NS |
| Arithmetic | | | | 0.42 | 0.01 |
| Durrell Analysis of Reading Difficulties | Same as above | Philadelphia, Pa. | 63 | | |
| Oral Reading | | | | 0.38 | 0.01 |
| Silent Reading | | | | 0.33 | 0.01 |
| Flash Words | | | | 0.42 | 0.01 |
| Word Analysis | | | | 0.41 | 0.01 |
| Spelling | | | | 0.38 | 0.01 |
| Handwriting | | | | 0.46 | 0.01 |
| Number of Words Called | | | | 0.44 | 0.01 |
| Comprehension | | | | 0.41 | 0.01 |
| Slosson Intelligence Test | Same as above | Philadelphia, Pa. | 63 | 0.31 | 0.05 |
| Pintner-Cunningham Primary Test | Same as above | Chester, Pa. | 42 | 0.32 | 0.05 |

Adapted from Colarusso, R. P., & Hammill, D. D. *MVPT, Motor-Free Visual Perception Test Manual,* Novato, California: Academic Therapy Publication, 1972.
*NS = Not significant.

child is shown a complete geometric figure and asked to point to the one of four incomplete figures that would, if completed, match the original geometric shape. On the ITPA the child points to hidden common objects in a complex array; the test is timed. Harber found a moderate correlation of .41 for the administration to normal subjects, and one of .43 for the administration to learning-disabled subjects. These correlations indicate that although the tests have some commonality, a good deal of the variance was unaccounted for.

Sexton (1977) studied auditory and visual perception, sex, and academic aptitude as predictors of achievement in first-grade children. The strongest association was between the MVPT and language achievement; there was also a relationship, to a lesser extent, to mathematics as measured by the Science Research Associates Achievement Series. Sexton stated that, "Visual perception added significantly to prediction of achievement beyond that which is already known through knowledge of the subjects' sex and academic aptitude score" (p. 6162A).

The MVPT has a solid theoretical base. Standardization information is somewhat lacking, although overall it is adequate. The test is reliable except perhaps in applications to children four years of age. Combining material from the literature with data in the manual, one would conclude that the test is valid.

**REVISED VISUAL RETENTION TEST (RVRT)**

(Benton, A. L., 1974, Psychological Corporation)

According to Benton (1974) the instrument is "designed to assess visual perception, visual memory, and visuoconstructive abilities" (p. 1). Despite this rather general description, the interpretive information focused on discriminating normal persons from brain-disordered individuals. Four modes of administration, A to D, are provided. However, only mode A will be discussed here because it is the one mode that has norms for children. Even though norms are not available in the other modes, Benton (1974) discusses their use with children. The norms provided for mode A are for children eight through fourteen years of age, grouped according to IQ (below 70, 70–109, above 109). Brook (1975) found that neither the number-correct nor the errors scores of forty-one subjects, seven through seventeen years of age, seen in a midwestern child guidance center, differed from those in the original standardization.

In mode A each design is exposed for ten seconds, and the subject is asked to reproduce the design from memory. There are ten designs in each of three forms, C, D, and E. The first two designs are single figures. The other designs are each made up of three geometric figures—two relatively large, central figures and a third, smaller figure located either to the right or the left of the other figures. Mode A takes about 5 minutes to administer. The scoring system is fairly complex, but clear instructions and six examples at each level are provided as guidelines. Designs are first scored as either correct or incorrect. The incorrect designs are then scored according to six types of errors: (1) omission, (2) distortion, (3) perseveration, (4) rotation, (5) misplacement, and (6) size. Norms are provided for number of correct reproductions and errors by age and general intellectual level. Benton (1974) makes recommendations regarding specific cutoff points.

*Reliability.* Because of the detailed scoring system, interscorer reliability is very important. Benton (1974) reported a coefficient of .95. Unfortunately, most research studies using the RVRT did not report interscorer reliability. Test-retest reliability and internal reliability were not reported.

*Validity.* Validity of the RVRT is generally based on its ability to discriminate between patients with organic and those with nonorganic diseases. Brilliant and Gynther (1963) found that the RVRT also discriminated subgroups within these broad categories. The combined scores (number-correct and error) on the RVRT correctly classified 81% of the subjects, in terms of both organic and nonorganic diagnosis. Within the nonorganic group, the combined RVRT scores classified 98% correctly. Subjects in this study ranged from seventeen to eighty-four years of age, with a median of forty years eight months.

Bobele (1976) investigated the effects of group administration of the RVRT; mode A was administered to children in grades one through three. No significant differences between group and individual testing formats were found. Performances of subjects in grades one and two were not different, but the performance of subjects in both grades as a whole was different (having more errors) from the performance of subjects in grade three. An issue not discussed in this research is the fact that many of these subjects were undoubtedly less than eight years of age, the youngest group in the standardization sample.

Benton (1963) noted that in a group of twenty subjects, nine to eleven years of age, with a reading disability, only two performed in the defective range. However, in an investigation of dyslexia in children eight to eighteen years of age, Mattis, French, and Rapin (1975), and Mattis (1979) found that a RVRT score at or below the border-line level could be used as one of three criteria for classification in a visuospatial perceptual-disorder syndrome. The percentages of children thus classified ranged from 5% to 17% across their groups in both studies. That relatively few were seen to have visual-perceptual disorders is consistent with Benton's earlier finding.

In a study of RVRT performance of black adolescents grouped according to age, sex, and ethnic identity, Knuckle and Asbury (1986) found that, of twelve- and thirteen-year-olds, male subjects made significantly more distortion and rotation errors on Administration A than did females of the same age. Subjects with high measured ethnic identity made significantly more total errors, distortion errors, and total right errors than did students with lower measured ethnic identity. These data suggest that the RVRT should be used with considerable caution with twelve- and thirteen-year-old black males.

## ASSESSMENT OF AUDITORY PERCEPTUAL-MOTOR SKILLS

### Theoretical Considerations

Gibson's (1969) three trends in perceptual development, discussed at the beginning of this chapter, apply to auditory perception or to any of the sensory modalities, as well as visual perception. Briefly they are (1) "increasing specificity of discrimination" (p. 450), (2) "optimization of attention" (p. 456), and (3) "economy in the extraction of information from the stimulus" (p. 463).

Woodcock (1976) presented a diagram (Figure 6-4) to illustrate the relationships among several components of auditory processing. This concept is consistent with Myklebust's (1954) and Chalfant and Scheffelin's (1969) definitions of auditory perception. Kirk, Kleiban, and Lerner (1978) separated auditory abilities into peripheral auditory functions and central auditory functions. The abilities included in the latter category are auditory discrimination, reception, association, closure, memory, and sound blending.

In Figure 6-4, the major area of interest for this chapter is the functions of auditory perception. Chalfant and Scheffelin (1969) described seven auditory processing tasks that can be classified under Woodcock's auditory acuity and auditory perception components. The first is "attention to auditory stimuli" (p. 11). Attention is obviously important in the assessment of any ability, but it is especially important in the auditory modality because of the fleeting nature of the stimulus. Chalfant and Scheffelin (1969) suggested that lack of attention "might be related to (a) low level or absence of hearing acuity; (b) distractibility involving competitive visual or auditory stimuli; (c) hyperactive behavior; (d) severe emotional disturbance; (e) severe mental retardation; or (f) inability to obtain meaning from auditory stimuli" (p. 11). Determination of the reason for lack of attention is important in the establishment of instructional priorities. Kirk, Kleiban, and Lerner (1978) treat attending as a thinking skill rather than a perceptual skill.

The second task, according to Chalfant and Scheffelin (1969), is assessing whether the person is receiving "sound versus no sound" (p. 12). It is clear from Woodcock's model (Figure 6-4) and from common sense, that assessment of auditory processing should not be started

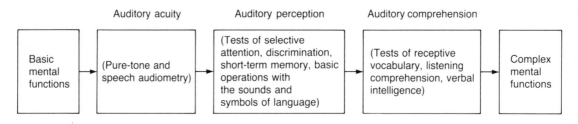

**Figure 6-4**

Auditory processes and measures along a continuum of mental functioning.
(From Woodcock, R. W. *Goldman-Fristoe-Woodcock auditory skills test battery, technical manual.* Circle Pines, Minn.: American Guidance Service, 1976.)

until the status of auditory acuity is determined. Unfortunately, that first step is not always done. In such cases, no interpretation of auditory processing tests can be made until acuity is checked. Kirk, Kleiban, and Lerner (1978) equated auditory acuity with peripheral auditory functions as opposed to central auditory functions.

The third task is "sound localization" (p. 12). Chalfant and Scheffelin noted that they found no reference in the literature to the assessment of sound localization.

"Discriminating sounds varying on one acoustic dimension" (p. 12) is the fourth auditory processing task listed by Chalfant and Scheffelin. Although this task can include the discrimination of non-speech sounds, most typically in educational assessment the focus is on speech sound discrimination. Also included is the ability to analyze a series of sounds and identify the separate components and synthesize separate components into wholes. Kirk, Kleiban, and Lerner (1978) do not list auditory analysis as a separate function, although they do include sound blending (synthesis of sounds) and auditory discrimination as separate functions. In contrast, Woodcock (1976) treated analysis and synthesis of sounds as separate functions, different from auditory discrimination.

The fifth task named by Chalfant and Scheffelin (1969) is "discriminating sound sequences varying on several acoustic dimensions" (p. 15). Essentially, this task deals with rhythm, pitch, and their combination, melody. They noted that this is a significant variable in the development of oral language, but the wider implications have not been the subject of a great deal of research. Much of the literature in this area has dealt with possible neurological sites, or with systems causing a deficit.

The sixth auditory task is "auditory figure-ground selection" (p. 16). Woodcock (1976) described a similar function that he refers to as "selective attention." Basically the task requires the ability to attend to and differentiate relevant sounds, generally speech sounds, from irrele-

vant sounds, which could include both speech and nonspeech sounds.

The seventh auditory processing task is "associating sound with sound sources" (p. 16). They referred to a difficulty in this area as "auditory agnosia." The auditory-reception function described by Kirk, Kleiban, and Lerner is a subcategory of this task. They refer to disability in this function as "receptive aphasia" or "learning disability." The person with receptive aphasia does not obtain meaning from language but does comprehend the meaning of other sounds. Persons with auditory agnosia cannot attribute meaning to any sounds in the environment (Myklebust, 1954).

Kirk, Kleiban, and Lerner listed, in addition to the auditory tasks described by Chalfant and Scheffelin, the following functions: *auditory association*—ability to relate concepts presented orally; *auditory closure*—ability to fill in the missing parts of units when only parts of the units are presented; *sound blending*—synthesis of isolated sounds into words; and *auditory memory*. Woodcock's (1976) list of auditory perceptual skills, around which the Goldman-Fristoe-Woodcock Auditory Skills Battery was developed, included selective attention, auditory discrimination, auditory memory, sound analysis, sound blending, sound-symbol associations, ability to associate two events received by different modalities, and sound-symbol translations, which include "grapheme-to-phoneme translations (phonics) and phoneme-to-grapheme translations (spelling)."

The reason that there is such variance between these authors is that they are using theoretical constructs to describe certain behaviors. Whether these constructs can be related to neurophysiological events in any direct way awaits further research. However, several tests that purport to tap these constructs have been developed.

The relationship of auditory-perceptual skills and reading ability was studied by Hammill and Larsen (1974b) and Kavale (1981), with differing results. Hammill and Larsen (1974b) concluded that "auditory skills are not sufficiently related to reading to be particularly useful for school practice" (p. 40). Whereas Hammill and Larsen used an integrated review procedure, Kavale conducted a meta-analysis of the literature on auditory-perceptual skills and reading ability. The auditory-perceptual skills included in this analysis were auditory discrimination, auditory blending, auditory memory, auditory-visual integration, and auditory comprehension. General reading achievement, word recognition, reading comprehension, vocabulary, and oral reading were the reading factors that were analyzed. Kavale found that when IQ was omitted, "The five auditory-perceptual skills accounted for approximately 25% of the variance in four reading skills . . . , while four of these skills were found to account for 17% [of the] variance in oral reading" (p. 544). However, Kavale concluded that, "Since the proportion of explained variance in reading skills was contingent on the combination of variables, no standard battery of auditory perceptual measures should be administered routinely" (p. 545).

Before diagnosticians undertake the assessment of central auditory functions, they must ensure that peripheral auditory function, that is, hearing acuity, is intact. Generally, as with visual acuity, this evaluation is conducted by a nurse. However, it is important that the diagnostician be able to interpret an audiogram and understand the implications of certain types of hearing loss. Omer (1976) has developed a very helpful book that describes the symbols used on the audiogram. Several audiograms, characteristic of the various types of losses, are shown. A section on interpretation describes certain auditory processing behaviors.

### AUDITORY DISCRIMINATION TEST (2ND ED.) (ADT)

(Reynolds, W. M., 1987, Western Psychological Services)

The ADT is one of the best-known tests of auditory discrimination. Originally developed in 1958 and revised by Wepman in 1975, the test is designed to measure a child's ability to discriminate words that differ only by a single phoneme. The role of speech-sound discrimination in articulation and in some areas of academic achievement has been studied extensively over the last twenty-five years. The results have often been contradictory (Locke & Kutz, 1975). Comparisons of assessment instruments designed to measure auditory discrimination have also produced conflicting results. For example, Bountress and Laderberg (1981) and Bountress (1984) studied the relationships among the ADT (Revised edition), the Goldman-Fristoe-Woodcock Test of Auditory Discrimination (Goldman, Fristoe, & Woodcock, 1970) and the Boston University Speech Sound Discrimination Test (Pronovost, 1974). Their results indicated that these tests cannot be considered equivalent measures of speech-sound discrimination. Much more research is needed to determine what these tests are measuring.

The ADT is designed for children aged four through eight years, who speak standard English. Two forms of the test (1A and 2A) are available. Each consists of thirty pairs of different words and ten pairs of identical words. In the thirty pairs of words, the differing phoneme may be either a beginning consonant, a medial vowel, or a final consonant. The word pairs are presented to the child in such a way that the child cannot see the examiner's mouth or the words on the test form. Any response that conveys the message that the two words presented are the same or different, is all that is required. The raw score is the number of different word pairs correctly identified as different. Test performance is considered invalid as a measure of auditory discrimination if the score on the different pairs part of the test is less than ten or the score on the same pairs is less than seven.

Administration time is approximately 10 minutes. From the raw scores, percentile ranks, T scores (Mean = 50, SD = 10), and a qualitative score are derived. The qualitative scale is a 5-point scale that ranges from +2 (good) to −2 (poor).

*Validity.* Several studies of various aspects of validity are presented in the manual (Reynolds, 1987). Correlations among the ADT, speech and language measures, intelligence tests, and academic achievement ranged from −.82 to +.85. Scores are shown to increase over the limited age span of the test. A significant threat to validity for applications to four- and five-year-olds is the need to ensure that these young children understand the concepts of *same* and *different.* According to the Boehm Test of Basic Concepts-Revised (Boehm, 1986), the concept of *different* was misunderstood by children at the beginning of kindergarten, by 43% of children from the low socioeconomic level and by 20% of children from middle and high socioeconomic levels. The standardization sample appears to be representative of the U. S. population. The sample of 1885 children is stratified by age, sex, ethnic background, parent's occupation, size of community, and geographic region.

The results of the ADT or indeed any test of speech-sound discrimination need to be very cautiously interpreted. These tests should never be used interchangeably nor should they be used to make critical decisions about a child's placement.

*Reliability.* Only internal-consistency reliabilities are reported in the manual. The median correlation for form 1A was $r = .75$. For Form 2A the median reliability was $r = .79$. These reliabilities are minimally adequate. Kruel, Bell, and Nixon (1969) found that the difficulty in tests of speech discrimination changes significantly with changes in examiner. They concluded that "the tests ought not be thought of as written lists of words but as recordings" (p. 287). Even if the reliability coefficients cited were adequate, those administered by other examiners might not be. This is a strong argument for local studies of reliability based on recorded word lists.

### GOLDMAN-FRISTOE-WOODCOCK AUDITORY SKILLS TEST BATTERY
(Woodcock, R. W., 1974, American Guidance Service)

The Goldman-Fristoe-Woodcock Auditory Skills Test Battery consists of four tests that measure a wide range of auditory skills in subjects from four years of age and upward. The tests and subtests are listed in Figure 6-5. Test materials are taped.

*GFW Auditory Selective Attention Test.* This test assesses the subject's ability to attend to a specific auditory stimulus (a word) in the presence of other auditory stimuli that are systematically varied in intensity (signal-to-noise ratio)

GFW *Auditory Selective Attention Tests*
  Quiet Subtest (11 items)
  Fanlike Noise Subtest (33 items)
  Cafeteria Noise Subtest (33 items)
  Voice Subtest (33 items)
GFW *Auditory Discrimination Tests*
  Part I  (100 items)
  Part II  (100 items)
  Part III (100 items)
GFW *Auditory Memory Tests*
  Test 1 Recognition Memory (110 items)
  Test 2 Memory for Content (16 items)
  Test 3 Memory for Sequence (14 items)
GFW *Sound-Symbol Tests*
  Test 1 Sound Mimicry (55 items)
  Test 2 Sound Recognition (30 items)
  Test 3 Sound Analysis (28 items)
  Test 4 Sound Blending (33 items)
  Test 5 Sound-Symbol Association (55 items)
  Test 6 Reading of Symbols (70 items)
  Test 7 Spelling of Sounds (50 items)

**Figure 6-5**
GFW Auditory Skills Test Battery.

and type (fanlike noise, cafeteria noise, and meaningful speech). This ability is often described as *auditory figure-ground perception.* Smyth (1979) found that in a sample of 300 youngsters, five to twelve years of age, 45.3% made errors in speech discrimination in the presence of classroom noise. The effect was greatest for the younger subjects. According to Woodcock (1976) the distraction potential of background auditory stimuli relies on three variables:

1. *Intensity:* The higher the intensity of the background noise, the more potent it is as a distractor.
2. *Variability:* The greater the variability, or intermittent character, of the background noise, the more potent it is as a distractor.
3. *Meaningfulness:* The greater the meaningfulness and/or personal significance of the background noise, the more potent it is as a distractor.

Components of the test were designed to assess the effects of these factors. However, only noise intensity is variable in all four subtests. As each subtest progresses, the signal-to-noise ratio shifts: the signal is initially louder than the noise but finally the noise is louder than the signal. The first eleven items are presented with no background noise. Subsequent items are presented with three different backgrounds: a constant fanlike noise, variable cafeteria noise played in reverse to remove any meaningful sounds, and a voice reading a meaningful story.

The subject's task is to point to the one of four pictures as directed by the speaker on the tape. The distractors have some common sounds with the correct response, but the required discriminations are not so difficult as those on the Auditory Discrimination Tests.

Answers are recorded on a response form that provides space for raw scores and percentile scores on each subtest and the total test. Age equivalent scores, standard scores, and stanines can be obtained from tables in the test manual. A space for recording Auditory Discrimination, Part I, scores is provided so that making comparisons is convenient. A comparative analysis of the attention and discrimination tasks is provided in the technical manual (Woodcock, 1976). A performance profile for raw scores and percentiles is also available for subtest and total scores.

*GFW Auditory Discrimination Test.* This test, designed to measure the subject's ability to discriminate between specific speech sounds, consists of three parts of 100 items each. Part I is composed of pairs of words that are likely to be confused. If performance on Part I is inadequate, Parts II and III are administered. In taking each of the three parts, the individual is required to point to one of two pictures that represents the word that the subject hears on the audio tape. The pictures represent words that vary in a "minimal" number of distinctive features.

One section of the response form for Part I is the Sound Confusion Inventory (SCI). If a subject has difficulties with auditory discrimination, the errors are plotted on the SCI. The SCI makes it possible for the diagnostician to "analyze the pattern of a subject's errors and determine whether they seem to be generalized, associated with certain sounds, or associated with certain sound clusters or target-lure combinations" (Woodcock, 1976, p. 8). The SCI contains twenty-five sound clusters. Sound clusters 5 and 12 are shown in Figure 6-6. As can be seen in cluster 12, for example, if the subject missed many of the items associated with /b/, one might suspect that he or she has difficulty with this sound in a wide range of contexts. If most or all errors with cluster 12, /b/, are with the lure /v/ and the only errors with cluster 5, /v/, are with the lure /b/, one would probably conclude that the subject does not discriminate between /b/ and /v/ but is able to discriminate /v/ from /f/ and /w/, and /b/ from /p/, /d/, and /m/. Interestingly, the failure to discriminate /v/ and /b/ could occur

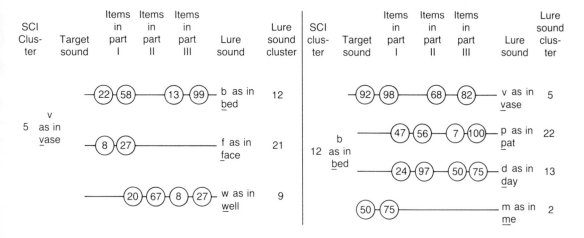

**Figure 6-6**

Sound confusion inventory (SCI) items 5 and 12. Complete the SCI by shading in the circle representing each item. (Adapted from response form—GFW Auditory Discrimination Test. Goldman, R., Fristoe, M., & Woodcock, R. W. *Goldman-Fristoe-Woodcock Auditory Skills Test Battery.* Circle Pines, Minn.: American Guidance Service, 1974.)

with a young child who is bilingual (Spanish-English), because in Spanish there is no difference in the sounds represented by the letters *v* and *b*.

The SCI permits the diagnostician to make a criterion-referenced interpretation of the results as well as a norm-referenced interpretation. On the basis of data obtained from the SCI, instruction in this area can be planned.

Also included in the response form for Part I are the summary scores for Parts II and III. The response form for Parts II and III has no space for derived scores. In addition, space is provided for the Sound Mimicry subtest of the GFW Sound-Symbol Tests. Comparative analysis of these tests is provided in the technical manual (Woodcock, 1976).

*GFW Auditory Memory Tests.* Test I, Recognition Memory, is a continuous memory task that measures the subject's ability to recognize whether or not a word has been previously

spoken. The subject is required to indicate only *yes* or *no*. The test has a total of 110 words divided into five lists of twenty-two words each. If the child is performing so poorly that he meets specified criteria (for example, fifteen errors in twenty-two words), the test can be terminated at the end of that group of twenty-two words. Each word occurs twice, and the range of separation between the first and second occurrences is zero (3 seconds) to eight words (24 seconds). The words were selected from a pool of 1200 words selected according to the criteria of familiarity, concreteness, length, and number of syllables (Fristoe & Blanton, 1970).

A table in the test manual provides estimated total-test raw scores for use when the entire test is not taken. Apparently this estimate is required because the norms are based on subjects who took the entire test. However, the requirement for use of this table is mentioned *only* in a footnote in the response form. No explanation of tables is found in the test manual.

Test 2, Memory for Content, according to Woodcock (1976) "measures the [subject's] ability to recognize a set of elements that occurred in a recent auditory event, without regard for the sequence of those events" (p. 10). Items are presented at the rate of one word every 2 seconds and the complexity of sequences ranges from two words presented with four pictures, to nine words presented with eleven pictures. Subjects are given credit for each of the two pictures correctly identified. When the subject points to more than two pictures, only the first two responses are scored.

The test can be terminated after items 6, 10, and 14 if the number of incorrect responses meets the specified criteria. To obtain an estimated total test raw score, the user is referred to a table in the test manual.

Test 3, Memory for Sequence, measures the child's ability to remember a list of words that is presented on tape while the child sees only a blank page. As soon as the oral list is completed, a page of movable picture cards corresponding to the spoken words is shown to the subject. The task is to place the cards in the order in which the corresponding words were given on the tape. Words are presented at the rate of one every 2 seconds. The lists increase from two to eight words in length. One point is given for correctly placing the first card, the last card, and for correctly sequencing any two cards. The total number of points possible ranges from three on item 1 to nine on item 14. Use of this rather complex scoring system is greatly simplified by the response form (Figure 6-7).

**GFW Sound-Symbol Tests.** Test 1, Sound Mimicry, measures the subject's ability to repeat nonsense words given orally. According to the test manual (Woodcock, 1976), this ability requires discrimination and echoic memory. Each word is presented twice before the subject is asked to repeat it. The test includes fifty-five nonsense words, one to three syllables in length.

Test 2, Sound Recognition, is a rather complex task that measures higher cognitive functions rather than recognition of sound. While the subject views a set of four pictures, the name of one of the pictures is presented on tape as a series of isolated phonemes. The subject then points to the picture named. The technical manual (Woodcock, 1976) suggested that most subjects use some combination of a sound blending-word identification strategy and a process of elimination, in which inappropriate pictures are rejected after each phoneme is spoken. The distractor pictures were selected to reduce the likelihood of a subject's giving a correct response on the basis of one phonemic element.

Test 3, Sound Analysis, measures the child's ability to identify and repeat as directed the first, middle, or last phoneme of two- and three-phoneme nonsense words. The test has twenty-eight items, but testing is terminated when eight or more consecutively incorrect responses have been given. The derived scores are obtained from tables entered with the actual number of items correct rather than with an estimated total raw score, as is used for the Memory tests.

Test 4, Sound Blending, measures the subject's ability to blend two to seven isolated sounds into real words. The rate of presentation is not specified. There are thirty-three items on the test, but testing is discontinued after five or more consecutive errors.

Test 5, Sound-Symbol Association, evaluates the child's ability to learn paired associations between unfamiliar auditory and visual stimuli. The subject is shown a new visual stimulus, and a nonsense word is presented orally. The examiner then presents a page of twelve abstract designs, and the subject is asked to select the correct design when the examiner says the nonsense word. The number of sound-symbols is progressively increased (one to ten). When an error is made, the examiner gives the correct response and has the subject repeat the correct label. To reduce the effects of difficulties in auditory and visual discrimination, each nonsense word and abstract design is made to be clearly different from the others.

**Figure 6-7**
Memory for sequence.
Response form for item 14.
Item 14's taped sequence:
shoe—wing—mail—
bag—lawn—cat—
rake—key. (Adapted from
response form—GFW
Auditory Memory Test.
Goldman, R., Fristoe, M., &
Woodcock, R. W.
*Goldman-Fristoe-Woodcock
Auditory Skills Test Battery.*
Circle Pines, Minn.: American
Guidance Service, 1974.)

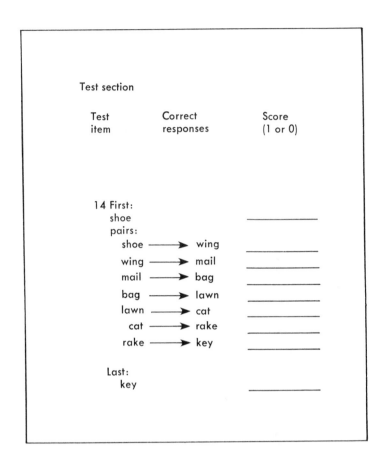

Test 6, Reading of Symbols, assesses the child's ability to read nonsense words. The seventy nonsense words "contain all the major spellings of English phonemes. Each phoneme is represented an average of four times" in different positions in the words (Woodcock, 1976, p. 12). The nonsense words are from one to three syllables long. The items were obtained from a pool of items also used in the Word Attack Test of the Woodcock Reading Mastery Tests (Woodcock, 1973). (See Chapter 7 for a discussion of this test.) Because the same norming statistics were used in both tests, the scores can be used interchangeably. Norms are available only for school-aged youngsters. Grade equivalent scores, in addition to the derived scores provided for all tests in the battery,

are available. Errors on this test can be recorded on a Reading Error Inventory (REI) included in the response form. Portions of the REI are shown in Figure 6-8. The REI permits the evaluation of a subject's performance on eighteen single-consonant sounds, five consonant digraphs, seventeen two-consonant blends, and five three-consonant blends. In the vowel section of the REI, nine single-vowel sounds and five vowel digraphs are included. A multisyllabic section provides an analysis of both syllabication and pronunciation. As does the SCI, this test enables a diagnostician to assess the specific skills in these reading areas and suggest appropriate starting points for instruction. The REI makes this test a criterion-referenced measure of word attack skills.

Single consonants and digraphs:

| REI cluster | Pronun- ciation | Items 1 to 40 | | | | Spellings | Items 41 to 70 |
|---|---|---|---|---|---|---|---|
| 1 | b | (4) b | (18) b | (32) b | (40) b | (55) b | |
| 2 | d | (1) d | (5) ed | (23) d | (31) d | | |

Consonant blends:

| REI cluster | Pronun- ciation | Items 1 to 40 | | | | | | | | | Spellings | | Items 41 to 70 | | | | | | | |
|---|---|---|---|---|---|---|---|---|---|---|---|---|---|---|---|---|---|---|---|---|
| 24 | Two- consonant blends | (12) nd | (18) tw | (19) x | (20) nk | (21) fl | (23) pl | (26) fs | (37) sp | (38) cks | (41) bl | (43) qu | (43) x | (44) st | (46) tr | (48) sl | (52) lf | (53) nch | | |
| 25 | Three- consonant blends | | | | | | | | | | (53) spl | (56) scr | (57) squ | (59) mps | (68) scr | | | | | |

Vowels:

| REI cluster | Pronun- ciation | Items 1 to 40 | | | | | | | Spellings | Items 41 to 70 | |
|---|---|---|---|---|---|---|---|---|---|---|---|
| 26 | a | (2) a | (6) a | (9) a | (23) a | | | | | | |
| 27 | e | (10) e | (12) e | (22) e | (26) e | (32) e | (35) e | (39) e | | (45) e | (62) e |

Multisyllabic words:

| REI cluster | Syllabication skills | Items 1 to 40 | | | | Spellings | Items 41 to 70 | | | | | | | |
|---|---|---|---|---|---|---|---|---|---|---|---|---|---|---|
| 40 | Word division | (30) –/– | (34) –/– | | | | (42) –/– | (54) –/– | (54) –/– | (58) –/– | (61) –/– | (61) –/– | (63) –/– | (63) –/– |
| 41 | Pronunciation | (30) lun | (30) dy | (34) rem | (34) bay | | (42) vit | (42) nap | (54) wub | (54) fam | (54) bif | (58) cig | (58) bet | |
| | | | | | | | (61) pel | (61) nid | (61) lun | (63) baf | (63) mot | (63) bem | | |

**Figure 6-8**

Portions of the Reading Error Inventory (REI) of the GFW Reading of Symbols subtest. Diagnostician completes the REI by shading in the circles representing the subject's word part errors in Test 6—Reading of Symbols. (From Goldman, R., Fristoe, M., & Woodcock, R. W. *Goldman-Fristoe-Woodcock Auditory Skills Test Battery.* Circle Pines, Minn.: American Guidance Service, 1974.)

Test 7, Spelling of Sounds, evaluates the child's ability to make phoneme-to-grapheme associations; this is the reverse of Test 6, which measures the child's ability to make grapheme-to-phoneme associations. Although the fifty "words" are nonsense words, they reflect the "psycholinguistic restrictions of phoneme groupings in English" (Woodcock, 1976, p. 13). The subject is required to listen to a taped nonsense word, repeat the word aloud, and then write it. Credit is given both for correct pronunciation and spelling.

*Norms.* Subjects for the normative group were selected from California, Florida, Maine, and Minnesota (Woodcock, 1976). However, the majority of subjects came from Minnesota. Subjects ranged from three to eighty years of age, but "concentrated in the age range three to twelve years because the most rapid development of auditory skills takes place during that time" (p. 19).

The technical manual gives the numbers of normative subjects grouped by test, age, and race. Unfortunately, the data for age are combined into three groups: three to eight years of age, nine to eighteen years of age, and nineteen years of age and older. Furthermore, data for race are given in percentages of the total sample used for each test in the battery rather than of each age group.

Data were also collected from subjects with "mild" speech and learning problems who were maintained in regular classrooms, and from "educable and trainable mentally retarded individuals" (p. 21). Such an effort is commendable, but again the researchers grouped the subjects by age, and the groupings are different from one another and from the normal sample. Consequently, evaluation of the adequacy of norms for any one age group is impossible.

*Reliability.* Internal-consistency estimates were obtained by the split-half method, corrected "to estimate of full-length test reliability by using the Spearman-Brown formula" (Woodcock, 1976, p. 23). Partial correlation procedures were used to remove the effect of age. For testing of subjects three to eight years of age, coefficients ranged from .76 on Selective Attention to .97 on Reading of Symbols and Spelling of Sounds. For testing of subjects nine to eighteen years of age, coefficients ranged from .46 on Selective Attention and Auditory Discrimination—Part I to .96 on Reading of Symbols. For testing of subjects nineteen years of age and over, coefficients ranged from .73 on Selective Attention, Auditory Discrimination—Part I, and Memory for Content, to .97 on Reading of Symbols. The test authors attribute the relatively low reliabilities in the middle age group to the fact that many subjects obtained perfect or near-perfect scores on these tests. Even so, correlations overall for this age group are unacceptably low. Test users should consult this table when they are preparing interpretations of test performance. Internal consistency reliabilities for testing of the clinical sample of mildly handicapped youngsters ranged from .74 to .98. Only two subtests exceeded the .90 level. However, for tests of the more severely mentally handicapped sample, no reliability coefficients were lower than .93.

Standard error-of-measurement data "derived from the error statistic associated with the log-ability scores obtained from a Rasch analysis" (Woodcock, 1976, p. 24) are presented for various points in each subtest. For the Selective Attention test, data are given for various subparts. This information is especially useful because the internal consistency estimates are lowest in this test.

*Validity.* The technical manual (Woodcock, 1976) offered as support for content validity a series of tables that describe the verbal content of the task, the primary memory store utilized, the size of linguistic unit in the stimulus and response, and the mode of the test stimulus and response. Although this information is interesting and useful from a clinical perspective, it falls far short of the rigorous controls described previously in Chapter 2 for the generation of test items.

Using the theoretical notion that the square root of a test's reliability coefficient is the maximum validity coefficient possible for that test, Woodcock (1976) argued that if two tests are measuring different traits, the correlations between them should be much lower than the square root of the reliability coefficient. Overall this argument is true, and the higher correlations are found to be between subtests that one would subjectively expect to be related. For example, in testing of subjects nine to eighteen years of age, the square root of the reliability coefficient for Sound Blending is .93. The two highest correlations with Sound Blending are Sound Recognition (.68) and Sound Analysis (.52).

In a comparison of normal subjects and mildly handicapped subjects, the handicapped uniformly obtained lower scores, but the differences on the Discrimination and Sound Mimicry tests were not significant.[66] "Age within group was generally a more significant source of variance than type of subject" (Woodcock, 1976, p. 29). With the mentally handicapped subjects, all scores were significantly lower than those of the normal subjects.

No studies of criterion-related validity are reported.

## PROFILES OF LEARNING-DISABLED READERS

Rather than present a case study with limited generalizability, we present in Figure 6-9 a series of profiles of eleven- and twelve-year-old learning-disabled readers. This series was derived from a cluster analysis of 102 subjects (Lyon, Reitta, Watson, Porch & Rhodes, 1981). Discussion will focus on the tests discussed in this text and on those that contributed most to discriminating between the groups.

Subjects in Subgroup 1 showed deficits in oral receptive language (Token), visual-motor integration (VMI), and visual-spatial functions (Ravens) and visual-memory functions (Memory for Design, MFD). Subgroup 1 scored lower than all other groups on the VMI and MFD. They showed no offsetting processing strengths. Con-

sequently, it was not surprising to find that they were the most severely retarded readers in the sample.

Deficits in oral receptive language, visual-motor integration, and visual-spatial functions characterized readers in Subgroup 2 ($N = 12$). Although similar to Subgroup 1 in deficits, they were unlike that group in that they showed average performance in naming, auditory discrimination, and visual memory. They had the third highest reading scores of the six groups.

Subgroup 3 ($N = 12$) was characterized by deficits in oral receptive language comprehension, auditory attention span, syntactical development, and sound-blending ability. However, they had average to above-average performance in naming, auditory discrimination, visual-motor integration, and visual-spatial and visual memory functions. They performed lower in reading recognition than did those in Subgroups 2, 4, and 6. In reading comprehension, Subgroups 2 and 3 had identical means, which were lower than those of Subgroups 6 and 4.

Subgroup 4 contained thirty-two subjects, at least twice as many as any other group. This group is characterized primarily by very poor visual-motor integration skills and by lesser deficits in auditory attention and sound blending. Receptive language functions were above average. Cluster 4 had the next to highest performance in reading recognition and comprehension.

A severe deficit in receptive language characterized Cluster 5 ($N = 12$). The only average performance was in the MFD. Only Cluster 1 scored lower on the reading measures. Both groups showed pervasive deficiencies on the test battery.

Cluster 6 ($N = 16$) was unique in that all scores were within the normal range. Auditory attention span and sound blending were relatively low. This group had the highest reading scores in the sample. However, they were at least two years behind in reading. The performances of this group demonstrate that there are some poor readers whose deficits are related to vari-

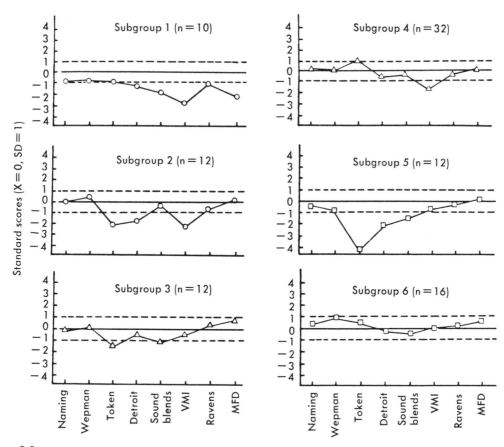

**Figure 6-9**
Profiles of subgroups of learning-disabled readers. (Adapted from Lyon, R., Reitta, S., Watson, B., Porch, R., & Rhodes, J. Selected linguistic and perceptual abilities of empirically derived subgroups of learning disabled readers. *Journal of School Psychology,* 1981, *19,* 157. Copyright 1981, *Journal of School Psychology,* New York.)

ables other than language and perceptual-motor processes.

## SUMMARY

In summary, several measures of visual and auditory perceptual-motor measures have been reviewed. Research with these measures has been integrated as possible in the analysis. The results indicate, as have most test authors, that these instruments generally do not meet rigor-

ous standards of reliability and validity and hence cannot be considered to be definitive diagnostic measures. This does not mean that they are not useful for clinical purposes and research, as this usefulness is demonstrated by the profiles of learning-disabled readers.

# CHAPTER 7

# Academic Assessment

## OUTLINE

Achievement tests
Diagnostic reading tests
Diagnostic arithmetic tests
Summary

**A**ssessment of academic perfor- mance has four basic purposes: (1) screening, (2) diagnosis and least restrictive placement, (3) instructional planning, and (4) program evaluation. School districts often are interested in economical screening for children who are at risk for school failure as well as those who have exceptional ability. To meet this need, group achievement tests are a first step in the screening process. Table 7-1 lists a number of achievement tests and the grades and subject areas for which they are designed.

Two major problems with this use of group achievement tests is the possible lack of a match between the curriculum of the school district and the content of the test (Gickling & Thompson, 1985; Neisworth & Bagnato, 1986), and the possible lack of a match between the students in the local school district and subjects in the normative sample. Children at-risk for failure in a district with superior programs might appear to do well on a test normed on subjects in programs of varying quality; these children consequently might not qualify for the assistance needed to prevent failure in their school curriculum. Mismatch can also occur in both content and sequence of content. For example, a particular comprehension skill might be presented at grade five in a local school curriculum, but be tested by a group achievement test at the end of grade four. Obviously these problems can occur with any achievement test, but group achievement tests are designed for global assessments, and consequently these problems occur more frequently with group achievement tests. Gifted and talented children might be penalized if they are evaluated on content not included in their school's program. However the publishers of most major group achievement tests devote considerable effort to the ensuring of content validity. The latest volume of the *Mental Measurements Yearbook* describes most of these efforts in great detail. Also, see Chapter 2 for a more comprehensive discussion of criterion- and curriculum-based assessment.

In addition to group achievement tests, there are several individually administered screening tests. Generally, however, these tests do not satisfy two major requirements for screening instruments: economy and ease of administration.

In addition to screening, the identification of learning problems is also made with academic tests. Teachers and parents recognize that the child's performance is far below (or far above) grade placement; the child is not achieving his or her maximum performance in the present program. A particular sort of test is needed to accurately determine the nature of the problem and the type of program that will be most appropriate, whether it involves special-education placement or modifications of in-class programs. Because the results of the testing have potentially far-reaching consequences for the individual, the reliability and validity of the measures is far more important than considerations of whether the tests can be administered economically and easily. Tests for these purposes should be norm-referenced, and the standardization sample should include persons similar to the child to be tested. If the child is from a minority group, especially if he or she uses a different dialect or language, every effort must be made to provide a nonbiased assessment. For more information on multicultural assessment, see Chapter 13.

Frequently a regular education teacher recognizes that the range of performance of individual students is so great that instruction must be given individually or in small groups. Even with a smaller class, the special-education teacher faces the same need: At what level do I begin instruction? This is a question that must be answered, so that the child who has already mastered material is not bored and the child who lacks the prerequisite skills to achieve the objective at hand is not discouraged. Ideally, what would be used is a test referenced to the curriculum objectives of the school, of sufficient length to serve a diagnostic function, and with

**Table 7-1**

Group achievement tests.

| Test | Grades | Academic areas | Selected references |
|---|---|---|---|
| California Achievement Test, Forms C & D (1977, CTB-McGraw Hill) | K–12.9 | Reading, spelling, language, mathematics, reference skills | Crowell, Hu-pei, & Blake (1983); Knochnower, Richardson, & DeBennedetto (1983); Price (1984); Swartz & Walker (1984) |
| Comprehensive Test of Basic Skills, Forms U & V (1983, CTB-McGraw Hill) | K–12.9 | Reading, spelling, language, mathematics, social studies, reference skills | Croft & Franco (1983); Slavin, Leavey, & Madden (1984) |
| Curriculum Referenced Tests of Mastery (1983-1984, Merrill) | 1–12 | Reading, spelling, language, mathematics, geometry, pre-algebra (school can design their own custom edition) | Kamphaus (1985); Ligon (1985) |
| Iowa Test of Basic Skills, Forms 7 & 8 (Hieronymus, Lendquist & Hoover, 1982, Riverside Publishing) | K–9 | Reading, spelling, language, mathematics, reference skills | Day (1983); Hoover & Kolen (1984) |
| Metropolitan Achievement Test: Sixth Edition (MAT6)-Survey Battery (Prescott, Balow, Hogan & Farr, 1985, Psychological Corporation) | K–12.9 | Reading, spelling, language, mathematics, social studies, science; Diagnostic tests of reading, mathematics, and language | Meyer, Gersten & Gutken (1984); Silliphant (1983) |
| Science Research Associates Achievement Series (Naslund, Thorpe, & Lefever, 1981, Science Research Associates) | K–12 | K–8: Reading, mathematics, language arts 9–12: Reading, mathematics, language arts, reference skills, social studies, science, survey of applied skills | Darakjian & Michael (1983) |
| Stanford Achievement Test Series, 7th ed. (Gardner, Rudman, Karlsen, & Merwin, 1986, Psychological Corporation) | K–13 | K–3: Reading, language, mathematics, environment 4–13: Reading, language, mathematics, science, social science 8.0–12.9: Task 1—Reading, language, mathematics, science, social science 9.0–13.0: Task 2—Reading, language, mathematics, science, social science | Caskey & Larson (1983); Voeltz (1983) |
| Stanford Diagnostic Mathematics Tests, 3rd ed. (Beatty, Gardner, & Karlsen, 1983, 1984, Psychological Corporation) | 1.5–12 | Number system and numeration, computation, application | Horodezky & Lebercane (1983); Ysseldyke (1985) |
| Stanford Diagnostic Reading Tests, 3rd ed. (Karlsen, Madden, & Gardner, 1983, 1984, Psychological Corporation) | 1.5–12 | Comprehension, decoding, vocabulary rate | Shepard (1985) |

empirically derived mastery-nonmastery cutoff scores. Unfortunately such instruments are rarely available. Consequently, school personnel must make a judgment: to select the test that is most closely related to local curriculum objectives, and that also has adequate reliability and validity.

Another purpose of academic assessment is to evaluate both individual progress and instructional programs. Again the purpose of the testing determines the characteristics of the test used. If school personnel want to evaluate individual progress in terms of local curriculum objectives, and instructional programs in terms of progress made by students in those programs, the same type of test can be used for both purposes. That test is the curriculum-based or criterion-referenced test described in the previous paragraph.

However, if the school's personnel want to know whether students who complete their curriculum are as knowledgeable as the students in other parts of the country who have completed similar but not identical curricula, the test should be one whose content is very broadly based. Some individual and group achievement tests serve this purpose well.

Although the four purposes of academic assessment have been discussed separately, tests that serve one purpose can probably also be used clinically for other purposes. Testing is only a brief, standardized *observation* of behavior. Whether the test is intended to determine placement or to aid in the planning of instruction, the administration of that test is observing behavior. Even though what is observed cannot always be verified by the test being administered, that observation can be identified as the focus of later assessment. For example, if a youngster writes *bise* for *vice* on a carefully devised, norm-referenced placement test, there probably will not be a sufficient number of items for the examiner to determine whether the *b-v* and *s-c* substitutions are a consistent problem that occurred because the child could not per-

form the task correctly, or a function of some internal or external event, such as a bell ringing and the child thinking that it is time for recess. Also, the examiner won't be able to tell whether the error results from a problem in auditory discrimination, a second-language discrimination problem, or the fact that the child's allergy was acting up and he did not hear well. All the examiner knows is what was observed. However, the possibilities just suggested and probably many others can become hypotheses (Wedell, 1970) to be investigated at another time with a different type of test.

Some issues involved in testing also transcend the specific purposes of academic assessment. For example, because of the influence of the medical model, oftentimes the examiner focuses exclusively on pathological characteristics. In psychological and educational evaluation, a careful description of the subject's strengths as well as weaknesses is important. In planning instruction, one can determine the starting point by noting where successes end and errors begin. The approach or model used to plan instruction will determine to some extent the effectiveness of the remediation.

Only a few of the many measures available in academic assessment are presented in this chapter. We believe that the tests presented are the most useful for some of the purposes just discussed. By citing some of the research with various groups and for various purposes, we will also point out possible problems as well as the potential benefits of the instruments. A number of group achievement tests are described in Table 7-1. Additional, individually administered achievement tests are listed in Table 7-2.

## ACHIEVEMENT TESTS

### PEABODY INDIVIDUAL ACHIEVEMENT TEST (PIAT)
(Dunn, L. M., and Markwardt, F. C., 1970, American Guidance Service)

The PIAT is a "screening measure of achievement" (Dunn & Markwardt, 1970, p. 1) in mathematics, reading recognition, reading comprehension, spelling, and general information. The authors emphasized that the test was not designed for diagnostic purposes. A multiple-choice format is used in all subtests except General Information, which requires a short-answer response. The PIAT is an untimed power test that takes approximately 30 to 40 minutes to administer. However, Davenport (1976) reported that an average time of 45 minutes was needed for administration to normal children in grade three and that up to 1 hour was needed for administration to children with learning disabilities.

The examiner has the choice of age or grade-equivalent scores for each subtest and the composite score. Percentile ranks are provided for both age and grade equivalents. Normalized, standard-score conversions are given for age and grade; these conversions are based on the percentile ranks for those norms. Age or grade equivalents or their percentile ranks may be profiled in the Individual Record booklet. In addition, current age, grade-placement level, grade-median level, age-median level, IQ level, and mental age may be plotted, according to the comparisons the examiner wishes to make.

Starting points for the average student are indicated on the Mathematics subtest for grades one through twelve. However, the test manual indicates that the examiner is to consider the age and ability of the subject. Subsequent starting points correspond to the subject's raw score on the preceding subtest. However, Wikoff (1979), in a study of subjects referred for learning problems in grades one to nine, found an average difference of 8 to 12 points between raw scores and adjacent subtest basals. He suggested that, for children with learning problems, to determine the starting point for the next subtest, examiners subtract eight points from the raw score. This is an especially helpful suggestion for those examining children with a history of school failure, high test anxiety, and low self-concept. Testing backward is an immediate clue to failure and probably depresses motivation.

Although the test is consistently termed a screening test rather than a diagnostic test, data are provided to help administrators examine the relationships between pairs of subtests. Such a procedure is highly questionable (Kaufman, 1979; Reynolds & Gutkin, 1980; Silverstein, 1980). Using a more appropriate method, Reynolds and Gutkin provided data on differences in standard score points required for significance, at the .05 and .01 levels on each subtest at grades one, three, five, eight, and twelve. However, Silverstein suggested a modification of the Reynolds and Gutkin procedure. Silverstein stated that their data could be used "but the differences that they cite as significant at the .01 level should be interpreted as significant at the .05 level instead" (p. 13).

*Standardization.* Subjects from kindergarten through grade twelve were regarded to be in the "mainstream of education" (Dunn & Markwardt, 1970, p. 26). The samples of each grade except kindergarten (N = 159) contained more than 200 subjects; each sample contained approximately equal numbers of boys and girls. Total sample size was 2889. The sample included 84.4% white, 11.3% black, and 4.3% other. This is significantly different from the Census Bureau (1967) data, because the sample data reports Spanish-Americans, Native-Americans, and Orientals under the "Other" category, whereas census figures only include Orientals in this category. Dean (1977) questioned the adequacy of the representation of Mexican-Americans in the standardization sample.

Subjects for the standardization were selected from the nine geographic subdivisions used by the census bureau; however, the distributions for the standardization were significantly different from those used for the census data. The differences were quite small and ranged from a −2.73% discrepancy in the Middle Atlantic states to a +1.16% discrepancy in the Pacific

**Table 7-2**

Individually administered tests of educational achievement.

| Test of basic skills | Age or grade | Domains/subtests |
|---|---|---|
| Adult Basic Learning Examination, 2nd ed. (Karlsen & Gardner, 1986, Psychological Corporation) | Adult | 3 levels based on years of education; vocabulary, reading comprehension, spelling, language, number operations, problem solving |
| Basic Achievement Skills Individual Screener (1983, Psychological Corporation) | 1–12 Past high school | Reading, Mathematics, Spelling, Optional Writing exercises |
| Brigance Diagnostic Comprehensive Inventory (English and Spanish) (Brigance, 1983, 1984, Curriculum Associates) | K–9 | Objective-based multiple measures of readiness, reading, listening, research and study skills |
| Brigance Diagnostic Inventory of Basic Skills (Brigance, 1976, Curriculum Associates) | K–6 | Objective-based multiple measures of readiness, reading, language arts, mathematics |
| Brigance Diagnostic Inventory of Essential Skills (Brigance, 1981, Curriculum Associates) | 4–12 | Objective-based multiple measures of reading, language arts, mathematics, and life skills |
| Criterion Referenced Curriculum Reading | K–6 | Criterion-referenced tests of 267 reading-skill objectives |
| Mathematics (Stephens, 1982, Psychological Corporation) | K–6 | Criterion-referenced test of 378 mathematics-skill objectives |
| Diagnostic Achievement Test for Adolescents (Newcomer & Bryant, 1986, Pro-Ed) | 7–12 | Word identification, reading comprehension, mathematics calculations, mathematics problem solving, spelling, writing composition, science, social studies, reference skills |
| Diagnostic Reading Scales (Revised Edition) (Spache, 1981, Technical Report, 1982) | 1–7 | Oral reading (word lists and passages) silent reading, passage comprehension, listening comprehension |

region. Distribution by type of community—urban, suburban, rural—was not significantly different from that of the census data.

The standardization's distribution of subjects by parents' occupation (U.S. Department of Labor, 1965) was also significantly different from that of census data. Again the differences were small and ranged from $-4.4\%$ in the Armed Services category to $+6.3\%$ in the Craftsmen and Foremen category. Although there are some minor discrepancies between census data and some of the categorical distributions, this test has one of the most adequate standardization samples of tests reviewed in this book.

*Reliability.* According to Dunn and Markwardt (1970b), "split-half reliability techniques were rejected as likely to result in spuriously high estimates of reliability for a test on which items have been carefully ordered in difficulty and on which the basal and ceiling procedure is utilized" (p. 43). Test-retest reliability coefficients and standard error of measurement are reported for kindergarten and grades one, three, five, eight, and twelve (Table 7-3).

Dean (1977) also compared Mexican-American and white children 6 to 16 years of age matched according to age, sex, socioeconomic status, educational placement, and reason for referral. He reported split-half reliabilities

**Table 7-2**

*continued*

| Test of basic skills | Age or grade | Domains/subtests |
| --- | --- | --- |
| Durrell Analysis of Reading Difficulty, 3rd ed. (Durrell & Catterson, 1980, Psychological Corporation) | 1–6 | Decoding, comprehension |
| Enright Diagnostic Inventory of Basic Arithmetic Skills (Enright, 1983, Curriculum Associates) | Below grade 7 | 13 areas of mathematical computation; wide range placement test, skills placement tests, basic facts test, skills tests |
| Gray Oral Reading Tests-Revised (Weiderholt & Bryant, 1986, Pro-Ed) | 7–17 yrs. | Passage (oral reading); Oral reading comprehensive |
| Multilevel Academic Survey Tests   Grade Level Tests (norm-referenced)   Curriculum Level Tests   (criterion-referenced) (Howell, Zucher, & Morehead, 1985, Psychological Corporation) | K–12 K–8 | Reading, mathematics |
| Tests of Academic Progress (Adams, Erb, & Sheelow, 1987, Psychological Corporation) | K–12 | Mathematics, reading, spelling |
| Test of Early Mathematics Ability (Ginsburg & Baroody, 1983, Pro-Ed) | 4 yrs., 0 mos.–8 yrs., 11 mos. | Informal mathematics (3 subtests); Formal mathematics (4 subtests) |
| Test of Early Reading Ability (Reid, Hresko, & Hammill, 1981, Pro-Ed) | 3 yrs., 0 mos.–7 yrs., 11 mos. | Alphabet knowledge, comprehension, conventions of reading |
| Test of Early Written Language (Hresko, 1988, Pro-Ed) | 3–7 yrs. | Written language |
| Test of Mathematics Ability (Brown & McEntire, 1984, Pro-Ed) | 3–12 | Attitude toward mathematics, general information computation, story problems, vocabulary |
| Test of Reading Comprehension (Brown, Hammill, & Wiederholt, 1986, Pro-Ed) | 7–17 yrs. | General vocabulary, syntactic similarities, paragraph reading, sentence sequencing |
| Test of Written Language (Hammill & Larsen, 1983, Pro-Ed) | 7 yrs., 0 mos.–18 yrs., 11 mos. | Vocabulary, thematic maturity, thought units, spelling word usage, style |
| Test of Written Spelling (Larsen & Hammill, 1986, Pro-Ed) | 1–12 | Predictable words, less predictable words |

and standard errors of measurement somewhat higher but not significantly different from the reliabilities reported in Table 7-3. Although the Total Test and Reading Recognition reliabilities are adequate, little confidence can be placed in the Reading Comprehension and Spelling subtests. Reliabilities for the Mathematics and General Information subtests are marginal. It is noteworthy that the highest reliabilities occur for the Reading Recognition and General Information subtests, which do not use a multiple-choice format.

*Validity.* Information on content and item validity, and concurrent validity, is given in the test manual. Content validity is claimed because the subtests were based on comprehensive reviews of school curriculum materials and consultations with subject-matter experts. This rather weak claim is weakened further because items were retained not on the basis of their criticalness to a content area but on whether or not they were answered correctly by 50% of the standardization sample at each grade level. The procedure is subject to all the shortcomings

**Table 7-3**
Test-retest reliability coefficients and standard errors of measure for PIAT raw scores, by selected grade levels.

| Grade | N | Mathematics | Reading recognition | Reading comprehension | Spelling | General information | Total test |
|-------|---|-------------|---------------------|-----------------------|----------|---------------------|-----------|
| K  | 75 | .52(2.75)* | .81(1.66) | —         | .42(3.42) | .74(2.40) | .83(6.50) |
| 1  | 60 | .83(2.63)  | .89(1.74) | .78(2.48) | .55(3.16) | .70(3.51) | .89(7.29) |
| 3  | 54 | .68(5.14)  | .94(2.21) | .73(4.90) | .78(4.16) | .77(5.71) | .91(12.0) |
| 5  | 51 | .73(4.63)  | .89(3.90) | .64(6.51) | .53(6.38) | .88(4.21) | .89(14.7) |
| 8  | 68 | .76(5.38)  | .87(4.54) | .61(7.39) | .75(5.51) | .83(4.69) | .89(16.3) |
| 12 | 60 | .84(4.83)  | .86(4.08) | .63(6.77) | .75(4.94) | .73(4.83) | .92(12.1) |

Based on material from Dunn, L. M., & Markwardt, F. C. *Manual for the Peabody Individual Achievement Test.* Circle Pines, Minn.: American Guidance Services, Inc., 1970, p. 44.
*Standard errors of measurement are in parentheses.

discussed in Chapter 2. However, the authors of the test are to be commended because they described their procedure very clearly.

When subjects were retested for reliability data, they were also administered the Peabody Picture Vocabulary Test (PPVT). Correlation coefficients between PIAT raw scores and PPVT standard scores ranged from a low of .29, in Spelling at grade twelve, to a high of .76, in General Information at grade five. Overall the highest correlations are with General Information (Median = .68) and Reading Comprehension (Median = .66), and the lowest are with Spelling (Median = .525) and Reading Recognition (Median = .545).

Since its publication, the PIAT has been the subject of a considerable number of validity studies, made with a wide range of subjects. Possibly the most important of these is a factor analytical study (Reynolds, 1979) based on the standardization sample. A two-factor solution was retained at each grade level. Factor 1 in grades one, three, and five was made up of Reading Comprehension, Reading Recognition, and Spelling, which Reynolds interprets as measuring primarily verbal comprehension and reasoning skills. Factor 2 was composed of the Mathematics and General Information subtests and was regarded as measuring acquired fac-

tual knowledge. At grades eight through twelve the factor structure changed somewhat. At these levels, Factor 1 was made up of the Reading Comprehension, General Information, and Mathematics subtests, and Factor 2 was made up of the Reading Recognition and Spelling subtests. Although the structure was changed, the factors measured the same underlying abilities across grade levels.

Reynolds (1979) stated that for a test to be an "interpretable profile, the separate subtests must (a) have sufficient specificity (greater specific variance than error variance), (b) be reliable, and (c) measure distinct factors" (p. 270). The Reading Recognition and General Information subtests show sufficient specificity at all grade levels. Again, as was shown in studies of test-retest reliability, the two tests that do not use the multiple-choice format give the most accurate information. The specific variance is in excess of error variance for the Mathematics subtest at all grades except grade three. The Spelling subtest shows adequate specificity only at grades three, eight, and twelve. The Reading Comprehension subtest does not show sufficient specificity at any grade level.

Reynolds (1979) concluded that "achievement profiles intended to provide specific diagnostic information . . . when compared to I.Q.

measures, should be viewed with extreme caution when based upon scores from individual PIAT subtests" (p. 274). According to Reynolds, the PIAT is best used to provide an overview of a subject's educational achievement.

Several studies have evaluated relationships between intelligence tests and PIAT scores. Dean (1976) reported moderately high correlations between the WISC-R subtest of Information and PIAT General Information (.89, Mexican-American sample; .76, Anglo-American sample) and WISC-R Arithmetic and PIAT Mathematics (.89, Mexican-American sample; .69, Anglo-American sample). Davenport (1976) obtained a similar correlation (.77) between PIAT General Information and the Otis-Lennon Mental Abilities Test, administered to normal children in grade 3. Dean (1976) also found poor discrimination validity for the PIAT subtests in both samples, as evidenced by moderately high intersubtest correlations. White (1979) found that the PIAT Mathematics subtest and the Total Test correlated most highly with IQs on the WISC-R (.70 to .84). The subjects were seven to nine years of age. Lowest correlations of the PIAT were with Spelling (.51 to .62). Overall-performance IQ had lower correlations with PIAT test scores than with Verbal or Full-Scale IQ. Correlations between the PIAT and the Draw-A-Man scores ranged from a high of .47, with Total Test, to a low of .40, with Reading Recognition and Spelling.

Several studies have examined differences between PIAT and Wide Range Achievement Test (WRAT) scores, and the results of these studies tend to show moderate to high correlations across subtests (Baum, 1975; Davenport, 1976; Wettler & French, 1973). However, all of these studies used the 1965 WRAT norms. Using the 1976 WRAT norms, Walden (1979) analyzed WRAT-PIAT relationships for subjects in grade four. Mean achievement was one to three grade levels above grade placement and mean IQ (PPVT) was 117.3 (SD = 11.25). Correlations for PIAT Mathematics and WRAT Arithmetic were .63; for PIAT Reading Recogni-

tion and WRAT Reading, .61; and for PIAT Spelling and WRAT Spelling, .63. Although these relationships are significant at the .01 level, they are generally lower than those reported in earlier studies. Despite these moderate correlations, mean grade equivalents for the WRAT subtests were considerably higher than the PIAT grade equivalents. In testing clients in a learning disability center, Harmer and Williams (1978) found similar results. WRAT Arithmetic scores were significantly higher than PIAT Mathematics scores at grade four and above. Reading and Spelling scores from the two tests showed more similarity.

In a study of subjects with learning disabilities, Scull and Branch (1980) reported that PIAT Mathematics scores were significantly higher than WRAT Arithmetic scores, while Reading and Spelling scores did not differ on the tests. Caskey (1985) obtained a similar result with children who were learning-disabled, when he compared scores from the PIAT Reading Comprehension subtest and the Passage Comprehension subtest of the Woodcock Reading Mastery Test. Although the subtest scores were found to be highly correlated, they were also found to be significantly different. The PIAT Reading Comprehension subtest produced the highest scores.

In one of the few studies with mentally handicapped subjects, Ysseldyke, Sabatino, and La Manna (1973) investigated the convergent and discriminant validity of the PIAT. *Convergent validity* refers to relationships between tests of similar content. Adequate convergent validity was established for the PIAT Mathematics and Reading Recognition subtests with their counterparts on the Metropolitan Achievement Test (MAT) and the WRAT. Discriminant validity (stronger relationships with measures of similar content than with measures of supposedly different content) was supported for the PIAT Mathematics subtest and to a lesser extent for the Reading Recognition subtest. According to Ysseldyke, Sabatino, and La Manna (1973), "scores that children (mentally handicapped) earned on the Spelling subtest were primarily a function of the method used to measure this behavior" (p. 204). The validities of the PIAT Reading Comprehension and the General Information subtests were not determined, because they have no equivalent on the WRAT or MAT.

Publishers of the PIAT have announced the publication of a revision (PIAT-R) (Dunn & Markwardt, 1988), which will be available about the same time as this text is available. According to prepublication material the PIAT-R will contain new items and will be based on new norms. In addition to the subtests in the current edition, a Written Expression subtest will be added. The age range has been extended to adults and the administration time is 60 minutes. Also new in the revision is a total reading score.

*Summary.* The PIAT is a well-standardized screening instrument, but subtest specificity is inadequate for diagnostic purposes. Correlations with the WRAT are moderate to high, but grade-equivalent scores at some levels are significantly different on the two tests. Test results for handicapped samples need to be interpreted in light of research with such subjects.

### WIDE RANGE ACHIEVEMENT TEST (WRAT)
(Jastak, J. J., & Jastak, S., 1978; Jastak, S. & Wilkinson, G. S., 1984, Jastak Associates)

The WRAT contains Reading, Spelling, and Arithmetic subtests. Each subtest has a pre-academic section that is administered to young children and to individuals who do not reach specified criteria on the academic portion of each subtest. The academic portion of the Reading subtest requires the subject to read a list of words. On the Spelling subtest, the individual writes the words dictated by the examiner. The subject completes arithmetic calculations on the Arithmetic subtest. Obviously the test samples very limited aspects of the areas of reading and arithmetic. Each subtest is divided into two levels. Level I is designed for children from five to eleven years of age, and Level II is used with persons from twelve to seventy-four years of age.

Portions of the test are timed. The test manual indicated that the entire test is usually completed in 20 to 30 minutes.

Three types of scores are provided: grade equivalent, percentiles, and standard scores. In addition to a standard score with a mean of 100 (SD = 15), other standard scores include $T$ scores, scaled scores, and stanines.

The test was revised in 1984 (Jastak & Wilkinson, 1984). Levels 1 and 2 have been slightly lengthened, and the upper age limit of the test-takers has been extended to seventy-four years. For the first time, apparently a stratified national sample was obtained. However, other than indicating that 2% of the sample was mentally retarded, no mention is made of stratification by educational placement. Despite these improvements, Witt (1986) noted that in many instances a small change in raw score resulted in significant changes in standard scores. Because the 1978 revision (Jastak & Jastak, 1978) is still being widely used and reported in the literature, information on the older version is included in our discussion.

*1978 Standardization.* Jastak and Jastak stated that the effect of the scaling procedures applied to the 1978 norms was significant as compared with the 1976 norms. Contrary to that statement, Silverstein (1980) found little effect at the preschool levels but rather large differences (five to seven grades) at the upper end of the distribution. Earlier, Silverstein (1978) had noted that the 1976 norms tended to underestimate the Reading score for average and above-average readers and to underestimate the score at all levels in Arithmetic (Level II especially); these estimates were compared to performance of a representative national sample (Hitchcock & Pinder, 1974; Schaie & Roberts, 1970). Because the upper end of the distribution is more compressed in the 1978 norms, these norms should even more strongly underestimate relative to the national samples.

Despite an implication that the 1978 test was administered to individuals in several states, the sample sizes, raw score means, and standard deviations of the 1976 and 1978 standardization samples are identical.

The 1976–1978 norms have a minimum of 400 and a maximum of 600 subjects in each age grouping. Half are males and half females at each age level. At numerous age levels, there are significant ·differences in favor of females. The only exception is for two age groups in Level II Arithmetic. According to the test manual (Jastak & Jastak, 1978), "the samples represent(s) appropriate proportions of average, superior, and inferior persons" (p. 43), and all ethnic groups are included in proportions representative of the national population. However, no data are presented to support these statements.

In regard to socioeconomic status, Jastak and Jastak (1978) stated that "the means of representative samplings of disadvantaged groups on all three subtests vary between a standard score of 88 and 95, indicating the degree of effect of deprivation on test results" (p. 15). They recommended the addition of 5 to 12 points to the obtained score, based on the examiner's estimate of deprivation. They also suggested that both the obtained and corrected scores be reported. A table of Ratings of Standard Scores by classification (Defective–Very Superior) and estimated deprivation (None–Severe) is included in the test manual. Without additional supporting information and research, examiners would probably do well to avoid this highly subjective procedure.

*Reliability.* The 1978 test manual presents split-half reliability coefficients and standard errors of measure for the 1965 norms. In fact the only new information in the 1978 reliability chapter is a section on reliability coefficients based on unique variances and a comparison of the 1946 and 1965 revisions. The section on unique variance does not indicate which set of normative data is being analyzed. Consequently one must conclude at least from the test manual that there are no reliability data on the 1976–1978 norms. In addition, a review of the literature

failed to turn up any reliability studies of the 1976–1978 WRAT.

In the 1984 revision, the authors have improved their procedures for assessing reliability. Overall, the test appears to be adequately reliable. Test-retest reliability coefficients range from a low of .79 (Arithmetic, Level 2) to .97 (Spelling, Level 1). Most coefficients exceed .92.

*Validity.* Again, the chapter on validity in the 1978 test manual does not include a single study using the 1978 norms. A factor analytical study is presented, but no reference is made as to which set of norms was used. Furthermore, the report on this study is so enmeshed in jargon unique to the authors (for example, *cobals, obals*) as to be virtually uninterpretable.

To investigate the predictive validity of the Stanford-Binet, Bossard and Galusha (1979) used the WRAT (1978 revision) as a criterion. Using a sample of students referred for psychological evaluation, they reported correlation coefficients of .79, .81, and .77 between the Stanford-Binet and the WRAT Reading, Spelling, and Arithmetic subtests, respectively. Intercorrelation coefficients between the WRAT subtests ranged from a high of .93 between WRAT Reading and WRAT Arithmetic to a low of .83 between WRAT Reading and WRAT Spelling. Because of these high intersubtest relationships, the user should exercise caution in assuming that the subtests are measuring unique abilities. Prasse, Siewert, and Breen (1983) found that WRAT Reading subtest scores were significantly higher than the Word Identification and Total Reading scores from the Woodcock Reading Mastery Test, for both learning disabled and regular education students. Such differences must be considered if placement decisions are involved.

Several studies (Brock, 1982; Grossman & Johnson, 1982; Wright, 1987) have investigated the factorial structure of the WISC-R and various achievement tests, including the WRAT. One finding of interest was that the traditional third factor on the WISC-R, or the freedom from distractibility factor (Arithmetic, Coding, and Digit Span), perhaps is not unitary. Wright's findings suggest that one aspect of the factor is numerical. The WRAT Arithmetic subtest weighted most heavily on that factor. The other possible component of the factor was written language, and the WRAT Reading and Spelling subtests weighted most heavily on that factor. An additional finding of these studies was that although there is substantial overlap between measures of intelligence and achievement, they are not identical constructs.

*Summary.* The 1984 revision appears to be considerably improved over previous versions. However the usefulness of the test is reduced because only limited aspects of reading and arithmetic were sampled.

### KAUFMAN ASSESSMENT BATTERY FOR CHILDREN —THE ACHIEVEMENT SCALE

(Kaufman, A. S., & Kaufman, N. L., 1983, American Guidance Service)

The Kaufman Assessment Battery for Children (KABC) is an individually administered test of intelligence and achievement. The test of intelligence, which is made up of the Mental Processing Scales, is discussed in Chapter 4. The purpose of the Achievement Scale is to "assess factual knowledge and skills usually acquired in a school setting or through alertness to the environment" (p. 33). Six subtests make up the Achievement Scale.

The Expressive Vocabulary subtest was designed for children aged two years, six months through four years, eleven months. In this subtest the child is required to name an object shown in a photograph.

The Faces and Places subtest requires children aged two years, six months to twelve years, five months, to name photographs and drawings of well-known places, people, or fictional characters.

The Arithmetic subtest is for use with children aged three years through twelve years, five months. It assesses knowledge of numbers, counting, computational skills, and mathematical concepts. All the items are cleverly presented in a zoo setting.

The Riddles subtest requires the children to infer the name of a concrete or abstract concept from a list of its characteristics. Riddles given to children aged two years through twelve years, five months.

The Reading/Decoding subtest is given only to children five years through twelve years, five months of age. They are asked to identify letters and read words.

The Reading/Understanding subtest demonstrates the children's comprehension as shown by their ability to follow commands given orally by the examiner.

Each of the subtests and the Global Achievement Scale provide a standard score with a mean of 100 and standard deviation of 15. Percentile ranks and stanines, based on the national norming group, are available. For the Global Achievement Scale and all achievement subtests except Expressive Vocabulary, sociocultural percentile ranks for a sample of 1569 whites and 807 blacks are also available. These norms take into consideration the child's race (black or white) and socioeconomic background (the parents' educations are indicated as being on one of three levels). Supplementary norms for out-of-level testing at ages 4½ and 5 years are also provided.

*Standardization.* The KABC was standardized on 100 children at each half-year of age between two years, six months and twelve years, five months. These 2000 children were stratified on the variables of sex, ethnic group, parental education, geographic region, community size, and educational placement. About 7% of the total sample (138 children) were attending full- or part-time special education classes. Six categories of handicap are represented in the normative sample. These categories represented the educational-placement stratification.

*Reliability.* Internal consistency was evaluated with split-half procedures. For the Achievement subtest and the Global Achievement Scale means, split-half reliabilities for the preschool sample ranged from a low of .77, on Faces and Places, to a high of .87, on Arithmetic. For the school-age sample the mean coefficients ranged from a low of .84, on Faces and Places, to a high of .92, on Reading/Decoding. Most coefficients for both groups were in the .80s and .90s. Test-retest reliabilities, with a mean inter-test interval of eighteen days, ranged from .72 (Riddles) to .87 (Arithmetic) for students ages two years, six months through four years, eleven months; for administrations to those aged five years through eight years, eleven months, the coefficients ranged from a low of .87, on Riddles, to a high of .98, on Reading/Decoding. When the test was administered to those aged nine years through twelve years, five months, the range of coefficients was .90 (Riddles) to .94 (Reading/Decoding). Mean standard errors of measurement for preschool children ranged from 5.4 (Arithmetic) to 7.2 on Faces and Places. For school-aged children the mean standard errors of measurement ranged from 4.0 (Reading/Decoding) to 5.9 (Faces and Places).

*Validity.* The manual reports numerous studies in which the KABC is shown to have substantial relationships with the WISC-R and the Stanford-Binet. Subjects in these studies included a wide age range of normal subjects, handicapped children, and culturally different children.

In the studies with the WISC-R, the Global Achievement Scale score correlated highest with the Verbal IQ. A number of predictive validity studies of the relationship between the Global Achievement score and achievement tests such as the PIAT, Iowa Test of Basic Skills, and the California Achievement Tests obtained correlations that ranged from .67 (Total PIAT) to .89 (Composite Iowa Test of Basic Skills). Intervals between the administration of the KABC and the criterion tests ranged from six to twelve months. Naglieri (1985), in a study of predictive validity, administered the KABC and the McCarthy Scale of Children's Ability. Three months

later the PIAT was administered to the same group of normal subjects. The KABC Achievement Scale was the best predictor of the PIAT Total score ($R = .75$). Murray and Bracken (1984) evaluated the ability of the KABC to predict scores on the PIAT in a group of normal subjects. They found that after an eleven-month interval, there were high and significant correlations between the Global Achievement score and all the PIAT subtests. They also found the mean scores to be nearly identical.

A concurrent-validity study of the KABC Achievement subtests, the Passage Comprehension subtest of the Woodcock Reading Mastery Test, and the Written Computation subtest of the KeyMath Test, shows that the Passage Comprehension subtest is highly related to both the Reading/Decoding and Reading/Understanding subtests. Interestingly the KeyMath Written Computation subtest has a slightly lower correlation with the KABC Arithmetic subtest than does the Woodcock Passage Comprehension subtest.

Naglieri and Haddad (1984) analyzed learning-disabled children's performance on the KABC, PIAT, and WRAT. KABC Global Achievement score was significantly related to all PIAT and WRAT subtests, and the mean KABC Achievement score did not differ significantly from the mean PIAT Total score or those of any of the WRAT subtests. Zins and Barnett (1983) studied the relationships between the KABC Achievement subtests and the WRAT subtests in a group of nonreferred subjects. The correlations were generally significant but somewhat low, except for the reading subtests of both scales. The KABC Arithmetic score had a lower correlation with the WRAT Arithmetic score than with the WRAT reading score. The difference was not significant, but it suggests that perhaps the Arithmetic subtest is not measuring number concepts specifically.

Hooper and Hynd (1986) evaluated the ability of the KABC to discriminate between normal and matched dyslexic readers. Normal readers produced significantly higher scores on each

Achievement subtest, and on the Global, Sequential, and Achievement scores.

**Computer-Assisted Scoring.** The Automated System for Scoring and Interpreting Standardized Tests (ASSIST) is available for the KABC. The program, available from American Guidance Services, provides standard scores, confidence intervals on standard scores, national and/or sociocultural percentile ranks, percentile intervals corresponding to the confidence intervals, age equivalents, classifications and global scale comparisons (Krug, 1987).

**Summary.** The KABC Achievement Scale is well standardized. The manual presents more studies on various aspects of reliability and validity than most tests acquire after years of availability. Users can evaluate the adequacy of the test for use on nearly any group they wish to assess.

### KAUFMAN TEST OF EDUCATIONAL ACHIEVEMENT (KTEA)

(Kaufman, A. S., & Kaufman, N. L., 1985, American Guidance Service)

The KTEA is a norm-referenced test of school achievement of children and adolescents in grades one through twelve. This individually administered test provides both age-based (six years through eighteen years, eleven months) and grade-based norms. A Brief Form evaluates performance in the global areas of reading, mathematics, and spelling. The focus of this discussion will be on the Comprehensive Form, which offers subtests in Reading Decoding, Reading Comprehension, Mathematics Applications, and Spelling. Various combinations of subtest scores offer reading, mathematics, and battery-composite scores. These standard scores have a mean of 100 and a standard deviation of 15 and are available for both fall (August–January) and spring (February–July) testing. In addition to standard scores, age equivalents, grade equivalents, and percentiles, normal-curve equivalents are also provided. In addition to the norm-referenced scores, criterion-referenced assessment is provided in

the analysis of student's errors on the various subtests. These analyses should provide insight into the precise nature of the child's errors.

**Standardization.** The standardization program was conducted in 1983, in school districts in twenty-five sites. The sample consisted of 2476 children; 1270 were females and 1206 were males. In the spring testing there were 1409 subjects and in the fall, 1067. The stratification variables included grade, sex, geographic region, parental education level, and race or ethnic group. Secondary stratification variables were age and educational placement. Students in special-education classes were included in the pool of students eligible for standardization testing. However, no effort was made to determine the actual percentage of children in special-education classes who were included in the standardization sample.

**Reliability.** Split-half reliability coefficients were used to determine the degree of internal consistency. Mean coefficients for all ages and all grades were .90 or higher. Coefficients for the composite scores were even higher. Test-retest reliability was also excellent. Data for grades one to six and grades seven to twelve were combined. For the subtests all coefficients exceeded .82. For the composites all coefficients exceeded .92.

Standard errors of measurement are in the 3- to 5-point range for the separate subtests. Standard errors of measurement for the Reading and Mathematics composites are in the 3- to 4-point range whether grouped by age or by grade, and the error of measurement for the battery composite for grade and age does not exceed 2.4 points. These data strongly support the reliability of this test.

**Validity.** Considerable effort was made to ensure the content validity of the test; however, the match between the content of the test and individual school curricula is the key consideration for content validity. The test authors have done their work; now the test users must do theirs. Criterion validity was assessed by the examination of the relationships between the KTEA and the KABC, PIAT, and WRAT. For additional analysis, current scores on the Stanford Achievement Tests, Comprehensive Test of Basic Skills, and Metropolitan Achievement Test were available for relatively small samples. Correlations between the KTEA and the WRAT were lowest for testing of normative subjects in grades one to three; the highest correlations were between the WRAT Reading scores and KTEA Reading Decoding (.67), Reading Comprehension (.62), and Reading Composite (.65). Correlations were higher in tests of higher grade groups. For example, with testing of subjects in grades ten to twelve, the correlations with Reading Decoding were .90, Reading Comprehension (.78), and Reading Composite (.89). Trends were similar with the Mathematics subtests; however, correlations were consistently lower than the reading correlations at all levels. Spelling correlations were consistently high beyond grade three.

The sample of subjects who were administered the PIAT and KTEA was small and ranged across grades one to twelve. Correlations between the mathematics subtests on both instruments ranged from .63 to .75. Between Reading Recognition and Reading Comprehension subtests, correlations ranged from .73 to .84. The correlation between the spelling subtests was .78. Correlations of the PIAT General Information subtest with the KTEA subtests and composites ranged from .41 (Mathematics Computation) to .88 (Reading Composite).

Subjects who were administered the KTEA and KABC were divided into two age groups: ages six to eight years, and ages nine to twelve years. Correlations of Global Achievement scores from the KABC and the KTEA subtests and composites for both age groups ranged from .51 (Mathematics Computation and Spelling, group aged nine to twelve years) to .84 (Battery Composite, group aged six to eight years and Reading Composite, group aged nine to twelve years). Results for the group tests are similar to the individual tests. Reading correlations were highest between the KTEA and the Stanford Achievement Test. In Mathematics the correlations were highest with the Comprehensive Test of Basic Skills.

*Summary.* The KTEA appears to be a well-constructed, well-standardized test of educational achievement. Overall reading scores appear to have the highest correlations with other selected tests. The test would have been strengthened considerably, if it had included language subtests and a language composite. Reliability appears to be excellent. As with the other achievement tests, the key question about its validity for most school districts will be answered by determining how well the test's content matches the local school curriculum.

### WOODCOCK-JOHNSON PSYCHO-EDUCATIONAL BATTERY (WJA)

(Woodcock, R. W., & Johnson, M. B., 1977, DLM-Teaching Resources)

The WJA is a multitest battery that integrates tests of cognitive ability, scholastic aptitude, academic achievement, and interest. Part Two, Tests of Academic Achievement, is the focus of this discussion.

Part Two consists of ten subtests that assess five areas or clusters of academic achievement. The Reading Cluster consists of the Letter-Word Identification, Word Attack, and Passage Comprehension subtests. The Calculation and Applied Problems subtests make up the Mathematics Cluster. The Written Language Cluster is made up of two subtests, Dictation and Proofing. The Knowledge Cluster includes the Science, Social Studies, and Humanities subtests. The Skills Cluster is made up of the Letter-Word Identification, Applied Problems, and Dictation subtests, all of which are also part of other clusters. According to Hessler (1984) the Skills Cluster subtests assess preschool level skills, but they are also suitable for older subjects as well. The subtests were normed on subjects aged three to adulthood (aged 57 years and more).

A large number of derived scores are available for the WJA. These include part and cluster scores, grade and age equivalents, instructional range, percentile rank scores, and relative-performance index scores (this index will be discussed in detail in the review of the WRMT-R), standard scores ($M = 100$, $SD = 15$, $M = 50$, $SD = 10$), stanine scores, and normal-curve equivalent scores. The examiner is not required to use all of these scores, but one criticism of the WJA has been the significant amount of time necessary for calculation of the scores that are necessary for an adequate analysis of performance (Estabrook, 1983).

One solution is the use of Compuscore for the Woodcock-Johnson Psycho-Educational Battery (Deemer, 1985). According to the manual, one protocol can be computer-scored in about five minutes, not including the time needed for the entry of raw scores. The result is a two-page printout containing personal information and a complete analysis of each cluster.

*Standardization.* The WJA was standardized with use of a three-stage, stratified, random-sampling design. The stratification variables included race, sex, parental occupational status, type of community, and geographic region. Educational placement was not a major consideration in selecting subjects; this decision is unfortunate because the WJA is frequently used in the making of placement decisions. Although the match with 1970 U.S. Census data is close, persons designated as nonurban and living in the South and Northeast were underrepresented in the normative sample. To achieve a more precise match with the census data, the authors used a proportional weighting procedure. Testing of the normative sample occurred between April, 1976, and March, 1977. The sample included 4732 subjects in 49 communities. Of the total sample, 555 were preschoolers, three to five years of age; 3577 were school-age children, six to seventeen years of age; 503 subjects were eighteen to sixty-four years of age; and 97 were over sixty-four years old.

*Reliability.* Split-half reliabilities, corrected by the Spearman-Brown formula, were used to assess internal consistency. Median correlations ranged from .78 on Capitalization, a subsection of the Proofing subtest, to .92 on the Word Attack subtest. The clusters' reliabilities are higher, with median reliabilities in the .90s. Unfortunately the technical data are not in the manual, but in a separate publication (Woodcock, 1978).

*Validity.* Content validity is claimed primarily on the basis of careful construction of the test and item-selection procedures. Hall, Reeve, and Zakreski (1984) examined the concurrent validity of the WJA used with two independent samples of learning-disabled subjects. Subjects were given the WJA, PIAT, and WRAT. Correlations with the PIAT ranged from .51 to .93; and with the WRAT subtests, from .49 to .92. Highest correlations were found among the reading subtests. These authors concluded that, according to their results, the WJA was technically adequate in regard to concurrent validity.

In another study of concurrent validity, Breen, Lehman, and Carlson (1984) administered the WJA reading and mathematics subtests, Key-Math, and WRMT to a group of thirty-two elementary-aged, learning-disabled subjects. They obtained significant correlations among both grade-equivalent and standard scores (range, .79 to .93). Mean grade-equivalent scores were significantly different for the two reading tests and the mathematics tests. However, the reading tests' standard scores were not significantly different. Because the KeyMath manual does not describe conversions from raw to standard scores, it was not possible to assess the difference in mathematics standard scores. Examiners should be cautious in treating these subtests as equivalent.

Woodcock (1978) also reported concurrent-validity studies with the PIAT, WRAT, WRMT, KeyMath, and the total reading score of the Iowa Test of Basic Skills across four groups of subjects. Most of the coefficients are in the .70s to .90s across the Reading, Mathematics, and Written Language Clusters. One study with severely learning-disabled subjects was reported. The subjects were given the WJA, PIAT, KeyMath, and WRAT Spelling subtest. Overall correlations are somewhat lower than in the studies with nonhandicapped subjects, but the highest coefficients were between the subtests with similar content, as would be expected. They ranged from .59 to .84.

*Summary.* The WJA appears to be generally a well-standardized test. Reliability and validity are satisfactory. However, examiners must understand that no two tests measure exactly the same thing. Again, the usefulness of this test to a particular school district in assessing student progress and determining program quality depends on the extent to which the content of the test matches the curriculum of that school district.

# DIAGNOSTIC READING TESTS

### WOODCOCK READING MASTERY TESTS-REVISED (WRMT-R), FORMS G AND H

(Woodcock, R. W., 1987, American Guidance Service)

WRMT-R is a comprehensive battery of tests of reading achievement. This revision of the 1973 edition was renormed on students in grades from kindergarten to college senior and with adults to age seventy-five years. Form G contains four tests of reading achievement (Word Identification, Word Attack, Word Comprehension, and Passage Comprehension), a readiness section (Visual-Auditory Learning) and Letter Identification, a two-part Supplementary Checklist. Form H only contains the four reading achievement subtests. Forms G and H provide a record form to be used if both Forms G and H are administered, so that greater precision and more material for error analysis are obtained.

The Test Record includes not only a place in which the subject's responses and scores but also three types of profiles (Instructional Level, Diagnostic, and Percentile Rank) can be recorded. Also included are a Word Attack Error Inventory and a Summary of Scores.

*Types of Scores.* "W scores are the result of a mathematical transformation of raw scores into Rasch-based ability scores. The W score has been so designed that users will not need to

work with negative numbers" (Woodcock, 1987, p. 38).

A difference score is based on the level of the subject's W score in relation to the W score that is the reference score for the particular grade or age with which the subject is being compared. The difference score is obtained by subtracting the subject's W score from the reference W score.

The grade equivalent (GE) score is the median score earned by subjects in the norming group in a particular grade. These scores are made more useful by the addition of an extended GE scale. Subscripts that indicate the percentile rank are added to extend the scale, beyond the beginning kindergarten (K.O) and college-senior level (16.9) GE scores. A superscript is attached to a kindergarten GE when a below-average performance is beneath the normal range; a superscript can also be attached to a college-senior GE score, when above-average performance places a score beyond the grade scale. Like the GE scores, age equivalent (AE) scores are the median scores made by norming subjects at a particular age level. An extended AE scale also provides AE scores for the youngest and oldest subjects who perform below or above those ages, respectively. Traditional scores such as percentile ranks (and extended percentile ranks), standard scores ($M = 100$, $SD = 15$), T scores, stanines, and normal curve equivalents are also available.

A relative performance index (RPI) indicates the percentage of mastery by a particular subject on a group of tasks that a specified reference group (generally average individuals at the same age or grade level as the subject) would perform at 90% mastery. This score is presented as the subject's percentage "over" 90% (e.g. 40/90). The RPI in the example indicates that the subject could be expected to perform at 40% mastery on a task that age or grade peers would perform with 90% mastery.

An Automated System for Scoring and Interpreting Standardized Tests (ASSIST), a scoring program designed for minicomputer use, is available. Data on the subject and the raw scores are entered into the program, which computes all the derived scores. Such programs are useful in reducing clerical errors and they reduce substantially the time required to complete the scoring.

*Subtests/Clusters.* In addition to the individual subtest scores, five cluster scores (Readiness Cluster, Basic Skills Cluster, Reading Comprehension Cluster, Total Reading—Full Scale Cluster, and Total Reading—Short Scale Cluster) may be obtained; these are useful for more global interpretation.

The Visual-Auditory Learning subtest, one of two tests included in the Readiness Cluster Score, is found in Form G only. In this subtest the subject learns a vocabulary of rebuses (unfamiliar visual symbols), which represent familiar words. Then the subject must translate sequences of rebuses into sentences.

Also included only in Form G, the Letter Identification subtest assesses the subject's ability to identify letters presented in both upper and lower cases and in various typestyles including cursive. The examiner may ask the child to respond either with the name of the letter or its most common sound, or both in separate administrations.

Form G includes the complete test battery of four tests of reading achievement (Word Identification, Word Attack, Word Comprehension, and Passage Comprehension), a readiness section that includes two readiness tests (Visual-Auditory Learning and Letter Identification), and a Supplementary Letter Checklist (Capital Letters and Lowercase Letters). Form H contains only the four reading achievement subtests; the readiness tests and the supplementary checklists are not included.

The Basic Skills cluster includes the Word Identification and Word Attack subtests. On the Word Identification subtest the subject is required to provide the correct reading of the word. The Word Attack subtest is made up of nonsense words and words with a very low frequency of usage in English. To pronounce

the words correctly, the child is consequently forced to use phonetic and structural analysis skills, in the absence of semantic content. Errors may be analyzed on the Word-Attack Error Inventory, which is similar to the GFW Sound-Symbol subtest, Reading of Symbols error inventory, described previously. Administration of both the Form G and Form H increases the reliability of the Inventory.

Word Comprehension and Passage Comprehension make up the Reading Comprehension Cluster. Word Comprehension includes three subtests: Antonyms, Synonyms, and Analogies. Theoretically these subtests measure reading vocabulary at three different levels of complexity, with Analogies at the highest level and Antonyms at the lowest level of complexity. Raw scores may be calculated for four specific reading vocabularies: general reading vocabulary, science-mathematics vocabulary, social studies vocabulary, and humanities vocabulary. Word Comprehension is a very comprehensive measure of vocabulary.

Passage Comprehension uses a modified cloze procedure. The subject is required to read a short passage silently and identify a word that has been omitted. The first one-third of the items contain only one sentence and include pictures that convey information helpful to the subject. These items make it possible to assess reading comprehension as it is taught in the early grades.

The total reading–short-scale cluster score provides an estimate of global reading ability, based on the scores of the Word Identification and Passage Comprehension subtests.

The total reading–full-scale cluster score is a combination of the four reading achievement subtests (Word Identification, Word Attack, Word Comprehension, and Passage Comprehension) and can be regarded as a global measure of reading ability. Administration of these subtests takes about 30 minutes.

A report to parents is available. It contains test results, an explanation of the subject's performance, and a brief description of the WRMT-R subtests and clusters. This report should be very useful in helping the parents understand the test and their child's performance. Chapter 4 in the manual includes a step-by-step procedure for the analysis of the subject's performance in relation to instructional planning.

Seven case studies are also included in the manual. Appendix 2 presents a criterion-referenced scale of selected items by subtest and by grade. Our discussion and Appendix 2 should be important aids for the diagnostician conveying test results and their implications for instruction to the child's teacher.

*Standardization.* Normative data for the WRMT-R are based on the performance of 6089 subjects, 4201 in the K through 12.9 sample, 1023 subjects in the college/university sample, and 865 subjects in the adult sample. The school-aged sample was stratified according to census region, community size (outside-urban subjects but no rural subjects were included), sex, and race. Educational placement was not one of the stratification variables. This is unfortunate because it is likely that the WRMT-R will be used extensively with handicapped children. Stratification variables for the college sample included census regions, sex, race, college (public or private) and college (universities, other 4-year, and 2-year). The adult sample included all of the variables except college in the stratification. Data on school-aged subjects were collected continuously over a two-year period, data on college/university subjects were collected from March to November, and data on adults were gathered from February to November, so that continuous-year data were collected. This procedure minimizes the error variance that is due to the combining of data collected over a period of time within a particular grade or year of age.

Because the various profiles can include data from the GFW Sound-Symbol Test and the Woodcock-Johnson Psycho-Educational Battery, 600 of the norming subjects were given these tests as well as the WRMT-R. Such equating studies make it possible for examiners to make direct comparisons between the scores from these tests.

*Reliability.* Internal-consistency reliabilities were calculated by use of the split-half (odd-even) procedure and corrected for length by use of the Spearman-Brown formula. Reliabilities were obtained on all forms and for all subtest and cluster scores, of subjects in grades one, three, five, eight, and eleven, in college, and for adults. Coefficients ranged from .68 to .99 on all subtests and clusters, except Letter Identification at grade five (.34); this coefficient undoubtedly is the result of a ceiling effect. Most coefficients were in the .90s. Standard errors of measurement also appeared to be satisfactory. No test-retest reliabilities are reported in the manual and none were found in the literature.

*Validity.* Claims for content validity are based on the fact that experienced teachers and curriculum specialists were consulted in the selection and evaluation of content, and that classical item-selection procedures were used in the early stages and the Rasch model of item selection was used in the later stages. Only one study of concurrent validity using the WRMT-R is included in the manual.

The Word Identification subtest scores of subjects in grades one, three, five, and eight were correlated to scores from the Woodcock-Johnson tests of Letter-Word Identification, Word Attack, Passage Comprehension and Total Reading. These correlations ranged from .48 (Grade 1, Word Attack) to .86 (Total Reading, Grade 3). The WRMT-R Word Attack subtest scores were also correlated to scores from the Woodcock-Johnson tests; correlations ranged from .57 (Letter-Word Identification, Grade 1) to .90 (Word Attack, Grade 5). Overall the correlations between the Word Attack and the Woodcock-Johnson tests' scores were only moderate. For Word Comprehension the correlations with Woodcock-Johnson tests ranged from .27 (Word Attack, Grade 8) to .82 (Passage Comprehension, Grade 1). Correlations among Passage Comprehension scores and Woodcock-Johnson scores ranged from .25

(Word Attack, Grade 8) to .71 (Total Reading, Grade 3). Most of these correlations were moderate to low. Correlations of or between the Full-Scale and Short Scale scores ranged from .48 to .91. Most correlations exceeded .70.

*Summary.* The WRMT-R appears to be well normed, and the test has many useful features to aid in the planning of instruction. The error analyses and the criterion-referenced interpretation available on selected items are among the most useful features. Test-retest reliability is unknown, and this unknown is a major shortcoming. Concurrent validity studies are also needed. The study included in the manual is only moderately supportive.

## DIAGNOSTIC ARITHMETIC TESTS

### KEYMATH DIAGNOSTIC ARITHMETIC TEST (KEYMATH)

(Connolly, R. G., Nachtman, W., and Pritchett, E. M., 1976, American Guidance Service)

The KeyMath (Connolly, Nachtman, & Pritchett, 1976) is one of the tests described in Chapter 2 as a criterion-referenced test. Because standardization data are also available, it must also be considered a norm-referenced test. The fourteen subtests of the KeyMath are divided into three general areas (Table 7-4).

According to the test manual, four levels of diagnostic data are provided. Total-test performance provides grade-level placement information. Organization of the subtests into three major categories purportedly allows the examiner to obtain information on area performance. Data are obviously available for each subtest, and subtest items are also grouped into instructional clusters. Unfortunately, items in the cluster often cover a wide range of difficulty, and consequently the clusters are not especially useful to the planning of instruction. Finally, item information is provided by a description of each item in a behavioral-objective format. This information is most helpful for the formulation of instructional procedures.

The test items use an open-ended format. Oral responses are required except in the computation subtests of addition, subtraction, multiplication, and division. Approximately 30 minutes are required to administer the test.

Subjects' responses are recorded directly on the Diagnostic Profile, which has several helpful characteristics. The Profile makes it possible for the examiner to see at a glance the grade placement of each item. Standard errors of measure for each subtest's raw score are provided on the Diagnostic Profile. A brief description of each item is also included. This allows the examiner to evaluate the items passed and failed without having to turn back to the test kit each time. Only grade equivalent scores are provided.

*Standardization.* The original item pool was drawn from the doctoral dissertations of the three authors of the test. Subjects were educable, mentally handicapped children. To expand

Table 7-4
Organization of the KeyMath Diagnostic Arithmetic Test.

| Content | Operations | Applications |
|---|---|---|
| Numeration | Addition | Word Problems |
| Fractions | Subtraction | Missing Elements |
| Geometry and Symbols | Multiplication | Money |
| | Division | Measurement |
| | Mental Computation | Time |
| | Numerical Reasoning | |

this item pool, the authors consulted ten major textbook series in mathematics. Each item met five criteria. The item had to "possess a wide range of difficulty . . . minimize the effect of guessing . . . minimize reading and writing . . . focus on functional mathematics . . . possess a maximum of instructional utility" (Connolly, Nachtman, & Pritchett, 1976, p. 22).

The final item pool of 400 questions was tested on 320 children in kindergarten and grades one, three, and five. Data from this study were analyzed by the Rasch-Wright procedures (Rasch, 1960; Wright, 1968). The calibration study included 951 subjects in kindergarten through grade eight, from five states. The norming study with a subset of the calibrated items included 1222 subjects in kindergarten through grade seven, from eight states in four of the nine census divisions (Bureau of the Census, 1967). Data are presented on race and community size. When these data deviated from the census proportions, variables were weighted to bring them into conformance. Grade-equivalent scores are provided up to and beyond grade 9.5 on the Diagnostic Profile. Placement beyond grade seven should be interpreted cautiously, because there were no subjects beyond grade eight in the calibration study and none beyond grade seven in the norming study.

*Reliability.* Split-half reliability coefficients are given in the test manual for testing of subjects in kindergarten through grade seven. Subtest coefficients range from .23 to .90. Median coefficients by subtest across grade level ranged from .64 for Mental Computation and Word Problems to .84 for Measurement. However coefficients by grade ranged across subtests from .94 to .97.

In most cases the low reliabilities are a result of the small number of appropriate items at a particular grade level. For example, the .23 reliability coefficient is at grade two on the Division subtest. The three problems necessary to establish a ceiling are located between preschool level and grade three.

The test authors recommend that "bands of confidence" be used in interpretation. Instructions are given in the test manual for plotting these standard-error-of-measurement "bands of confidence." No test-retest reliabilities on the final version of the test are reported in the test manual or in the literature.

*Validity.* Claims for content validity are based primarily on the fact that 3000 youngsters were tested at various stages of test development and that many item and procedural revisions were based on the results of these assessments. Colorful materials, a variety of tasks, and basal and ceiling procedures are cited as evidence of face validity.

A few concurrent validity studies have been reported in the literature, but they have generally involved handicapped youngsters. Tinney (1975) found that total scores on the California Achievement Test (CAT) (Arithmetic) and KeyMath were significantly related in a learning-disabled sample. Some support for the major areas (Content and Application combined) was indicated, although the results were inadequately reported and conclusions are difficult to draw from the narrative.

Greenstein and Strain (1977) also conducted an extensive study of KeyMath with learning-disabled adolescents from special-education schools. Subjects ranged from twelve to seventeen years of age with an equal distribution across the ages. In addition, Greenstein and Strain had access to protocols from the standardization sample for purposes of comparison.

A factor analysis revealed two factors. Factor one included all the Operations subtests plus the Content subtest, and Geometry and Symbols. Factor two included all the Applications subtests, and Numeration and Fractions subtests from the Content area. The most significant finding of this study is the identification of error patterns listed in Figure 7-1. The errors of learning-disabled subjects are seen to be significantly different from the errors of normal subjects.

The psychometric properties of the KeyMath test were examined in testing of a large sample of young, educable, mentally handicapped students (Goodstein, Kahn, & Cawley, 1976). Support was found for the sequence-of-item difficulties within the subtests; only 13 of 209 items were improperly placed by this sample. The Geometry and Symbols, and Time subtests showed the most deviations from the standardization sample. Although the sequencing appeared appropriate for this group, Goodstein, Kahn, and Cawley reported "numerous gaps in difficulty between subtest items" (p. 68). Fourteen unique factors were derived from a factor analysis supporting the fourteen subtests. This finding is widely at variance with the Greenstein and Strain (1977) factor analysis with learning-disabled adolescents. Although there is no means of comparing the data, to obtain a factor per subtest when only one test is used is quite unique. Only minimal support was obtained for the major concept areas of Content, Operations, and Applications.

Powers and Pace (1976) investigated the relationship between KeyMath and the Level 1 Arithmetic subtest on the WRAT, in thirty young, educable, mentally handicapped youngsters. The fourteen KeyMath subtests accounted for 91% of the variance of the WRAT Arithmetic subtest.

Correlations between individual subtests of the KeyMath and WRAT ranged from .40 (Missing Elements) to .86 (Numeration). Obviously, the WRAT Arithmetic subtest does not contain the counterparts of some KeyMath subtests (Powers & Pace, 1976).

Despite the test manual's suggestion that data on area performance would provide diagnostic information, the results of these studies overall do not support training based on the Content, Operations, and Applications subtest groupings.

In a study of the predictive validity of the KeyMath, Kratochwill and Demuth (1976) studied the performance of mainstreamed six-year-olds

| Defective algorithm | $\begin{array}{r} 66 \\ +4 \\ \hline 1010 \end{array}$ |
| Computational error | $\begin{array}{r} 94 \\ -42 \\ \hline 42 \end{array}$ |
| Spatial error | $\begin{array}{r} 34 \\ +31 \\ \hline 5 \\ \\ 6 \end{array}$ |
| Subtraction problem reversal | $\begin{array}{r} 25 \\ -16 \\ \hline 11 \end{array}$ |
| Detail | $\begin{array}{r} \$5.09 \\ -2.00 \\ \hline \$3\ 09 \end{array}$ |

**Figure 7-1**

Types of errors by learning-disabled adolescents on the KeyMath Diagnostic Arithmetic Test. (Adapted from Greenstein, J., & Strain, P. S. The utility of the KeyMath Diagnostic Arithmetic Test for adolescent learning disabled students. *Psychology in the Schools,* 1977, *14,* pp. 275–282. Copyright 1977 Clinical Psychology Publishing Company, Inc., Brandon, Vermont.)

in a Title I program. KeyMath and the WRAT Arithmetic subtest were administered in the fall, and the arithmetic subtests from the Metropolitan Achievement Test (MAT) were given in the spring. Correlations between the WRAT and MAT were not significant, while the KeyMath correlated .63 with the MAT. Word Problems (.53), Numerical Reasoning (.45), and Money (.44) demonstrated the highest subtest correlations.

*Summary.* The KeyMath is a very useful tool for identifying specific mathematical difficulties in samples of handicapped children. Although the data are limited, it would appear to be more useful with learning-disabled than with educable, mentally handicapped subjects.

## KEYMATH-REVISED, A DIAGNOSTIC INVENTORY OF ESSENTIAL MATHEMATICS (KEYMATH-R)

(Connolly, 1988, American Guidance Service)

American Guidance Service has announced a revision of the KeyMath (KeyMath-R), which will be available in 1988. The revision is designed to assess the subject's understanding and application of important mathematical concepts and skills, in three content areas: Basic Concepts, Operations, and Applications. Basic Concepts includes the Numeration, Rational Numbers, and Geometry subtests. Addition, Subtraction, Multiplication, Division, and Mental Computation subtests make up the Operations area. The Applications area consists of the subtests of Measurement, Time and Money, Estimation, Interpreting Data, and Problem Solving. These thirteen subtests can be individually administered in a total of 35 to 50 minutes.

Diagnostic information is available for total test, area, subtest, and domain. Information about the student's strengths and weaknesses is provided by a careful analysis of performance in the domains. Standard scores ($M = 100$, $SD = 15$), age and grade equivalents, percentile ranks, stanines, and normal-curve equivalents are provided for the three area composites and the total test. For the subtests, scaled scores ($M = 10$, $SD = 3$), percentile ranks, stanines, and normal-curve equivalents are provided.

To reduce the time needed and possible errors made in calculating the derived scores, an optional KeyMath-R ASSIST software package is available. In less than five minutes, the program will produce a score summary and profile, and a descriptive report of the subject's strengths and weaknesses.

KeyMath-R includes a number of changes and improvements over the earlier edition. The range of the test extends from kindergarten through grade nine. Fall and spring norms, which allow a more accurate assessment of beginning- and end-of-school-year performance, are included. Also, the revision is available in two forms (A and B) that make the test more useful for research requiring pre- and post-testing.

Standardization was done in the fall of 1985 and spring of 1986. To ensure a nationally representative sample, selection was based on the latest U.S. Census. The normative sample was stratified on the variables of geographic region, grade, sex, socioeconomic level, and race. Educational placement was not one of the stratification variables. This is unfortunate because the test will probably be used extensively with handicapped subjects.

## SUMMARY

A number of new and revised tests of academic achievement have been published since the first edition of this book. In general these tests represent an improvement in quality. The value of a test is dependent on whether it measures the material to which the subject has been exposed, whether it is administered correctly, and whether interpretation is consistent with the purpose and within the limitations of the instrument. Examiners must keep in mind that a test is no more than a brief observation of behavior in a standardized but contrived situation.

# CHAPTER 8

# Behavioral Assessment

## OUTLINE

Levels of inference
Key generalizations
Contingent relationships
Observing and recording
Phases of behavioral assessment
Summary

**B**ehavioral assessment, broadly conceived, is the identification of meaningful child-response units and their "controlling variables (both current environmental and organismic—individual differences produced by physiology and past learning) for the purposes of understanding and altering human behavior" (Nelson & Hayes, 1979, p. 49). Implicit in the notion of assessment is that it is a purposeful process directed at some intervention goal rather than an end in and of itself (Kampus, 1987). From this conceptualization comes the basic reason for assessing or diagnosing children: to obtain information that can be used to plan a treatment program. Our focus, then, is on the consideration of the kinds of data that help teachers develop and guide treatment programs.

Several authors (Coulter, 1980; Ollendick & Hersen, 1984) have noted that behavioral assessment and traditional assessment (diagnostic-prescriptive) share similar techniques (for example, observations, informal testing, questionnaires, interviewing). However, as noted in Chapter 1, the two approaches differ radically in their assumptions and levels of inference (Hawkins, 1979; Keller, 1986). In traditional assessment, behavior is viewed as a sign of rather stable intraorganismic variables (perceptual-motor), whereas behavioral assessment views behavior as a sample of responses made in a particular assessment situation (Ollendick & Hersen, 1984; Mash and Terdal, 1976; Lentz & Shapiro, 1986).

In assessment these distinctions refer to two types of test behaviors: those that are in themselves representative of the criterion behavior (for example, spelling words as a sample of achievement ability) versus test behaviors that have no intrinsic or necessary relationship to the criterion (for example, projective information). Test behavior scored for thematic content, for example, is topographically dissimilar from the criterion behaviors subsequently needed for change (actual spelling performance). In behavioral assessment, the sample of responses has meaning only in a particular assessment situation. Unless the interaction between individual children and program variables is assessed, little can be done toward determining the child's problem and how to change it for the better.

## LEVELS OF INFERENCE

Direct analysis of behavior, as noted by Goldfried and Kent (1972), must take into account the three levels of inference associated with the explaining of behavior. The first level of inference is the conclusion that the recorded observation reflects the occurrence or nonoccurrence of some response. For example, is the child's test score a true score? Behavioral assessment would consist of viewing the child in a number of settings or situations that elicit the particular behavior under consideration. In contrast, a "true" sample from a traditional assessment orientation would include samples of hypothetical populations with related responses. Most current behaviorists consider all child activity to be behavior. Thus their behaviors may include (1) actual motor behavior (for example, jumping out of seat), (2) physiological responses indicative of responding, and (3) cognitive behavior— verbal responses recorded in questionnaires. Behavioral assessment includes several measures in various settings, so that a broad assessment is ensured.

The second level of inference is the responses that are measured in reference to some larger population; that is, the criterion behavior(s) selected from observation reveal relevant aspects of the true response(s) in question. In behavioral assessment, criterion behaviors are derived directly from a defined classroom analysis (for example, classroom interaction with teacher and peers), whereas traditional measures consider test responses, but not as consisting of samples of the criteria themselves but only as signs. Goldfried and Sprafkin (1976) have summarized behavior assessment as stimulus-organism-response-consequence (SORC), in which it is assumed that (1) individual differences are affected by past learning and physiology, and

(2) behavior results from the interaction between the current situation and those individual differences. Because child behavior is variable, behaviors are selected not only on the basis of face validity, but also in terms of their ability to differentiate the child from the groups in that context.

The third level of inference is the theoretical assumptions that describe the relationship between the behavior in question and the criterion behavior. Behavioral assessment is directed toward conceptual validity (understanding of environment-controlling variables) and treatment validity (contribution to treatment). From a behavioral-assessment perspective, once the criterion behaviors have been derived through the ignoring of inductive and deductive theoretical assumptions, psychometric measures can then be implemented. In contrast, traditional assessment uses a standardized measure, samples specific behavioral interactions, and then selects procedures for measuring criterion behaviors (for example, direct measurement). The comparison of the two approaches in terms of level of inference is oversimplified; nevertheless, it underlies a crucial difference in assessment orientation (see Goldfried & Kent, 1972; Ollendick & Hersen, 1984, for a comprehensive review).

## KEY GENERALIZATIONS

Mash and Terdal (1976) summarize several key characteristics of behavioral assessment:

1. Assessment is based on the assumption that intraindividual variability occurs across time and situations.
2. The situation (classroom) defined in a controlled variable setting (predicted antecedents, behaviors, and consequences) is somewhat stable.
3. Measurement must include contextual variables in relation to those stimuli that are present (either symbolically or directly) while the behavior is occurring. Development of an

instrument to describe situational variables is a needed refinement in the field.
4. Focus of assessment is on providing information that can be utilized in the design, implementation, and evaluation of programs.
5. Assessment should replicate naturally occurring conditions.
6. Assessment is ongoing and self-corrective; measurement is repeated on a consistent, time-sampling basis.
7. Assessment is oriented not toward pathology but toward contextual strengths, assets, and deficiencies (pp. 20–21).

To further help you conceptualize a behavior-assessment orientation, a summary of behavioral contingencies (relation of behavior to its antecedents and consequences) follows.

## CONTINGENT RELATIONSHIPS

Table 8-1 presents an overview of procedures, behavioral effects, and related learning principles influencing the strength or weakness of behavior. As shown in the table, behaviorists view the control on behavior (B) as being stimuli (S) and consequences (C). Contingent relationships between behavior and consequences are defined specifically in terms of the direction of target-behavior change. When contingent pairing of behavior and consequences is intended to increase a target behavior, the pairing is called *reinforcement.* Behavior increases occur when the behavior causes either positive consequences or a reduction in aversive consequences. If target behavior decreases because of either the presentation of aversive stimuli or the reduction of positive consequences that the child has in his or her possession, the procedure causing the decrease is called *punishment.*

*Extinction* occurs when behavior is reduced by the removal of the reinforcing contingencies that have supported the child's behavior. Extinction requires that the reinforcing consequences that have maintained the behavior be removed abruptly. *Shaping,* on the other hand, requires a

**Table 8-1**
Behavioral contingencies.

| Operant concepts—direction of target behavior | Contingency | Probable effects | Example of events |
|---|---|---|---|
| I. Behavior increases | | | |
|   A. Positive reinforcement | Behavior (B) followed (→) by positive consequence (C +) = B→C + | Increase in strength of target behavior | Teacher praise for appropriate math performance |
|   B. Negative reinforcement | = B→Reduction ( ↓ ) in negative consequence (C −) | Same as above; escape or avoidance | Reduction of teacher criticism improves percent correct on math performance |
| II. Behavior decreases (punishment) | | | |
|   A. Presentation of aversive con-sequence | = B→C − | Decrease in strength of target behavior; escape or avoidance | Presentation of teacher criticism decreases percent of error on math performance |
|   B. Removal of obtained and possessed positive con-sequences | = B→ ↓C + | Same as above; response cast | Removal of tokens or free time decreases math error performance |
| III. Extinction | = B→No C + | Same as above | Removal of teacher verbal attention decreases math error performance |

reinforcement of only those behaviors that approximate a terminal behavior. Once behavior is maintained on one step of the hierarchy, behavior-extinction procedures are administered to that step and reinforcement contingencies are applied to the next step on the behavior hierarchy.

*Generalization* refers to a person's tendency to perform a response in a situation similar to that in which the response has been reinforced. The stimulus situation must be changed, for some degree of generalization to occur. *Discrimination,* on the other hand, is the person's tendency to respond differently to two situations in which different reinforcement contingencies are in effect. Contingencies are given to one stimulus and not another during discrimination procedures; performing a generalization requires that contingencies be made on varying stimulus environments.

## OBSERVING AND RECORDING

Behavior assessment depends on keen observation and precise measurement. Therefore it is necessary for psychologists and teachers to understand the fundamental aspects of measurement, so that they can interpret records and

**Table 8-1**

*(continued)*

| Operant concepts—direction of target behavior | Contingency | Probable effects | Example of events |
|---|---|---|---|
| IV. Shaping | $= B_2 \to C+$ or $\downarrow C-$ $= B_1 \to$ No C | Increase strength of $B_2$ and decrease strength of $B_1$ | Teacher only reinforces for 80% correct on math and now provides no consequence for 70% correct |
| V. Generalization | Two stimuli, $S_1$ and $S_2 \to B \to C+$ or $(\downarrow C-)$ | Increase strength of B occurring in $S_1$ and $S_2$ | Resource room teacher reinforces math performance; regular classroom teacher reinforces math performance |
| VI. Discrimination | $= S_1 \to B_1 \to C+$ or $(\downarrow C-) = S_2 \to B_1 \to$ No C; $\downarrow C+$; $C-$ | Increase strength of $B_1$ occurring in $S_1$, but weaken strength of $B_1$ occurring in $S_2$ | Teacher reinforces correct math performance on school work by having child get answer sheet and correct answers; child is not reinforced by getting answer sheet on standardized math test |

Based on material from Swanson, H. L., & Reinert, H. R. *Teaching strategies for children in conflict.* St. Louis: The C. V. Mosby Co. 1982

techniques that have been used in the classroom. More importantly, psychologists and teachers must be able to understand and use measurement procedures if they are to apply behavior modification techniques in the classroom. Observing and recording behavior involves five steps.

*Step 1* determines the setting in which the behavior will be observed. Maladaptive behavior is observed in the situation in which the behavior is to be modified.

*Step 2* involves deciding on a method by which to code behavior. Observational data are usually coded in a manner efficient to record

and use. According to Becker and co-workers (1967), in establishing coding categories, teachers should follow these rules:

1. Categories should reflect behaviors that interfere with classroom learning (for example, time on task).
2. Categories should involve behaviors that violate the rules for permissible behavior established by the teacher.
3. Categories should reflect particular behaviors a teacher wants to change (for example, thumbsucking).
4. Categories should be comprised of behaviors

that are topographically similar in some important way.

5. Categories should be mutually exclusive.
6. Categories must refer to observable behavior and not involve inferences.
7. The number of categories should not exceed ten.

As Table 8-2 indicates, coding categories can be used for groups or individuals. If the teacher is using more than one observer, the percentage of interobserver agreement should be computed to determine the consistency of ratings. When event, duration, or permanent products are recorded, the percentage of interobserver agreement is found by dividing the lesser number or time by the greater and multiplying by 100. When data are recorded in intervals, the records of two observers are compared interval by interval, so that percentage agreement can be obtained for one session or day. The total number of intervals is divided by number of intervals for which they disagree, and this quotient is multiplied by 100 (Hall, 1974). Behaviors coded in step 2 must be observable, repeatable, and countable, in order for high interobserver agreement to be obtained.

*Step 3* is used to determine the interval of time during which the behavior is observed each day and the number of days in which observation will take place, once a method of coding has been devised. O'Leary and O'Leary (1977) report that typically a 5-day baseline observation period is used, with approximately a 45-minute observation period.

*Step 4* involves observing and recording a baseline level. The baseline phase is the performance of an individual or group during a period before any special teaching procedures are employed.

*Step 5* involves plotting the behavior data on a graph that depicts the entire project. Usually, behavior is charted on a line graph in which the vertical axis denotes dependent measures (for example, number of outset behaviors, rate of errors on math problems) and the horizontal axis represents the time of the behavior project. Observation and recording of the deviant behavior continue until the desired behavior change has taken place.

A classroom study by Hall and co-workers (1977) illustrates procedures for recording and observing behavior. According to the teacher in this study, for ten days students in a class for the emotionally disturbed roamed around the room so much that academic development was impaired. Each time a child left his or her seat without permission during reading and math periods, the teacher placed a mark next to the child's name on a paper attached to a clipboard. Baseline data collected before intervention (Figure 8-1) show that the children were out of their seats twenty-three times per session. The teacher's strategy, which required each child to remain after school for 5 minutes every time he or she got out of the seat without the teacher's permission, was then implemented. During the ten sessions that this contingency was in effect, the mean number of out-of-seat behavior for the class dropped to 2.2. Following the teaching strategy, a 5-day reversal phase was instituted. The children were given 5-minute detentions for getting out of their seats, and the incidence of behavior quickly increased to 15.8. The graph in Figure 8-1 indicates that a reimplementation of the teaching strategy is necessary to keep out-of-seat behavior at desired low levels.

## PHASES OF BEHAVIORAL ASSESSMENT

As noted by Craigheid, Kazdin, and Mahoney (1981), Nelson and Hayes (1979), and Ollendick and Hersen (1984), behavioral assessment may be categorized in any of several schemata. The most popular schema distinguishes between the assessment of children (individual) and the assessment of treatment. Hawkins (1979) describes these stages in terms of (1) screening and general disposition, (2) definition and general quantification of the problem or achievement, (3) pinpointing and designing interven-

**Table 8-2**
Coding categories.

| Symbols | Class label | Class definitions |
|---|---|---|
| **Behaviors incompatible with learning: general categories** | | |
| X | Gross motor behaviors | Getting out of seat, standing up, running, hopping, skipping, jumping, walking around, rocking in chair, disruptive movement without noise, moving chair to neighbor |
| N | Disruptive noise with objects | Tapping pencil or other objects, clapping, tapping feet, rattling or tearing paper; do not include accidental dropping of objects or noise made while performing X above |
| A | Disturbing others directly; aggression | Grabbing objects or work, knocking neighbor's book off desk, destroying another's property, hitting, kicking, shoving, pinching, slapping, striking with object, throwing object at another person, poking with object, attempting to strike, biting, pulling hair |
| O | Orienting responses (¼-second duration) | Turning head or head and body to look at another person, showing objects to another child, attending to another child; not rated unless seated |
| ! | Blurting out, commenting, and vocal noise | Answering teacher without raising hand or without being called on, making comments or calling out remarks when no question has been asked, calling teacher's name to get teacher's attention, crying, screaming, singing, whistling, laughing loudly, coughing loudly; must be undirected to another child but may be directed to teacher |
| T | Talking | Carrying on conversations with other children when it is not permitted; must be directed to a particular child or children |
| | Other | Ignoring teacher's question or command, doing something different from that directed to do (includes minor motor behavior such as playing with pencil when supposed to be writing); to be rated only when other ratings not appropriate |
| **Relevant behavior** | | |
| / | Relevant behavior | Time on task, for example, answering question, listening, raising hand, writing assignment; must include whole 20 seconds except for orienting responses of less than 4-seconds duration |

Based on material from Becker, W., et al. The contingent use of teacher attention and praise in reducing classroom behavior problems. *Journal of Special Education,* 1967, *1,* pp. 287–307.

tion, (4) monitoring progress, and (5) follow-up. Each phase will be discussed.

## Screening and General Disposition

A preliminary formulation occurs when a child first enters an educational or clinical setting. An account is taken of the extent of the child's behavioral repertoire that is nonproblematical or that represents behavioral excesses, deficits, and assets. Hawkins (1979) suggests that, in an educational environment, quick screening devices may include the Wide Range Achievement Test, an AML (Cowen et al., 1973), Scholastic Testing Service, Youth Inventory (1971), or Mooney Problem Checklist (Mooney & Gordon, 1950).

Other means of screening have relied on single, behavior-rating scales. Assumptions behind rating scales are that (1) overt-behavior

**Figure 8-1**

The number of out-of-seat behaviors exhibited by the entire class during the mathematics and reading periods. Baseline₁—before experimental procedures performed after school for out-of-seat behavior. Student had to remain after school 5 minutes for each out-of-seat behavior. Baseline₂—return to baseline conditions. (Based on material from Hall, V. and others. The effective use of punishment to modify behavior in the classroom. In K. O'Leary & S. O'Leary (Eds.), *Classroom management: The successful use of behavior modification* (2nd ed.). New York: Pergamon Press, 1977.)

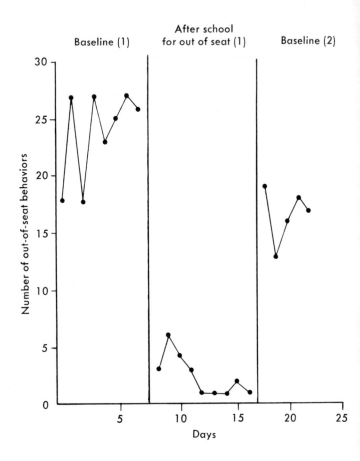

items are better predictors than traits or items requiring the teacher to infer behavior, (2) overt items rate teacher-student interaction and require no special observation procedures, and (3) items are representative of the classroom and not the psychiatric clinic. In the field of delinquency, the Glueck Prediction Scale (Kvaraceus, 1966) is widely used and the best known. Currently, the public school rating scales include such popular instruments as the Behavior Rating Profile (Brown & Hammill, 1978), as well as the Burks (1968), Cassel (1972), Quay and Peterson (1967), and Walker (1969) behavior checklists. To provide examples of behavioral ratings, we describe the Walker Problem Behavior Checklist, Burks' Behavior Rating Scales, and the Cassell Child Behavior Rating Scale.

## WALKER PROBLEM BEHAVIOR IDENTIFICATION CHECKLIST (WPBIC)

(Walker, H., 1970, 1976, 1983 Western Psychological Services)

This is a 50-item checklist for identification of children with behavioral problems. For use in the elementary grades by a classroom teacher, it is designed as a supplement in the total identification process. It is composed of observable, operational statements about classroom behavior furnished by a sampling of elementary school teachers.

The 1983 form is designed for students in pre-school through grade six; it has separate forms for males and females. The 1983 revision uses the same items as were used on previous tests. It was standardized on a sample of 469 preschool/kindergartners, 852 primary-grade students, and 534 intermediate-grade (grades 4–6) students, from Eugene, Oregon, and Battleground, Washington. Separate norms have been established for males and females.

A 2-month observation period is required, to increase the reliability and validity of the teacher's ratings and also to reduce the probability that high-magnitude, low-frequency behaviors are not missed. The scoring sheet has a profile-analysis chart to help the teacher in interpreting the raw scores. This test should be seen as a screening device, not a classification device. Sample items include:

- Habitually rejects the school experience through actions or comments
- Has temper tantrums
- Does not obey until threatened with punishment
- Reacts with defiance to instructions or commands
- Does not engage in group activities
- Is overactive, restless, and/or continually shifting body positions
- Utters nonsense syllables and/or babbles to himself/herself

This checklist was standardized on 534 children in grades four, five, and six. All the children in twenty-one classes were used. The mean score for the normative sample was 7.76, and the standard deviation was 10.53. The distribution of raw scores was positively skewed and did not represent a normal distribution. To normalize the data and establish separation points within the distribution, the raw data were converted to a $T$ score distribution. A $T$ score of 60 was established as the separation of disturbed from nondisturbed. A raw score of 21 indicates the need for further evaluation or behavioral analysis. Validity is described in four parts:

1. *Contrasted-groups validity:* The difference between the means of the two groups was significant beyond the .001 level of confidence. The disturbed group received significantly higher scores than the nondisturbed group, but no coefficient was given.

2. *Criterion validity:* Biserial correlation between checklist scores and criterion yielded a correlation of .68 with a standard error of .039. The index of predictive efficiency is .33.

3. *Factorial validity:* The test was determined to involve five factors—acting out behavior, withdrawal, distractibility, disturbed peer relations, and immaturity.

4. *Item validity:* The detailed analysis confirmed the hypothesis that the WPBIC items are measuring separate functions of the same behavior domain. The correlations of each item with the total test ranged from .03 to .67; four items were below .10. It was suggested that the items other than these constitute a homogeneous set of behaviors.

The reliability was estimated by use of the Kuder-Richardson method, and the coefficient was found to be .98, with a standard deviation of 10.53 and a standard error of measurement of 1.28. This indicates that 97% of variance was true-score variance and 3% was error variance. Doubling and tripling the length results in an improvement of only .01. Actual administration time is less than 5 minutes. The items are to be circled only if present, and the items are pre-weighted so the score could reach 100. There are five subscores for each subgroup, and the total of these gives the total score.

### BURKS' BEHAVIOR RATING SCALES (BBRS)
(Burks, H., 1968, Arden Press)

The Burks' Behavior Rating Scales are specifically designed to identify patterns of pathological behavior shown by children already showing behavioral difficulties in the classroom or home. It is suitable for children in grades one to nine. It is not suitable for the routine screening of large groups of children who are performing adequately in school settings. The BBRS is meant to be a preliminary device to gauge the severity of negative symptoms as seen by outside persons—ordinarily teachers or parents. The 110 items used as criteria for the instrument's ratings describe behaviors that are infrequently observed among normal children.

The scales consist of a four-page booklet and a profile sheet. To perform a quantitative judgment, the rater determines the degree to which each behavior listed in the booklet is seen in the child being rated (score of 1, behavior not noticed; score of 5, behavior noticed to a very large degree). The results are scored by a professional person (other than the rater) and graphed on the profile sheet. The profile sheet, rather than the booklet, is used for diagnostic purposes. Factor analysis found the 110 items to cluster in 19 groupings. Each grouping measures a particular conduct:

1. Excessive self-blame
2. Excessive anxiety
3. Excessive withdrawal
4. Excessive dependency
5. Poor ego strength
(1 to 5—considered, learned defense mechanisms against outward stress)
6. Poor physical strength
7. Poor coordination
8. Poor intellectuality
9. Poor academics
(6 to 9—strong genetic roots; learns at slower rate)
10. Poor attention
11. Poor impulse control
(10 and 11—may suffer some form of neurological handicap or may outgrow in early adolescence)
12. Poor reality contact
13. Poor sense of identity
14. Excessive suffering
(12 to 14—unwilling constructive involvement with environment)
15. Poor anger control
16. Excessive sense of persecution
17. Excessive aggressiveness

18. Excessive resistance
19. Poor social conformity
(15 to 19—express hostility, resistance to goodwill of others; nonacceptance of social standards of conduct)

The test takes approximately 10 minutes to administer.

Item reliability was established by having ninety-five disturbed children from grades one to six rated and rerated within a period of ten days by their teachers. Considering the small sample employed, all items demonstrated high correlation coefficients, ranging between .60 and .83. The average item/item retest correlation coefficient was .705. Constructed over a period of four years, items on the scale were selected from clinical observations of children and from evidence in literature. Extensive use of the scales for eight years established that they do possess content validity, as judged by 22 school psychologists and over 200 teachers of normal, educationally handicapped, speech and hearing handicapped, orthopedically handicapped, and retarded pupils. Other topics of investigation include criterion-related validity, contrasted-groups validity, factorial validity, and construct validity.

### CHILD BEHAVIOR RATING SCALE (CBRS)

(Cassell, R., 1972, Western Psychological Services)

The CBRS is a 78-item instrument to measure some aspects of child behavior. Its range includes kindergarten, grades one to three, and/or children who are unable to read or who are handicapped in conventional areas such as self-adjustment, home adjustment, social adjustment, school adjustment, and physical adjustment. The CBRS provides basic information through observation. The test kit consists of a manual and protocol. The CBRS takes approximately 5 to 10 minutes to administer. On each CBRS item, the child is rated on a six-point scale as to the degree he or she presents specific aspects of a behavior. Scoring is easily completed and usually takes a few minutes.

Sample items under self-adjustment include:

|  | 1 | 2 | 3 | 4 | 5 | 6 |
|---|---|---|---|---|---|---|
| 15. Often tends to be on the go and can't relax | Yes | | | | | No |
| 16. Often is very nervous and excited about things | Yes | | | | | No |
| 17. Often has trouble controlling temper | Yes | | | | | No |
| 18. Often is not very tactful with others | Yes | | | | | No |
| 19. Often does things that later regrets having done | Yes | | | | | No |
| 20. Often behavior goes in cycles of good and bad | Yes | | | | | No |
| Number checks | | | | | | |
| Weighted values | | | | | | |
| Total weighted score | | | | | | |

The CBRS provides a Personality Total Adjustment Score (PTAS) that indicates an overall adjustment of the child. The PTAS can be converted to a $T$ score by use of test tables and can assist in the comparing of normative data. The test has two types of validity. The first is construct validity (.66), obtained directly from summary case reports made by a trained person in the different disciplines dealing with child behavior. The second validity, status, is determined when scores on the CBRS differentiate well-adjusted ("typical") children from those diagnosed as maladjusted, by professionals working with maladjusted children. The Spearman-Brown odd-even reliability ranged from .59 for the maladjusted group to .87 for the normal group.

The CBRS items were obtained by a study and screening of over 2000 case studies of elementary school pupils referred for psychological or psychiatric services.

*Other Rating Scales.* Spivack and Swift (1973) have provided the classroom teacher with a critical review and evaluation of behavioral rating scales that have been developed to assess the overt classroom behaviors of children. These rating scales have been used in screening and identifying disturbed children. Table 8-3, which is adapted from Spivack and Swift, provides the teacher with dimensions, grade levels, and norms to assist in selection of the appropriate scale.

Several behavioral rating scales appear on the market. However, particular ones that offer the greatest utility include the Behavior Problem Checklist (Quay & Peterson, 1979), Child Behavior Checklist (Achenback & Edelbrock, 1979), and Eyberg Child Behavior Inventory (Eyberg, 1980). Several reviews can be consulted for information concerning other behavioral rating scales (e.g., Humphreys & Ciminero, 1979; Ollendick & Hersen, 1984).

Screening instruments currently available for use on young children include the Preschool Behavioral Classification Project Scale (Baker & Dryer, 1977), Kohn Social Competence Scale and Kohn Symptom Checklist for the Preschool Child (Kohn, 1977), and the Preschool Behavior Questionnaire (Behor, 1977). A behavioral rating scale for differentiation at the junior high and high school level is the Hahneman High School Behavior Rating Scale (Spivack & Swift, 1977). Rating scales are most useful when they are used to identify and differentiate among dimensions of deviance in children and adolescents. Bower's study (1960) has suggested that teacher ratings, self-descriptive data, and peer ratings, when combined, give a clear picture of the general disposition of children.

*Behavioral Coding.* Craigheid, Kazdin, and Mahoney (1981), Hawkins (1979), and Kanfer

## Table 8-3
Behavior scales (authors and grade-level applicability).

| Dimensions measured | 1 Kellam and Schiff (1st grade) | 2 Pimm (1st grade) | 3 Cassell (K-3rd grade) | 4 Kim et al. (2nd grade) | 5 Cowen et al. (3rd grade) | 6 Walker "Checklist" (4th-6th grades) |
|---|---|---|---|---|---|---|
| **Group 1** | | | | | | |
| Aggressive, destructive, disobedient | X | | | | | X[a] |
| Restless, cannot sit still | X | | | | | |
| External blaming, does not assume responsibility | | | | | | |
| Irrelevant verbal responding | | | | | | |
| Passive resistant, sulking | | | | | | |
| Impatient | | | | | | |
| Dogmatic, inflexible | | | | | | |
| Expressed inability in schoolwork | | | | | | |
| **Group 2** | | | | | | |
| Socially withdrawn, timid | X | | | | | X[a] |
| Immature | X | | | | | |
| Anxious | | | | | | X[a] |
| Worried, fearful, neurotic symptoms | | | | | | X[a] |
| **Group 3** | | | | | | |
| Good general school adjustment | | | | X | | |
| Enthusiastic, creative, interactive | | | | | | |
| Positive relationship to teacher | | | | | | |
| Socially outgoing, friendly | | | | X | | |
| Emotionally controlled and sensitive | | | | X | | |
| **Group 4** | | | | | | |
| Reasoning, comprehending | | | | | | |
| Cognitively disoriented | | | | | | |
| Inattentive, distractible | | | | | | |
| Reliant on external support, lacks intellectual independence | | | | | | |
| **Group 5** | | | | | | |
| Poor work habits, careless, quits easily | X | | | | | |
| Evidence of neglect at home | | | | | | |
| Factor analysis employed[d] | | | | X | | X |
| Total adjustment score available | X | X | X[e] | | X | X |

Based on material from Spivack, G., & Swift, M. The classroom behavior of children: A critical review of teacher administered rating scales. *Journal of Special Education*, 1973, 7, 55–89.
[a]No validity or reliability provided for individual factor scores.
[b]Data only available on total scores of scales in question.

| 7<br>Walker BRS (4th-6th grades) | 8<br>Davidson and Greenberg (5th grade) | 9<br>Rutter (elementary grades) | 10<br>Rubin et al. (elementary grades) | 11<br>Deitcher (elementary grades) | 12<br>Dayton (elementary grades) | 13<br>Dayton (high school grades) | 14<br>Quay and Peterson (elementary grades) | 15<br>Quay and Peterson (7th-8th grades) | 16<br>Ross et al.; Miller (elementary grades) | 17<br>Spivack and Swift DESB (elementary grades) | 18<br>Swift and Spivack HHSB (7th-12th grades) | 19<br>Vinter et al. (7th-12th grades) |
|---|---|---|---|---|---|---|---|---|---|---|---|---|
| X[a] | X[b] | X | X |  | X[b] | X[b] | X | X | X | X | X[c] | X[b] |
|  |  |  |  |  |  |  |  |  |  | X | X |  |
|  |  |  | X |  |  |  |  |  |  | X |  |  |
|  |  |  |  |  |  |  |  |  |  | X |  |  |
|  |  |  |  |  |  |  |  |  | X |  |  |  |
|  |  |  |  |  |  |  |  |  |  | X |  |  |
|  |  |  |  |  |  |  |  |  |  |  | X |  |
|  |  |  |  |  |  |  |  |  |  |  | X |  |
| X[a] |  |  | X |  |  |  |  |  |  |  | X | X |
|  |  |  | X |  |  |  | X | X |  |  |  |  |
|  |  |  |  |  |  |  |  |  |  | X | X |  |
|  | X | X |  |  |  |  | X | X | X |  |  |  |
|  | X |  |  |  |  |  |  |  |  | X | X[c] | X[c] | X |
|  |  |  |  |  | X | X |  |  |  | X | X |  |
|  |  |  |  |  |  |  |  |  |  | X | X | X[f] |
|  |  |  |  |  |  |  |  |  |  |  |  |  |
|  |  |  |  |  |  |  |  |  |  |  |  |  |
|  |  |  |  |  |  |  |  |  |  | X | X |  |
|  |  |  | X |  |  |  |  |  |  |  |  |  |
| X[a] |  |  |  |  |  |  |  |  |  | X |  |  |
|  |  |  |  |  |  |  |  |  |  | X | X |  |
|  |  |  |  |  | X[b] | X[b] |  |  |  |  | X |  |
|  |  |  | X |  |  |  |  |  |  |  |  |  |
|  | X |  | X |  | X | X | X | X | X | X | X | X |
| X |  | X | X | X |  |  |  |  |  | X[c] | X[c] |  |

[c]Dimension measured by considering total behavior profile type.
[d]For scales when factor analysis was not employed, items were grouped into dimensions through clinical judgment.
[e]This score available only as part of the total scale score, but not independently.
[f]As worded, this factor probably measures overcloseness with, or excessive need for, the teacher.

255

and Saslow (1969), have suggested a need for general codes for the screening and general disposition phase. This screening and disposition phase requires a broad-bond assessment "capable of detecting any likely kind of problem, even if it does not satisfactorily specify the nature of the problem" (Hawkins, 1979). In general, most behaviorally oriented assessments do not give a child a diagnostic classification derived from standard nomenclature (for example, anxiety neurosis, learning disability). To meet the needs for a standardized system that will classify behavioral difficulties and relate to intervention, Cautela and Upper (1973) have developed a behavior coding system that includes 283 specific, maladaptive behaviors, divided into twenty-one major behavioral categories. The categories and examples of each follow.

1. *Thinking:* thoughts (covertly talking to oneself) that lead to inappropriate affect or inappropriate overt behavior (recurring thoughts accompanied by anxiety or fear, recurring thoughts about harming oneself)

2. *Intellectual performance:* deficits in the areas of reasoning, problem solving, and/or memory (inadequate problem-solving ability, inadequate recall of facts or events)

3. *Imagery:* covert sensing or experiencing sensations not related to present environmental stimulation (sensory experiences with no external cause accompanied by the belief that the source is outside the individual)

4. *Addictions:* behaviors that occur at a high frequency (ingestion of substances that have a short-term pleasurable effect)

5. *Eating:* eating behavior that occurs with inappropriate frequency or involves inappropriate objects (overeating, eating inadequate amounts)

6. *Sex:* inappropriate sexual object and/or performance (choosing younger children as sexual objects)

7. *Fears:* exaggerated fears (behavioral avoidance, sympathetic nervous system arousal, verbal reports of fear in the presence of relatively innocuous stimuli, such as fear of heights, fear of hurting others)

8. *Locomotion:* locomotion that occurs at an inappropriate rate or in an inappropriate manner (lack of locomotion)

9. *Socially inappropriate behaviors:* physical behaviors that are likely to result in disapproval by others (thumbsucking)

10. *Inadequate hygiene:* behaviors involving personal cleanliness that occur at such a low frequency as to result in detriment to health and/or disapproval from others (not washing or bathing regularly)

11. *Inappropriate dress:* behaviors involving personal dress that may result in detriment to health and/or disapproval from others (repeatedly wearing soiled clothing)

12. *Vocational adjustment:* behaviors related to vocational adjustment (not following directions, slow performance)

13. *Inappropriate habits of daily living:* behaviors that involve activities of daily living and that are likely to result in aversive consequences (physical isolation from other human beings)

14. *Sleep:* problems involving sleep duration or inappropriate behaviors occurring during sleep (excessive sleeping)

15. *Emotional behavior:* verbal reports of an inappropriate (to the situation) experience of sadness, happiness, anger; inappropriate overt behavior involving laughing or crying

16. *Speech:* inappropriate vocal behaviors (mutism, high rate of repeating what others say)

17. *Repetitive tasks:* task-oriented behaviors that occur at a frequency higher than is necessary for adaptive functioning, or repetitive behaviors without functional significance (excessive arranging of objects or putting in order, performing an ordered sequence of behaviors as a prerequisite to performing another behavior)

18. *Organic impairments influenced by psychological factors:* organic problem for which there is anecdotal or experimental evidence that the problem can be alleviated or eliminated by behavior-modification techniques
19. *Self-injurious behavior:* behavior that results in immediate physical damage to the organism
20. *Antisocial behavior:* behavior that is likely to result in injury to others or that involves depriving others of their property (physical assault on people, arson)
21. *Inappropriate body movements:* repetitive body movements that have no adaptive function (rocking, assuming unusual postures)

The behavior coding system helps determine those areas of adjustment in which the child may have sufficient difficulty that further inquiry is warranted. The kind of output needed for screening and dispositions is simple. The assessment must simply classify the child as appropriate or inappropriate for educational intervention and identify further assessments that may be useful.

For the teacher, behavior assessment, at least the screening and general disposition stage, becomes a matter of asking good questions about the learner. By quantifying behaviors to be measured, the asking of appropriate questions provides a good framework for the observation process. A behavioral assessment approach provides a systematic process for observation, task analysis, class structure, and reinforcement factors. Sample questions in such an assessment might include*:

I. Observation
   A. Is the behavior observable?
   B. Can it be reliably measured (high amount of interobserver agreement)?
   C. Is the behavior repeatable?

---

*We thank Drs. Jack Little and Annette Tessiers, California State University at Los Angeles, for suggested questions.

   D. Does the academic behavior occur often enough for:
      1. Instruction?
      2. Reliable assessment?
      3. Daily progress
   E. Is the behavior directly related to the overall instructional objective of the class?
   F. Is the behavior of high priority?
   G. If the behavior is a deceleration target, has an incompatible behavior been identified that will improve at the same time (for example, modality strengths)?
   H. Under what circumstances is the behavior occurring? How often?
   I. What environmental contingencies in the classroom are keeping the child from learning?
II. Instructional objectives
   A. Are objectives stated in terms of the desired terminal behavior?
   B. What are the stated standards of performance desired of this child (level of allowable error)?
   C. Under what conditions can the task be accomplished successfully (for example, speed, neatness)?
   D. Are some behaviors dependent on another for successful completion (for example, pencil grip before writing)?
   E. Is the objective within the child's capability?
   F. Is a lower-level task needed first?
III. Task Analysis
   A. Are the current educational objectives stated as a series of specific tasks for this student?
   B. Is every concept that is needed for successful performance of the task noted?
   C. Are the tasks that teach these concepts specific enough for the student?
   D. Does each task have a concept open to only one interpretation?
   E. Does the child learn one concept at a time?

F.  Does the child's program meet various criteria of performance specified by the objectives?

G.  What are the elements or components of the total task that lead to successful completion of the task?

H.  At what level of learning hierarchy is the task?

I.  Are the steps of learning for the student appropriately incremented?

J.  Are the steps in a logical sequence for the child?

K.  How much work can the child do in an allotted time?

L.  How much work is on a single page?

IV.  Class and student structure

A.  What is the child's preferred seating and which is to his or her best advantage?

B.  Do movement patterns within the room interfere with the child's work?

C.  Is the child in proximity to the necessary materials, activity centers, and storage centers?

D.  Does the child respond to contingency management and/or social reinforcement?

E.  Have teachers in the past planned ways to eliminate negative reinforcement?

F.  Is the child field dependent or independent?

G.  Does the child know what the objectives are and what is expected?

H.  Does the child know that misbehavior will not be tolerated and is not expected from him or her?

I.  Has the child helped in setting his or her own goal and the planning of learning tasks?

J.  Can the child make a commitment as to what he or she can do, how much can be done, and how long it will take?

K.  Can the child help to keep progress records so that he or she can see improvement?

L.  Have the child's previous assignments been arranged so that success occurs between 80% and 90% of the time?

M.  What other means have been used to help move the child from a failure syndrome to a success syndrome (for example, monitor, helper, chances to show strengths to the class)?

N.  Have previous regular classroom assignments been dropped to a simple enough level so that the child can succeed?

O.  What alternate-response levels does the child use if he or she fails with a specific type of task?

P.  What has been the reason in the past for assigning the child to a particular task?

V.  Reinforcement

A.  Does the child respond positively to direct reinforcements?

B.  What type of reinforcement does the child respond to most readily (for example, tangible items, tokens, one-to-one teaching, verbal reinforcement for task completion, knowledge of results)?

C.  Will the child respond to a contracting or contingency-based program?

D.  Can the child make choices and determine a course of action or must the teacher direct the action?

E.  Is the child self-structuring?

F.  At what task and learning level is the child (for example, attention, response, order, exploratory, social mastery, achievement [see Chapter 9])?

*Summary.* The function of the screening assessment phase is a crude sorting of children into "serve or send elsewhere and assess for X or do not assess for X" (Hawkins, 1979, p. 53). The identification of skill or problem areas that require educational remediation, the quantification of general level of skill in relevant areas, and the determination of situational variables are accomplished in the next phase.

## Definition and General Quantification

The definition and quantification of child responses may be conceptualized as a procedure by which behaviors are designated into one of three general categories: behavioral excess, behavioral deficit, and behavioral asset (Coulter, 1980; Ellis, 1980; Haynes, 1978; Ollendick & Hersen, 1984).

Behavioral excess is defined as problematical if the frequency, intensity, duration, or occurrence of the behavior is deemed inappropriate, depending on the vantage point from which the behavior is observed. In other words, the designation of behavior as excessive or deficient is based on its consequence to other people. Behavioral deficits are described as problematical if the behavior fails to occur with sufficient frequency, with adequate intensity, with appropriate form, or under socially accepted conditions; a child with problematical behavior is the child not performing well in school, a withdrawn child, or the child with few friends. As noted by Haynes (1978), this category also includes children who are retarded in the development of skills. Behavioral assets are considered non-problematical behavior, because the areas described are areas in which the child has already acquired competence.

Clarification of problematical behaviors is done in terms of excesses and deficits. Groups objecting to these behaviors, and related consequences, are identified, as well as the conditions in which the problematical behaviors occur (physiological, social, symbolic, vocational). Maintaining factors (for example, reinforcement) are also considered. Behavioral assessment in this phase can employ a variety of methods: behavioral coding systems, assessment guides and checklists, probing procedure, and precision measurement (teaching).

***Behavioral Coding System.*** Behavioral coding systems (Cautela & Upper, 1977; Keller, 1986) are functional guides for measurement of behavior only when they specify (1) the behavior's beginning and ending, and (2) the observable action, activity, or measurement of the child. A coding system may be characterized as a measurement procedure (for example, time sampling, duration recording) that uses a permanent product (for example, paper-and-pencil format, videotape, tape recorder) to represent the categorical classroom activity of children. The behavioral code must be discrete enough so that interactions of children in the classroom are not missed. Several authors (Becker et al., 1967; Greenwood and others, 1979) provide examples of student code categories that incorporate not only common student behavior but also teacher responses in the classroom context:

### Student code summaries (what the student is doing)

*Attending (AT):*
   A. Looking at the teacher when the teacher is talking
   B. Looking at materials in the classroom that have to do with the lesson
   C. Engaging in other looking behavior appropriate to the academic situation

*Working (WK):* Working on academic material without any overt verbal components, either in a group or in individual seatwork situations

*Volunteering (VO):* Responding to teacher requests by volunteering information of an academic nature

*Reading aloud (RA):* Reading aloud either individually or as a part of a group recitation

*Appropriate behavior (AB):* Includes asking or answering questions, raising hand for help, acquiring or passing out materials

*Interaction with peer about academic materials (IP+):* Interacting with a peer or peers about academic materials and not violating classroom rules (for example, talking, handling materials, working together on academic materials)

*Interaction with peer about nonacademic materials (IP−):* Interacting with a peer about academic materials inappropriate for the period in which the observation occurs (unless this has been approved by the teacher) or about nonacademic material

*Don't know (DK):* Verbal or nonverbal manner indicates that he or she does not know the answer

*Inappropriate locale (IL):* Without the teacher's approval, child in a classroom area not appropriate for the academic activity

*Look around (LA):* Looking away from the appropriate academic task at hand

*Inappropriate behavior (IB):* Situations in which the child calls out an answer when a question is directed to another student or interrupts the teacher or another student who is talking

## Teacher code summaries (what the teacher does)

*Approval (AP):* Gives clear verbal, gestural, or physical approval to the student or the group

*Disapproval (DI):* Gives clear verbal, gestural, or physical disapproval of the child's behavior either individually or as part of a group

*No response (NR):* Does not respond to the student either as a part of the group or individually

*Verbal interaction (VI):* Verbalizations, directed at the subject or his or her group, that are not approvals or disapprovals

## Class code summaries (what the class does)

*Appropriate behavior (AB):* Entire class (all students) is engaged in activities that are appropriate to the situation according to the teacher's rules and the activity at hand

*Inappropriate behavior (IB):* Student in the class is engaged in activities that are not appropriate to the situation according to the teacher's rules and the activity at hand

Before a method of direct observation of these classes of behaviors can be recommended for widespread use in the classroom, instruments must be (1) sufficiently inclusive of general classes of behavior to be relevant to child and program evaluation, (2) simple enough to be used by various other individuals (teacher aides, counselors), and (3) sensitive enough to be responsive to differences and changes in child and/or program.

Cautela and Upper (1973) have developed the most comprehensive coding system (discussed earlier), as an alternative to traditional classification models. To determine excesses and deficits, a separate form (Figure 8-2) can be

| Name _____ | | | | Date _____ |
| Code no. | Specific behavior | Date behavior first observed | Present frequency | Duration at present frequency |
|---|---|---|---|---|
| | | | | |
| | | | | |
| | | | | |
| | | | | |
| | | | | |

**Figure 8-2**
Behavioral coding system cover sheet.

used: on it can be listed all the problematical behaviors in terms of code numbers, but more importantly, how often those behaviors occur, when they begin, and how long they last. Cautela and Upper (1973) suggest several uses for the cover sheet: (1) summary of pretreatment problematical behaviors and frequencies, a standard for the determination of treatment effectiveness and evaluation, (2) part of a contingency contract procedure for motivating a child, and (3) system with which coded behaviors can be grouped into related classes. Besides the coding system developed by Cautela and Upper (1973), similar coding systems have been developed by Keller (1986).

In behavior-coding procedures, behaviors are measured in the natural context, and reflect the social expectations of that context. One disadvantage of coding systems is their inability to classify behavior into discrete skill areas. Another weakness in behavior-coding or -rating procedures is the influence of reactivity—the influence of the observer's presence on the behavior of those being observed. One difficulty in observing children's behaviors is that children may react to the presence or absence of an observer. To reduce this effect, Haynes (1978) has suggested using product measure (for example, worksheet output) or participant observers, providing instruction to those observed (for example, act natural), or decreasing conspicuousness of observation procedure. In making behavioral observations in which information is coded and tabulated, multiple observers (for example, parent, teacher's aide) might improve the accuracy of the observation procedure.

*Assessment Guides and Checklists.* Another approach within behavioral assessment is to quantify information within a criterion-referenced format (see Chapter 2). Such assessment guides vary in sophistication, reliability, and validity. Many checklists or behavioral guides rely on the earlier works of Bayley, Binet, Cattell, Doll, and Wechsler. However, recent trends have

noted that these earlier scales tend to concentrate on only one or two factors of the developmental domain; their administration also requires considerable time and training. These scales are therefore lacking in efficiency and comprehensiveness (Harrison, 1987; Smith & Snell, 1978).

Two popular instruments currently used are the American Association on Mental Deficiency (AAMD) Adaptive Behavior Scale for use in institutions (Nihira, Foster, Shellhaas, & Leland, 1974) and the Vineland Social Maturity Scale (Doll, 1965). The AAMD also has a public-school version (Lambert & Windmiller, 1981). Research on the adaptive behavior scales has been extensively reviewed (Harrison, 1987). Harrison's review includes the following common measures:

- ☐ Adaptive Behavior Checklist (Schwartz, Allen, & Cortazzo, 1974)
- ☐ AAMD Adaptive Behavior Scale (Nihira, Foster, Shellhaas, & Leland, 1975)
- ☐ AAMD Adaptive Behavior Scale, Public School Version (Lambert, Windmiller, Cole, & Figueroa, 1975a)
- ☐ AAMD Adaptive Behavior Scale, School Edition (Lambert & Windmiller, 1981)
- ☐ Adaptive Behavior Inventory for Children (Mercer & Lewis, 1978)
- ☐ Adaptive Functioning Index (Marlett & Hughson, 1971)
- ☐ Balthazar Scales of Adaptive Behavior (Balthazar, 1973)
- ☐ Behavior Development Survey (Arndt, 1981)
- ☐ Behavior Rating Inventory for the Retarded (Sparrow & Cicchetti, 1978)
- ☐ Behavior Rating Profile (Brown & Hammill, 1978)
- ☐ Cain-Levine Social Competency Scale (Cain, Levine, & Elzey, 1963)
- ☐ Children's Adaptive Behavior Scale (Richmond & Kicklighter, 1980)
- ☐ Client Development Evaluation Report (California State Department of Developmental Services, 1978)

☐ Minnesota Developmental Programming System (Bork & Weatherman, 1975)

☐ Personal Competence Profile (Greenspan, 1982)

☐ Personal Competency Scale (Reynolds, 1981)

☐ San Francisco Vocational Competency Scale (Levine & Elzey, 1968)

☐ Scales of Independent Behavior (Bruininks, Woodcock, Weatherman, & Hill, 1984)

☐ Social and Prevocational Information Battery (Irvin, Halpern, Raffeld, & Link, 1975)

☐ Vineland Adaptive Behavior Scales, Interview Edition, Survey Form (Sparrow, Balla, & Cicchetti, 1984a)

☐ Vineland Adaptive Behavior Scales, Interview Edition, Expanded Form (Sparrow, Balla, & Cicchetti, 1984b)

☐ Vineland Adaptive Behavior Scales, Classroom Edition (Sparrow, Balla, & Cicchetti, 1985)

☐ Vineland Social Maturity Scale (Doll, 1935, 1966)

☐ Vocational Adaptation Rating Scale (Malgady, Barcher, Davis, & Towner, 1980a)

☐ Weller-Strawser Scales of Adaptive Behavior (Weller & Strawser, 1981)

### AAMD ADAPTIVE BEHAVIOR SCALE

(Nihara, K., and others, 1974, American Association of Mental Deficiency)

The AAMD Adaptive Behavior Scale is a set of 111 items covering twenty-four areas of social and personal behavior. It is intended to evaluate a subject's effectiveness in coping with environmental demands. Its classification of mentally retarded individuals is based on the way in which the individual maintains personal independence and meets social expectations. The scale is divided into two parts, one to be used with persons three to twelve years of age, and the other to be used with persons thirteen years of age and over. The test consists of two scales (one for each part of the test), two answering sheets (child and adult), and one manual. Administering the first part of the scale takes 20 to 25 minutes and the second part, 25 to 30 minutes. Part I tests independent functioning, economic activity, physical development, language development, number and time concepts, occupation-domestic, occupation-general, self-direction, responsibilities, and socialization. Part II tests violent and destructive behavior, such as withdrawal and hyperactive tendencies, and maladaptive behavior related to personality and behavioral disorders. Although the AAMD Adaptive Behavior Scale was designed primarily for mentally retarded persons, it can also be used with emotionally maladjusted and other handicapped persons. Below is a sample item.

F. Stereotyped behavior and odd mannerisms
   (23)   Has stereotyped behaviors
   Check "No" or "Yes." If "Yes," select *all* statements that are true of the child.
   a. Drums fingers
   b. Taps feet continually
   c. Has hands constantly in motion
   d. Slaps, scratches, or rubs self continually
   e. Waves or shakes parts of the body repeatedly
   f. Moves or rolls head back and forth
   g. Rocks body back and forth
   h. Paces the floor
   i. Other

Part I is designed to assess the individual's skills and habits in twenty behavior domains that are considered important to the maintenance of personal independence in daily living. The ten behavior domains and twenty-three subdomains are:

I. *Independent functioning:* Eating skills, toilet use, cleanliness, appearance, care of clothing, dressing and undressing, locomotion, general independent functioning

II. *Physical development:* Sensory development, motor development

III. *Economic activity:* Money handling and budgeting, shopping skills

IV. *Language development:* Speaking and writing, comprehension, general language development

V. *Number and time concept*
VI. *Occupation-domestic:* Cleaning, kitchen duties, general occupation-domestic
VII. *Occupation-general*
VIII. *Self-direction:* Sluggishness in movement, initiative, persistence, planning and organization, self-direction (general)
IX. *Responsibilities*
X. *Socialization*

Part II is designed to provide measures of maladaptive behavior related to personality and behavior disorders. It consists of the following fourteen domains:

Violent and destructive behavior
Antisocial behavior
Rebellious behavior
Untrustworthy behavior
Withdrawal
Stereotyped behavior and odd mannerisms
Inappropriate interpersonal manners
Inappropriate vocal habits
Unacceptable or eccentric habits
Self-abusive behavior
Hyperactive tendencies
Sexually aberrant behavior
Psychological disturbances
Use of medications

The scale can be administered by psychologists, teachers, nurses, social workers, daycare center instructors, ward attendants in residential institutions, and others who have observed closely or personally know the daily behavior of the individuals to be rated.

There are two methods of scoring IQ on the AAMD Adaptive Behavior Scale. The first is to use computer systems. This method can be used by those examiners who have access to computers. The second method is hand scoring. To use this method, the examiner must have the appropriate answer sheet provided by the publisher. When this sheet is being completed, all items with negative meanings must be converted to the positive. To do this, the scorer

subtracts the number of negative responses from the maximum number of responses. The hand-scoring sheet provides further specific instructions for scoring.

The manual presents, in addition to instructions for scoring the answer sheet, specific instructions for recording individual responses. There are two steps involved in the recording of behaviors for this test. The first step consists of the examiner's making the decision as to whether the specific behavior observed directly applies to the general category or if it is merely a repetition or interpretation of another behavior previously mentioned. Only behaviors directly related to a category are included in the score.

The second step involves three different types of times and their related scorings. The first requires that the number of the most applicable statement be circled. The second type allows for multiple responses; however, in scoring the item, the examiner records the number of circled responses. The third requires the examiner to check all applicable statements in either an "occasionally" or "frequently" column. One point is given for each item in the "occasionally" column and two points for each item in the "frequently" column. The total score for one item is the sum of the points in both columns.

After scoring each item and adding the items to find the different subdomain scores, the examiner may refer to Table II in the manual. This table relates scores to broad categories of intelligence levels. There are six levels: 0 = IQ of 84 or above; 1 = IQ of 83 to 68; 2 = IQ of 67 to 52; 3 = IQ of 51 to 36; 4 = IQ of 35 to 20; and 5 = IQ of 19 to 0.

Face validity of the AAMD Adaptive Behavior Scale suggests that it is an instrument that would describe the critical behavior on which crucial decisions about the mentally retarded may be based. Factor analysis of domain scores results in three dimensions: (1) personal independence, (2) social maladaption, and (3) personal maladaption. Each of these dimensions was used in the construction of factorial analysis.

Interrater reliability of the scale was estimated through the application of the adult form to twenty-six male and twenty-one female retarded patients. Reliabilities ranged from .86 for "independent functioning" to .40 for these three domains: withdrawal; stereotyped behaviors and odd mannerisms; and inappropriate interpersonal manners. Part I of the scale had a mean reliability of .74, while the mean reliability for Part II was .61. The mean reliability for the entire scale was .67.

The scale was standardized on a sample consisting of approximately 2800 patients from sixty-three residential institutions for the mentally retarded throughout the United States. Of the number sampled, none was from a "noninstitutionalized" population. The standardized sample was stratified by sex, intelligence, and age.

### VINELAND SOCIAL MATURITY SCALE (VSMS)
(Doll, E., 1965, American Guidance Service)

This scale (for ages birth to maturity) provides an outline of performances, showing children's progressive capacity for looking after themselves and for participating in those activities that lead toward ultimate independence as adults. The examiner interviews a person intimately familiar with the subject and determines the subject's demonstrated performance on the 117 items covered by the scale. Arranged in order of increasing difficulty, the items of the scale represent progressive maturation in self-help, self-direction, locomotion, occupation, communication, and social relations.

Each item within the age range involved is scored either plus, plus F (temporary failure under certain conditions), plus NO (no opportunity), plus minus (items that are occasionally but not ordinarily performed with full success), or minus. To calculate the total score, the sum of these scores, the examiner adds the basal score and the additional scattered credits beyond the basal score, and expresses this sum as the total number of items passed. The results can be used to determine social competence—the number of tasks the child can perform. This score is converted into a social age, useful in classifications for necessary care and training.

As this is a scale rather than a test, there are few quantitative terms. The child either has the skill, has no opportunity to do it, or cannot perform it. Numerical values have meaning in the computation of a social age and then a social quotient: $SQ = (SA \div LA) \times 100$. The LA is the child's chronological age.

Standardization data were obtained from ten normal subjects of each sex, from birth to thirty years of age; there was a total of 620 subjects. Extensive research has been done with the scale; the manual itself reports fifty-nine studies selected as being representative. The Vineland norms are currently outdated.

***Review of Instruments.*** Walls, Werner, and Bacon (1977) have provided an annotated bibliography reviewing 157 different behavior checklists. Table 8-4 provides a brief review of some other assessment guides.

Two issues of importance to educators emerge from an examination of the behavioral assessment guides. First, many assessment guides are too general to provide information on specific target behavior, because they do not provide either the conditions in which a particular behavior occurs, or the criteria by which behaviors are scored (see Harrison, 1987; Sailor & Horner, 1976, for a review). These omissions are important to two major goals of the assessment: determining the presence or absence of behaviors, and determining the success or failure of behaviors. For example, a strict interpretation of whether behavior is present or absent provides no information on that behavior's frequency. Furthermore, some scales rely on verbal reporting procedures, which, under conditions of nebulous specification of correlations on criteria, could cause one to question how accurately the scale represents the individual's behavior.

A well-known example of the error in an assessment that is too loosely constructed is the "halo effect"—the tendency of raters to be unduly influenced by a single behavior. One way to avoid this, of course, is to select assessment guides that define behaviors in terms of behavioral objectives. Also, whenever feasible, child behavior should be evaluated by more than one rater. The rating process can also be improved by the training of raters. In spite of some limitations, once the behaviors have been rated and translated into a behavior definition (which is then accurately measured), a program can be readily identified and developed for each deficient behavior.

*Probing Procedures.* Probing is a process in which brief samples of a pupil's performance are placed under standard, timed conditions (Haring & Gentry, 1976). Testing material consists of learning sequences, which are placed in a task-analysis format so that their uniformity is maintained. Because these probing materials control the uniformity of response, they also help control the conditions and amount of time under which a child performs. Haring and co-workers (Haring & Gentry, 1976) identify several steps that must be completed before probing procedures can be implemented:

1. Identify sequence of tasks to be taught; for example, arithmetic—rote counting, counting objects, addition, subtraction, multiplication; reading—grapheme, phoneme correspondence, word families, word analysis skill.
2. Divide each sequence into further component parts; for example, addition—basic facts, two-column problems without carryovers, two-column problems with carryovers, multiple-column problems without carryovers.
3. Develop scoring keys for the counting of correct answers and errors.
4. Administer probing devices within uniform time periods; for example, 30 seconds, 2 minutes.

Following is a probe series that includes rationale, subtest names, objectives, and other administrative directions for English Composition, grade four.

## General introduction to parts of speech and general directions for administration

I. Rationale
   A. This test is a criterion-referenced tool.
   B. This test follows the behavioral objectives listed in *English Composition Grade 4,* by John H. Treanor.
   C. This test has been correlated with the English Composition Series (see II below).
   D. This test can be administered to all students, grade 4 and above, who speak English.

II. Subtest names correlate with *English Composition* skills, and related grade levels.

| Subtest name | English Composition chapter | Grade level |
|---|---|---|
| A. Nouns—common | Chapter 5 | 4 |
| B. Nouns—proper | Chapter 5 | 4 |
| C. Pronouns | Chapter 5 | 4 |
| D. Adjectives | Chapter 5 | 4 |
| E. Verbs | Chapter 5 | 4 |

III. Objectives
   A. The learner will identify common nouns as told, to underline them, when presented with 10 phrases, at a rate of 90% correct in 5 minutes.
   B. The learner will identify proper nouns as told, to underline them, when presented with 10 phrases, at a rate of 90% correct in 5 minutes.
   C. The learner will identify pronouns as told, to underline them, when presented with 10 phrases, at a rate of 90% correct in 5 minutes.
   D. The learner will identify common adjectives as told, to underline them, when presented with 10 phrases, at a rate of 90% correct in 5 minutes.
   E. The learner will identify common verbs as told, to underline them, when presented with 10 phrases, at a rate of 90% correct in 5 minutes.

**Table 8-4**

Behavioral assessment guides and scales.

| Name | Description/Characteristic | Standardization | Publisher |
|---|---|---|---|
| Educational Evaluation and Planning Package | Focus on daily living, motor development, early language development, math, later language development, and social development; includes a breakdown of specific skills, specific level of assistance needed to perform each skill (e.g., verbal prompt, physical prompt), and parameters of performance (e.g., duration, setting, frequency) | Not standardized | Massachusetts Center for Program Development and Evaluation, 10 Hall Ave., Medford, Mass. |
| Santa Cruz Behavioral Characteristics Progression Observation Booklet | Checklist divided into 59 areas (e.g., daily living—toilet habits, hygiene; auditory and visual processing—language, academic behaviors; math, spelling, reasoning). | Not standardized | Vort Corporation, P.O. Box 1132, Palo Alto, Calif. |
| Lexington Developmental Scale | Items (452) evaluate five major areas: motor, language, personal and social, cognitive and emotional; areas except emotional are scored in terms of development of age | 3yr., 7 mo. to 7 yr., 4 mo. | United Cerebral Palsy of the Bluegrass, P.O. Box 8003, 465 Springhill Dr., Lexington, Ky. |
| Teacher's Guide Performance Inventory | Checklist on toilet training, behavior problems, dressing and grooming skills, mealtime skills, helping skills, and understanding and speaking skills; contains specific breakdown of the component skills in each task | Not standardized | Research Press, Box 3177, Champaign, Ill. |
| Progress Assessment Chart | Measures skills in four areas: self-help, communication, occupation, and socialization | Not standardized | USA Distribution Center, AUX Chandelles, PAC Department, P.O. Box 398, Bristol, Ind. |

IV. Materials needed for test administration
   A. Stopwatch or kitchen timer for timing testing sessions
   B. Sharpened pencils with erasers
   C. One chart for recording results for each student
   D. One set of 10 tests for each student to be tested

V. Directions for test administration
   A. Each student is allowed 5 minutes to complete each subtest.
   B. Explain the subtest to each student. Be sure students understand all directions. They must read the item, comprehend the item, and identify the part of speech requested.

   C. Score the students' responses in the recording booklet. Keep scores for each day they are tested.
   D. If students finish before time is up, they should return to the beginning and check responses.
   E. The examiner records and scores students' responses in the recording booklet.
   F. The number of attempted answers should equal one per 30 seconds of total time allotted. Answers to at least 50% of the total items must be correct, to continue testing.
   G. Test on 3 consecutive days. Average the best two out of three scores; multiply by 2. Record date and score for each test.

**Table 8-4**

*continued*

| Name | Description/Characteristic | Standardization | Publisher |
|---|---|---|---|
| TARC Assessment System | Four-stage system focusing on self-help, motor communication, social skill; stages include (1) assessment, (2) profiling, (3) derivation of instructional objective, and (4) curriculum selection | Items gathered from 283 severely handicapped children of various ages | W. Sailor, & J. Mix, TARC Assessment System, H & H Enterprises, Lawrence, Kan. |
| Cain-Levine Social Competence Scale | Number of items in each domain is either 10 (initiative, social skills, and commmunication) or 14 (self-help); interviewing and scoring formula similar to Vineland | 5 to 14 yr. | L. Cain and others, Consulting Psychologists Press, Palo Alto, Calif. |
| Balthazar Scales of Adaptive Behavior | Section I includes scales in (1) eating , (2) dressing and undressing, (3) toileting questionnaire; Section II includes (1) unadaptive self-directed behaviors, (2) unadaptive interpersonal behaviors, (3) adaptive self-direct, (4) adaptive interpersonal, (5) verbal communication, (6) play activities, (7) response to instructions, and (8) personal care; primary emphasis given to information obtained by direct observation | Severely and profoundly retarded individuals, 5 to 57 yr. | E. E. Balthazar, Research Press, Champaign, Ill. |
| Portage Project Checklist | Checklist of behavior normally occurring in children from birth to 5 yr; checklist is pooling of items from several inventories and scales; cognitive, self-help, motor, language, and socialization; deficient behavior in the checklist is referred to in cards that state the instructional goal in behavioral terms and suggest materials and methods for teaching the skill | Not standardized | Sheares and others, Portage Guide to Early Education: Instructional Checklist, Cooperative Educational Agency, No. 12, Portage, Wis. |

VI. Acceptable examples of parts of speech
The following list provides examples of the different parts of speech that the learner is to identify:
A. Common noun—names a general person, place, or thing (doctor, man, kitchen, train)
B. Proper noun—names a specific person, place, or thing (Aunt Ann, San Francisco, George)
C. Pronoun—takes the place of a noun (I, she, we, they)
D. Adjective—modifies a noun or pronoun (brave, frozen, blue, cloudy)
E. Verb—action or mode of being (run, talk, is, are)

VII. Recordkeeping
A. Pretest
1. Record pretest date and child's grade for all subtests administered. Begin with subtest Nouns—Common.
2. Record percent of correct answers for each subtest.
B. Mastery level (see objectives)
1. If pretest indicates mastery, do not remediate. Record pretest data and percent correct for mastery.
2. For those in remediation, record date. Date will vary for each student and for each subtest.
3. To determine mastery for each remediated subtest:

    a. Give test on 3 consecutive school days (unless mastery is achieved).

    b. Take the best 2 out of 3 scores.

    c. Average the scores.

    d. Record the subtest score and date under Mastery.

C. Follow-up

    1. Give 3 days at the end of school.

    2. Include mastery and remediated subtests.

    3. Follow same procedures for recording as used for pretest and mastery.

**Sample item**—probe for learning objective 1

1. A hungry, black bear
2. The yellow paint
3. Empty boxes
4. A hot, sandy desert
5. Fluffy, playful kittens
6. The huge, foreign ship
7. A bicycle, rusty and broken
8. The fire, warm and bright
9. The soft, cheery quilt
10. A savage tiger

Because probing materials are often adapted from existing classroom curriculum, we suggest that those selecting material to be used in assessment, attend to these requirements:

1. Instructional materials should have the same content as the learning objectives the teacher selected.

2. Instructional materials should provide for overt or active response.

3. Instructional materials should separate a learning task into small, sequential steps appropriate to the learner.

4. Curricular materials should allow for immediate correction and feedback to the learner.

5. Materials must allow individualization of performance, so that each child is allowed to respond individually at his or her own level.

6. Instructional materials should specify the knowledge prerequisite for entrance into the program.

7. The format of instructional materials should be clear, so that pupils' performance errors are not due to misunderstanding of instructions.

8. Instructional materials should provide for various overt responses so that the child is not locked into certain responses.

*Precision Measurement (Teaching).* Precision measurement (teaching) is a system of monitoring, charting, analyzing, and evaluating behavioral acceleration and deceleration rates. Precision measurement, as developed by Lindsley (1964), is not a new system of assessment for teaching within a particular behavioral teaching method, but is a set of procedures to be used with *any* method of teaching. According to Lindsley (1971), a teacher's problem is not to discover a new universal teaching method, but to use the excellent teaching methods already available within a daily measurement procedure. These procedures are based on the concepts of measuring and recording each child's progress. The system of precision measurement operates on the premise that each child is different, and the method is, therefore, designed to enable the teacher to find the abilities of each child and allow each child to advance at his or her own rate (Haring & Bateman, 1977; Howell, Kaplan, & O'Connell, 1979).

The steps involved in the use of precision-measurement techniques to evaluate pupil performance are:

1. Pinpoint behavior (academic and behavioral)

2. Record (frequency or movement cycles per minute)

3. Compute performance rate (number of movement cycles ÷ minutes recorded)

4. Chart performance on six-cycle semilog graph paper

5. Change rate (either acceleration or deceleration)

The purpose of measurement is to find out what has been learned and the exact conditions that produced learning, so that the effective condition can be used again (Howell, Kaplan, & O'Connell, 1979). A movement cycle is a pinpointed behavior stated in a form that can be assessed for reliability. It has the following three characteristics: (1) it is controllable by the child, (2) the behavior has movement, and (3) it is repeatable. For example, drawing a circle is a behavior that one can make or not make; therefore, it is controllable. Someone pushes the pencil so it has movement. Another circle can be made when the first one is finished; therefore, it is repeatable. The frequency and observation time of the pinpointed behavior can be recorded.

The basic measure in precision teaching is rate—the number of movement cycles divided by the number of minutes the teacher observed. For example, if 10 circles are made in 1 minute, the rate would be determined by dividing 10 by 1. Because many devices for counting are available (tally sheets, wrist counters, hand tally), any procedure that accurately keeps track of behavior and time (later converted to movement cycles per minute) can be used.

Step 1 begins a process called the "Is-Does" formula. This is a method by which precise information about what is happening in the classroom is gained. The "Is" part of the formula is a description of what is going on currently; it refers specifically to the planning and describing of environmental events that might have an effect on classroom behavior. It consists of five components: (1) program, (2) programmed event, (3) movement cycle, (4) arrangement, and (5) arranged event. Haring and Gentry (1976) explain these components and give an example of how to set up the "Is" part of the formula:

*Program (P):* overall classroom setting (includes subject taught, seating arrangement— Sullivan Program, Math Book #2, 11:00– 11:30)

*Programmed event (PE):* event that occurred before desired or undesired behavior emissions (instruction, material, teasing from another child)

*Movement cycle (M):* behavior under change— the controlling stimuli or consequences are unknown at this stage (two-digit addition problems, talking, writing name)

*Arrangement (A):* the ratio of times a desired or undesired behavior is emitted and the consequences that occur (1:1 would mean that for every behavior, M, emitted, a subsequent event, teacher verbalization, occurs); arrangements usually set up by the teacher

*Arrange event (AE):* specified environmental consequences used to determine the effects of reinforcement on a movement cycle (praise, allowed to leave room, points earned)

The "Does" formula represents a teaching strategy that has been proved effective with a particular child. "Does" is identical in structure to "Is" except that it consists of those events identified as having an effect on the pinpointed behavior. When the programmed event is changed and there is a change in the movement cycle, a functional relationship has been demonstrated. The reason for the terminology change is to help differentiate between an environmental event that is being tried and an environmental alteration that *does* work. As indicated, environmental events that do influence the movement cycle are applied only after the teacher has collected and analyzed pinpointed behaviors. Therefore, in the "Does" analysis (P) becomes disposition (D), (PE) becomes stimulus (S), (M) becomes response, (A) becomes contingency (K), and (AE) becomes consequence (C). Understanding the "Is-Does" formula enables a teacher to analyze the classroom environment, and thereby provides information needed for change procedures. After learning to pinpoint and count movement cycles and to analyze the classroom environment, the teacher is ready to record data.

Steps 2, 3, and 4 involve recording the rate of behavior on six-cycle semilog paper (Figure 8-3). The horizontal lines represent the rate of frequency, divided into cycles; the vertical lines are daily lines. The dark vertical lines are Sunday lines, while the vertical sequence of numbers to the left of the lines represents the number of movement cycles per minute. Again, movement cycles per minute are the number of recorded behaviors divided by the time in which the behavior was re-

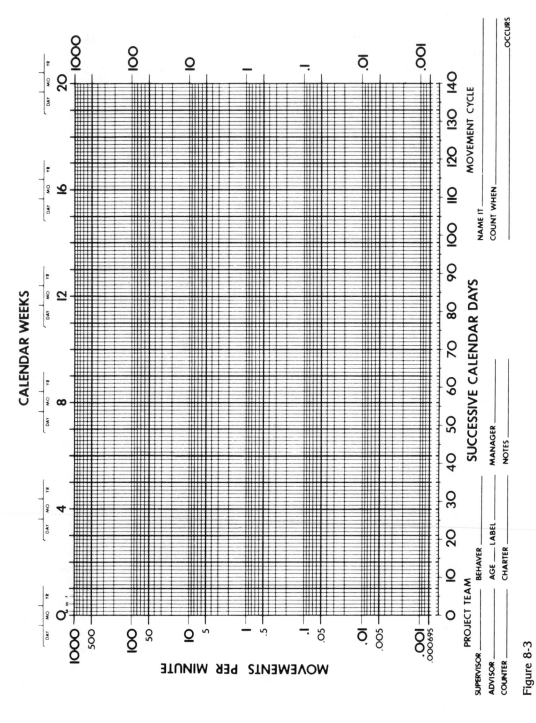

Figure 8-3

Six-cycle semilog paper. (Reprinted by permission of Behavior Research Co., Box 3351, Kansas City, KS 66103.)

corded. The cycles on the vertical line are in "multiple" arrangements of 1 to 1000 on the top half of the chart, to 1 on the bottom. On the top half of the chart (1 to 1000), lines begin from 1, 2, 3, ... 10 times per minute. The next group of lines means 10, 20, 30, ... 100 times per minute. The next cycle means 100, 200, ... 500, ... 1000 times per minute.

The purpose of the bottom half of the chart (below 1, to 0.001 or 0) is to record movement cycles that happen less frequently than once in 1 minute. For example, from 1 to 0.1, movement cycle per minute is divided by 10, and each rate line decreases by one tenth (0.9, 0.8, 0.7, ... 0.1). The next cycle (0.1 to 0.01) is divided by 100, and each rate line decreases by one hundredth. The final cycle is divided by 1000 from 0.01 to 0.001, and each line decreases by one thousandth. The advantages of six-cycle charting are that (1) all behavior can be recorded (high frequency and low frequency), and (2) the proportion or ratio of changes is related over time and compared with other recorded behaviors. Also, on this logarithmic scale, there is never an absolute zero point, so that the location of any given datapoint, which indicates movement cycles per minute, varies as the amount of time varies. All pertinent administrative information is recorded in the appropriate space as a permanent record. For a more detailed analysis, see Howell, Kaplan, and O'Connell (1979).

Step 5 focuses on changing movement-cycle rates. Discussion of this stage relates directly to the earlier discussion on procedures designed to increase and decrease behaviors (see Table 8-1). The use of continuous recording enables teachers to provide a uniform measurement of a pupil's daily progress. The curriculum, type of materials, and content of program must be included in the "Does" part of the plan. A procedure for analyzing the graphed data was outlined by White and Haring (1976); this procedure is called a trend analysis. Data on the graph must be divided into two parts with equal numbers of datapoints; the median and mid-middle points (point half-way between median) of each half are then established.

The trend line is the connection of the mid-middle points on each half. The trend line shows if pupil performance is increasing, decreasing, or remaining constant.

General behavior-assessment procedures stress the use of reinforcers; precision teaching also stresses the use of measurement and the more traditional change-procedures from curriculum. In essence, the system calls for the daily charting (on standard behavior charts) of the rate of any specified behavior. Precision measures provide the teacher with a way of comparing and evaluating daily teaching effects.

*Summary.* The definition and general quantification stage can be summarized as a phase in which a series of assessment activities takes place (each with its own validity requirement), to accomplish at least the following: (1) identification of skill and problem areas, (2) quantification of general levels of skills, and (3) determination of the "where and how" of needed learning (Hawkins, 1979). Strategically, this phase represents a period of hypotheses-formation and measurement of the presence or absence of hypothesized factors. The variety of measurement may include direct assessment in controlled environments (for example, probing), direct methods in natural environments (for example, checklists), or indirect assessment of behaviors.

### Pinpointing and Designing Intervention

*Objectives.* Behavioral assessment in the classroom usually involves six steps. Step 1 simply involves *defining the specific target behaviors.* Within step 1, the following questions have to be answered:

1. What observable behavior do you want to increase or decrease?
2. Has the behavior been defined in objective terms (for example, conditions and performance)?
3. What do you want the child ultimately to do (criteria)?

4. Does your definition of behavior generate between 80% and 100% agreement among different observers (does it achieve interobserver agreement)?

Once the general target behavior has been defined, decisions concerning the objectives of a particular course of intervention and appropriate teaching-learning strategies can be made. Before teaching strategies can be made operational, instructional objectives must be written. General statements in terms of the child's deficits are based on the purpose and direction or, more accurately, the statement of conditions or "states of being" the teacher wishes to have exist in the future. Such a general statement includes conditions in which the task is to be performed, how well the child must perform to be considered successful, and the amount of time spent on the task. Thus, educational intervention is based on Mager's (1972) concept of behavioral-instructional objectives.

A behavioral-instructional objective is a "teaching plan-of-action" describing intended outcomes in relation to a terminal behavior expected of the learner. The *terminal behavior* is a goal behavior whose achievement requires the learner to make a reasonable change. Instructional objectives are based on the following elements: (1) performance-based terms (what the learner will do physically to demonstrate achievement), (2) conditions or situation in which behavior is to occur, and (3) criteria of acceptable performance, used to evaluate the success of the teacher's daily objectives. Criteria of acceptable performance usually state degrees of time (two lessons), accuracy (90% correct responses), and difficulty level (second-grade basal reader). Instructional objectives identify a specific direction and goal for each type of behavior.

A sample objective would be: Given the *Sullivan Programmed Mathematics Division* (Behavioral Research Laboratories) *Book Number 27* (problems with one-digit quotients, no remainders), the student will write correct answers in 5 minutes, at a rate of 30 digits per minute, with no errors. The word "write" represents a performance-based term. The condition under which writing is to occur is prescribed by the Sullivan materials. Criteria of acceptable performance used to evaluate this objective are time (5 minutes), accuracy (30 digits per minute with no errors), and difficulty level (book 27: problems with one-digit quotients, no remainders).

*Measurement procedures.* Step 2 is *deciding on an appropriate measurement procedure.* Step 2 is crucial in the quantification of information. Once behavior has been pinpointed, it becomes necessary to maintain accurate measurement so that behavior can be charted for analysis. The target behavior that has been selected will influence the type of measurement used. Questions related to this step include:

1. What is the time, period, interval, for measuring the target behavior?
2. What measurement techniques will be used (time sample, permanent products)?
3. What type of material will be used in data collection (worksheet, stopwatch)?
4. Who will be the other observers?
5. How will data be charted (percentage, rate, frequency, proportion)?
6. What evaluation design should be used (reversal, multiple baseline, criterion changing)?

Measuring and recording behavior are commonly achieved through the use of two methods: direct measurement of permanent products, and observational recording. Behaviors of children sometimes result in permanent products. These products are tangible and can be observed and counted. A technique that allows the teacher to measure the tangible output of a student's work is called *direct measurement of permanent products.* Examples include written answers to math problems, the written spelling of words, or the writing of alphabet letters (Figure 8-4). Teachers can translate permanent products into numerical terms of percentage, rate, or frequency of occurrence.

Name _____ _____

Subtraction facts

| 12 | 16 | 9 | 10 | 14 | 12 | 9 | 14 | 10 | 12 |
|----|----|---|----|----|----|---|----|----|----|
| 7  | 9  | 2 | 5  | 7  | 4  | 1 | 8  | 6  | 9  |
| 5  | 7  | 7 | 4  | 8  | 7  | 8 | 7  | 4  | 3  |

Time began _____    Time ended _____

Interobserver _____    Teacher _____

**Figure 8-4**
Illustration of form for direct measurement of permanent products.

A major advantage of measuring permanent products is that student behavior can be measured after its occurrence. Other advantages include the precision with which records can be kept, the availability of permanent records that can be translated into numerical terms, and the development of products that represent the end product of academic behaviors. Teachers can translate permanent products into numerical terms (see Figure 8-4), in terms of (1) percentage (Scott worked 60% of the problems correctly), (2) frequency (Scott incorrectly calculated four problems), and (3) rate (Scott calculated one problem per minute).

Teachers concerned with social behaviors that do not result in permanent products can produce records of that behavior as it occurs. *Observational recording* is the recording of behavior as it happens. Five major observational techniques are available for the classroom context: (1) continuous recording, (2) event record-

ing, (3) duration recording, (4) interval recording, and (5) time sampling.

*Continuous recording,* also called anecdotal recording, requires the teacher to write down everything as it happens. Continuous recording produces a written narrative of behavior for a specified period. Continuous recording techniques contain the following common elements:

1. A specified time sequence: the sequence to be reported may be in short or long units of time.
2. Target behaviors are not pinpointed.
3. Data are narrative descriptions of behavior, that include a three-term contingency of (a) events that occur before a behavior is emitted, (b) the behavior, and (c) consequences or events that occur after the emission of the observed behavior.

The purpose of continuous recording is to produce as complete a description as possible of a child's behavior in the classroom. Teachers use continuous recording techniques to (1) aid in assessing and pinpointing target behaviors, (2) identify antecedent and consequent events maintaining behavior, and (3) observe and record a large range of behaviors for pre- and post-measurement of teacher effectiveness.

Bijou, Peterson, and Ault (1968) report an example of continuous recording with Timmy, a preschool child (Figure 8-5). To produce a clear impression of the time relationships among antecedent stimulus-events, responses, and consequent stimulus-events, we present the objective aspects of the narrative in a columnar format. As stated by Bijou, Peterson, and Ault, a response event ("5 ... says, 'Mrs. Simpson, watch me' ") may be followed by a consequent social event ("6. Mrs. S. turns toward Timmy"), which may also be the antecedent event for the next response ("7. T. climbs to top of apparatus"). Note that only the child's responses are described. Inferences about feelings, motives, and other presumed internal states are omitted. Even words such as *ignores* and *disappointed* do not appear.

*Durational recording* is used if it is important to know how long a particular behavior lasts. Durational recording is an appropriate measurement tactic for the recording of behavior that occurs at very high rates (rocking, tapping, or twisting objects) or of behaviors that occur for extended periods (task-oriented behavior). Measures of duration are usually reported as the percentage of total episodic time in which a behavior continues. If a teacher wishes to know how long a temper tantrum lasts, for example, he or she would merely have to record with a watch how many minutes the child engages in that particular behavior, as part of a specified observation period. To determine what percentage of total time is spent in the specified behavior, data reporting follows the formula:

$$\% = \frac{\text{Duration of target behavior}}{\text{Duration of class or observation period}} \times 100$$

A major problem in durational recording is that the teacher must continuously attend to the child of concern. For example, if a teacher is concerned with the amount of time a student takes to begin an academic task, the teacher will have to attend to the particular student's behavior for the full duration. For this type of objective, durational recording can be adapted to determine how much time elapses before a certain behavior is emitted (for example, taking seat to begin school work). If we measure the time that elapses between the teacher giving the instruction ("take your seat") and the time when the appropriate behavior is begun or is carried out, we can measure the latency of the behavior.

A stopwatch is usually the most efficient tool for making durational recordings. *Event-recording* procedures make a cumulative record of discrete events of a certain behavior classification (for example, number of times a student gets out of seat). Numerical data may be expressed in terms of rate, frequency, or percentage. Devices such as a wrist golf-counter, hand-tally digital counter, wrist tally board, masking tape attached to the wrist, or a tally with buttons or paper clips may facilitate making tallies of frequency counts. The amount of time during which a particular child or group can be observed, can vary from situation to situation, but time durations should be consistent for that particular situation. Further, frequency-count report forms can be expanded to include many behaviors.

Event-recording procedures are a good measurement procedure for short-duration behaviors, such as out-of-seat, hitting, and academic error behaviors. Long-duration behaviors, such as temper tantrums, would not be appropriate pinpointed behavior for event-recording procedures.

Event and durational recording generates data on student behavior occurring during one time period; *interval recording* is used to measure the occurrence or nonoccurrence of behavior within specified time intervals. Each observation period is divided into equal time periods,

**Setting:** Timmy (T.) is playing alone in a sandbox in a play yard in which there are other children playing. T. is scooping sand into a bucket with a shovel, then dumping the sand onto a pile. A teacher, Mrs. Simpson (S.), stands approximately 6 feet away but does not attend to T.

| Time | Antecedent event | Response | Consequent social event |
|---|---|---|---|
| 9:14 | | 1. T. throws bucket and shovel into corner of sandbox. | |
| | | 2. ... stands up. | |
| | | 3. ... walks over to monkeybars and stops. | |
| | | 4. ... turns toward teacher. | |
| | | 5. ... says, "Mrs. Simpson, watch me." | |
| | | | 6. Mrs. S. turns toward Timmy. |
| | 6. Mrs. S. turns toward Timmy. | 7. T. climbs to top of apparatus. | |
| | | 8. ... looks toward teacher. | |
| | | 9. ... says, "Look how high I am. I'm higher than anybody." | |
| 9:16 | | | 10. Mrs. S. says, "That's good, Tim. You're getting quite good at that." |
| | 10. Mrs. S. says, "That's good Tim. You're getting quite good at that." | 11. T. climbs down. | |
| | | 12. ... runs over to tree. | |
| | | 13. ... says, "Watch me climb the tree, Mrs. Simpson." | |
| | | | 14. Mrs. S turns and walks toward classroom. |
| | 14. Mrs. S. turns and walks toward classroom. | 15. T. stands, looking toward Mrs. S. | |
| 9:18 | 16. Girl nearby trips and falls, bumping knee. | | |
| | 17. Girl cries. | | |
| | | 18. T. proceeds to sandbox. | |
| | | 19. ... picks up bucket and shovel. | |
| | | 20. ... resumes play with sand. | |

**Figure 8-5**

An example of continuous recording. (From Bijou, S., Peterson, D., & Ault, M. A method to integrate descriptive and experimental field studies at the level of data and empirical concepts. *Journal of Applied Behavior Analysis,* 1968, *1,* 179–180.)

varying in seconds depending on the behavior to be observed. Data are usually reported in terms of frequency and duration (behavior across time intervals).

Figure 8-6 shows a data sheet for interval recording of attending behaviors on an academic task (for example, eye contact with SRA Reader assignment) and talking aloud. The teacher records the occurrence or nonoccurrence of each target behavior during 10-second

intervals of a 10-minute observation period. If at any time during the 10-second interval the child engages in the target behavior, the student interval is scored A or T.

An advantage of interval recording is that it gives the teacher an indication of both frequency and duration of single and multiple categories of behaviors. Interval recording also generates information concerning the times at which a behavior is likely or not likely to occur.

**Figure 8-6**

Illustration form for internal recording of talking/nontalking and attending/nonattending for every 10 seconds.

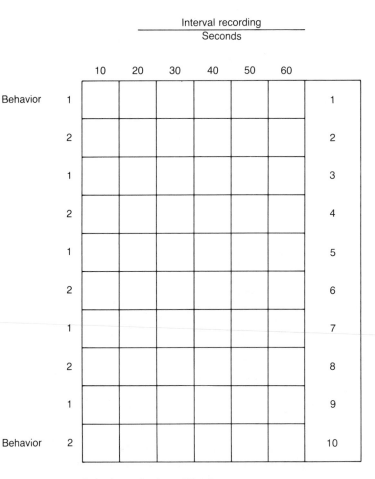

Behavior code:  A  = Attending
N  = Nonattending
T  = Talking
NT  = Nontalking

Time of observation session _____

Interval recording is also useful when more than one behavior or the behavior of more than one subject at a time is being recorded. In such cases, additional rows of squares may be used for recording the additional behaviors.

Time sampling is similar to interval recording except that the teacher observes only what the child is doing at the end of the interval. Time sampling is a useful measurement procedure for obtaining numerical estimates of group or student behavior that occurs while the teacher is engaged in instruction or other activities. Although time samples are frequently made in equal intervals, it is sometimes practical to sample at irregular intervals throughout the observation sessions. The length of the intervals between observations is determined by the frequency of behavior. If the behavior is of relatively short duration, frequent samples must be made. Intervals on a time-sampling procedure are usually recorded in minutes.

Another procedure that is sometimes used to sample the behavior of groups is called *placheck*. The "placheck" (Planned Activity Check) technique requires that the observer:

1. Specify in observable terms the behavior(s) to be recorded in the classroom.
2. Within specified intervals (minutes), tally how many children are involved in the specific behavior.
3. Tally the number of children within the classroom or area of activity.
4. Divide the number of children engaged in the specified behaviors by the number of children in the class or area of activity, and multiply by 100. The endproduct of the procedure is the percentage of children engaged in the specified time interval at a particular time

*ABC Analysis.* In step 3 the teacher begins to take a baseline and develop an ABC analysis. *Baseline* is merely a record of behavior under the existing classroom conditions. The reason for taking baseline measurement is to provide a basis by which the behavior under normal con-

ditions can be compared with behavior under conditions in which a special technique is being applied. An *ABC procedure* involves analyzing the *antecedent* stimuli (A) and *consequences* (C) maintaining the target *behavior* (B). Information for this analysis can be gathered by the use of a continuous-recording technique. The ABC analysis helps the teacher formulate behavioral strategy for the identification of suitable consequences, while identifying stimulus cues that set the occasion for inappropriate behavior.

*Teaching Strategy.* In step 4 the teacher *implements the teaching strategy.* The teacher identifies an appropriate reinforcer (or punisher), criterion for the consequence, and details of the contingency. Procedures for the teaching strategy are detailed so that they can be repeated.

*Effectiveness of the Contingencies.* In step 5 the teacher evaluates the *effectiveness of the contingencies.* Essentially, step 5 asks the question, "Did the teaching strategy substantially affect the baseline rate?" Information is given to the teacher to either modify or continue teaching procedures, schedules, or details of the student contingencies.

*Generalization/discrimination.* In step 6 the teacher develops *a generalization and/or discrimination procedure.* It sometimes happens that a new behavior is learned in one situation (for example, a special-education classroom) but not transferred to another (for example, regular classroom), or that behavior learned in one situation is not appropriate in another. To avoid or reduce difficulties of generalization, the teacher should attempt to (1) increase similarities between the training setting and other settings in which the behavior is expected to occur, (2) practice new behaviors in numerous settings, (3) train people in the natural environment to use discriminative and reinforcing events, and (4) teach the child to manage his or her own behavior. Step 6, then, includes a process for the communication of results, to ensure that behavior success is programmed.

## Monitoring Progress

Hawkins (1979) states that the primary function of assessment in this phase is the "determination of the current level of performance so that the intervention can be evaluated and changed as needed" (p. 508). A secondary function is the determination of the "palatability" of intervention to the learner. To address these two functions, this section will briefly review evaluation designs.

*Evaluation Designs.* A distinguishing feature of a behavioral assessment is the careful evaluation of the current educational program. All evaluations of behavioral programs can be summarized by the question: Does the teaching strategy substantially affect the baseline rate of a student's academic and/or management behavior? Special-education programs contain various evaluative procedures that are used to (1) assess the learner's progress toward attainment of terminal objectives, and (2) provide evidence on the direction of behavioral change that results from intervention. The demonstration of experimental control in behavior assessment has been achieved primarily through the use of single-subject designs, in which the effects of successive experimental conditions on the performance of children are observed. Several alternative single-subject designs for modifying children's behavior in applied settings have been developed. The precise, daily evaluation procedures have many advantages over global, norm-referenced, or infrequent measurement (Kampus, 1987). Each design has, however, limitations and advantages that make it suitable for particular classroom problems.

A review of simple designs indicates that classroom application of baseline logic often employs a procedure called "A-B analysis." *A* represents repeated measures of the baseline period, and *B* represents the application of instructional strategy. This design is most useful in providing information on when to change

instruction, for if the *B* condition does not differ from the baseline condition, then the instructional material should be modified, tasks should be in smaller steps, or the reinforcement of behavior needs to be changed.

Although this procedure can indicate the magnitude of change, it cannot establish the effectiveness of the teaching, because it does not provide controlled demonstrations of causality. A design adopted to extend and control the limitations of the AB format is the *reversal,* or withdrawal, *design.* Conditions of the reversal design include an ABAB format in which an experimental variable, *B,* is alternately introduced and reversed or withdrawn. If the teaching strategy is causally related to the behavior under observation, the behavior should be alternately increased and diminished according to the manipulation of the instructional or environmental variable (Kratochwill, 1978).

Three variations on the reversal design have appeared in literature. These variations can be classified as (1) noncontingent reinforcement as a control condition, (2) contingent reinforcement to a polar behavior, and (3) differential reinforcement of other behaviors (DRO). Noncontingent reinforcement, a control factor, is best suited for demonstration of causality if the contingent application is social reinforcement (for example, verbal praise, smiling). The design prototype is best represented as *ABCBC,* where *B* represents noncontingent reinforcement (reinforcement given regardless of student behaviors) and *C* the reinforcement-given contingent for a specific behavior. The second variation, the application of contingent reinforcement to a polar behavior (for example, talking/nontalking, writing *21* for *12*), is represented as an *ABCB* design, where *B* represents the reinforcement of the target behavior and *C* represents the differential reinforcement of any or every occurrence of behavior except the target behavior. Limitations of the reversal designs and their variants are usually related to the classroom situation (for example, an aggressive-destructive behavior-reversal procedure may be physically harmful to others); certain behaviors may continue even after the teaching procedure is withdrawn.

Using an alternative strategy to reversing or withdrawing contingencies, a teacher may record several baselines and introduce a teaching variable in each baseline in succession. A *multiple-baseline design* is based on the assumption that each baseline will change in the same direction when a teaching variable is applied only *if* that variable is in fact functionally related to the behavior. The multiple-baseline design can be applied to (1) multiple but conceptually related behaviors of a child or group of children under the same conditions, (2) several children or groups who are under the same conditions, and whose similar behaviors are compared, and (3) multiple conditions (for example, resource room, regular classroom) in which the identical behaviors of a child or group occur. Intervention strategies are implemented on only one behavior (or child) after simultaneous records of other behaviors under similar or different conditions have been made. After a behavior change is generated for the first intervention, the same procedure is applied to the second baseline behavior. If change is generated, the teaching strategy is applied to the third baseline behavior, and so on. A major advantage of the multiple-baseline strategy is that reinforcement procedures do not have to be withdrawn. In the multiple-baseline procedures, the second condition, behavior, serves as a control condition. A limitation of this design is a "generalization effect," in which the teaching strategy affects not only the teaching behavior, but also other target behavior in baseline status (Kratochwill, 1978).

Another type of design is a *changing-criterion design*. After a baseline period, the intervention program is introduced; a specified response level must be attained before a specific reinforcement can be applied. This design requires the specification of successive criteria for performance as new responses are acquired, or a hierarchy of steps in the improvement of skills. Again, a major advantage of this design is that it does not require reversal or withdrawal of reinforcement; a disadvantage is that when a dramatic change is desired, a changing-criterion design is of little value. Unfortunately, changing-criterion designs have been used infrequently in special education.

*Multielement designs* (Ulman & Sultzer-Azaroff, 1975) intersperse baseline conditions and intervention strategies throughout the evaluation procedure. Treatment and baseline condition are presented alternately within sessions and from one session to the next. For example, the effects of three contingencies (no consequence, staying after class, reinforcing a competing behavior) on the completion of math assignments, could be alternated from day to day. The design involves measurement of behaviors under alternating conditions that can provide a clear discrimination of independent variables. The outcome of each contingency could be identified and evaluated after a reasonable number of sessions. The design permits the comparison of (1) the effect of one or more independent variables, (2) dependent variables whose rates are not likely to be reversed, and (3) the demands of time on the behavioral assessor. The multielement design is best adapted for use on complex behavior (such as written composition) and not simple operant behaviors such as talking aloud, out of seat, and attending.

## Follow-Up

Hawkins (1979) notes that a primary function of a follow-up assessment is "evaluation of the durability of sufficiency of behavior changes" (p. 510). Follow-up evaluation is achieved through the continuation of measurement procedures discussed earlier. Because these evaluation designs affect a narrow context that is constant over time, they may limit follow-up assessment in terms of producing desired change in key situations. Recently (e.g., Garbarino & Kapadia, 1986; Ollendick & Hersen, 1984; Lentz & Shapiro, 1986), there has been a bridging of ecological-related variables in behavioral procedures. Unfortunately, the ecological perspective does not provide a cohesive body of information, nor does it define any particular methods of assessment. Rather, its perspective provides a context in which assessment questions can be generated.

*Common features.* Earlier, Willems (1974) provided some distinctive features held in common by ecological and behavior-modification orientation:

1. *Empiricism and objectivity:* Emphasis for much of their theoretical orientation is placed on empirical data.
2. *Environment as selective:* Emphasis for both is placed on the transaction of behavior within an environmental context.
3. *Importance of site specificity:* Emphasis for both is placed on site specificity of behavior. A strong linkage is made between the place and the behavioral occurrence.
4. *Baseline data on behavior:* Emphasis for both is placed on the gathering of reliable, frequent, and relatively atheoretical data, as a beginning point.
5. *Environmental measurement:* Emphasis for both is placed on extensive documentation, measurement, and recording of the environment.
6. *Commonplaceness:* Both accept commonplace behavior such as eating, talking, resting, reading, as primary phenomena to be documented and modified.
7. *Common sense and principles of behavior:* Both accept common-sense principles of behavior change while at the same time pursuing principles that are counterintuitive.
8. *Intervention and its effects:* Emphasis for both is placed on creating conditions for the maintenance or shaping of a particular level of function, on a case-by-case basis (pp. 157–160).

Willems (1974), Carlson, Scott, and Elclund (1980), and Wahler, House, and Stambough (1976) have noted many areas in which behavioral analysts and ecologists tend to differ in their interpretations of data and arrive at different objectives for intervention. Behavioral assessment tends to restrict itself to an intervention in what the therapist considers to be a direct and immediate characteristic for behavior changes. The ecologist tends to focus on the context of interventions and the possible indirect effects of intervention (for example, unanticipated complexities, or indirect stimulus control—one set of behaviors can be maintained or affected by a reinforcer applied directly to other behaviors). A review of general points of contention between the two approaches may provide specific direction for behavioral assessment follow-up. Among the central themes for behavior assessment within a behavioral ecology are:

1. Child behavior is to be studied at levels of complexity beyond simple ABC-analysis procedures.
2. Complex relations that link behavior, social environment, and physical environment variables are to be assessed in a child.
3. Interrelations of social and physical environment are to be appropriately conceptualized (not piecemeal).
4. Behavior-environment systems are to be studied over time so that important properties can be discovered.
5. Tampering with only one part of a child's ecosystem does not necessarily relate to other parts of the system or to its whole.
6. Simple intrusion can produce unintended effects, and indirect harm (short-term goals) may follow a narrowly defined assessment, in terms of long-term goals.
7. Focus of assessment is on interventions and planned changes designed in a comprehensive fashion.

Taking into account these points of divergence, we can conclude that success in monitoring must be linked inextricably to interdependent systems of the child. For example, behavioral assessment might consider the classroom activity's (1) format, (2) proxemics, (3) mutual delivery of interpersonal reinforcers and punishers, and (4) shape, in the distribution of the furniture in the classroom.

*Classroom Variables.* An ecological frame-work can be used in the assessment of some physical variables, so that a positive follow-up is ensured. Some valuable working guidelines for classroom application follow.

1. Determine the optimal organizational space in the classroom. This includes consideration of variables such as closed versus open cubicles. Some children are more likely to be social isolates when closed cubicles are used.
2. Determine child-to-child, teacher-to-child physical and functional distance. For example, it is important in determining seating arrangements, to consider which distance is functional for the control of extraneous behavior and which distance is functional for the development of teacher-student relationships through close formal contact. Halahan and Seagart (1973) offer a continuum for chair and furniture arrangements based on the effects of arrangement on social contacts. The arrangements are "sociofugal-seating," with seats placed along the walls and tables in the center of the room; "sociopetal-seating," with seats clustered around tables in the center of the room; mixed (some seating near wall and some near tables); and free (asking individuals to arrange chairs as they please). Less positive social interaction was found in the "sociofugal" and free settings.
3. Determine how the overall design of the classroom may facilitate or inhibit teacher-child interaction. Getzel (1974) found that particular architectural arrangements of the classroom imply certain "images" to students. Rectangular classrooms, with straight rows and the teacher's desk in front, imply the image of an "empty organism," in which the child learns only from the teacher. The square classroom, with movable chairs and the teacher's desk in the corner, is congruent with images of an "active organism," in which the child participates in the learning process. Classrooms that do not contain a teacher's desk and have pupils' desks placed in a trapezoid or circle, next to the teacher, imply the image of a "social organism," in which learning is primarily obtained from peers. The open classroom with several activity centers is congruent to the image of a "stimulus-seeking organism," in which the child discovers or experiences the learning process.
4. Determine if the provision of amenities (wall decorations, posters, colored tables, radio music) increases or decreases incongruent behavior. The purpose is to have the child associate these amenities with familiar home and community environments.
5. Determine the child's body-buffer zones that signal the need for personal space. When the child's space is invaded, he or she may verbally or physically defend this space.
6. Determine the various negative and positive reactions to noise in the classroom. Children habituate differently on classroom noise. Different thresholds of noise can affect how children attend to the task at hand.

*Monitoring Behavioral Assessment.* Willems (1977) makes some practical suggestions: For the maintenance of behavior-assessment procedures that will ensure positive outcomes of follow-up,

1. Increase the number of settings in which observations are made (complex effects occur across different settings).
2. Increase the length of observation time (complex effects are often obscured by short lapses of time).
3. Increase the number of persons other than the target person who are observed.
4. Increase the number of behavioral categories.
5. Increase the number of observations on uncontrolled stimuli (e.g., reaction to intervention that was not targeted) (p. 53).

## SUMMARY

This chapter reviewed basic distinctions between traditional and behavioral assessment. These models were contrasted on their levels of inference. Five phases of behavioral assessment were suggested: screening and general disposition, definition and general quantification, pinpointing and designing intervention, monitoring progress, and follow-up. The contributions of behavioral analysis to classroom variables, as well as some possible observational systems, were identified.

# CHAPTER 9

# Assessment of Affective Competence

## OUTLINE

**A**ffect, in contrast to other domains of assessment, is difficult to quantify, yet very few educators and psychologists would deny its existence. *Affect* connotes a process of internalization (Krathwohl, Bloom, and Masia, 1964). *Internalization* is viewed as the adaptation of social values and products as one's own; only an incomplete adaptation of positive behaviors is made at first, followed by a more complete adaptation (Dogge, Pettit, & Brown, 1986; Eisenberg & Harris, 1984; Erickson, 1964; Kohlberg, 1964; Krathwohl, Bloom & Masia, 1964). *Competence* connotes the existence within a personality of particular capabilities for coping with social situations (Carlson, Scott, & Elclund, 1980; Furman, 1980; Gresham & Elliot, 1984, 1987; Scott, 1980; Wicker, 1979). Both concepts are necessary to the process by which the individual problems of a child are linked to the characteristic demands of a social system. The purpose of this chapter is to (1) provide a theoretical base for affective-competence assessment, and (2) review test instruments applicable to this assessment.

## AFFECTIVE COMPETENCE DEFINED

In reviewing construct systems used for children who might be classified as having affective difficulties, several authors (e.g., Gresham & Elliot, 1984, 1987; Jackson & Pavnonen, 1980) have noted a growing need for assessment of the child's competence. However, the term *competence* itself is vague; it denotes such things as social skills, interpersonal actions, social judgments, and affective objectives for educational programs. For competence to be adequately assessed, the assessment procedure must be embedded within an ecological framework (Swap, 1973; Thurman, 1977; Wicker, 1979). As pointed out by Popham (1978), a child's affective development is related to many separate, though interrelated, environmental systems (ecosystems). It is becoming increasingly clear that affective development is not separate from the biological, psychological, and social needs of children. In addition to the interaction of cognitive and affective development (Erickson, 1968; Kohlberg, 1964; Piaget, 1970), school, family, and a variety of social interactions are involved.

Three general definitions of social competence are generally evidenced in the literature (see Gresham & Elliot, 1984, for a review). One definition focuses on *peer acceptance*. According to this definition, students who are accepted by their peers are assumed to be socially competent. Gresham and Elliot (1984) argue that although it is feasible to obtain objective measures of social acceptance, use of a peer-acceptance definition in assessment does not result in data that target the specific behaviors that enhance acceptance among peers. Therefore, even if behavior is accurately assessed, the assessment does not provide information useful to the next step, the improvement of behavior. A second definition provides a *behavioral* definition of competence. Competence is described as specific behaviors that maximize the probability of reinforcement being maintained in a social context. Unfortunately, this definition does not ensure that the social behaviors that are assessed are socially important. A third definition reflects an *ecological or social* interpretation. Competence is defined in terms of those behaviors that focus on (1) peer acceptance, (2) the judgment of significant others and, (3) the correlation of peer acceptance and significant-others' judgment. This definition allows competence to be conceptualized as an exchange between the child and a responder (school, community, family).

If we gather information about both the child's affective development and ecology (social setting), then we can more adequately conceptualize the child's affective competence. Some indications of a child's affective competence can be obtained through the answering of these questions:

1. What sociocultural conditions are most likely to produce disturbances in affective behavior?

2. Why do children continue disturbing behavior despite control brought to bear on them by community, family, or school?
3. What determining factors cause a child to be set apart?
4. To what extent do children realign their self-concept in accord with the labels given them?
5. What changes in peer-group membership result from the behavior disturbance?

Most children function in an ecology system that can be defined as adaptive, or congruent; that is, most children are in harmony with the social norms of their environmental contexts (Dodge, Pettit, & Brown, 1986; Gresham & Elliot, 1984; Brion-Meisels & Selman, 1984). However, when congruence with the ecological system no longer exists, the child is viewed as either deviant (out of harmony with social norms), incompetent (lacking means to achieve expected goals), or an aggravator to the tolerance level of the community (Carlson, Scott & Elclund, 1980).

## DETERMINING AFFECTIVE DEVIANCE

In earlier writings, Becker (1963) and Gove (1975) state that the concept of deviance is created by "social definition." Affective disturbance arises not when persons commit certain kinds of acts, but when a person commits an act that becomes known to some other person(s) who then defines (or labels) that act as inappropriate. The inappropriate behavior is seen, therefore, as a relative phenomenon (Szaz, 1970). If a deviant act is an act that breaks a norm and if norms vary from social group to social group, an act considered deviant in one setting might not be deviant in another situation or another social ecology. Therefore, judgment about a particular child's behavior or set of characteristics can only be made relative to the social context in which it occurred.

If a specific behavior is neither good nor bad, neither competent nor incompetent, the labeling

process demands that an examination be made of (1) the effect of the behavior on the perceiver, (2) the viewpoint of the perceiver, and (3) the specific "behaver" and his or her behavior. Becker (1963) illustrates this point:

> ... social groups create deviance by making the rules whose infraction constitutes deviance, and by applying those rules to particular people and labeling them as outsiders. From this point of view, deviance is not a quality of the act the person commits, but rather a consequence of the application by others of rules and sanctions to an "offender." The deviant is one to whom that label has successfully been applied; deviant behavior is behavior that people so label (p. 9).

## CONSTRUCT SYSTEMS FOR THE LABELING OF AFFECTIVE DEVIANCE

Underlying any practice of labeling is the need for a language describing individuals and situations. Descriptions, classifications, and labeling of individuals are made for the following reasons: (1) Scientists believe that descriptions and classifications must precede explanation and will in fact aid in the process of explanation. (2) The disposition of deviancies in affective behavior presents society with practical problems, and solutions to these problems will be achieved more efficiently if large numbers of individuals can be reduced to small categories. (3) Diagnosticians assume that the process of classification lends itself to appropriate disposition and treatment. Most clinical systems or classifications rely heavily on standardized tests. Testing provides classifications that are attractive because they tie into diagnosticians' preconceptions of the instruments and the "dispositional" alternatives. In other words, construct systems are most helpful when they relate society's notions about affective processes to specific measures for making decisions about children.

The most common construct system is the psychiatric diagnostic nomenclature that classifies people rather than behaviors or traits. The psychiatric descriptive approach incorporates the general and personality factors of a child within a clinically descriptive classification (Jackson & Pavnonen, 1980; Kendell, 1975).

An example of a clinically descriptive classification system is the *Diagnostic and Statistical Manual* (DSM), published by the American Psychiatric Association over the years: DSM-I (1952), DSM-II (1968), and DSM-III (1980). Extending beyond preceding editions, DSM-III specifies more precisely the criteria used for clinical diagnoses. Whereas DSM-I had 60 categories and DSM-II had 145, DSM-III has 230. DSM-III uses a multiaxial classification system, which implies that children are classified not into one category, but in terms of a number of factors. Axis I codes all psychiatric syndromes (e.g., attention deficit disorders, anxiety, depression), except developmental or personality disorders. Axis II covers specific developmental disorders in children (e.g., developmental reading disorders) and personality disorders in adults. Axis III refers to current physical disorders or conditions relevant to the psychological problem. Axis IV provides a rating of the severity of any psychosocial stress related to the disorder. Severity is rated on a scale of 1 to 7, ranging from *0/none* to *catastrophic.* Axis V codes the assessment of the child's adaptive functioning. Ratings again are made on a 7-point scale, ranging from *superior* to *grossly impaired.* A sample DSM-III diagnosis of a child follows:

Axis I: 314.01 Attention-deficit disorder with hyperactivity
Axis II: 315.00 Developmental reading disorder
Axis III: Asthma
Axis IV: Psychosocial stress (divorce of parents) severity (5 = severe)
Axis V: Highest level of adaptive function in past year (4 = fair)

The application of the DSM classification system to special education has been extensively critiqued (Forness & Cantwell, 1982). The system does have limitations, in terms of predicting differential responses to treatment. Use

of this system also implies acceptance of the medical model, the attribute model (discussed in Chapter 1).

Another approach has been used to classify behavior disorders in children. The Committee on Child Psychiatry of the Group for the Advancement of Psychiatry (GAP) has proposed an alternative to the DSM, which is designed primarily for categorizing adult psychopathology. The DSM-III's only provision for children's psychotic disorders without organic etiology is the category of "Schizophrenic Childhood Type." An ideal classification scheme would include a clinical description, and psychodynamic and psychosocial factors. The GAP committee (1966) opted for a "clinical-descriptive" system and has proposed ten major categories for children's behavior. These categories and a brief clinical description follow.

1. *Health responses:* Normal state of appropriate behaviors
2. *Reactive disorders:* Acute reactions to environmental stress, that apparently are not caused by underlying psychopathology (e.g., child's reaction to death in family)
3. *Developmental deviations:* Hereditary, constitutional, and maturational precocities, or unevenness in developmental patterns (e.g., disturbances in particular functions of motor development, or in psychosexual development, speech development)
4. *Psychoneurotic disorders:* Intrapsychic conflicts (e.g., anxiety, phobia, conversion, obsessive-compulsive state, and depressive type problems resulting from repression of basic drives)
5. *Personality disorders:* Deeply ingrained personality traits that harmonize with the child's ego (e.g., sexual deviation, antisocial personality, subcultural delinquent)
6. *Psychotic disorders:* Disorders of emotional responsiveness, self-identity, speech, and cognitive process (e.g., childhood autism, schizophrenia)
7. *Psychophysiological disorders:* Predisposing biological factors affecting psychologi-

cal functioning (e.g., disorders of the respiratory, cardiovascular, or nervous system)

8. *Brain syndromes:* Impairment of brain tissue (e.g., minimal brain dysfunction syndrome)
9. *Mental retardation:* Degrees of intellectual impairment (e.g., impairment caused by biological or environmental factors, or by an interaction of both factors)
10. *Other disorders* (category for future differentiation of disorders)

The preceding clinical descriptions indicate that the classification procedures for a psychiatric diagnosis of childhood disorders lack precision. Furthermore, the present diagnostic classifications are only tentative schemes by which a wide variety of children's behaviors can be ordered. Psychiatric classifications reflect the many gaps that exist in the knowledge of childhood psychopathology; different systems tend to classify children according to a variety of different criteria. For example, one might conclude from a diagnostic appraisal that the child exhibits psychotic behavior but also personality and/or psychophysiological disorders. Such classifications are limited in scope and contribute relatively little to an understanding of how to educate these children.

Another popular approach views children's overt affective disorders as consisting of clusters of highly correlated behaviors. Behaviors that cluster together (are correlated or related to each other) yield certain factors or dimensions. The chief statistical technique used in these studies is called a factor analysis (discussed in Chapter 4), although a related technique, known as cluster analysis, may also be used. Factor analysis determines the correlations of every item with every other item. Therefore, items or characteristics are subject to quantification.

Although discussion of the statistical techniques used in this approach is beyond the scope of this chapter, it should be noted that they permit independent confirmations of dimensions or categories established by statistical analysis. For example, Quay (1975) has identified four pervasive dimensions among children with behavior disorders: "personality problems" (hypersensitivity, lack of self-confidence, anxiety, "under-behaves" as compared with misbehaves), "conduct problems" (impulses against society, physical and verbal aggression, hyperactivity), "inadequate maturity factor" (preoccupation, daydreaming, inattention, passivity), and "socialized delinquent factor" (delinquent peer group, truancy, failure to abide by middle-class school ethics). Support for these dimensions has come from case data, behavior ratings, and personality questionnaires obtained on populations from public schools, correctional institutions, and child guidance clinics. Of these dimensions, personality problems constitute a small incidence of childhood problems.

Quay (1975, 1977) suggests that differential assessment can be developed from his classification system, but one of the difficulties with this approach is that children are seldom "pure" examples of any category. Distractibility, for example, is common to all four dimensions. Thus, in deciding the category in which a child belongs, the diagnostician must consider the general list of symptoms rather than a single symptom.

In sum, classification of affective development has purpose only when treatment is linked with prognostic statements. As discussed in Chapter 3, further criteria for the evaluation of affective or behavioral classification systems would include reliability, face validity, and predictive validity. Classification systems should also include the child's potential competencies (assets).

## CLASSIFICATION VARIABLES OF SOCIAL COMPETENCE

The ecological perspective suggests that there are specific contingencies that influence the labeling process (Carlson, Scott, & Elclund, 1980; Gresham & Elliott, 1987; Thurman, 1977). Gresham and Elliot (1984) provide a classification scheme that categorizes social competence into four general areas: skill deficits, performance deficits, self-control deficits, and self-control performance deficits. The classification into the four categories rests on the child's knowing how to perform the skill and the existence of emotional arousal responses (e.g., anger). *Skill deficits* reflect the child's limited acquisition of behavior that allows him or her to interact with peers. *Performance deficits* reflect the child's inability to spontaneously use the skills he has in his repertoire in the context in which it is expected. *Self-control deficits* characterize a child for whom an affective response (e.g., anxiety, anger, phobia) has hindered the ability to acquire a social skill. *Self-control performance deficits* characterize a child who has a specific skill in his or her behavior repertoire but does not use the skill because of an affect response.

The possession of certain skills increases the avoidance of labeling, while a lack of appropriate resources increases the likelihood of false labeling. Thus, children with affective lags (lacking skills and resources) are more adversely affected by false labeling (Becker, 1963; Gove, 1976). On the other hand, children with certain skills (such as, being able to avoid social conflict) are more likely to be classified on the basis of desirable traits. Furthermore, the beliefs that particular traits exist in a child may in fact be the result of discrepancies between the child's behavior and another individual's expectations. If a child is labeled as emotionally disturbed, for example, certain behavior is expected of the child (Algozzine, Mercer, & Counteronine, 1977). Some of the variables that contribute to social expectations about children's adaptability are the developmental, moral, social, cognitive, and attribution skills of the child. We will briefly review each of these contributors.

### Developmental Adaptability

Developmental contributors to affective competence have been outlined extensively in Eisenburg and Harris (1984). An understanding of developmental changes, particular with aspect

to the child's needs and those of the child's interaction with society, is an important foundation for the assessing of competence. Consider the classical theory of Erickson as a reference point. Erickson (1963, 1968) stated that children develop within their culture in such a manner as to satisfy not only basic needs but also a sense of competency about their interaction with people, things, and events. Developmental competence, according to Erickson, includes:

1. *Infancy:* The bases for trust versus mistrust of self and others are related to physiological processes and social pressures (weaning and toilet training), the achievement of a sense of security and order in the environment, and a mastery of communication of feelings and concepts through the use of language.
2. *Early childhood:* Beginning feelings of autonomy and independence versus dependence are related to the achievement of appropriate sex-role behavior, the internalization of roles into conscience and superego, and mastery of physiological and language skills.
3. *Juvenile era:* The bases for initiative and competency are achieved through mastery of motor skills, the assumption of responsibility for one's actions, and the adjustment of peer group expectations and standards.
4. *Early adolescence:* Identity is established through independence from parents and other adults, acceptance of behavioral role in society, and comfort in intimacy with another individual.
5. *Youth culture:* Foundations of intimacy, responsibility, and integrity are established through attachments to members of the opposite sex, participation in adult social and sexual roles and career choices, and acquisition of a set of values and an ethical system appropriate to a future lifestyle.

Children entering school whose growth has been arrested at any particular stage may exhibit a wide range of affective difficulties. Some do not negotiate successfully at critical points in their development and therefore manifest patterns of behavior that are disruptive, inappropriate, or exaggerated compared with that of other children their own age. Because of these developmental imbalances, a certain aggravated exchange exists between the child and his or her ecosystem.

A direct application of Erickson's theory by Swap (1973, 1974) within an ecological framework has been suggested. Swap's framework is appropriate not only for assessment, but also for direct intervention. A brief discussion of some school-age problems addressed within this framework follows.

*Autonomy Versus Shame and Doubt.* A developmental lag at the autonomy-versus-shame-and-doubt stage yields behaviors such as an inability to complete tasks, compulsive rituals, disruptive outbursts, intolerance or frustration, defiance of authority, distractibility, and destruction of products. As discussed by Swap (1973, 1974), disturbances at this stage are variable; for example, a child, demonstrating his power and autonomy, manipulates others to disruptive behavior but complies himself. Another child may indicate self-doubts through an inability to complete the work, perhaps by a perfectionistic destruction of any product marred by error (Swap, 1974). The unifying factor of behaviors displayed during a developmental lag at this stage is the child's inability to control himself or herself or to tolerate control from others. Adaptive environmental responses include providing a structural learning environment, setting clear expectations for student behavior, requiring finished products, establishing a firm one-to-one relationship, and setting up peer activities of a simple design.

*Initiative Versus Guilt.* The triggering behavior at this stage is the child's guilt over goals contemplated and enjoyment of perceptual-motor and cognitive activities. Swap (1974) notes:

> Children who have been inhibited in developing their sense of initiative may reflect their discour-

agement through a lack of zest and disinterest in exploring the activities and stimulation offered by the school environment. ... On the other hand, a child may exhibit behaviors which trigger maladaptive responses in the environment by overzealous exploration (p. 168).

Remediation of behavioral lags in the initiative-versus-guilt stage is carried out by the emphasis of order, exploration, and activities that will increase the likelihood of affective transfer to the next stage.

*Industry Versus Inferiority.* Lags in the industry-versus-inferiority stage are manifested in low self-esteem, isolation, difficulty with sharing and competition, aggression, and overdependence on others' approval or initiative. An important consideration at this stage, as stated by Erickson (1963, 1968), is that the child may feel inadequate or inferior in relation to others and not gain pleasure from work efforts. Two important components necessary for assessment at this stage are the (1) child's needs to acquire academic skills and produce quality products, and (2) child's needs to achieve those skills in conjunction with others. Swap (1974) suggests that remedial strategies at this stage should include educating children about their own values and attitudes, providing communication exercises, providing a wide range of group projects and learning activities, and encouraging self-evaluation by the children.

*Summary.* The theoretical and practical applications of Erickson as interpreted by Swap (1974) suggest that children have difficulty negotiating developmental crises within a social context. Although Erickson's concepts of development are not without challenge (Ausebel, 1952; Bijou, 1968), they can be applied to the assessment of affective competence. If a developmental lag in affect occurs, the interaction between the child and critical persons in the labeling process may become more apparent. For example, an assessment perspective may focus on the contingencies outside the child's affective lag that lead to the labeling. Prominent among these contingencies are the type, degree, amount, and visibility of the act; the power and social distance of the individual child in relation to the agents of control in the child's ecology; and the availability of alternative roles for the child.

## Adaptability in Moral Judgment

Moral judgments or social decisions may also contribute to assessment of a child's affective competence (Eisenberg & Harris, 1984). Since Piaget's studies in the 1930s (see Chapter 4), studies of the development of children's social play and moral judgment have provided valuable information on how children prescribe, evaluate, and justify socially good and right action. Based on Piaget's earlier work (1928), Kohlberg (1958, 1964) established a typology of six stages in the development of moral judgment. Obtained from several sources, the six stages are provided below.

*Stage 1:* Obedience and punishment orientation. Egocentric deference to superior power or prestige, or a trouble-avoiding set; objective responsibility.

*Stage 2:* Naively egoistic orientation. "Right" action is that instrumentally satisfying the self's needs and occasionally those of others; awareness of relativism of value to each actor's needs and perspective, naive egalitarianism, and orientation to exchange and reciprocity.

*Stage 3:* Good-boy orientation. Orientation to approval and to pleasing and helping others; conformity to stereotypical images of majority or natural role behavior; and judgment by intentions.

*Stage 4:* Authority and social-order maintaining orientation. Orientation toward authority, fixed rules, and maintenance of the social order; "right" behavior consists of doing one's duty, showing respect for authority, and maintaining the given social order for its own sake; morality is not based on individual or personal values and judgments.

*Stage 5:* Contractual legalistic orientation. "Right" action is defined in terms of individual rights and of standards that have been initially examined and agreed on by the whole society; emphasis is on procedural rules for reaching consensus and ensuring general welfare; concern with establishing and maintaining individual rights, equality, and liberty; distinctions are made between values having universal, prescriptive applicability and values specific to a given society.

*Stage 6:* The universal-ethical-principle orientation. "Right" is defined by the decision of conscience in accord with self-chosen ethical principles appealing to logical comprehensiveness, universality, and consistency; these principles are abstract, not concrete moral rules; they are universal principles of justice, of the reciprocity and equality of human rights, and of respect for the dignity of human beings and individual persons.

The factors that determine a child's current stage in moral development are the perspective ways in which the child evaluates or justifies judgments. Kohlberg's (1964) Heinz dilemma permits the elicitation of different ways in which moral judgments can be justified, in relation to conscience, life, punishment, or law. The dilemma represented is that Heinz's wife is dying of cancer and only a new drug can cure her. Unfortunately, Heinz cannot afford it. The dilemma for Heinz is whether to try to save his wife's life by stealing the drug or obey the law and let his wife die. As expected, young children focus on the immediate or perceptual actions justifying their moral actions. In other words, their actions depend on whether they get caught or the severity of the punishment. Little understanding is given to the intentionality of action from a social perspective. In the example, if Heinz is caught, the child does not seem to consider that the judge would consider the husband's reasons for stealing the drug. Moral judgment as applied to affective competence would be viewed as a decision-making capacity.

This decision-making capacity would of course depend on the child's level of cognitive development and perspective-taking ability. Only perspective-taking abilities of children will be discussed here.

*Perspective-Taking Skills.* Flavell (1974) proposed a model of social cognition (perspective taking) involving four components. First, to abandon egocentrism children must learn that the psychological processes of others (whatever they represent) are not necessarily like their own "existence." In other words, children must learn that different psychological processes may exist in others. The second component, "need," focuses on the child's spontaneous ability to use the potential knowledge he or she possesses concerning the psychological processes of others. In other words, can the child perform in social situations with the knowledge gained from the first component? The third component, "inference," is the child's ability to obtain impressions about the psychological states of others. Can the child use information that is involved in personal perception? The fourth component, "application of knowledge," reflects more directly what the child does with what he or she knows. Flavell's model, although preliminary in nature, may provide a useful guide for the assessment of affective competence. For example, examination of the need component may suggest that children are not using the full extent of their knowledge, while an examination of inference would direct our assessment to the information that children pick up in relation to others. It thus becomes necessary to determine how children become skilled in perception and prediction of others' behaviors, emotions, and intentions.

An earlier study by Walker (1980) suggests that there can be no gain in the intervention of moral problem-solving behavior unless the cognitive and perspective-taking development is considered. Table 9-1 provides the parallel stages of perspective taking, moral judgment, and intellectual functioning. Children's behaviors can also be related to the child's attribution or the difference between others' perceptions specifically as they affect their own self-perception.

**Child Attributions**

*Attributions* are defined as the perceived causes of a person's behavior. Attributions show how our "perceptions affect our feelings about past events and our expectations about future ones, our attitudes toward other persons and our reactions to their behavior, and our conceptions of ourselves and our efforts to improve our fortunes" (Kelley & Michela, 1980, p. 489). A central concept of the study of child attributions is *locus of control*—the perceived internal or external source of responsibility for an outcome or event. Children who have high external control perceive that their behaviors are controlled not necessarily by themselves but by other persons (teachers, parents, others in the community), chance, or forces outside themselves. *Internal control* is a person's taking responsibility for the fact that his or her own abilities and efforts lead to success or failure. In essence, the child with strong internal control recognizes that he or she determines or controls his or her own destiny.

An assessment of a child would benefit from a focus on the child's perception or inference concerning the cause of behavior. As suggested by several studies (Rice, 1975; Ruble & Boggiano, 1980), the majority of children labeled as having trouble adapting in an appropriate affective manner have high external control. According to the earlier work of Thibaut and Riecken (1955), attribution has both antecedent and consequence aspects. Certain information about a behavior and the circumstance of its occurrence is used by human beings as an antecedent with which they infer a cause. A child's antecedent information is certainly affected by information about the particular behavior, beliefs about what others would do in this situation, and the child's motivation (the impact of the behavior on the child) (Nowicki & Strick-

**Table 9-1**
Parallel stages in cognitive, perspective-taking, and moral development.

| Perspective-taking stage | Moral stage | Cognitive stage |
| --- | --- | --- |
| **Stage 1 (subjectivity)** There is an understanding of the subjectivity of persons but no realization that persons can consider each other as subjects. | **Stage 1 (heteronomy)** The physical consequences of an action and the dictates of authorities define right and wrong. | **Preoperations** The "symbolic function" appears but thinking is marked by centration and irreversibility. |
| **Stage 2 (self-reflection)** There is a sequential understanding that the other can view the self as a subject just as the self can view the other as subject. | **Stage 2 (exchange)** Right is defined as serving one's own interests and desires, and cooperative interaction is based on terms of simple exchange. | **Concrete operations** The objective characteristics of an object are separated from action relating to it; and classification, seriation, and conservation skills develop. |
| **Stage 3 (mutual perspectives)** It is realized that the self and the other can view each other as perspective-taking subjects (a generalized perspective). | **Stage 3 (expectations)** Emphasis is on good-person stereotypes and a concern for approval. | **Beginning formal operations** There is development of the coordination of reciprocity with inversion; and propositional logic can be handled. |
| **Stage 4 (social and conventional system)** There is a realization that each self can consider the shared point of view of the generalized other (the social system). | **Stage 4 (social system and conscience)** Focus is on the maintenance of the social order by obeying the law and doing one's duty. | **Early basic formal operations** The hypothetico-deductive approach emerges, involving abilities to develop possible relations among variables and to organize experimental analyses. |
| **Stage 5 (symbolic interaction)** A social system perspective can be understood from a beyond-society point of view. | **Stage 5 (social contract)** Right is defined by mutual standards that have been agreed upon by the whole society. | **Consolidated basic formal operations** Operations are now completely exhaustive and systematic. |

From Walker, L. Cognitive and perspective-taking prerequisites for moral development. *Child Development,* 1980, *51,* p. 132. Copyright 1980 by The Society for Research in Child Development, Inc. Reprinted by permission.

land, 1973; Weiner, 1974). In determining a consequence, a subject must evaluate the behavior in terms of its compliance or noncompliance. For children this evaluation would of course be related to their environment (for example, feedback, skills, intention). Differences will obviously occur in children's ascriptions of causality in behavior as they adapt to their social context. When they view their behavior as determined by chance or with little hope of being changed, children may question the value of persistence or effort in adapting to community goals. On the other hand, if behavior is considered to be determined by the child's own abilities and effort, change in behavior becomes more readily remedial.

## NOWICKI-STRICKLAND LOCUS OF CONTROL SCALE

(Nowicki, S., and Strickland, B., 1973, *40,* 148–154, *Journal of Consulting and Clinical Psychology*)

This is one of many scales that assess a child's locus of control. The scale can be administered individually or in groups. The subject must answer yes or no to each of forty questions read aloud by the examiner. Each question concerns reinforcement situations in a variety of areas. Sample question (and answers that indicate high external control) include:

☐ Do you feel that you have a lot of choice in deciding who your friends are? (No)
☐ If you find a four-leaf clover, do you believe that it might bring you good luck? (Yes)
☐ Do you often feel that whether you do your homework has much to do with what kind of grades you get? (No)
☐ Do you feel that when a kid your age decides to hit you, there's little you can do to stop him or her? (Yes)

Means and standard deviations are reported for males and females in grades three to twelve. The normative sample consisted of 1017 students, in elementary and high school, from four predominantly white communities. Samples were drawn from various socioeconomic groups. IQs ranged from 101 to 106. The higher the scale score, the more external the child. The test authors report correlations between scale scores and achievement test scores. The Nowicki-Strickland correlates at a significant level with three other locus of control scales: Potter, Bailer-Cromwell, and Intellectual Achievement Responsibility. Split-half reliability ranges from .63 to .81. Test-retest reliability ranges from .63 to .71, with 6-week intervals.

## Community Tolerance

As stated earlier, the evaluation of affective competence is determined by norms in the child's ecology (Carlson, Scott, & Elclund, 1980). Determining which norms should be taken as the standards for evaluation within the child's community becomes difficult. However, from an ecological perspective, certain kinds of questions concerning the child's ecosystem can provide definitions and propositions that tentatively describe the boundaries of assessment.

1. Which adult and peer members in the child's ecosystem represent norms?
2. Which social norms within the child's ecosystem are the bases of evaluation by the child and others?

3. What expectations of the child are accompanied by variations in the degree of adaptability to community demands?
4. Which children have different ecosystems and present different standards for conduct (for example, excessive classroom conformity may become deviation, rule violations may be highly supported by the child peers)?
5. The lack of which adaptation skill in the child's ecosystem may cause the child to become labeled?
6. What tolerance level in the child's community can serve as a stimulus for specific negative and positive reactions in the child?

When considering assessment, as well as the means by which tolerance levels in the child's ecosystem can be changed, the diagnostician can draw some insights from research (Carlson, Scott, & Elclund, 1980; Thurman, 1977):

1. Tolerance levels of a child are assessed more readily during the process of group participation (for example, as behavior is rewarded for changed situation) than during isolated behavior (for example, viewing responses to change within the child).
2. If only one agent (for example, school) is attempting to exercise control of the child, the effect of group responsibility is decreased.
3. A child's resistance to adapting can be avoided by dissemination of information about the child, to the community.
4. Education is not limited to a particular time frame but must take place continuously.
5. Community participation should be encouraged in the making of educational decisions for a child's normalization within that community.
6. Focus of normalization process is better placed on comprehensive coordinated service rather than isolated services.

The emphasis shifts from the professional assessment of and intervention in the child's behavior to assessment and provision of support and community care of the child and the family. Certain values, those attaching importance to success, are widely accepted in the child's ecosystem. A child's failure to distinguish social expectations and competencies depends on the child's community expectations, but more specifically on the family in which he or she is being socialized.

### Family Tolerance

The family is probably the most important factor in the success or failure of the child's adaptive process. A logical point for beginning the assessment of a child's adaptation would be an interview with the child's family. From the beginning of assessment, the parents' emotions, marital status, religious beliefs, and expectations for the child must be considered. Parents or guardians must be interviewed so that a complete psychosocial history of the child can be made.

Most current procedures that gather psychosocial information follow a model developed by Mercer (1972). This model identifies family networks and social agencies in the child's ecosystem. A parental interview form is used to guide the diagnostician in assessing the family network. Ecological assessment would include determination of the parents' marital status, child's relationship to parents, sex of head of household, child's friends' activities, internal organization of family, cultural background, religious affiliation, adaptive behavior rating of child, child's health history, and preferred spoken language.

After the ecological information is gathered, participation and cooperation by the parents is emphasized. An initial commitment from the family should be established, to ensure that they will work with the school staff to the extent determined by the needs of the child and their own capabilities.

Parents should also be involved in goal setting for their child. They should develop a better understanding of the child's disability, and thereby develop more realistic expectations for the child. They should be involved in the assessment and treatment of their child through demonstration, observation, implementation, and direction from the teacher. Parents should also become involved in community activities affecting their child, such as parents groups, extended family situations, and auxiliary agencies.

### Agency Contacts

Other variables in the child's ecosystem must also be considered in development of an assessment strategy. Contacting appropriate agencies within the community is necessary so that treatment alternatives can be determined, information can be disseminated, intervention assessed, and goals modified. For example, the classroom teacher may be required to interact with the police department, YMCA, and a wide variety of other agencies. Agency concerns are considered in the establishment of priorities and goals for the achievement of community adaptation. Assessment also includes the identification of high-risk groups in the community who might not otherwise seek or receive services.

### Classroom Labeling

After information is gathered from community sources, attention should focus on classroom adaptation. Hargreaves, Hester, and Mellar (1975) identified five major constructs that appear early in the process by which a child is labeled deviant in the classroom. Although this study was done mostly in British schools at the secondary level, application to the public school is readily apparent. Children who exhibited positive aspects of the following constructs were not labeled as deviant:

1. *Conformity to behavioral roles:* Negative constructs are disruptive, argumentative, and uncooperative behavior in group situations; child does not obey until threatened with punishment; fights, and reacts with defiance to instructions.
2. *Conformity to academic values:* Negative constructs are underachieving, slow, lethargic, inattentive characteristics; child who performs below demonstrated level, is poor reader, for example.

3. *Likability:* This label relates to general positive feelings of liking the child. Sample negative constructs are, does not initiate relationships, does not respond to teacher approval, complains about teacher unfairness.
4. *Peer group relations:* Although these were fairly infrequent at the early stages of the labeling process, negative constructs are being aggressive with peers and continually seeking attention from children.

According to Hargreaves, Hester, and Mellar (1975), labeling by the teacher results from an interaction with classroom social control. Beyond the mere interchange of the labeling process, such an assessment may focus on (1) a continuum of affective expectations, and (2) expected behavior for classroom competence. The following factors are involved in assessment:

1. Certain norms or classroom expectations should exist.
2. Children and teachers must both know the rules or expectations.
3. Certain acts constitute conformity or deviance.
4. The teacher as a strategist must act against deviant conduct.
5. The child as a strategist should develop concealment or reactive behaviors.

*Affective Taxonomy.* To determine a continuum of behaviors within the classroom, one can assess the child's achievement in meeting affective objectives. The utility of an affective continuum is based on two factors. First, affective development is comparable in importance to academic skills. Second, because the affect area has been imprecisely defined by such terms as attitude or appreciation, a continuum must be provided to operationalize observations. Perhaps the earliest and most ambitious affective continuum for classroom instruction is that developed by Krathwohl, Bloom, and Masia (1964). They identified five categories, each of which has several subdivisions:

**1.00** *Receiving (attending)*
The willingness of the learner to receive or to attend to stimuli; this is the beginning step if the learner is to respond to instruction.
**1.10** Awareness
**1.20** Willingness to receive
**1.30** Controlled or selected attention
**2.00** *Responding*
The willingness of the learner to attend actively; this describes the child's "interest" objectives.
**2.10** Acquiescence in responding
**2.20** Willingness to respond
**2.30** Satisfaction in response
**3.00** *Valuing*
The willingness of the learner to recognize that a thing, phenomenon, or behavior has worth; the learner develops his or her own domain criterion of worth.
**3.10** Acceptance of a value
**3.20** Preference for a value
**3.30** Commitment (conviction)
**4.00** *Organization*
The willingness of the learner to successively internalize values encountered in situations for which more than one value is relevant; development includes organization of the values into a system, determination of the interrelationships among values, and establishment of the dominant and pervasive values.
**4.10** Conceptualization of a value
**4.20** Organization of a value system
**5.00** *Characterization by a value or value complex*
The willingness of the learner to integrate beliefs, ideas, and attitudes into a total philosophy or world organized into an internally consistent system.
**5.10** Generalized set
**5.20** Characterization

Each of these behaviors can be represented as a basis for the assessment of and instruction in adaptability within the educational context.

*Classroom Competence.* Internalization involves the development of self-management and voluntary self-control. Self-control can be classified within a behavioral framework (Furman, 1980) as (1) *self-assessment*—the child's ability to examine his or her behavior and decide whether or not it has occurred, (2) *self-recording*—the child's ability to collect information on his or her behavior such as its frequency, (3) self-determination of reinforcement—determining what the desirable outcome should be for behaving in a certain manner, and (4) self-determination of consequences—providing own reinforcement for appropriate responses. These behaviors follow a progression in response and represent a close approximation to Krathwohl, Bloom, and Masia's taxonomy of internalization.

A more direct system for the assessment of the child's affective competence for regular classroom placement is provided by Taylor and Soloway (1973). Their standards for the child are based on the following categories:

1. *Preacademic competence:* The child's progress or readiness level for learning. Abilities include paying attention, starting assignment, following task directions, taking part verbally in discussion, and getting along with others.
2. *Academic competence:* Abilities include being right, neat, efficient, and well-organized, as related to basic school programs of reading, writing, spelling, and arithmetic. (Academic skills relate to proficiency in language and perceptual-motor functioning.)
3. *Setting competence:* Instructional setting found in regular classrooms. Developmental instruction includes situations in which the student is working alone with teacher, independently with teacher readily available, independently within small group, or independently among entire class while teacher is instructing a small group of students or standing in front of the entire class.
4. *Reward competence:* Child's reinforcement hierarchy. Reinforcement continuum varies from concrete tangible rewards (prizes) to traditional classroom rewards.

## Assessing Child Tolerance

As indicated in the study by Hargreaves, Hester, and Mellar (1975), control of the child is a crucial aspect of the labeling process. Lack of control is related to the extent that internalization (affect) of the regulatory norms of the child's ecosystem has not taken place. The degree to which a child possesses affective competence is reflected by his or her actions. The psychological variables involved are the child's expected goals, the way the child actively behaves, and the tolerance of these behaviors by others within their ecosystems. Some measures that have been favorably reviewed are provided below. *Ratings by others (teacher and/or peer ratings):*

1. Social Behavior Assessment Guide (Stephens, 1980)
2. Walker Social Skills Curriculum Scale (Walker, McConnel, Holmes, Todis, Walker, & Golder, 1983)
3. Guess Who Scale (Gottlieb, Semmel, & Veldman, 1978)
4. Progress Assessment Chart of Social Behavior Rating Scales (Gunzberg, 1980)
5. Pupil Behavior Rating Scale (Lambert, Hartsough, & Bower, 1979)
6. Kohn Social Competence Scale (Kohn, Parnes, & Roseman, 1979)

*Behavioral role play (provide situations that encourage behavioral enactment of a skill):*

1. Role play tests for assessing social skills (a review by Bellack, Hersen, & Lampmarski, 1979)

*Self-report (children report on own social skills):*

1. Children's Assertative Behavior Scale (Michelson & Wood, 1980)
2. Matson Evaluation of Social Skills with Youngsters (Matson, Esvedlt-Dawson, & Kazdin, 1983)

Several other measures are available that assess children's behavior in terms of their interactions with the regulatory norms of society. For example, *self-concept* ratings incorporate three perspectives: (1) the point of view of an adult group leader such as a classroom teacher, (2) the point of view of the child's peers, and (3) the point of view of the child. Following is a discussion of several such self-concept rating instruments. Some of these ratings have rather controversial reviews and are only presented as examples of possible ways in which affective competence might be assessed.

### PROCESS FOR IN-SCHOOL SCREENING OF CHILDREN WITH EMOTIONAL HANDICAPS

(Bower, E. M., and Lambert, N. M., 1962, Educational Testing Service)

This screening process is directed toward helping the regular classroom teacher discern children who might have an emotional handicap. The procedure uses three reference points: (1) perception of the child by the teacher, (2) perception of the child by peers, and (3) perception of the child by himself or herself. These references are used only for screening, not for diagnosis, classification, or as a way of finding causation. The screening device can be used on children in grades from kindergarten through grade twelve; different materials are used at different levels. Administration time is 1 to $1\frac{1}{2}$ hours.

Each grade level has a Behavior Rating of Pupils that is completed by the classroom teacher and includes his or her perceptions of each child in the class. Items in the teacher rating subscale include fights with other pupils, has difficulty in learning school subjects, makes unusual or inappropriate responses during normal school activities, behaves in ways that are dangerous to self and others, and is unhappy or depressed. The rating of the pupil by peers uses many devices: a class picture—each child says who in the class is most like the person in the picture; a class play—each child picks classmates to play different parts in the play; or a student survey—each student says which classmate is best described by a particular statement. The rating of oneself is done with a picture

game for kindergarten through grade three; a series of questions, Thinking About Yourself, for grades three through six; and a Self-test for grades seven through twelve. These ratings attempt to measure the discrepancy between a wanted self and a perceived self. They provide scores that the teacher can use in screening those students whose scores stand out at the extremes of the class. Scores that are extreme in reference to the rest of the class in two of the three areas are then referred to someone in the field of mental health for further screening.

Data on validity and reliability are being gathered, but because of the nature of this screening procedure, these data will not necessarily reflect the usefulness of the materials.

### PERCEIVED COMPETENCE SCALE FOR CHILDREN

(Harter, S., 1979, 1982, Department of Psychology, University of Denver)

The perceived competence scale assesses a child's feelings of competence in three skill domains: (1) cognitive or intellectual skills (the major focus is on school performance), (2) social skills (involve peer interaction and popularity), and (3) physical skills (sports and outdoor activities). A fourth subscale assesses the child's feelings of self-esteem. Overall, items refer to the child's general feelings about the way he or she is. Each of the four subscales contains seven items. Half of the items are worded so that the first part of the statement reflects high perceived competence and the second part reflects low perceived competence. After each item is read aloud, the child is asked which kind of kid is most like him or her and then asked whether this is only sort of true or really true. Special emphasis has been placed on the instrument's factor validity because each subscale defines a factor structure stable across normed aged groups. Unlike the Bower and Lambert screening device, no assessment is done with peer ratings.

The complete scale, instructions for administration, and scoring key are included in the manual. Harter devised a "structured alternative format" to be used with the scale, in which the child is presented with the following type of question:

|  | Really true | Sort of true |
|---|---|---|
| Some kids often forget what they learn | ☐ | ☐ |
| but | | |
| Other kids can remember things easily | ☐ | ☐ |

Each item is scored on a scale from 1 to 4, 1 indicating low perceived competence and 4 high perceived competence. In the example, the child who first indicates that he often forgets what he learns and then describes this as really true for him would receive a 1. The child for whom this part of the statement is only sort of true would receive a 2. The child who indicates that he can remember things easily, though describes this as only sort of true for him, would receive a 3, and the child for whom this part of the statement was really true would receive a 4.

**Sample Items**

|  | Really true | Sort of true |
|---|---|---|
| Some kids feel that they are very good at their school work | 4 | 3 |
| but | | |
| Other kids worry about whether they can do the work assigned to them | 1 | 2 |
| Some kids find it hard to make friends | 1 | 2 |
| but | | |
| For other kids it's pretty easy | 4 | 3 |
| Some kids do very well at sports | 4 | 3 |
| but | | |
| Other kids don't feel they are very good when it comes to sports | 1 | 2 |

|  | Really true | Sort of true |
|---|---|---|
| Some kids aren't very happy with the way they do a lot of things | 1 | 2 |
| but | | |
| Other kids think the way they do things is fine | 4 | 3 |

To assess the degree of convergence between a child's perception of his or her competence and the teacher's perception, a teacher rating-form is completed. The form contains the same 28 items, ordered as they are on the child's form. The same scoring procedure is used on the teacher's form as is used on the child's form.

The scale is designed for children in grades three through six. Earlier versions were individually administered to approximately 300 children in Colorado. Factor validity of the scale has been generalized on a sample of 133 9- to 12-year-old children from California to whom the scale was group-administered. Norming of the scale has been extended to a combined Connecticut-California sample of 341 children in grades three through six, a New York sample of 714 children in grades three through six, three separate Colorado samples of 740 children in grades three through six, and a California sample of 746 children in grades three through nine. Samples are drawn primarily from middle- and upper-middle-class populations. For every sample, there were approximately the same number of boys and girls at each grade level. The estimates of reliability were based on a measure of the internal consistency within each subscale, specifically, the Kuder-Richardson formula (KR-20). These values were .76, .78, .83, and .73, for the cognitive, social, physical, and general subscales, respectively. Test-retest reliabilities over a 3-month period are also within this range.

### INFERRED SELF-CONCEPT SCALE (ISCS)
(McDaniel, E. L., 1973, Western Psychological Services)

The ISCS focuses on children's self-concepts as learned through behavioral observation by teachers, counselors, or other educated observers. The test kit includes one manual and one form; instructions are given for each form. Administration time is 10 minutes. To describe their perceptions of a student's self-concept, the observers rate thirty items on a five-point scale: never, seldom, sometimes, usually, or always. To obtain the actual ratings, the scorer circles the appropriate number for each item. To obtain the total score the scorer adds the circled numbers in each column and then totals the columns.

Validity and reliability on this type of scale are variable. For example, correlations between the ratings of teachers and counselors on independent items ranged from .07 to .58. Such a coefficient suggests that different observers will not see children the same way. The test was normed on 30 socially undesirable, 150 socially desirable, and a group of 180 other children in elementary schools in Austin, Texas. Ratings on the children were done by fifty teachers and one school counselor.

### CAIN-LEVINE SOCIAL COMPETENCY SCALE
(Cain, L., Levine, S., and Elzey, F., 1963, Consulting Psychologists Press)

The Cain-Levine Social Competency Scale is a rating scale based on information obtained from parents, house parents, or teachers; it is intended to measure the social competence of trainable mentally retarded children from five to thirteen years of age. The scale consists of 44 items divided into four subscales: self-help, initiative, social skills, and communication. Each of the 44 items is followed by four or five descriptive statements that represent varying degrees of independence. The interviewer introduces each item with a general question about the child's behavior and selects the appropriate descriptive statement that is most typical of the child's behavior, as indicated by the answers to specific questions that he or she asks the parents or caretakers.

Face validity is based on the criteria of expert judges and an item analysis. Reliability has been reported at .98 for the total scores and subscores, and the coefficients vary from .88 to .97

for the subscales. The standardized group consisted of 716 trainable mentally retarded children (414 males and 302 females) from California. The subjects had IQs ranging from 25 to 59, mental ages from 2 to 7 years, and chronological ages from 5 to 13 years. Tables for the chronological ages permit the user to determine a child's percentile rank relative to his or her age group. Norms are listed at 2-year intervals.

### CHILD BEHAVIOR CHECKLIST
(Achenbach, T., and Edelbroch, C., 1980–1983, Thomas M. Achenbach)

The Child Behavior Checklist (CBCL) is designed to be administered individually to children ages four to sixteen years. There are four forms available: the Child Behavior Checklist, to be completed by parents of children aged four to sixteen years; Teacher's Report Form, for children aged six to sixteen; Direct Observation Form, for ages four to sixteen; and a Youth Self-Report Form for ages eleven through sixteen. This checklist is based upon a review of the literature and empirical studies, and pays much more attention to psychometric properties than is usually given.

The CBCL consists of 118 items assessing, in a standardized format, behavioral problems and social competencies of children. Test re-test reliabilities of mothers' ratings were reported at .89; some differences between mothers' and fathers' individual ratings were found. The CBCL was normed on a sample of 1300 children and T-scores were derived so that a child's profile could be compared to the scale norms. Norms are available for age groups four to five, six through twelve, and twelve through sixteen, combined male and female.

The Teacher's Report Form, Direct Observation Form, and Youth Self-Report Form are currently being evaluated with the same psychometric analyses as were used in evaluation of the CBCL. These supplemental forms can provide cross-sectional data, to counter the inherent problems in sole reliance on a parental report form. Although the CBCL and its related forms are fairly new and as such are still undergoing reform and development, it promises to become a standard assessment instrument for use with child behavior problems.

### BEHAVIOR RATING PROFILE, 1983

(Brown, L., and Hammill, D., 1983, Pro-Ed)

The Behavior Rating Profile is a norm-referenced scale consisting of a battery of five rating scales (teacher, parent, student, home, school and peer) and a sociogram. Each scale is normed individually so that they can be used separately as a rating scale or administered as a battery to produce a profile. Each component generates a standard score and a percentile rank.

The BRP was normed on an unselected sample of 1966 students six to eighteen years of age, 955 teachers, and 1232 of the students' parents. The sample was representative of the United States population in the 1980 census, in term of sex, race/ethnicity, and parental education and occupation. Test-retest reliability was in the .80s and validity was checked by correlations of the BRP with similar behavior scales. The manual provides questions to help administrators interpret the results of the profile.

### TEST OF EARLY SOCIO-EMOTIONAL DEVELOPMENT

(Hresko, W., and Brown, L., 1984, Pro-Ed)

The Test of Early Socio-Emotional Development (TOSED) is designed as a downward extension of the Behavior Rating Profile, for children aged three to seven years. It can be administered individually or as a battery and has four components: a student rating scale, teacher rating scale, parent rating scale, and a sociogram. Oral administration is used for the student rating scale. Scales are designed to elicit perceptions of students' personal behavior, behavior in interpersonal relationships, and behavior with authority figures.

The TOSED was standardized on the rating of 1606 children, 1773 parents, and 1006 teachers from fifteen states. Reliability coefficients are reported for each one-year interval and are reported to be between .70 and .90. Validity has

been established by correlations of the TOSED with similar behavior scales. Scales yield both standard scores and percentile ranks.

## PROJECTIVE TECHNIQUES

Projective techniques continue to be used widely by testing practitioners despite controversy over their validity, reliability, and general usefulness (Jackson & Pavnonen, 1980). A common feature of projective techniques is that rather ambiguous stimuli are presented to the child; these are assumed to permit responses that mirror characteristics of the child's personality. The applicability of this procedure in the determination of adaptability in various settings of the child's ecosystem is questionable (Jackson & Pavnonen, 1980), because the multitudes of hypotheses advanced with these techniques await vigorous verification. Basic problems of reliability and validity have not been conclusively answered (Nelson & Mitchell, 1976). Instruments commonly used to evaluate children having difficulty adapting within their environment include (1) Rorschach Psychodiagnostic Plates, (2) Educational Apperception Test, (3) Children's Apperception Test, (4) Draw-a-Person Test, and (5) Rohde Sentence Completion Test. *The Mental Measurement Yearbooks* (Buros, 1978) is the reference for the discussions of these instruments.

### RORSCHACH PSYCHODIAGNOSTIC PLATES

(Rorschach, H., and Huber, H., 1921–1954, Grune & Stratton)

There are thirteen currently available Rorschach materials, including the Rorschach Method, Rorschach Test, Rorschach Ink Blot Test, and Rorschach Psychodiagnostic Plates, which are used most frequently. The plates consist of ten carefully chosen, bilaterally symmetrical inkblots originated by Rorschach. The plates, used with persons three years of age and older, are used to describe aspects of the human personality—cognitive, emotional, and motivational—in both normal and psychiatric subjects. Historically Rorschach himself concentrated on diagnosis, quality of perception, ego capacity, personality mechanisms, sexual thought, and psychosexual level. The primary purpose of the plates is the formulation of psychiatric diagnosis and prognosis.

Training for administration of the test usually takes 1½ years. The test takes approximately 45 to 60 minutes to administer; the exact length depends on the productivity of the subject and the thoroughness of the examiner's inquiry and testing of the limits. Scores are interpreted in terms of configurations or combinations with other Rorschach scores. Supplementary materials, which relate typical example interpretations to various scores, are available. Formal scores entering into the interpretation are the subject's language, content and sequence of responses, and reaction time to each card.

The reliability of the scoring depends on the training of the examiner. Reports have ranged from .64 to .91. Split-half reliability estimates have yielded reliabilities ranging from .33 to .91 and averaging .54. Test-retest reliability ranges from about .10 to about .90, depending on the test-retest interval and the particular score. Parallel-form reliability has been determined by use of the Behn-Rorschach, a set of similar blots that approximate the psychometric criteria of the Rorschach. Correlations for various scores range from about 0 to .86, with a mean of .60. Examiner and situational influences are recognized as contributors to the variance of Rorschach scores. The Rorschach has been shown at present to have neither satisfactory validity nor invalidity. Of course, distinctions are made between experimental and clinical types of validation studies. Experimental studies have reported validity correlations between .20 and .40, and most such correlations have not stood the test of cross validation. Norms were originally derived in large part from adult groups. In an effort to extend the empirical framework for Rorschach interpretation to other age groups, researchers have also made available norms on children between two and ten years of age, adolescents between ten and sixteen years of age, and persons seventy years of age and older.

## EDUCATIONAL APPERCEPTION TEST

(Thompson, J. M., and Somes, R. A., 1973, Western Psychological Services)

This test measures a child's perceptions of school and the educational process. Four major areas are assessed: (1) reaction toward authority, (2) reaction toward learning, (3) peer relationships, and (4) home attitude toward school. An assumption is made that the child will respond to pictures in a unique manner, reflecting a particular style of behavior and personality organization.

The test consists of eighteen pictures depicting children in school and school-related situations. Children portrayed are of the middle elementary school age. Various responses can be obtained from the pictures. Following is a sample response from a 13-year-old student in a self-contained classroom for emotionally disturbed children. The child's response was recorded verbatim.

Well, this is me here talkin' about the teacher. Sometimes when I ask him a question he listens but he doesn't understand right what I'm saying. And, uh, then I tell him sometin' that I don't understand one problem—he tells me the whole thing when I just want to know about one little bitty mistake, that's all. See, so, kind of having a little hard trouble. And then when, uh, I'm doing my work right, now I get one mistake wrong, he's telling me, he's like he's telling me to do it all over again. Then when I tell em I'd doing it over, den, he us, we both get angry at each other. See, so he kinda talks a lot when he—the—he talks the same time I'm talking so we can't hear each other. So, that's why. And, he doesn't understand my math right. So—and sometimes he makes me confusing, by all different ways.

Validity of the test is based on its content and constructed validity. Specific research studies have not provided information concerning its validity and reliability because no one method of interpretation is proposed. Several aspects that are helpful in interpretative analysis include (1) main theme, (2) attitudes toward other figures, (3) identification, (4) main character, (5) nature of anxieties and conflicts about the educational process, (6) reaction toward the learning situation—self in student-role, and (7) outcome of stories. No information on norms is provided.

### CHILDREN'S APPERCEPTION TEST
(Bellak, L., and Bellak, S. S., 1949, Consulting Psychological Services)

This test requires the child to respond to a series of pictures. It is assumed that under this free-response condition, the child projects manifestations of personality characteristics and organization that can, by suitable methods, be scored and interpreted to yield a description of his or her basic personality structure. There are two sets of stimuli cards—human figures and animal figures. The pictures are divided into sets of ten pictures each. The pictures of the second series are more unusual, dramatic, and bizarre than those of the first set. The two sets of pictures are shown to the child on two separate occasions, usually with a 1- or 2-day interval.

The test can be administered individually or to a group. Administration time is 30 to 40 minutes. The test is used with children nine to ten years of age. The administrator must have clinical experience. Knowledge of psychoanalysis and some practice in translating the imagery of dreams and ordinary speech into elementary psychological components are needed. Scoring is done by recording everything the child says about each picture. Specific scoring categories include main theme—restate the gist of the story, main hero, main needs and drives of the hero, concept of the world, figures seen as . . . (withdrawn, aggressive), significant conflicts, nature of anxieties, main defenses against conflicts and fears, adequacy of superego as manifested by "punishment" for "crime," and integration of the ego. Ego functions that the test claims to measure include reality; judgment; sense of reality; regulation and control of drives; object relations; thought processes; defensive, stimulus, autonomous, synthetic, and integrative functioning; mastery; and competence.

Because responses reflect a fleeting mood as well as the present life situation of the subject, reliability of the test is not high. Reviews (Buros, 1970) have stated that no data regarding reliability were available. "Not a single study clearly supports the alleged supremacy of the CAT over pictures with humans . . . the majority show a clear superiority for figures employing humans" (p. 206). "The CAT continues to be difficult to evaluate. As with other projective techniques, the kind of data one gets using the CAT is not easily translated into statistical measurement language" (p. 207). Attempts are being made within personality theory to discover if the facts of a child's given story reflect a factual or wishful state of affairs. A Recording Analysis Booklet is available to facilitate the interpretation of responses. Of course, any results must be predicated on clinical experience with projective instruments and a theoretical knowledge of psychodynamics (content analysis, formal analysis, Gestalt functioning, body image or self-image, and analysis of choice). No information was provided on the norming sample.

### DRAW-A-PERSON
(Urban, W. H., 1963, Western Psychological Services)

This test is a popular projective technique for use with persons five years of age and older. The test assumes that a person's drawing represents an unconscious projection of self-image. Certain features and body parts are considered "signs" of qualities such as aggression and anger. The test consists of a manual, record booklet, and interpretative booklet. Administration time is 5 to 10 minutes. The subject is given paper and pencil and told to "draw a person"; then the subject is told to draw a person of the opposite sex. The subject may also be asked to tell a story about each person drawn. The examiner observes the order in which the body parts are drawn and notes any comments made by the subject while drawing. Clinical judgments are recorded in the interpretative booklet according to five categories: qualities to be inferred or concluded (aggression, dependency, perseveration), drawing characteristics (dim lines, eyes, shoes), diagnostic categories (obsessive-compulsive, paranoia, schizophrenia), behavioral characteristics (reluctance to draw), and subject matter of drawings (nudes, stick figures, themes). Little research is available on the validity of this test. A reliability intercorrelation is reported from .33 to .71.

### ROHDE SENTENCE COMPLETION TEST

(Jensen, A. R., 1967, Western Psychological Services)

This test requires the subject to complete sixty-five sentences. Space is provided for the subject to write "anything that seems important." A certain level of literacy in English is a prerequisite for this test. The test is suggested for children twelve years of age and older and consists of a manual, protocol booklet, and scoring booklet. Following are sample items:

I suffer _____ .
Friends _____ .
My mother _____ .
There are times _____ .
Eating _____ .
My mind _____ .

Administration time is 30 to 40 minutes. The test can be administered individually or in groups. Mention is made of standardization procedures carried out for an earlier (1940) edition, but this information is not included in the current manual. Face validity is supported by the manual's inclusion of comparative items from other sentence-completion tests. It is claimed that the stimulus items have become "more or less standardized" in both content and wording. No reliability measures are reported.

## PERSONALITY ASSESSMENT AND OBJECTIVE TECHNIQUES

Other instruments that are more reliable measures of personality include inventories or scales. Many of the scales, however, rarely include items directed toward community-adaptation skills (Jackson & Pavnonen, 1980). Popular scales and inventories for children include (1) Early School Personality Questionnaire, (2) Children's Personality Questionnaire, (3) California Psychological Inventory, and (4) Tennessee Self-Concept Scale.

### EARLY SCHOOL PERSONALITY QUESTIONNAIRE

(Coan, R., and Cattell, R. B., 1966, 1972, Institute for Personality and Ability Testing)

This questionnaire consists of two parts and evaluates thirteen factors that purportedly describe personality dimensions that extend into adult life. The thirteen factors are reserved versus warm-hearted, dull versus bright, affected by feeling versus emotionally stable, undemonstrative versus excitable, obedient versus dominant, somber versus enthusiastic, disregards rules versus conscientious, shy versus venturesome, tough-minded versus tender-minded, vigorous versus circumspect individualism, forthright versus shrewd, self-assured versus guilt-prone, and relaxed versus tense. The test is administered orally in two sessions. Administration time is 1 to 1½ hours. Sample questions include:

☐ When your mother is angry, do you: (A) feel happy anyway, or (B) feel like crying?
☐ If another child has your coat, do you: (A) take it away from him, or (B) tell the teacher?
☐ If you get upset or sad, do you: (A) get happy again pretty soon, or (B) stay sad for a long time?
☐ Would you rather: (A) look at a picture book by yourself, or (B) look at it with another boy or girl?

The test's authors discuss factor validity (reconfirmation of the original factor structure) of children's verbal self-reports in the manual. Self-report scores can, however, have little relationship to other behavioral measures. For this reason, the test should be considered a research instrument until empirical investigation can relate its results to a larger body of theoretical knowledge. The test's reliability estimates in the range of .50 lack some stability. The test was normed on over 1600 children with separate norms for boys and girls, six through eight years of age. Scales are rated for equivalence and intercorrelations.

### CHILDREN'S PERSONALITY QUESTIONNAIRE
(Porter, R. B., and Cattell, R. B., 1968, Western Psychological Services)

To provide a general assessment of personality, this questionnaire measures fourteen traits of personality. Designed for children eight to twelve years of age, the test can be given either individually or to a group. The test requires one class period for administration. The test has two forms and is a forced-choice format. There are seventy questions on the test. Hand-scoring keys are available.

Construct validity, theoretically based in factor analysis, is vague, and little information is used outside the test data itself. Test-retest reliabilities after two days ranged from .47 to .72 on Form A, .42 to .71 on Form B, and .56 to .80 on a combination of the forms. Homogeneity coefficients (KR-20 for internal consistency) ranged from .25 to .68 on Form A. Reliability of Form A with Form B ranged from .27 to .54. Reliability coefficients are in a middle range, which the test authors claim reflects their broad sampling of behaviors. The test provides norms for each form of the test according to sex. There are also tables combining scores for both sexes. Approximately 2800 children were tested. A table of means and standard deviations for children 10 ½ years of age is included as well as several tables of percentile scores.

### CALIFORNIA PSYCHOLOGICAL INVENTORY
(Gough, H. G., 1969, Consulting Psychologists Press)

This test consists of 480 items presented in a true-false format (for example, "I enjoy social gatherings just to be with people"). The items measure character traits that are assumed to be relevant to the prediction of social behavior in all situations. In other words, "folk concepts" that are culturally universal. The test is also available in Dutch, French, German, Italian, and Spanish. The test used persons thirteen years of age and older and requires 45 to 60 minutes to administer.

Scales were based on external criteria and an internal strategy. Validity of each derived score was determined by a comparison of groups that the scale presumably identifies (for example, psychotic) and cross validities on sizable samples. Validity is based largely on differences between extreme groups; a large middle group is omitted. Test-retest reliability of 200 male prisoners retested after one to three weeks ranges from .49 to .87, with a median of .80. For high school subjects retested after one year, the median test-retest correlation is .65 for males and .68 for females. Reliability estimates based on a single administration are not available.

The inventory has eighteen derived scores and transfers to a profile, with conversion to standard scores with a mean of 50 and a standard deviation of 10. Norms are based on over 6000 male and 7000 female subjects. Samples include a wide range of ages, socioeconomic groups, and geographical areas. The male groups ranged from machine operators to military officers, and the female groups ranged from prison inmates to medical-school students. Separate profiles for college and high-school subjects of each sex are available. The test is one personality inventory for which enough research has accumulated that the user can evaluate the probable utility of predictions in industrial, clinical, and educational settings.

### TENNESSEE SELF-CONCEPT SCALE
(Fitts, W. H., 1965, Counselor Recordings and Tests)

This scale is a 100-item instrument that purportedly measures a person's self-concept. It can be used with individuals twelve years of age and older, provided they have at least a sixth-grade reading level. The test kit includes the manual, test booklet, and scoring sheet. The test requires 10 to 20 minutes for administration.

The items on the scale include three statements: "This is what I am. This is how I feel about myself. This is what I do." For each item, the subject chooses one of five responses ranging from "Completely false" to "Completely true." Scores derived from these subtests include a total positive score (overall level of self-esteem), variability score (consistency from one area of self-perception to another), distribution score (measures of extreme response style), true-false ratio (measure of response style), net conflict score (empirical scales for groups of discriminations of various sorts), and number of deviant signs score (number of deviant features on all other subtests). The test's author suggests that people who have high scores tend to like themselves, while people with low scores have doubts about their own worth.

Content validity is provided by the agreement of judges on the items. The scale suggests validity through discrimination between groups (for example, normal and psychotic). Concurrent validity was measured by correlations with other personality measures. The Taylor Anxiety Scale correlates .70 with the total positive score. Correlations from .50 to .70 are common with the Cornell Medical Index and the Inventory of Feelings. Correlations with various Minnesota Multiphasic Personality Inventory scales are frequently in the .50s and .60s.

Test-retest reliability is in the high .80s. The test was standardized on 626 people from various geographical locations and social, economic, and intellectual levels. The manual includes tables of scores for norm groups.

In summary, the objective inventories and scales discussed here can be useful if they are presented in a competence orientation. Some of the inventories have caused critics to question both the content and actual sampling of behavior (Goldfried, 1977). Items may represent racial, ethnic, and sexual biases. Because of these biases, inventories or scales are rarely integrated into an assessment of children's communications skills. However, the California Psychological Inventory and possibly some others (Mercer, 1972) represent a move toward a competence orientation.

## INTERVIEWING

Interviewing methods have been discussed from a behavior-assessment orientation in this text. However, many of the behavioral-assessment procedures are not adaptable to a study of competence of ecological orientation (Carlson, Scott, & Elclund, 1980). Interviews concerning affective competence should assess such areas as child support systems, interests, perceived opportunities, and skills. Questions used to obtain general information from individuals in the child's community include the following:

A. Community interaction
 1. What are the expectations of the people in the community on the behaviors in question?
 2. How do they use their leisure time?
 3. How do they work?
 4. What is most valued?
 5. What are the community expectations (outcome) for this child?
B. Child's family background
 1. What is the attitude of the parents and other members of the family toward school?
 2. What is the status of the family in the community?
 3. What is the economic status of the family?
 4. What is the educational status of the family as well as their perception of education?
 5. What is the role of the child in the family group?
 6. What is the nature of verbal interaction in the home?
 7. How many children are in the family?
C. Child as a school participant
 1. How does the child get along with others at school?
 2. Is the child accepted by other children?
 3. Is the child accepted by all children or just a few?
 4. If the child is rejected, is the child rejected by both sexes?

5. How does the child react to other children and adults?
6. Does the child come into conflict with rules of the class habits and values of others? If so, are the conflicts often or occasionally?
7. How widely does the child participate in activities?
   (a) In classroom activities?
   (b) In social activities, playing, talking to friends?
8. Does the child withdraw from the teacher or other children in certain situations?
9. Does the child feel a responsibility to a certain group?
10. Does the child defend friends even when they are wrong?

D. Child's interests
1. What are the child's main interests?
2. What doesn't the child like to do?
3. What does the child want to do when he or she grows up?

E. Child deviation from normal affect
1. What situations seem to aggravate the child's development?
2. What behaviors seem to hinder classroom growth or community adaptability?
3. Is there a particular type of reaction evident within the social context?

As can be seen from these questions and prior discussion, assessment of affective competence goes beyond simple procedures of testing and interviewing and combines various kinds of informing and communicating by which the child can better adapt to his or her ecosystem.

## SUMMARY

If the concept of affective competence is to be useful in the assessment of exceptional children, it must take into account several variables: analysis of the labeling process, child and community tolerance, psychosocial development, moral judgment, perspective-taking skills, child attribution, and the roles of community- and family-related agencies. Furthermore, the analysis of these variables is sensitive to rapidly changing social demands. Methods of assessing competence within an ecological perspective are at present somewhat fragmented and disjointed (Brion-Meisels & Selman, 1984). Several points of emphasis suggest a future direction:

1. Focus of assessment is on the child's entire community or ecological system. It is necessary to understand the impact of the environment from the child's perspective and to form an attitude toward children that recognizes their many potentialities, in contrast to forming judgments on normative-based information.
2. An effort must be made to synthesize information regarding a child's affective competence obtained from the child's different social situations. This synthesis may include developmental factors (psychosocial development, moral judgment), environmental skills (perspective taking), and social adaptation (labeling, community tolerance).
3. Individual adaptation and adjustment must be emphasized. The child must adapt not only to the physical environment (classroom, home), but also to the social environment. The child's ability to successfully interact with others provides the framework for his or her coping with the physical environment.
4. Information obtained from the various aspects of the child's environment can be used to facilitate a "congruent" environment. Assessment is designed to provide teachers and children with accurate and complete information about the existing environment and environmental choices.
5. Focus is placed on values. The plurality of cultural backgrounds and values and the development of appropriate assessment must be recognized. Although the child's response is culturally relative, the situation in which the child finds himself or herself reflects the internalized community values. The ecological habitats are connected with the

child and each system so that modification in any area causes a shift in values for the whole of the child's ecosystem.

Averting the labeling process and developing community tolerance for differences are significant steps in the process of assessing and assisting adaptation of children to their community. Many factors (sex, age, religion) determine the tolerance for differences with any system. A probable trend in future assessment of affective competence is the melding of ecological theory and the individual child's social perceptions.

# CHAPTER 10

# Assessing Vocational Abilities

## STAN SCARPATI

### OUTLINE

**A**ssessment to determine the careers that are available to special-needs children and adults, and the skills and personality traits that are needed to meet job demands, is especially challenging today as technology rapidly moves our society away from industry and manufacturing. Vocational assessment of special-needs individuals is in many ways similar to other types of evaluation. Measurements determine the current level of performance in cognitive, affective, and motor abilities; an additional purpose is the prediction of future functioning. The significant departure in vocational assessment is the view that work (employment) is pivotal to the assessment process. Vocational evaluators intend to estimate under conditions of typical work situations, the exhibited behavior patterns that indicate the potential for the acquisition of specialized skills. This estimate is usually accomplished through formal and informal testing. Formal vocational testing collects and organizes data from psychometric tests, interest and attitude surveys, and work samples, to name a few examples. Informal assessment would most likely occur while students explore work opportunities; they are then evaluated in terms of their curriculum. This chapter focuses on formal assessment rather than on techniques used during informal curriculum-based data-gathering.

Evaluation must not only identify the levels of individuals' attitudinal, motivational, and prerequisite skills, but must also coordinate these outcomes with specific work activities. The ideal analysis will produce a series of statements that will predict and organize an individual's future behaviors during both training and experiential learning in the work setting, and will closely match the person's abilities with the job requirements.

Special-education professionals have consistently specified vocational assessment as invaluable in the preparation of special-needs students. In recent years other professionals have also begun to recognize its importance (Cobb & Larkin, 1985). The development of a vocational program for special-needs individuals involves first the production of a systematic plan, implementing desired work and work-related objectives, methods for attainment, activities, and measurement criteria for success.

Surveys have shown that two-thirds of disabled people between ages sixteen and sixty-four years are unemployed, while two-thirds of these individuals want to work. Moving special-needs students from school to gainful employment has been designated as crucial to the solution of this problem. The Education for All Handicapped Children Act (P.L. 94-142) and the corresponding vocational educational legislation (P.L. 94-482) require that an Individualized Education Plan (IEP) be written for each handicapped student; this plan should outline the specific educational and related services, including vocational, that are needed. Also, the Rehabilitation Act of 1973 (P.L. 93-112) requires that an Individualized Written Rehabilitation Program (IWRP) be prepared for each person receiving vocational rehabilitation services. A heavy demand for school-based vocational assessors has evolved, as transition programs for special-needs adolescents have been authorized under P.L. 98-199 (amendments to P.L. 94-142) and corroborated by the Rehabilitation Act Amendments (P.L. 99-506) in 1986. The Carl D. Perkins Vocational Education Act of 1984 (P.L. 98-524) was enacted to ensure men and women equal access to quality, vocational education programs for special-needs (and others considered disadvantaged) persons. This law for the first time identifies vocational assessment as critical to the education process. Although transitional services are receiving increased attention, special-education workers continue to perceive the needs of these children not in terms of skills they will need as adults but in terms of more basic skills (Nadolsky, 1985). Although vocational assessment is becoming increasingly available within schools, state-level monitoring systems and professional-certification criteria differ nationally (Peterson, 1985).

For special-needs individuals to realize their work potentials and for professionals to identify existing patterns of feasible employment, evaluation must evolve from a focal point that systematically utilizes either real or simulated work experiences (Bitter, 1979). Logical and analytical approaches to assessment aid in career development when observed patterns of behavior are formulated into a plan that will assist in employment choice and success. When tests are the bases for the selection of individuals for particular occupations, there is always the risk that false negatives and false positives will be revealed, and that the selection will thereby become a process of exclusion rather than selection. It is essential that a system of assessment be established that identifies unique strengths and weaknesses and attempts to develop a comprehensive, viable work plan (Meister, 1976). The eventual goal is for special-needs individuals to become more productive and to adequately function in achievement-demanding work settings (Gellman & Soloff, 1976).

Accurate assessment and eventual career-development plans are formulated from information that reflects the medical, psychological, social, and vocational factors pertinent to the individual. The evaluation becomes the basis for (1) establishing the presence of the physical or mental condition that limits performance, (2) appraising current health status to determine limits and capacities, (3) determining the extent to which the handicapping condition may be expected to be corrected or minimized by rehabilitation services, (4) selecting employment objective(s) commensurate with the individual's capacities and limitations, and (5) developing a written plan (IEP, IWRP) that will enable the individual to enter the chosen field of employment.

The specific questions that are formulated during the analysis of particular work and work-related behaviors, will enable the examiner to predict an individual's potential for achieving goals. Gellman (1968) describes the ability to predict work behavior, training capacity, and response to treatment, as techniques, which will vary with individual work behaviors. He believes

that vocational assessment can be categorized as follows:

1. Determination of work behavior or functioning capacities—the observational techniques employing work as an assessment methodology (work-sample)
2. Estimates of learning capacity in a work situation—by confronting clients with work problems, these situational techniques permit the evaluator to observe the subject's reactions
3. Estimates of training capacity or ability to acquire skills
4. Analysis of psychosocial factors influencing the work personality

Gellman (1968), who based his studies on the child-development hierarchies described by Meir (1965), suggests that, when career-development plans based on vocational evaluation are implemented, the following principles of evaluation be considered:

1. Vocational evaluation is future-oriented and designed to enable a prediction of vocational development and behavior to be made.
2. Effective vocational evaluation results in client-specific treatment plans.
3. Vocational evaluation should be periodic, and regular assessment of progress and validity of prediction should be made.
4. Vocational evaluation requires the examiner to maintain a complete knowledge of available rehabilitation and training resources.
5. Vocational evaluation becomes an ongoing, parallel process to the rehabilitation of handicapped persons. It begins with the need for rehabilitation and continues to function until the client can operate at an optimal level. The examiner uses a continuous procedure outlining individual changes in vocational development, training, and job changes, and modification of environmental and vocational components.
6. Vocational evaluation requires professional procedure input from ancillary disciplines, to

answer questions about individual needs. These services typically include psychologists, workshop specialists, social workers, physician, rehabilitation counselor, and the client.

7. The value of a vocational evaluation is a function of the quality and value of the questions it poses. Hence the evaluation follows a rudimentary two-stage process: its applicability to the individual is first determined, then a restatement of the questions is made after the gathered data is analyzed.

The application of vocational-evaluation principles and assessment procedures to school-age exceptional children is difficult. By utilizing the IEP, vocational education is a multidisciplinary effort to decrease the separation between academic performance and vocational-skill development. Although the use of the IEP has had a positive influence on programming for special-needs students, the specific annual goals and short-term objectives generally are in the more traditional areas of instruction, for example, reading and math. There is little research to direct the vocational-assessment process in schools and to detail precisely the skills that should be measured by school-based assessors. Career development does not appear to occupy as important a place in program development as more traditional education. Meyen and White (1980) identify several factors that could contribute to the lack of career instructional plans for handicapped students. They suggest that career planning rarely exists as a separate programming option, few school districts have viable programming options, instructional content does not readily fall into a sequence of precise developmental hierarchies, and, most important, there are no normative reference data for individual comparisons— ongoing evaluation is required but is currently lacking.

The vocational-assessment process becomes a salient contributor to the establishment and implementation of career education pro-grams, and to the provision of these services to persons with special needs. Not only will the evaluation identify a student's specific skills and needs, but it will also augment the development of appropriate methods and materials. Sitlington (1979) suggests that the evaluation process can provide diagnostic information in the following areas:

1. General training needs in each component area, including values, attitudes, and habits; human relationships; occupational information; and acquisition of daily living, cognitive, and psychomotor skills

2. Specific occupational training needs that can be identified when students enter junior and senior high school and that can deal with areas of concentration

3. Identification of appropriate methods and materials to be used; begun on a formative basis in early elementary years and including learning modality preference (visual, auditory, kinesthetic) and effective methods, such as demonstration or verbal instructions, by which information can be conveyed

4. Best program options throughout and at the end of the program, such as high-school work experience, on-the-job training, or placement in a technical program after graduation

## CAREER DEVELOPMENT ASSESSMENT

For program planners to take full advantage of vocational-assessment information, they must have prior knowledge of specific occupational prerequisites. A job analysis (such as the determination of academic skills, and capabilities needed for a worker to label, sort, classify, or assemble), can provide information pertaining to the operations and skills required for a particular task. Such an analysis also yields information as to how these skills apply to actual job performance. These performance skills can be organized into a task-analysis procedure, hierarchically arranged from simplest skill to final objective (Sitlington, 1980). By analyzing patterns of work performed and workers' traits, job analysis systematically studies the worker (Bitter, 1979).

The United States Department of Labor offers a standardized form for the recording of occupational procedures in a uniform fashion. Sitlington (1980) recommends developing job-specific forms that will more efficiently analyze individual jobs. Completing such a form should require actual observation of the task while it is being performed, as well as interviews with those individuals associated with the job, such as supervisors, employers, and workers.

Bitter (1979) suggests that the study of several, specific components can assist in the designing of job-analysis strategies; these components include (1) the level of training or education required for a particular job, (2) the required aptitude for learning, (3) the required personal traits or temperaments, (4) the subject's interests in a particular job, and (5) the physical or environmental demands of the work, such as cold, heat, noise.

In selecting appropriate assessment tools and techniques, one must consider the type of information needed for each individual, whether the selected materials yield one or several types of data, and the relevance of the resulting data to the decision-making process. One must also consider the economic factors contributing to the cost of evaluation and the benefit of the information to the client. For instance, job-site evaluations or situational assessments (requiring workshops and supervisory staff) are more expensive to conduct than "homemade" or commercially produced evaluations of work samples (Botterbusch, 1978). Paper-and-pencil tests, although least likely to represent the actual skills necessary for job success, are economically feasible because they are usually inexpensive and are often group administered. Figure 10-1 depicts the relationships between various assessment techniques, the degree to which they reflect life, and their cost. Regardless of the approach used, the questions concerning a client's particular skills and abilities and that person's potential for occupational success, should serve as the basis for the vocational assessment. Test selection and application, therefore, becomes an ongoing procedure in which the information needed about the individual is compared to the suitability of a particular assessment approach for gathering those data. Sitlington and Wimmer (1978) suggest that the evaluation procedure should provide specific

**Figure 10-1**
Comparison of various assessment methods.

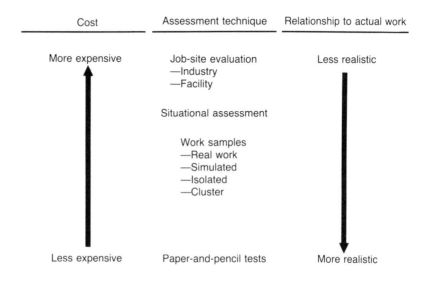

| Cost | Assessment technique | Relationship to actual work |
|------|---------------------|----------------------------|
| More expensive | Job-site evaluation<br>—Industry<br>—Facility | Less realistic |
| | Situational assessment | |
| | Work samples<br>—Real work<br>—Simulated<br>—Isolated<br>—Cluster | |
| Less expensive | Paper-and-pencil tests | More realistic |

information in the following areas: (1) medical, (2) educational, (3) personal/social, (4) interests, (5) work habits and attitudes, (6) aptitudes, and (7) learning style.

## JOB ANALYSIS

Before any systematic approach is undertaken to evaluate an individual's existing vocational abilities or potential for training and employment in a particular occupation, it is helpful to make a critical analysis of the job. Specific questions to be answered include, what are the tasks that make up the job, what are the beginning and end points of the job, and how precisely can the job be described. A job analysis is a systematic study of an occupation in terms of its specific methods and techniques utilized; its required equipment and tools, materials, products, and services; and the relationships between those characteristics, the demands on workers, and the optimal worker's traits. There is often confusion in how a *job, task,* or *position* is defined, and the near-interchangeability of these terms adds to the dilemma. The United States Manpower Administration has developed a set of definitions to assist in the process of analyzing jobs (U.S. Department of Labor, 1972):

*Element:* the smallest, practicable subdivision of any work activity without analyzing separate motions, movements, or mental processes.

*Task:* one or more elements of a distinct activity that are logical and necessary in the performance of the work. A task is created whenever human effort, physical or mental, is expected to accomplish a specific purpose.

*Position:* a collection of tasks constituting the total work assignment of a single work. Positions are in one-to-one correspondence with the workers.

*Job:* a group of positions identical in respect to their major or significant tasks and sufficiently alike to justify their being covered by a single analysis. One or many persons may function in the same job.

Each job analysis should represent a complete description of one job, with identification of all its components. Such analysis should include information pertaining to whether or not the worker (1) performs a specific sequence of tasks or cycle of operations, (2) frequently changes from one set of tasks to another, or (3) must be flexible and perform tasks not directly related to the primary job. These directives will assist in the decision whether there is to be one or more actual job analyses. In general, the information gathered from this analysis should specify the nature of the work performed (such as machinery used, products, or worker functions), and required personal traits of the workers (such as aptitudes, interests, temperaments, and physical demands) (U.S. Department of Labor, 1972).

Following is a review of several methods currently being used to gather vocational information about persons with special needs. The methods described are (1) situational assessment, (2) job-site assessment, (3) work sample techniques, and (4) commercially prepared paper-and-pencil tests.

## SITUATIONAL ASSESSMENT

This technique incorporates efforts to systematically observe a client's behavior—occupational assets and liabilities—during actual work or daily living situations (Sitlington, 1980). Most widely used in vocational evaluation in rehabilitation, this approach is most frequently conducted on job sites or in sheltered workshops; because the latter allows the observer to manipulate the work setting, it can provide a multitude of assessment situations (Bitter, 1979). Although almost any work environment, such as a clerical setting, a farm, or a laboratory can be utilized, the adaptability of the industrial job-site lends itself to the situational-analysis model (Poor et al., 1975). The primary difference "between situational assessment . . . and ordinary employment . . . is that [in situational assessment] it is possible to alter all of the customary conditions of employment without [affecting] the overriding concern for efficient production" (Neff, 1968, p. 207). In gathering information about a client, the examiner must repeatedly enforce the two critical concerns of situational analysis: (1) recreate actual work settings and environments, and (2) manipulate and modify as many work and work-related variables as possible, so that as many work behaviors as possible are elicited from the client. Only then can an individual's response to ongoing demands of the job, i.e., that person's work performance and work-related behaviors, can be determined. For example, to reveal all facets of his or her behavior, a worker must not only meet task requirements but also interact with other workers and with supervisors.

The need for unbiased data and a permanent product that truly reflects a client's performance is strong in situational assessment, whether it focuses on actual skill limitations and abilities, interests, or interactions between workers and supervisors. To assist in this process, Sitlington (1980) suggests that the instruments used for recording the data focus precisely on the behaviors and attitudes of concern. Also, these instruments should report the data as objectively as possible. Procedures for gathering situational data are more likely to be standardized than are the assessments themselves.

For persons with special needs, failure to demonstrate personal skills related to the work environment is as likely a cause for lost employment as is poor performance. The *Work Personality Profile* (Roessler & Bolton, 1985) is an example of an instrument that attempts to identify observable personality behaviors. Administered at the beginning of a situational assessment, the instrument rates workers' strengths and weaknesses on a 4-point scale of eleven personality dimensions.

Situational assessment relies more heavily on the observational skills of the examiner than on psychometrics. Dunn (1973) proposes several guidelines that facilitate the process of observation: (1) use measurable terms when describing behavior, (2) describe the situation in which the behavior occurred, (3) describe only what occurs, (4) report results in behavioral terms (ini-

tiating statements with action verbs), (5) describe a frequency, rate, or duration whenever possible, (6) write in a simple, direct style, and (7) record observations immediately.

The Materials Development Center at the University of Wisconsin-Stout offers a measurement device (*MDC Behavior Identification Format*, 1974) to assist observers in identifying, observing, and recording behavior during situational work evaluations. To aid evaluators in writing behavioral descriptions of their observations, the device lists, in addition to sample descriptions, examples, and definitions, twenty-two behavior categories: hygiene; grooming and dress; irritating habits; odd or inappropriate behaviors; communication skills; attendance; punctuality; work-coping skills; personal complaints; vitality; stamina; work consistency; distractibility; conformity; reactions to change in work assignments; reactions to monotonous or unpleasant tasks; social skills (relating to coworkers); required supervision; recognition-acceptance of authority; reactions to close supervision, criticism, and pressure from supervisors; need for assistance; and organizational skills.

The ability to perform job activities with minimal supervision, high yield of quality production, and optimum levels of client comfort and ease, is an obvious goal of situational evaluation because it pinpoints vocational promise. To assist in this process, the Work Adjustment Rating Form (WARF), primarily used by rehabilitation facilities, provides information concerning the determination of progress toward work readiness and adjustments in training procedures (Bitter, 1979). Eight subscales, identifying five levels of performance from high to low, describe behaviors in terms of the amount of supervision required, the display of teamwork, realism of job goals, rule/authority acceptance, work tolerance, perseverance, extent of assistance needed, and importance attached to job training. To control rate bias, a rating form with randomly presented WARF items (Bitter & Bolanovich, 1970) is used. Using more than one rating per client is also suggested.

# JOB-SITE ASSESSMENT

Because situational assessment usually occurs during the final stages of career development, it is closely related to job-site assessments in which actual job settings are the evaluation setting. This situation differs slightly from situational assessment because it attempts to view the global aspects of an individual with respect to the person's capacity to perform as a total person (Nadolsky, 1971). In a job-site assessment, all variables that influence an individual's ability to perform adequately interact freely, and true performance is thereby revealed. Situational assessments place certain constraints on these interactions. Poor and co-workers (1975) note, along with the obvious advantages of "real-life" evaluative techniques, other advantages of this procedure:

1. Business and industry are directly involved with the problems of helping special-needs individuals help themselves.
2. No additional financial investment is required for equipment or personnel.
3. Potential on-the-job evaluation [sites] are present even in small communities.
4. Work has an urgency and an immediacy about it that helps stimulate people to do their best.
5. A job tryout is eminently suitable for involving the client in determining the areas in which he or she wants to be evaluated and in providing feedback about likes and dislikes. The counselor may evaluate the client or the employer may evaluate the client—but the client evaluates the job.
6. The job tryout can be used to help the client develop better self-awareness and can contribute to the ultimate objective of more independent living.
7. In certain instances, the employer will hire the client [whom] he or she assisted in evaluating on a job tryout (p. 178).

Bitter (1967) maintains that the job-tryout process provides a forum for a functional analysis of behavioral dynamics and allows individual likes and dislikes to be ascertained. Also, this process presents no need for interests to be interpreted, as do more formal methods of assessment. In view of these advantages, the job-site tryout approach is a viable format for accurate vocational assessment.

But, as with any assessment device, one method of data collection does not provide all the information that is needed and there are inherent difficulties with all methods. Poor and co-workers (1975) advance several cautions and considerations for the observer to contemplate when utilizing on-the-job placements for evaluations:

1. Before placing a client for evaluation in a job-tryout situation it is essential to have already developed much information about a client, such as social, vocational, and medical data which will assist in anticipating problem areas, strengths and special considerations.
2. Since using job tryouts relies on the goodwill and existing resources of the community for success, careful attention to public education is essential.
3. The examiner must be skilled in employer-oriented communication.
4. The counselor should be alert for the employer who may be too sympathetic toward the client and thus limit the effectiveness of a real and objective experience.
5. Some employers, even with the best of intentions, do not have enough time available to give the close supervision that is necessary with many clients, particularly during the early stages of the experience.
6. Some kind of built-in system of feedback and rewards for job tryout is needed.
7. Insurance laws, safety hazards, and regulations regarding minimum wages may make it difficult to develop some situations [even though] employers would otherwise be willing to cooperate.
8. Job tryout opportunities in a particular setting with a specific employer, unique tasks, work environment, and other factors are not easily duplicated (p. 179).

Because of the diverse nature of job sites and the numerous variables involved in evaluations, few assessment instruments provide for accurate data recording. The Job-Site Evaluation Form was developed so that employers and those making the placement could determine a person's work potential while on the job. The employer compares the subject's performance with that of other workers, from poor to excellent, on such worker traits as listening to directions, accepting responsibility for work assigned, working independently, starting work on time, and adjusting to variations in work. The employer is also questioned as to whether or not the subject would be hired. The checklist takes approximately 15 minutes to complete, and the employer must respond to the question concerning hiring. The resulting information provides a fairly comprehensive picture of an individual's work habits and skills and readiness for competitive employment.

## WORK-SAMPLE TECHNIQUES

Work samples are self-developed or commercially prepared activities that represent one or several aspects of a particular work skill. The use of work samples is an evaluative technique in which a client's actual job skills are assessed in a simulated work situation before that client is placed in an actual competitive situation. By definition, a work sample is "a well defined work activity involving tasks, materials, and tools which are identical or similar to those in an actual job or cluster of jobs" (Vocational Evaluation and Work Adjustment Association, 1975, p. 52). The work-sample approach is most useful during the preparation and exploration stages of career development. They are assumed to more accurately assess individuals, particularly on performance, than do paper and pencil tests. They are limited, however, to entry-level jobs. Recent use of computer technology, although simple, has resulted in more sophisticated techniques.

Whether work samples are commercially prepared or individually developed specifically for the occupation and the individual, they have several advantages and disadvantages that must be considered before they are used. In general, work samples (1) closely approximate real work, (2) require minimum academic skills, (3) provide direct and immediate feedback, and (4) provide numerous opportunities for client exploration (Bitter, 1979). A major characteristic of commercially developed work samples is that they have undergone population and task standardization, which limits the subjectivity involved in the evaluation of personal traits. Self-developed work samples are, of course, economically more feasible, tend to reflect individual needs, and can be specifically related to the local marketplace. Also, self-developed work samples do not become obsolete because of rapidly changing technologies. But self-developed work samples do require continuous monitoring and reconstruction. They rarely provide statistical data supporting the predictive validity of the sample to community jobs (Bitter, 1979). It is this single issue (lack of performance criteria and norming precision) that makes work-sample assessment most useful in suggesting areas of client promise and occupational exploration (Meister, 1976).

Commercially made or self-developed work samples can be selected only after a critical analysis is made of the information needed and the interaction of that need with the variables of cost, need for standardized results, and applicability to local industry. Because work samples can be used in a multitude of diverse skill activities, Roberts (1969) suggests a taxonomy of samples that may be helpful to the examiner deciding what type of work sample to use:

1. *Real-work sample:* utilizes sample of work from an actual job in the locality, to determine the client's interest and potential.
2. *Simulated-work sample:* processes and operations of actual jobs are altered in structure; replication of the common critical factors of a job.
3. *Isolated-trait work sample:* assesses specific skill common to a larger group of jobs;

additional traits, difficult to remove from the trait of concern, often contaminate the measurement and make single-trait samples difficult to construct.

4. *Cluster-trait sample:* contains many traits inherent in a job or variety of jobs, and assesses an individual's potential to perform a variety of tasks.

## Developing Work Samples

As with any assessment methodology, the use of work samples should include every effort to obtain as much pertinent information about a client as possible—job skills and abilities, work attitudes, gross and fine motor skills, and physical attributes. In self-developed work samples, diagnostic questions should identify the sample construction process and assist in determining the priorities of job-related performance objectives. Sitlington (1979) proposes six basic steps for preparation of a work sample:

1. Decide on samples to develop. This involves conducting an informal survey of the community to determine which jobs are feasible for the specific special needs population being served, then ascertaining if work samples for some of these jobs have already been developed by someone else.
2. Conduct job analysis. After selecting a job, conduct an accurate analysis, including task description, work requirements, and environmental demands, which will provide content validity.
3. Design and construct work samples. [The selection of] tasks is related to their importance to the job and feasibility of replication. Performance criteria should be based on measurements of correct products produced, number of errors, quality of work, or time required to complete the sample.
4. Develop work sample manual. Systematic administration of work sample will require a manual for standardized implementation, [which] should include specific instructions

to be given to the individual and to be followed by the examiner.
5. Establish norms. As an ongoing process, norms should be updated and established so [that] individuals being evaluated are compared with the population with which they are competing. Percentile or standard scores are most commonly used in deriving norm tables.
6. Establish estimates of reliability and validity. While complex statistical calculations are not necessary, it is necessary to decide whether work samples actually measure what they intend to measure. Test-retest reliability analysis is considered most applicable in determining consistency. Validation of the work sample can be determined from careful and realistic considerations of the job itself if essential activities of the job are actually included in the work sample and if the individuals who perform well on the samples replicate their performance on the real job.

The development of work samples often becomes a time-consuming and therefore expensive project, when the use of available personnel and experienced staff is included as expenses. Evaluators are often unsure as to what types of samples to use. Do the samples actually relate to potential employment positions available in the community? Is prior training necessary before a job can be attempted? These perplexing questions often cause evaluators to consider commercially prepared evaluation systems that ideally will provide all the necessary information about an individual at one time. Although commercially prepared samples can provide a major savings of time over self-developed samples, they simply do not provide all the necessary information and must be supplemented by other techniques. However, it has been suggested that commercially prepared work samples, carefully selected from several systems, can be combined into a unified scheme specific to the needs of the facility and the particular individuals involved (Botterbusch, 1976). The use of commercially prepared systems is increasing, as the demand for standardization and limited staff time and experience have created a need for critical and accurate vocational evaluation.

Brolin (1973) lists ten questions that will help counselors to decide which system will provide the information they need.

1. Does the system take into account expectancy to fail?
2. Does the system take into account academic limitations?
3. Does the system take into account verbal limitations?
4. Does the system take into account limited experience?
5. Does the system allow for more than one trial on tasks?
6. Does the system allow for repeated instruction and check for comprehension?
7. Does the system have face validity?
8. Does the system allow for appropriate conditions for testing—pleasant surroundings, orderly administration, and fatigue?
9. Does the system use "spaced" rather than "massed" evaluation?
10. Is the system adequately normed on handicapped individuals and the workers who are doing the various types of tasks? Have follow-up studies been conducted on vocational prediction validity?

## COMMERCIALLY PREPARED SYSTEMS OF WORK SAMPLES

### MCCARRON-DIAL WORK EVALUATION SYSTEM

(McCarron, L. T., & Dial, J. G., 1972, McCarron-Dial System)

This system was developed to assess the functioning ability of mentally retarded and chronically mentally ill persons. The primary purpose was to combine measurement data from eighteen separate instruments (grouped into five factors), along with behavior observation, into one predictive measurement system. The system is organized into five groups:

1. Verbal-cognitive
   a. Wechsler Adult Intelligence Scale
   b. Stanford-Binet Intelligence Scale
   c. Peabody Picture Vocabulary Test
2. Sensory
   a. Bender Visual-Motor Gestalt Test
   b. Haptic Visual Discrimination Test
3. Motor skills
   a. Fine motor assessment
      (1) Beads-in-Box
      (2) Beads-on-Rod
      (3) Finger-Tapping
      (4) Nut-and-Bolt Task
      (5) Rod Slide
   b. Gross motor assessment
      (1) Hand Strength
      (2) Finger-Nose-Finger Movement
      (3) Jumping
      (4) Heel-Toe-Tandem Walk
      (5) Standing on One Foot
4. Social-emotional
   a. Observational Emotional Inventory (designed for use in sheltered work shops)
5. Integration-coping
   a. Behavioral Rating Scale (developed by Dial)
   b. San Francisco Vocational Competency Scale

It is recommended that the work-evaluation process follow a sequence, starting with a preliminary screening by means of an interview with the client and/or referral source. The subject is encouraged to participate and, when the system is completed, is counselled as to realistic work and goal expectations. The first three factors are administered in a formal setting and are usually completed in one day. To be tested for the last two factors, the client must be placed in a work setting and must undergo observation for two weeks. Little opportunity for the client to experience vocational exploration is available, although this exploration is possible during the observation period.

Normative data were derived from 200 adult "mentally disabled individuals" in sheltered and community employment. No reliability data are offered. Validity results are inconclusive because information was derived from inadequate procedures. Microcomputer software is available for scoring.

### TALENT ASSESSMENT PROGRAMS (TAP)

(Nighswonger, W. E., 1974, Talent Assessment Inc.)

This system consists of eleven tests designed to evaluate work in industrial, technical, and service areas; it emphasizes the measurement of dexterity, perception, gross and fine motor finger manipulation, and retention skills. Assessment should be limited to these areas.

The occupational clusters related to specific job titles in the *Dictionary of Occupational Titles* are (1) structural and mechanical visualization, (2) discrimination by size and shape (sorting), (3) discrimination by color (sorting), (4) tactile discrimination, (5) fine discrimination without tools, (6) gross dexterity without tools, (7) fine dexterity with tools, (8) gross dexterity with tools, (9) circuital visualization (using an electrical flow diagram), (10) retention of structural and mechanical detail, and (11) structural and mechanical visualization in greater depth. It is recommended that work sample Number 1 be given first and Numbers 10 and 11 last, but other samples may be administered in any order. The entire battery is usually completed in about 2 hours.

Normative information is available for junior and senior high school students of both sexes, as well as for mentally retarded adults and alcoholic males. Test-retest studies reveal a reliability coefficient of .85. No validity data are available.

### SINGER VOCATIONAL EVALUATION SYSTEM

(1971, Singer Education Division)

This system consists of twenty self-contained, independent work samples and includes an audiovisual presentation of the instructions for performing the task. Clients pace themselves through each work station; instructions are recorded on audio cassettes and synchronized with instructional filmstrips. The work samples include: (1) sample making, (2) bench assembly, (3) drafting, (4) electrical wiring, (5) plumbing and pipefitting, (6) carpentry, (7) refrigeration, heating, and air conditioning, (8) soldering and welding, (9) office and sales clerk, (10) needle trades, (11) masonry, (12) sheetmetal, (13) cooking and baking, (14) engine service, (15) medical service, (16) cosmetology, (17) data calculation, (18) soil testing, (19) photo lab technician, and (20) production machine operating.

Individuals' scores are derived from time (rated on a five-point scale) and error evaluation, and the scores are then compared with norms based on more than "100 individuals." Exactly who made up this sample is unclear. Another disadvantage is that no reliability or validity data are available. A major advantage of the Singer System is that it provides for career exploration and a functional analysis of vocational aptitudes and interests, and allows for client input through self-evaluation of performance.

### PHILADELPHIA JEWISH EMPLOYMENT AND VOCATIONAL SERVICE WORK SAMPLE SYSTEM (JEVS)

(1970, Vocational Research Center)

Developed in the late 1950s, the system consists of twenty-eight work samples that relate to ten groups of workers' traits. First identified in the 1965 *Dictionary of Occupational Titles,* these trait groups are sequenced according to increasing complexity:

1. *Handling:* nut, bolt, and washer assembly; rubber stamping; washer treading; bugette assembly; and sign making
2. *Sorting, inspecting, measuring, and related work:* tile sorting; nut packing; and collating leather samples
3. *Tending:* grommet assembly
4. *Manipulating:* union assembly, belt assembly, ladder assembly, metal square fabrication, hardware assembly, telephone assembly, and lock assembly

5. *Routine checking and recording:* filing by number, proofreading
6. *Classifying, filing, and related work:* filing by three letters, nail and screw sorting, adding machine, payroll computation, and computing postage
7. *Inspecting and stock checking:* register reading
8. *Craftsmanship and related work:* pipe assembly
9. *Costuming, tailoring, and dressmaking:* blouse making and vest making
10. *Drafting and related work:* condensing principles

Most instructions are given orally, and reading is required only when it is specific to a work task. Although each sample is administered (from easiest to more complex) individually, fifteen clients may be evaluated together at one time. The JEVS specifically outlines twenty-five work factors, and all factors associated with each sample are carefully defined so that observations, which are summarized on a daily basis, can be accurately recorded.

The norming sample is clearly identified as 322 clients who were predominantly black males. No test reliability data are available. Research (Nadolsky, 1973) indicate that the JEVS system is a valid predictor for the evaluation of immediate employment potential.

### VOCATIONAL INFORMATION AND EVALUATION WORK SAMPLES (VIEWS)

(1970, Vocational Research Center)

A modification of the JEVS evaluation system, the VIEWS system is specifically designed for mildly and moderately mentally retarded persons. The primary difference between the two systems is that VIEWS emphasizes training the individual in the work task before evaluation. Sixteen work samples, related to workers' traits as grouped in the *Dictionary of Occupational Titles,* are presented in an orientation-demonstration-training sequence under conditions of positive reinforcement (Bitter, 1979).

The workers' traits are clustered into categories of (1) element, including handling and feeding; (2) clerical, including routine checking, typing, and collating; (3) machine skills, such as use with hand tools and larger tools, for example drill-press operation; and (4) crafts. Although no reading is required, there is a required entry level of reading competence. The administration of the complete battery usually requires five to eight days. Results indicate such abilities as work skills, levels of occupational independence, and vocational interest.

### COMPREHENSIVE OCCUPATIONAL ASSESSMENT AND TRAINING SYSTEMS (COATS)

(1976, Prep Inc.)

Four major components contain work samples pertaining to those attributes associated with job-seeking and job-keeping, job matching, and living skills. Each component contains three program levels: (1) assessment and analysis, (2) prescription and instruction, (3) evaluation and placement. The work sample uses self-paced audiotapes to present twenty-seven actual job activities. The sample measures the client's aptitude and preference for jobs such as food preparation, drafting, metal construction, wood construction, medical services, travel services, barbering-cosmetology, and small-engine assembly. The Employability Attitudes component, using six audiovisual cassette cartridges, allows clients to express their attitudes concerning problem-solving skills needed for both employment searches and the eventual job. The Living Skills component identifies both the skills and knowledge necessary to the client's functioning in modern society, and the objectives by which his or her performance will be measured. Audiovisual cartridges allow clients to stop the work-sample instruction as they need to, both before and during actual performance. Evaluation is based not only on the examiner's ratings of skill proficiency and behavioral attributes, but also on the client's interpretations of job expectancies and interests. Computer scoring is available and each test component may be purchased separately.

## WIDE RANGE EMPLOYMENT SAMPLE TEST (WREST)

(Jastak, J. F., & Jastak, S. R., 1979, Guidance Associates)

This test was originally developed to assess mentally retarded and physically handicapped individuals employed in a sheltered workshop. The ten work samples reflect those tasks most commonly found in that type of setting: (1) single and double folding, pasting, and stuffing, (2) stapling, (3) bottle packing, (4) rice measuring, (5) screw assembly, (6) tag stringing, (7) scratch pasting, (8) collating, (9) color and shade matching, and (10) pattern making. Work samples are administered in sequential order from 1 to 10 and can be completed in 1 1/2 hours. Scores are based on errors and time of completion; the total score indicates the individual's efficiency in technical work. A disadvantage of this system is its inability to truly reflect a person's potential in the competitive job market. It is also an inefficient system for behavior observation. Males and females of various age groups but unspecified sources made up the norm group. Test-retest reliability data are high, but no validity information is offered.

## VALPAR COMPONENT WORK SAMPLE SERIES (VALPAR)

(1973, Valpar International)

This system was intended to contribute to comprehensive vocational evaluation and planning. The series consists of work samples that are coordinated with work-trait information in the *Dictionary of Occupational Titles*. These samples are (1) small tools (mechanical), (2) size discrimination, (3) numerical sorting, (4) upper-extremity range of motion, (5) clerical comprehension and aptitude, (6) independent problem-solving, (7) multi-level sorting, (8) simulated assembly, (9) whole-body range of motion, (10) tri-level measurement, (11) eye-hand-foot coordination, (12) electronic soldering and inspection, (13) money handling, (14) inte-

grated peer performance, (15) electrical circuitry and print reading, (16) drafting, (17) prevocational readiness battery, and (18) dynamic physical capacities.

In addition to time and error scoring, behavioral observations and ratings attempt to describe the client in terms of universal characteristics; job-related motor activities and cognitive skills are assessed as an integrated whole. Normative data are available on sheltered workshop employees, rehabilitation clients, and employed workers. Most test-retest reliability coefficients are reasonably high, but validity data are not available. To accommodate the special needs of visually handicapped persons, the VALPAR series has developed modifications (B-Kits) to the work samples. To evaluate the conceptual skills of visually impaired persons, a perfor mance-based battery (C.U.B.E.) measures perceptual-compensation abilities. Individual components include tactual perception, mobility discrimination, spacial organization and memory, assembly and package, and audible perception.

## TOWER SYSTEM (TESTING, ORIENTATION, AND WORK EVALUATION IN REHABILITATION)

(Rosenberg, B., & Usdane, W., 1963, ICD Rehabilitation and Research Center)

Originally developed by the ICD Rehabilitation and Research Center in New York City, the Tower system was designed for physically and emotionally disabled persons. The oldest work-evaluation system, it is often used as a guide for the development of other systems. Through a sequence of work tasks in fourteen occupational areas (arranged and presented in order from simple to complex), more than 100 work activities are available for client evaluation. Job-training areas include the following:

1. *Clerical:* business arithmetic, filing, typing, one-hand typing, payroll computation, use of sales book, record keeping, and correct use of English

2. *Drafting:* use of T square, triangle, compass; making working drawing; drawing to scale; and use of geometric shape
3. *Drawing:* use of perspective; forms, shapes, and objects; shading, tone, and texture; color; and free-hand sketching
4. *Electronics assembly:* color perception and sorting, running a ten-wire cable, inspecting a ten-wire cable, lacing a cable, and soldering wires
5. *Jewelry manufacturing:* use of saw, needle files, electric drill press; piercing and filing metals; use of pliers; use of torch in soldering; and making earrings and brooches
6. *Leather goods:* use of rulers, use of knife, use of dividers, use of paste and brush, use of scissors and bond folder in pasting, constructing picture frame, and production task
7. *Machine shop:* reading and transcribing measurements, blueprint reading, measuring with a rule, drawing to measurement, metal layout and use of basic tools, drill press operation, manipulation of fractions and decimals, measuring with the micrometer caliper, and mechanical understanding
8. *Lettering:* lettering aptitude, use of T square, use of pen and ink, and brush lettering
9. *Mail clerk:* opening, date-stamping, and sealing mail; sorting, delivering, collecting, folding, and inserting; mail classification; use of scale; and postage calculation
10. *Optical mechanics:* use of metric ruler, use of calipers, lens recognition, lens centering and marking, use of lens protractor, and hand beveling and edging
11. *Pantograph engraving:* introduction to the engravograph; setting up, centering copy, and determining specified ratios; use of workholder and adjustment of cutter; and setting up and running off a simple job
12. *Sewing machine operating:* sewing machine control, use of needle lift and needle chine control, use of needle lift and needle pivoting, tacking and sewing curved lines, upper threading, winding and inserting bobbin, sewing and cutting, and top stitching
13. *Welding:* measuring, making a working drawing, identifying welding rods, use of acetylene torch, use of rods and electrodes, use of torch and rod, measuring and cutting metal, and soldering
14. *Workshop assembly:* counting; number and color collation; folding and banding; weighing and sorting; counting and packing; washer assembly; inserting, lacing, and typing; and art-paper banding.

Although the tasks incorporate various training needs and reveal individual performance levels, clients are not required to experience the entire series. Areas are chosen according to the client's interests and the evaluation plan. Work samples within each occupational area are sequenced in degrees of difficulty, and poor performance on a simple task indicates that testing in this area should be discontinued. Although testing with the Tower System may require up to three weeks, the time and error scores formulate a thorough evaluative profile of an individual's personal characteristics and abilities in work performance. Although the work samples are useful for evaluations of handicapped persons' suitability for a narrow group of jobs, the realistic nature of the tasks is demonstrated by Towers' use for an extended period for assessment and training.

The system was normed on clients at the Institute for the Crippled and Disabled (former name of the ICD Rehabilitation and Research Center). Validation research comparing information from seven cities produced equivocal results. No reliability data are available.

The ICD Rehabilitation and Research Center has also developed the Micro-TOWER Battery of thirteen work samples that are actual job activities, for use in group evaluations. Vocational aptitudes are measured in the areas of (1) motor skills, (2) spatial-perceptual skills, (3) clerical perceptual skills, (4) verbal skills, and (5) numerical skills. To structure activities and stimulate group discussion and interaction, test administrators use audio cassettes and photographs, as work samples are compared with real work situations. The Micro-TOWER can be used with adults as well as disabled and disadvantaged adolescents, and can be completed in three to five days.

## Paper-and-Pencil Tests

A primary concern with any method of assessment is whether or not the results are truly accurate for a particular individual. In assessing a person's vocational potential in comparison with existing skills (reading ability, sensory skills, physical attributes), the most accurate method might not be the shortest or least expensive method (Botterbusch, 1978). Selection of an assessment technique should be based on whether or not the results will be worthwhile, applicable, and accurate in providing a true "vocational" picture of the individual being tested.

Because pencil-and-paper tests are furthest removed from real-life situations, they are least likely to reflect an individual's true ability, need for training, and vocational potential. However, they can provide valuable information. Compared with other procedures, the "psychometric" approach to vocational evaluation frequently evokes criticism and is less representative of a person's vocational ability than any other type of testing (Kulman et al., 1975). However, certain characteristics of these instruments, specifically their low cost and speed of administration, enable them to play an important, yet guarded, role when people are being prepared for meaningful career opportunities.

Several problems must be considered before paper-and-pencil assessments are used. Inherent in the characteristic of administrative ease is the problem of indiscriminate use, or the "everyone gets the same test (or battery)" syndrome. Indiscriminate usage of test instruments can provide results as uninformative as those produced by test overuse or poor test selection. Psychometric tests tend to be abstract, to rely on brief samples of behavior that are often removed from real work and training situations, and to employ methods applied to ensure optimum levels of motivation and concentration (Bervin, 1980).

However, the information derived from these devices can prove valuable if it is gathered with caution and from rational and realistic implementation of the tests. Sitlington and Wimmer (1978) list several safeguards to be considered when psychometric instruments are used. First, will the content and format of the results provide useful information? If information on vocational interest is sought, do the occupations selected on the test coincide with the individual's ability? Also, as must be asked of all standardized tests, is the test reliable and valid, and does the norming population represent the person(s) of concern? Finally, can the individual understand the questions, whether read or read to, and do his or her answers reflect true knowledge or feelings? The reading level for most paper-and-pencil tests approaches the sixth grade, and many special-needs individuals simply can not perform at this level. Also, physically challenged and sensory impaired students are limited in responding, so the examiner should not rely too strongly on the results of these tests.

## VOCATIONAL INTEREST INVENTORIES

The mental-abilities testing approach to vocational assessment focuses on functional academic skills revealed by achievement batteries and reading tests, character and personality assessment, measures of intellectual capacity, aptitude batteries, and vocational interest scales. The following section is limited to vocational-interest inventories, personality inventories, and scales of general vocational aptitudes. Inventories are an invaluable resource that provides the examiner with an understanding of a person's orientation towards work and level of vocational maturity. In addition, these instruments not only determine persons' attitudes and knowledge toward the career-choice process, but also toward themselves; their attitudes toward themselves might have been significantly affected by their particular disability (Harmon, Sharma, & Trotter, 1976).

### AAMD-BECKER READING FREE VOCATIONAL INTEREST INVENTORY

(Becker, R. L., 1981, Elbern Publications)

This test was designed as a systematic, non-reading, vocational preference test for use with mentally retarded males and females; it is particularly useful for high-school, educable, mentally retarded students. Information pertaining to occupational interest at the unskilled and semi-skilled levels is provided separately for males and females. The male scoring form provides interest scores in the areas of automotive services, building trades, clerical services, animal care, food service, patient care, horticulture, janitorial services, personal service, laundry service, and materials handling. Areas for females include laundry service, light industrial, clerical, personal service, food service, patient care, horticulture, and housekeeping.

Each interest area is portrayed by pictures that represent occupations in which mentally retarded individuals have demonstrated productivity. Verbal responses are not required, as subjects are required only to circle the activity they would most like to do. Test-retest reliability coefficients are reasonably high, as reported for six separate groups, and represent both test-retest correlations and internal-consistency coefficients.

### KUDER OCCUPATIONAL INTEREST INVENTORY (FORM DD)

(Kuder, F., 1970, Scientific Research Associates)

This test is designed to assist individuals in making vocational selections, identifying occupational fields of interest, and narrowing the field of exploration. It can be group administered in approximately 30 to 40 minutes and requires at least a sixth-grade reading ability. The survey contains 114 occupational scales, of which 37 were developed with female groups and 77 with male groups. Triads of occupations are presented, and the respondent selects the most preferred and least preferred activity. Included is a verification scale to assess carelessness and insincerity. Test-retest reliability coefficients computed over a two-week period are high, but there is no evidence that verifies the test's ability to predict future job success based on interest. The visually impaired may be given this test orally.

### MINNESOTA IMPORTANCE QUESTIONNAIRE (MIQ)

(Weiss, D. J., Davis, R. V., England, G. W., & Lofquist, L. H., 1964, Vocational Psychology Research)

The questionnaire consists of 210 items and measures twenty vocational needs; it is intended to identify job satisfaction. The first 190 items are paired statements, but the last 20 items are independent statements. The individual assigns degrees of importance to paired statements in the need dimensions of (1) ability utilization, (2) achievement, (3) activity, (4) advancement, (5) authority, (6) company policies, (7) compensation, (8) co-workers, (9) creativity, (10) independence, (11) moral values, (12) recognition, (13) responsibility, (14) security, (15) social services, (16) social status, (17) supervision/human relations, (18) supervision/technical, (19) variety, and (20) working conditions.

The MIQ is a self-administered group test and may be completed in less than 40 minutes. Oral administration can be used when respondents have less than the suggested fifth-grade reading ability. The test is normed on over 5000 individuals. Computer scoring is recommended. Test-retest reliability coefficients are high when the interval between tests is very short, but reliability diminishes significantly over a six-month interval. Detailed validity data provide reasonably good support for content, group differences, and concurrent validation.

### STRONG-CAMPBELL INTEREST INVENTORY (SCII)

(Strong, E. K., Hanson, J., & Campbell, D., 1974, Consulting Psychologist Press)

This inventory is intended to guide persons in making decisions about their life plans and in identifying occupations of greatest satisfaction. A long developmental history makes this instrument particularly attractive for the assessment of interest in professional, semi-professional, and managerial positions. Previously separate forms for men and women are combined in the 1974 revised edition. Most of the 325-item inventory is presented in a "Like-Indifferent-Dislike" format; the inventory is arranged in seven sections: (1) occupations, (2) school subjects, (3) activities, (4) amusements, (5) types of people, (6) preference between two people, and (7) personal characteristics.

Responses yield three types of scores: 6 general occupational themes (realistic, enterprising, social), 23 basic interest scales (nature, social service, sales), and 124 occupational scales. Final scores are tabulated and reported as percentages of agreement between subject responses and the particular scale composed of the norm groups. The SCII may be either individually or group administered, requires a sixth-grade reading ability, and takes approximately 30 minutes to complete. Only machine scoring is available. Most beneficial to persons over eighteen years of age, the SCII is useful in identifying goals that require post-secondary education.

### OHIO VOCATIONAL INTEREST SURVEY (OVIS)

(D'Costa, A., Winefordner, D., Odgers, J., & Koons, P., 1981, Psychological Corporation)

To assist students in grades eight through twelve in making vocational decisions, this survey utilizes a questionnaire. Results of the survey are most often applied to the world of business. Based on the "Date-People-Things" model in the *Dictionary of Occupational Titles*, twenty-four interest scales were developed: manual

work, machine work, personal services, caring for people and animals, clerical work, inspecting and testing, crafts and precise operations, customer services, nursing, skilled personal services, training, literary, numerical, appraisal, agriculture, applied technology, promotion and communication, management and supervision, artistic, sales representative, music, entertainment and performing arts, teaching, counseling, social work, and medical.

Because it is based on the *Dictionary of Occupational Titles*, the OVIS provides an extremely wide exposure to vocations and provides interest analysis for persons with a wide range of abilities and interests. Each item requires a response on a five-point scale ("likes very much" to "dislikes very much") and the test can be administered to those with limited reading ability. Because scoring is complex, it requires a machine. The OVIS II (2nd edition) can be used with individuals in grade seven through adult, can be either hand- or machine-scored, and is available in a microcomputer version.

### GIEST PICTURE INTEREST INVENTORY, REVISED

(Giest, H., Western Psychological Services)

This is a self-administered, pictorial inventory that is particularly useful for use with persons who have limited verbal skills or who are either culturally or educationally deprived. Instructions may be orally presented for persons with limited reading abilities, and they are required only to mark their responses on the answer booklet. Picture triads assessing eleven male and twelve female areas of general interest require only "most-liked" and "least-liked" responses. Test and re-test reliability coefficients are reasonably high and reflect individuals in remedial reading groups, trade schools, high schools, and Puerto Rican and Hawaiian high schools and colleges.

### CAREER AWARENESS INVENTORY (CAI)

(Fadale, L., Scholastic Testing Service)

A self-administered, untimed test, the inventory emphasizes career knowledge, social attitudes, and personal experiences. The target population is children in grades four through eight. The multiple-choice items can be read aloud by the examiner if reading ability is a concern. The instrument is categorized into nine parts: careers, workers, job occupations, awareness of educational requirements, personal acquaintance with workers, familiarity with occupations that produce products, high-prestige jobs, common clustering jobs, and job requirements.

### CAREER MATURITY INVENTORY (CMI)
(Crites, J. O., 1978, CTB/McGraw-Hill)

This inventory is designed to measure career-choice attitudes and competencies. The CMI is composed of an Attitude Scale and a Competence Test. The Attitude Scale surveys a person's response to involvement in the career-choice process, orientation toward work, independence in decision-making, preference for career-choice factors, and concepts of the career-choice process. These measures would indicate a level of vocational maturity. When used for screening, one form (A-2) yields the overall measure, while a counseling form (B-1) provides indicators of decisiveness, involvement, independence, orientation, and compromise. The Competence Test, which need not be given at the same time as the Attitude Scale, consists of five parts measuring other factors related to job selection: self-appraisal, occupational information, goal selection, planning, and problem solving. Whether the tests are administered to a group or an individual, the time needed to complete the Attitude Scale is 30 minutes and each part of the Competency Test takes 20 minutes. Oral directions may be given to subjects who have less than a sixth-grade reading level. Machine scoring is available.

### CAREER ASSESSMENT INVENTORY (CAI)
(Johansson, C. B., National Computer Systems)

The *Dictionary of Occupational Titles* was used in the development of most of the items for this inventory. In many ways other inventories that measure interest in nonprofessional occupations provide similar results. Scale I indicates an orientation towards six work themes, Scale II discloses academic strength and weakness, and Scale III draws a comparison between the person being assessed and workers currently on the job. Stable test-retest reliabilities are reported. When the test was developed, a concerted effort was made to present sexually unbiased occupations.

### SUPER'S WORK VALUES INVENTORY (WVI)
(Super, D. E., 1970, Riverside Publishing)

This test was developed to assess the intrinsic and extrinsic work values of adolescent and adult males and females. Subjects respond to forty-five value statements on a five-point scale ranging from "very important" to "unimportant." Measures of occupational choice and job satisfaction are obtained. The test consists of fifteen value scales: altruism, aesthetic, creativity, intellectual stimulation, achievement, independence, prestige, management, economic returns, security, surroundings, supervisory relations, associates, way of life, and variety. Extensive norms for grades seven through twelve are reported as percentiles for each scale. Comprehensive construct, content, and concurrent validity data are available as well as reputable test-retest reliability coefficients. The information obtained from this inventory is of invaluable assistance in the creation of career development curricula.

## PERSONALITY ASSESSMENT

Vocational interests are closely related to one's personality. Instruments that reveal information about a person's innate characteristics can be invaluable in assessments of job potential and success.

### THE VOCATIONAL PREFERENCE INVENTORY (VPI)
(Holland, J. L., 1985, Psychological Assessment Inventories)

This test is designed to gain information about a person's interpersonal relations, interests, values, self-concepts, and coping behavior. The inventory is composed of eleven scales, representing 160 occupational titles. The respondent indicates whether titles are liked or disliked. The eleven scales consist of these tendencies: realistic, intellectual, social, conventional, enterprising, artistic (oriented toward vocational interest), self-control, masculinity, status, infrequency, and acquiescence (personality-oriented). The VPI scale is self-administered, and subjects should be at least fourteen years of age, of average intelligence, and free of brain damage. High test-retest reliability values are reported.

### EDWARDS PERSONAL PREFERENCE SCHEDULE (EPPS)
(Edwards, A. L., 1959, Psychological Corporation)

This test is designed to provide quick and convenient percentile measures of the following personality variables: achievement, deference, order, exhibition, autonomy, affiliation, intraception, succorance, dominance, abasement, nurturance, change, endurance, heterosexuality, and aggression. The test is composed of 225 forced choice items beginning with "I". Most items use the verb "like" to present social situations. It is recommended that the test not be used with severely disturbed individuals or persons who have reading difficulties, because the reading level is fairly high. Male and female college students and adults were used when the test was designed. No norms are used, because the test-taker's characteristics are measured in terms of the influence of one need on another. Reported split-half and test-retest reliabilities for each scale are quite acceptable. Minimal validity study data with other personality tests are provided.

### MINNESOTA MULTIPHASIC PERSONALITY INVENTORY (MMPI) (GROUP FORM R)
(Hathaway, S. R., & McKinley, C., 1984, University of Minnesota Press)

The MMPI is designed to provide an objective assessment of some major personality traits that affect personal and social adjustment. Such traits are characteristic of a disabling psychological abnormality. The inventory consists of ten clinical scales: hypochondriasis, depression,

hysteria, psychopathic deviate, masculinity-femininity, paranoia, psychasthenia, schizophrenia, hypomania, and social. There are also three validation scales. Three test formats are available; all utilize a true-false response to statements about a personal characteristic, personality trait, feeling, or habit. The test requires at least a sixth-grade reading ability. Individuals sixteen years of age and older can complete the inventory in approximately 45 to 90 minutes.

Normative data were developed from comparison studies of "normal" adults and clinical cases. Three test-retest reliability studies provide coefficients that average in the middle .70s. Original predictive validity comparisons with clinical diagnosis reported 60% successful predictions. A substantial amount of research data on the MMPI provides additional support.

### SIXTEEN PERSONALITY FACTOR QUESTIONNAIRE (16PF) (FORM E)
(Cattell, R., 1980, Institute for Personality and Ability Testing)

This recent form of this questionnaire is composed of 128 forced-choice statements ("I like to watch team games" or "In a group task I would rather") and provides a quick battery for a person with limited educational and cultural experiences. Bipolar, primary personality factors include (1) reserved/outgoing, (2) less/more intelligent, (3) affected by feelings/emotionally stable, (4) humble/assertive, (5) sober/happy-go-lucky, (6) expedient/conscientious, (7) shy/adventuresome, (8) tough/tender-minded, (9) trusting/suspicious, (10) practical/imaginative, (11) forthright/shrewd, (12) self-assured/ apprehensive, (13) conservative/experimental, (14) group-dependent/self-sufficient, (15) undisciplined self/conflict-controlled, and (16) relaxed/tense.

The test can be administered to either groups or individuals and requires between a third- and sixth-grade reading ability. Earlier forms of this test are appropriate for use with the visually and hearing impaired, whereas this form is not. A lower reading level is Form E's main advantage.

# APTITUDE ASSESSMENT

Aptitude assessment is considered comparable to achievement assessment. Although they are quite similar, achievement tests typically measure ability to perform previously learned tasks and test items reflect a person's recall ability, whereas aptitude instruments assess a person's innate capacity to learn, ability to solve problems, and potential for skill and knowledge proficiency when training procedures are implemented (Parker & Hansen, 1976). Aptitude tests are helpful in the selection of those individuals with the potential for specific occupations and in the outlining of vocational plans for training.

### GENERAL APTITUDE TEST BATTERY (GATB)
(United States Employment Service, 1983, U.S. Department of Labor)

This test is a valuable assessment instrument for use in training and job selection as well as job placement, primarily because of its relevancy to actual work and training. The GATB is one of several assessment instruments provided by the office of the United States Employment Service of the Department of Labor. The test consists of twelve subtests made up of 284 multiple choice items, 150 same-difference items, and two dexterity form boards. It measures nine aptitudes:

1. *General learning ability*: ability to "catch on" or understand instructions and underlying principles, and ability to reason and make judgments
2. *Verbal aptitude*: ability to understand meaning of the words and ideas associated with them and to use them effectively, to comprehend language, to understand relationships between words, and to understand meanings of whole sentences and paragraphs
3. *Numerical aptitude*: ability to perform arithmetic operations
4. *Spatial aptitude*: ability to think visually of geometric forms, to comprehend two-dimensional representations of three-dimensional objects, to recognize relationships resulting from movements of objects in space
5. *Form perception*: ability to perceive pertinent detail in objects or in pictorial or graphic material, and to make visual comparisons and discriminations
6. *Clerical perception*: ability to perceive pertinent detail in verbal or tabular material, to observe differences in copy, to proofread words and numbers, and to avoid perceptual errors in arithmetic computation
7. *Motor coordination*: ability to coordinate eyes and hands or fingers rapidly and accurately, in making precise movements with speed
8. *Finger dexterity*: ability to move the fingers and to manipulate small objects rapidly with the fingers
9. *Manual dexterity*: ability to move the hands easily and skillfully, and to work with the hands in placing and turning motions

The GATB is group administered, timed, and takes approximately 2 1/4 hours to complete. It has proved successful with several special-needs groups, such as mentally retarded, deaf, and emotionally disturbed, as well as English-speaking minorities (Spanish and French versions are available). The norming sample consisted of 400 general working people, and additional data have been developed for students in grades nine and ten. Extensive and high reliability coefficients are provided, along with strong validity studies that were developed on over 600 occupations. Computer software is available to assist with scoring.

### NON-READING APTITUDE TEST BATTERY (NATB)
(United States Employment Service, 1982, U.S. Department of Labor)

Also developed by the United States Employment Service of the Department of Labor, the NATB is intended for illiterate and disadvantaged individuals. It measures the same nine aptitudes as the GATB. Many of the tests are similar or identical to the GATB but do not require the ability to read; this test instead uses (1) picture and word matching, (2) oral vocabulary, (3) coin matching, (4) design completion, (5) tool matching, (6) three-dimensional space, (7) form matching, (8) coin series, (9) name comparison, (10) mark making, place, turn, assemble, and disassemble. The NATB was standardized on over 800 high school students and is useful for studies of mentally retarded subjects. Recent research has proved disappointing, in that low correlations with the GATB inhibit equivalent-score interpretations.

### DIFFERENTIAL APTITUDE TEST (FORMS V AND W)

(Bennett, G. K., Seashore, H. G., & Wesman, A. G., 1982, Psychological Corporation)

This test provides information about a person's school and work abilities. It does not assess particular school subjects. The following areas are assessed:

1. *Verbal reasoning*: concept-formation items use thinking skills related to verbal association but do not rely on vocabulary recognition.
2. *Numerical ability*: numerical concepts, relationships, and computations determine a person's ability to manipulate quantitative material. A measure of general learning ability is determined when numerical ability scores are added to verbal reasoning scores.
3. *Abstract reasoning*: a series of diagrams, in which a principle determines sequential changes, is presented. The figure that would logically follow in the sequence, is selected by the subject. The response is nonverbal.
4. *Clerical speed and accuracy*: speed of response is measured, as individuals select similar combinations that are displayed in groups.
5. *Mechanical reasoning*: items consist of mechanical situations and simple questions.
6. *Space relations*: to construct an object from a picture, the subject must use visualization.
7. *Spelling*.
8. *Language usage*: language skills are assessed through punctuation, grammar, and capitalization error recognition.

An additional score may be obtained by a combination of the Verbal Reasoning and Numerical Ability scores. The test may be administered in two, four, or six sessions, and the entire battery will take slightly over 3 hours to complete. It may be used with students in grades eight through twelve. An optional Career Planning Questionnaire and alternate forms are available. The manual contains no information of its use with special-needs population but the DAT is clearly not appropriate for the visually impaired.

## VOCATIONAL MEASUREMENT OF MANUAL ABILITIES

### PURDUE PEGBOARD

(Tiffen, J., 1948, Science Research Associates)

This test measures gross motor activities usually associated with industrial occupations that require manual dexterity. Gross motor movements of hands, arms, and fingers, and specific finger manipulations are assessed. Four subtests are given independently. In taking the first three subtests, individuals must use the right hand only to place twenty-five pins into pegholes within thirty seconds; then only the left hand is used; and then both hands simultaneously. On the fourth subtest, the subject must assemble pins, washers, and collars within 1 minute. No reading is necessary. Obvious physical limitations of the upper body should be taken into consideration before test administration.

### BENNETT HAND-TOOL DEXTERITY TEST

(Bennett, G. K., 1910, Psychological Corporation)

This test measures functional proficiency in the use of standard mechanic's tools. Three wrenches and one screwdriver are used to remove nuts, bolts, and washers of three different sizes from a board. The process is then reversed, with the nuts and bolts refastened to the opposite side of the board. The time needed to complete the task is then compared with norm tables standardized on such groups as airline engine mechanics, apprentice welders, vocational high-school boys, and adult males at a vocational guidance center.

### CRAWFORD SMALL PARTS DEXTERITY TEST
(Crawford, J., 1956, Psychological Corporation)

The Crawford test places primary emphasis on fine eye-hand coordination. Part I of the test requires a person to use tweezers to place a pin in one of forty-two holes in a board, and then to use tweezers to place a collar over the pin. Part II requires the client to use a small screwdriver to place thirty screws into a plate. No reading is required, and the test can be completed in 15 minutes. Adaptations can make this test useful with the visually and auditorally impaired. Scores may be derived either from the total time needed to complete the task or from the amount of work completed within a specified time period. The time that male respondents need to complete Parts I and II is compared with norms established on factory workers, veterans, and high-school students. The time needed by females is compared with standardized values on assembly-job applicants, factory applicants, hourly employees, and employed assemblers. Split-half reliability coefficients between Parts I and II range between .80 and .95.

### STROMBERG DEXTERITY TEST (SDT)
(Stromberg, E. L., 1949, Psychological Corporation)

Various industrial occupations require specific prerequisite skills such as speed and accuracy of arm and hand movements. The SDT is designed to discern individuals with those abilities. The testing device consists of a collapsible board with fifty-four disks on one side. Using only one hand, the subject must transfer set patterns of colored discs from the form board to the open board. A subsequent trial requires moving the disks back to the form board. The first two trials are for practice, and the next two are timed. Norms were standardized on groups of trade-school students as well as male and female workers. Caution must be used with this test because its reliability and validity data are

questionable. The SDT should not be used as a single measure of manual skill.

## VOCATIONAL MEASUREMENT OF MECHANICAL ABILITIES

### BENNETT MECHANICAL COMPREHENSION TEST (BMCT)
(Bennett, G. K., et al., 1970, Psychological Corporation)

The BMCT is a group-administered test that assesses the subject's perception and understanding of mechanical principles. Each of the sixty-eight items contains questions, pertaining to two illustrations about the mechanical nature of such things as pulleys, gears, and levers. Norms were derived from groups of males who were industrial applicants, industrial employees, and students. Reported reliability coefficients are considered statistical overestimates, but a high face validity has made the BMCT a long-standing device for measuring mechanical comprehension. Oral and tape-recorded instructions are available in both English and Spanish.

### REVISED MINNESOTA PAPER BOARD TEST
(Likert, R., & Quasha, W. H., 1970, Psychological Corporation)

This test is designed to assist in the selection and placement of individuals in occupations requiring mechanical skills. A nonverbal measure of intellectual performance, the test assesses "spatial imagery" abilities. Each of the sixty-four items consists of two-dimensional diagrams separated into parts. For each diagram, there are five line figures "indicating the different shapes out of which [the diagram is] made." The respondent selects one figure constructed of the exact parts depicted in the original diagram. No reading is required. Both educational (grades ten through twelve) and industrial norms are provided. Considerably high test-retest and alternate-forms reliability correlations are reported.

### SRA MECHANICAL APTITUDES
(1950, Science Research)

Developed by Science Research Associates, this test measures mechanical aptitude. The mechanical-knowledge section requires the identification and use of forty-five common tools and implements. The space-relations test requires the mental construction of forty figures cut into two or three separate pieces. In the shop-arithmetic section are drawings pertaining to 124 problems. Reading level is estimated at grade five, and adequate visual skills are necessary. Norms are given for males and females in grades nine through twelve. Internal reliability ratings appear adequate, but no validity data are available.

## VOCATIONAL MEASUREMENT OF CLERICAL ABILITIES

### MINNESOTA CLERICAL TEST (MCT)

(Andrew, D. M., Paterson, D. G., & Longstaff, H. P., 1979, Psychological Corporation)

This test measures speed and accuracy in the performance of tasks associated with clerical work, and reveals characteristics useful to both employee selection and the identification of the individual's interest. Test items include letter, number, and symbol differentiation. Subjects compare names or symbols for identical features under timed conditions. The Number Checking and Name Scoring Section contains 100 identical and 100 dissimilar items. Reading level is not considered important because letter perception rather than word comprehension is the variable measured. Norms are available for males and females for grades eight through twelve, and for male and female employed clerical workers. Office supervisory ratings and test-score correlations are respectable.

### SRA TYPING SKILLS TEST

(Richardson, M. W., & Pedersen, R. A., 1975, Scientific Research Associates)

This test measures the subject's ability to use either mechanical or electrical typewriters. To obtain speed and accuracy scores, the subject types a 225-word, four-paragraph business letter from a clearly printed copy. Both experienced and inexperienced office workers were used to develop norms for manual and electrical typewriters. No reliability or validity data are available.

## OTHER INSTRUMENTS FOR VOCATIONAL EVALUATION

The McCarron-Dial Systems have developed the *Street Survival Skills Questionnaire* (SSSQ) (McCarron, L. T., & Dial, J. G., 1980, McCarron Dial Systems), which assesses adaptive-behavior levels. The questionnaire assesses the following areas: (1) basic concepts, (2) functional signs (ability to recognize basic signs and symbols), (3) use of tools, (4) domestic management, (5) health, first aid, and safety, (6) need for public services, (7) use of time, (8) responsibility with money, and (9) use of measurements. Nonverbal responses make the test applicable to the more disabled persons. Measures are recorded on a master planning chart designed to facilitate individual planning.

The *Social and Prevocational Information Battery* is designed primarily to predict the community preparation of educable, mentally retarded adolescents. True-false items are administered orally to ascertain the degree of employability, economic self-sufficiency, family living, personal hygiene and grooming skills, and communication. The results from this test appear to be realistic, because they are directly associated with community and school-based work-experience programs.

The American Association of Mental Deficiency intends that its *Adaptive Behavior Scale* (ABS) (Nihira, K., Foster, R., Shellhaas, M., & Leland, H., 1981, Publishers Test Service) be used to determine the personal independence of developmentally disabled, retarded, and emotionally maladjusted individuals (see Chapter 8). Divided into two parts, the test assesses general skills necessary for independent functioning; characteristics indicating maladaptive social or personal traits are evaluated. Evaluators may collect data from direct observations, interview those considered to be familiar with the person being assessed, or have those with considerable knowledge about the person fill out an ABS form. Part I reliabilities are relatively stable (.71–.93), while Part II coefficients are generally unacceptable. Evaluators should note that normative data were derived from an institutionalized population in 1968 and have not been revised to include a recent deinstitutionalized sample.

# TECHNOLOGY IN VOCATIONAL ASSESSMENT

The use of computer technology in vocational assessment is a relatively new development that will apparently become more closely infused as the technology itself becomes more sophisticated. The increased use of microcomputers in schools and rehabilitation facilities has necessitated that vocational assessors become "computer literate" and begin using hardware and prepackaged software for developing and managing assessments. For the most part, computers have gained a foothold in relieving the evaluator from repetitive and tiresome tasks and from activities that are prone to be mistakenly done. One convenient application has been computerized systems that match an individual's assessment data with appropriate competitive jobs (see Botterbusch, 1984, for a review of these programs). Computers cannot yet accurately simulate a wide variety of jobs, or interact with an individual so that ongoing analyses can be instantly calculated and profiled. Expert systems, that is, computer programs written to match the ability level of a human expert performing a job, have yet to emerge. For these reasons computers are more often used with paper-and-pencil tests than with work samples. The major advantage of computers in vocational assessment is that they provide immediate feedback to the assessor and to the individual taking the test.

Microcomputer software versions of paper-and-pencil tests, such as interest or aptitude surveys, can aid in administering and scoring the test, as well as with developing interpretive profiles from the results, and with report writing.

Microcomputers are also useful in training evaluators. One drawback, however, is that normative data for many instruments are based on the paper-and-pencil versions and not the computerized format. The use of computers to administer tests requires that an individual use a keyboard or, if that is not possible, an adaptive interactive device. Joy-sticks, voice-activated devices, and manual-switching devices are examples of keyboard interfaces designed by the test-giver and adapted to the test-taker.

## Computerized Vocational Assessment

Vocational assessors have taken the opportunity to adapt assessment techniques for computerized applications. Technology has created a potential that promises to enhance the accuracy with which special-needs persons are matched to occupations in which they are likely to succeed. Following are descriptions of two systems that represent, in structure and use, most of what is available.

The *Microcomputer Evaluation and Screening Instrument* (MESA) may be group or individually administered; group administration requires one terminal per person. This system, available in either Apple (64K) or IBM-PC (128K) environments, is said to be both criterion- and norm-referenced. Academic subtest scores are based on current criteria from national competency research, and the work-samples scores are compared to time-performance norms. The MESA consists of sections that 1) measure physical capacities and mobility, 2) make hands-on assessment of short-duration work samples, 3) individualized assessment, 4) provide independent perceptual screening, 5) survey vocational interests and vocational awareness (with slide/tape presentations of occupations), 6) assess tolerance for working conditions and specific vocational preparation, 7) determine talking/persuasive skills, and 8) measure skills in computer-assisted report-writing (with raw score conversions and profiles). Some subtests are listed as optional; the MESA may take anywhere from 1 1/2 to 4 hours to complete. Some subtests require using the computer (there are paper and pencil responses, and manual tasks, also) but typing skills are not necessary. Recent updates have added practice sessions, made academic testing optional, and provided limited tests of word-processing capabilities related to report-writing.

The *Computerized Career Assessment and Planning Program* (CCAPP) was designed to help high-school students define and select career occupations, and to aid them in developing plans for achieving their career goals. The *Dictionary of Occupational Titles* is used as the data base for 1200 specific occupations. The CCAPP is written for the Apple II (48K) operating system. Recorded on disks, all program information is divided into sections: an introduction, definition of CCAPP, description of how CCAPP works, counseling strategies for Module I—career assessment, counseling strategy for Module II—selecting strategies, counseling strategies for Module III—career planning, and career exploration. Modules I and II require students to rate their interests and abilities in school subjects and in job-related demands, such as dealing with others. Module III is unique in that it assists students in selecting the means by which they will reach their specified occupation, such as post secondary education, vocational training, or job hunting. Occupations are arranged into sixty-six clusters that assist in career planning, but several occupations indicate avenues of training that are not realistic for the particular job.

Deciding to purchase a computerized assessment system requires considering first if those assessed will benefit in ways unattainable with more traditional tests. The user must view the system not in isolation but in terms of the entire assessment process. Assessors must decide where the system will be used, how compatible the results will be with other data collected, to what extent the results will facilitate employment, and to what degree the improvement to the assessment process will justify the cost. As more tests are converted to software for com-

puter application, data base resources and bulletin boards are useful and provide assistance in test selection. COMPSYCH (Anderson & Hornsby, 1988) is a system of software reviews organized into assessment categories, levels of expertise, and equipment needed. Test reviews and publishers' addresses are accessible via modem.

### The Future of Technology and Vocational Assessment

Rapidly changing technological advances place an additional burden on the vocational assessor. Future employment trends are more difficult to predict as the society shifts from a manufacturing to an information and service marketplace. It's been suggested that this change may significantly alter over 45% of the existing jobs within the next two decades (Best, 1984). Some predict that by the year 2000, over 80% of the work force will be involved with information and services, and that manufacturing will require only 3% of the available work force (Feingold, 1984). Robotics, computer-assisted design and manufacturing, and non-domestic competition will eliminate many jobs once available to special populations. Special-needs individuals with limited or nonexistent skills will face additional barriers when trying to access the job market.

A major portion of current, commercial assessment instruments remains focused on manufacturing or manufacturing-related skills. These instruments require individuals to use a variety of tools, sequence events on a production line, or participate in actual production work. Assessment of work adjustment skills are also related to manufacturing and industrial job sites and their requirements. There is an emerging recognition that these tests, at least in their present forms, may very well be no longer applicable (e.g., Botterbusch, 1983).

However, there is clear evidence that people with special needs are finding gainful employment in service industries that appear to be not significantly affected by automation (e.g., Hasazi, Gordon, & Roe, 1985; Plue, 1984). Food service leads all others (i.e., construction, maintenance, recreation) yet few assessment devices and techniques have been developed with these areas in mind. Academic as well as performance standards for these jobs are needed, before assessments can properly predict how well the students will function. Although it is clear that most jobs will be entry level (Rumberger, 1984), they will also demand a high level of education and sophisticated skills (Honig, 1985), such as problem solving, communication, math and spelling. Vocational assessment must meet head-on the changing employment demands, with meaningful and thorough job analyses. Technology will hold more promise when evaluators use authoring programs with interactive video to realistically represent jobs. Regardless of how advanced the assessment "tools" become, however, the responsibility for accurate and dependable vocational assessment and employment planning will remain with those implementing the assessment process.

## STRATEGIES FOR EFFECTIVE EVALUATION: SUMMARY

Effective use of evaluation instruments does not always follow a logical pattern because assessment often proceeds in a haphazard manner. Although the examiner realizes that several pieces of information pertaining to someone's abilities or potential are needed, the examiner might not know how that information is to be determined and how separate pieces fit into the complete picture. The wide variety of available instruments, each with varying degrees of application to special-needs persons, will add to the confusion. The unique nature of the subject, whose interests and motivational and attitudinal levels might not inherently coincide with achievement or aptitude levels, could quite possibly make the evaluation process a futile experience.

A worthwhile and versatile vocational evaluation relies on one's knowledge of psychometric instruments (functional, statistical, technologi-

cal); ability to formulate hypotheses concerning the subject's skills, needs, and desires; and an understanding of occupational opportunities available in the community. Taken as a group, these three functions will answer the question of whether or not testing will provide the information that is needed. Ideally, the end result is a viable, comprehensive plan written with specific outcomes and plans for direct job entry or vocational training, or retraining. To allow for modifications and change, any strategic assessment plan should be dynamic in structure.

### Assessment Plan

Figure 10-2 depicts an evaluation plan that contains procedures and questions concerning the subject, the tests, and the available job market as identified before test administration. This figure summarizes the main topics of this chapter.

During Level A the evaluation process is concerned with determining whether formal assessment is a realistic procedure for the person of concern. Step 1 determines why the person has been referred for assessment. It asks the basic questions, Is this an initial evaluation for someone who has never entered the work world, Is it a re-evaluation of a special-needs person who is unable to maintain active employment for unknown reasons, or Has the individual recently become disabled as a result of trauma or disease? Hypotheses or questions concerning the subject's potentials, existing skills, or possible causes for lack of employment should be determined (Step 2). For example, an individual is unable to keep employment, yet observations and work samples reveal no definite lack of skills. Considerations could focus on the possibility of psychiatric or personality deficiencies, lack of motivation or interest, or intellectual deficits.

A beneficial approach is to sort behaviors into components that direct the assessment questions and assist in the predicting of work potentials. Bolton (1982) structures employability according to 1) prevocational skills—an individual's

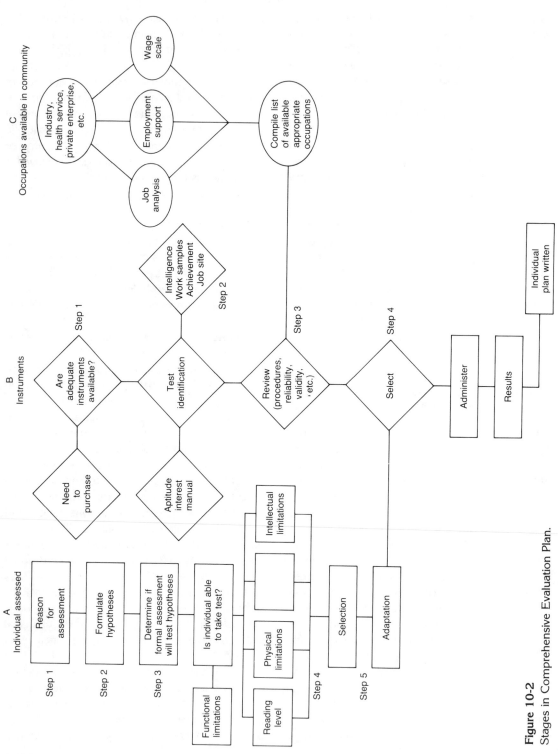

**Figure 10-2**

Stages in Comprehensive Evaluation Plan.

interests and knowledge about the need to work and what a job is, 2) job-seeking skills—what is needed to locate and apply for employment, 3) interview skills—understanding and responding to the job interview process, 4) job-related skills—behaviors associated with adjusting to a job, such as following rules, 5) work-performance skills—ability to arrive at work on time, use tools, avoid hazards, etc., and 6) on-the-job skills—sociability with co-workers, taking criticism. This analysis will partition the assessment process into measures that indicate whether someone is primarily ready for employment or ready for a particular job. Once these questions have been answered, a decision must be made whether or not formal assessment techniques are necessary (Step 3).

Step 4 requires identification of prevailing individual strengths and weaknesses. For instance, will sensory limitations, such as visual or auditory impairments, or certain physical or motoric problems, such as ambulation or speech deficiencies, affect the evaluation results? Also, the examiner must consider reading level, intellect, cognitive skills, and environmental limitations. Once these factors are determined and compared with the formulated hypotheses, the appropriate tests are selected, and adaptations to either the tests themselves or administrative procedures are made (Step 5).

Level B refers to the instruments themselves. Does the examiner have access to appropriate and current tests, or is purchasing them a feasible alternative (Step 1)? Step 2 allows for the identification of tests to be used, such as aptitude batteries, manual dexterity scales, or achievement tests. The instruments should be reviewed as to their applicability to the evaluation question, procedures (which need to be practiced), and the significance of the statistical data (Step 3). This review results in the selection of the appropriate tests. Considerations of computer hardware and prepackaged software would occur at this time. Although most schools and facilities now have computers, specific assessment programs can require additional hardware components, such as expanded memory, extra disk drives, adaptive devices, etc. not available to the examiner. Selections of software should be based on need, particularly as these products are constantly changing and there are no agreed-upon selection criteria.

Level C requires an active knowledge of the work resources currently available in the community, the personnel to be contacted, and specific occupations that are potential placements. An updated list of vocational alternatives, along with the individual's specific special needs or a combination of special needs, will have a major influence on what tests are selected. For instance, if the community is composed of a few light industrial facilities and many business offices, tests that measure clerical skills may form the body of the evaluation plan.

After assessments are completed, individuals receive recommendations for job training and/or job placement. Individuals may also receive preemployment and work-maturity skills training and, eventually, training in skills associated with specific tasks. To make effective recommendations, the counselor must know about company policies regarding the hiring of special-needs people, and whether tax incentives are available to the employer who hires special-needs people; the counselor should also know about insurance, employee benefits, and unions. Whether the evaluation plan is designed to determine a direct job placement or to identify training or retraining procedures, the final, written plan should specify the activities, objectives, and goals necessary for a special-needs individual to become an active, productive participant in the work world.

# CHAPTER 11

# Neuropsychological Assessment of Exceptional Children

G. REID LYON
JANE M. FLYNN

## OUTLINE

Purposes and measurement properties
Neuropsychological models and assessment batteries
Advances in neurodiagnostic technology and their applications
Summary and conclusions

**C** linical neuropsychology is a field of study that attempts to relate what is known about the functioning of the brain to what is understood about human behavior. More specifically, to define the role of the nervous system in thought and action, neuropsychologists study empirically the behavioral phenomena associated with neural changes induced by injury, disease, or dysfunction (Adams, 1973; Lyon, 1985a).

Within the past decade, clinical neuropsychological studies of children have been increasingly called upon to make relevant and informed contributions to the assessment and treatment of acquired (i.e., cerebral trauma) and putative (i.e., learning disabilities) neurologically based developmental disorders. This increase in the application of neuropsychological principles to the understanding and remediation of developmental disorders can be attributed to several factors. First, advances in the basic neurosciences have provided new technologies for investigating the means by which the brain develops and processes information, and the differences between individuals with respect to information processing.

Second, there has been a marked increase in the survival rates for youngsters who have received traumatic brain injuries. In addition, improvements in neonatal intensive-care practices have decreased the mortality rates of infants who are born with significantly low birth weight (<1500 grams) (Hynd & Obrzut, 1986). However, children recovering from such conditions frequently display persistent learning and behavior difficulties associated with their neurological history. As such, assessment practices that are based upon knowledge of brain development (and maldevelopment) and behavior, are useful for documenting the nature of the disorder, monitoring the recovery and/or development of cognitive, linguistic, perceptual, and motor skills, and delineating treatment options.

Finally, there is a growing awareness that some relatively subtle learning and behavioral difficulties frequently seen in school settings (i.e., dyslexia, attention deficit-hyperactive disorder) are referrable to intrinsic neurological differences in brain structures or functions that are responsible for linguistic processing, alertness, motor activity, and arousal levels (Duane, 1986; Rourke, Fisk, & Strang, 1986). Because a greater number of children are identified each year as manifesting neurodevelopmental learning and behavior disorders, one can expect that the need for specialists with expertise in neuropsychological assessment will also increase in the future.

With this information as background, the primary purpose of this chapter is to acquaint the reader with (1) the major purposes and measurement properties of neuropsychological assessment practices; (2) the different types of neuropsychological models and assessment batteries employed with exceptional children and their usefulness in contributing to remediation programs; and, (3) some recent advances in the application of neurodiagnostic technology to the understanding of developmental disorders.

There is a significant volume and complexity of literature and topics associated with neuropsychological assessment of exceptional children, so our review is necessarily selective rather than exhaustive. Readers are encouraged to peruse recent papers and texts by Boll (1981); Lyon, Moats and Flynn (in press); Obrzut and Hynd (1986); Rourke, Fisk, and Strang (1986); and, Tramontana and Hooper (in press), for comprehensive coverage of the concepts presented.

## PURPOSES AND MEASUREMENT PROPERTIES

One's purpose for conducting neuropsychological assessment obviously influences the means by which brain-behavior relationships are measured and assessment results interpreted. As Boll (1981) has pointed out, the primary initial purpose or goal of neuropsychology is to describe brain-behavior relationships in a reliable and valid manner. Boll also stated that the ultimate, but yet to be realized, purpose is "... the development of remediation and rehabilitation procedures based upon the empirically validated understanding of the behavioral consequences specific to the condition in question in each patient" (p. 582). It is clear, however, that the majority of neuropsychological measures and allied procedures have been designed to infer brain function from behavior rather than to be used in formulating treatment programs. This issue will be addressed throughout the chapter.

In the main, prominent neuropsychological assessment batteries and diagnostic procedures have been developed and refined over the past fifty years to (1) describe the impact of brain damage or dysfunction on a range of human abilities, (2) reliably differentiate individuals who present with brain damage and dysfunction from those who do not, and (3) discern the specific behavioral effects of different types of neuropathology (e.g., tumor vs. stroke vs. head injury) (Lyon, Moats, & Flynn, in press).

It is frequently reported in the neuropsychology literature that these clinical outcomes are realized most effectively when (1) the assessment procedures consist of objective, standardized, and quantitative measures of an individual's structure of neuropsychological ability (Alfano & Finlayson, 1987; Reitan, 1966; Reitan & Wolfson, 1985; Rourke, 1981; Rourke, Fisk, & Strang, 1986); (2) the assessment procedures include measures that are psychometrically scaled to measure abilities on a continuous scale rather than an interval scale (Golden, Hammeke, & Purische, 1978); (3) the assessment tasks and measures are valid and reliable reflections of cerebral dysfunction, and are not confounded by the effects of age and education (Finlayson, Johnson, & Reitan, 1977); and (4) the assessment tasks sample a broad range of abilities to include measures of general intellectual ability, the ability to retain verbal and nonverbal information, motor and psychomotor abilities, sensory-perceptual functions, receptive and expressive language skills, attentional skills,

analytical reasoning and concept-formation, and personality, behavioral, and emotional status (Alfano & Finlayson, 1986; Reitan & Wolfson, 1985).

A number of studies have shown that neuropsychological assessment batteries and allied procedures that have been developed according to these principles are valid for the purpose of identifying the presence of brain damage or dysfunction in both adults (Boll, 1981; Golden, Hammeke, and Purische, 1978; Reitan & Davison, 1974) and children (Hynd & Obrzut, 1986; Rourke, 1981; Rourke, Fisk, & Strang, 1986; Teeter, 1986). Further, there are data that indicate that widely used neuropsychological batteries (e.g., Halstead-Reitan, Luria-Nebraska) are capable of describing the nature of the neural insult (e.g., type of lesion, site of lesion, etc.), particularly when those batteries are applied to adult clinical populations and interpreted by skilled clinicians. There is also some evidence, albeit limited in scope, that the information derived from adult neuropsychological assessment batteries can be useful in constructing some remediation and rehabilitation programs, (Diller & Gordon, 1981a, 1981b; Diller & Weinberg, 1977; Finlayson, Gowland, & Basmajian, 1986; Luria, 1966b; Luria & Tzetkova, 1968; Rao & Bieliauskas, 1983).

## NEUROPSYCHOLOGICAL MODELS AND ASSESSMENT BATTERIES

In general, neuropsychological models of developmental disorders conceptualize a child's learning strengths and weaknesses as manifestations of efficient or inefficient brain regions and/or systems (Gaddes, 1980; Hartlage & Telzrow, 1983; Obrzut & Hynd, 1986; Rourke, Bakker, Fisk, & Strang, 1983). A variety of standard neuropsychological batteries as well as selected neuropsychological assessment procedures have been employed to elucidate such patterns of strengths and weaknesses. Selected batteries will be discussed in the following section. Emphasis is placed on elucidating the general properties and clinical contributions made by each battery, with respect to their diagnostic validity and ability to forge linkages to treatment. Space limitations preclude comprehensive descriptions of the tasks and tests employed in the batteries. For such details, readers are referred to Boll (1981); Golden, Hammeke, and Purische (1978); Reitan and Davison (1974); Rourke (1981); and Teeter (1986).

### THE HALSTEAD-REITAN NEUROPSYCHOLOGICAL TEST BATTERIES
(Reitan, R. M., 1979, Reitan Neuropsychology Laboratory)

The Halstead-Reitan assessment procedures (Boll, 1981; Hartlage & Tarnopol, 1977; Teeter, 1986) are a mainstay of clinical neuropsychological practice with children. The Halstead-Reitan tests have been reported to be sensitive to brain dysfunction in a number of developmental disorders, including asthma (Dunleavy & Baade, 1980), autism (Dawson, 1983), Gilles de la Tourette's Syndrome (Bornstein, King, & Carroll, 1983), and epilepsy (Herman, 1982). An abundance of data shows that the Halstead-Reitan batteries are valid for the differential diagnosis of brain damage in children (Boll & Reitan, 1970; Reed, Reitan, & Klove, 1965). Further, the batteries have been found useful for the neuropsychological classification of minimal brain dysfunction in young children ages five to eight years (Reitan & Boll, 1973) and learning disabilities in older children (Reitan, 1980; Selz & Reitan, 1979).

The tests and clinical-interpretation methods within the Halstead-Reitan Battery for adults have now been extended downward for children between the ages of five and eight years (Reitan, 1979) and ages nine to fourteen years (Reitan & Davison, 1974). Hartlage and Tarnopol (1977) have reported that the tasks, designed by Ward Halstead and expanded and revised by Reitan, now form the best and most comprehensive neuropsychological batteries available. In the main, the development and use of the Halstead-Reitan tasks are predicated on the belief that neuropsychological batteries must include procedures that are sensitive to the full range of human adaptive abilities that are subserved by the brain and that are predictably impaired when brain systems are deficient.

A critical element in all phases of the neuropsychological examination, from test selection to clinical interpretation, is the use of several inferential methods. These methods include (1) comparing an individual's performance on the tasks with the performance of an appropriate comparison sample, criterion group, or an absolute standard of expectation, (2) evaluating variations in performance within and between components of a task (e.g., comparing verbal and performance IQ's), (3) identifying pathognomonic signs that are highly predictive of brain impairment (e.g., aphasia), and (4) comparing the functional efficiency of the two sides of the body. Excellent discussions of these interpretive methods can be found in Boll (1981), Reitan and Davison (1974), and Rourke (1981).

In 1980, Reitan initiated formal attempts to explicitly relate neuropsychological assessment data to treatment, through the development of a program titled Reitan Evaluation of Hemispheric Abilities and Brain Improvement Training (REHABIT). According to Reitan (1979, 1980), the efficacy of REHABIT for remediation is dependent upon (1) a comprehensive neuropsychological evaluation (by use of the Halstead-Reitan procedures), which clearly identifies areas of brain-related strengths and weaknesses, and (2) a determination from the assessment data as to whether the particular neuropsychological deficits reflect specific neural-cognitive deficiencies or generalized cognitive problems affecting several functional systems.

According to Reitan (1980), direct linkages between assessment and treatment are forged by the training concepts inherent in the REHABIT model. For example, REHABIT proposes that the general area of neuropsychological deficit be directly treated by use of alternate forms of neuropsychological tests as training items. According to Alfano and Finlayson (1987), such an approach seems reasonable, because challenging the areas measured by neuropsychological tasks could provide direct stimulation of the wide range of neural functions that they assess. (Serious readers are referred to Mann, 1979; and Mann & Sabatino, 1985, for alternate points of view.)

Following this general form of deficit training, remediation in five specific areas (tracts) uses previously developed educational materials and tasks. The tracts include (1) Tract A, materials for the development of expressive and receptive language and verbal skills; (2) Tract B, materials to develop abstract language functions, to include verbal reasoning, verbal concept-formation, and verbal organization; (3) Tract C, materials designed to enhance general reasoning capabilities; (4) Tract D, materials for developing abstract, visual-spatial and temporal-sequential concepts; and (5) Tract E, materials designed to promote understanding of basic visual-spatial and manipulation skills. Thus, Tracts A and B are generally linked to left-hemisphere functions, Tracts D and E to right-hemisphere functions, and Tract C to general logical analysis and reasoning functions subserved by all functional systems.

Data to support the REHABIT rehabilitation and remediation concepts are difficult to find (Lyon, Moats, & Flynn, in press). Reitan (1979, 1980) does report a few case studies but the information provided in them can not be construed as empirical validation for the REHABIT model. In fact, reviews of similar neuropsychological process remediation models (Lyon & Moats, in press; Mann, 1979) have indicated that such practices suffer from a lack of both construct and ecological validity, particularly in their application to children who display academic achievement deficits but do not demonstrate brain injury. In the absence of empirical validation for the REHABIT model, the clinician is ultimately responsible for judging whether the time spent in assessment and training activities is in the best interests of the child.

## Rourke's Neuropsychological Assessment and Treatment Model

Rourke and his colleagues (Rourke, Bakker, Fisk, & Strang, 1983; Rourke, Fisk, & Strang, 1986) have argued convincingly that the aims, content, and style of neuropsychological assessments are improved significantly when a comprehensive battery of neuropsychological tasks is administered to children and the data interpreted according to several frames of reference (level of performance, pathognomonic signs, differential (pattern) score approach, comparisons of performance on two sides of the body, pre- and post-lesion comparisons). Rourke's (1975) orientation to assessment practices and the relationship between assessment data and treatment, is influenced significantly by Reitan's concepts of neuropsychological measurement and modes of clinical interpretation (see previous discussion and Rourke, 1981).

Rourke, Fisk, and Strang (1986) propose that linkages between assessment and remediation are best formed when a developmental, neuropsychological model is employed. Within the context of such a model, specific information related to the child's neuropsychological ability-structure is collected and interpreted in relation to (1) the immediate demands in the environment (e.g., school and social demands), (2) hypothesized long-range demands (e.g., occupational and social functioning), (3) specific short- and long-term behavioral outcomes that best characterize the child with respect to developmental status, information-processing strengths and weaknesses, and neuropsychological status, (4) based on the above information, an ideal remediation program for the child, and (5) the development of a realistic remediation program, taking into account the child's characteristics and the actual availability of remedial sources for family, school, and child. Rourke's developmental, neuropsychological remediation/rehabilitation model appears to have potential for linking assessment data to treatment, because it stresses a comprehensive analysis of the systematic interactions between the child's variables and environmental factors, and the pragmatics of clinical-service delivery (Lyon, Moats, & Flynn, in press).

## THE LURIA-NEBRASKA NEUROPSYCHOLOGICAL TEST BATTERIES
(Golden, C. J., 1987, Western Psychological Services)

A. R. Luria's (1973, 1980) seminal conceptualization of the human brain as composed of functional systems, has led to the development of standardized, neuropsychological assessment batteries for use with both adults and children. The first attempt to organize Luria's clinical assessment methods into a formal test battery was carried out by Anne-Lise Christensen (Teeter, 1986). Charles Golden and his colleagues further refined Luria's procedures into standardized batteries for adults (Golden, Hammeke, & Purische, 1980) and children (Plaisted, Gustavson, Wilkening, & Golden, 1983).

The Luria-Nebraska Neuropsychological Battery for Children (Plaisted, Gustavson, Wilkening, & Golden, 1983) consists of eleven scales, which assess motor skills, acoustico-motor organization, cutaneous and kinesthetic functions, visual functions, receptive language, expressive language, reading, writing, arithmetic, memory, and intellectual processes. The battery has been found to be sensitive to detecting demonstrable neuroencephalopathy in children (Teeter, 1986). Several recent studies have also shown that the battery can discriminate between learning-disabled children and normally-achieving students (Geary & Gilger, 1984; Noland, Hammeke, & Barkley, 1983).

To date, there have been no formal attempts to relate assessment data obtained from the Luria-Nebraska to structured remediation programs for children. However, Luria's (1973) concepts of brain-behavior relationships can be clinically useful if applied to intervention practices in an informed manner. This conclusion may be a reasonable one for at least two reasons. First, Luria's model incorporates concepts related to both brain systems and their development. As such, a dynamic theoretical basis exists from which predictions about outcome and potential for remediation can be made. Second, Luria's model argues that disturbances in complex cognitive functions can be related to a wide variety of brain-related deficiencies. For example, failure to learn to write could be attributable to deficits in any of several brain systems. Thus, different children who display written-language deficits might not each respond equally well to the same remediation procedure.

One additional point is in order. Luria (1963, 1973, 1980) advocated the use of dynamic, nonstandardized assessment methods that could vary across patients, according to the nature of the clinical question. He supported the use of these procedures with substantial data from clinical case studies. Further, Luria (1963, 1980) presented a rationale for the application of assessment procedures directly to the treatment and rehabilitation process, and reported case-history data to substantiate his point of view. It is possible that attempts to standardize Luria's dynamic assessment methods could reduce their power in relating assessment findings to treatment-program planning. The reader should keep in mind that this possibility remains an open question.

## THE KAUFMAN ASSESSMENT BATTERY FOR CHILDREN (K-ABC)
(Kaufman, A. S., & Kaufman, N., 1983, American Guidance Service)

Another standardized assessment tool that relies on neuropsychological constructs is the Kaufman Assessment Battery for Children, K-ABC (Kaufman & Kaufman, 1983). Emphasizing a dual-processing model of cognition, the K-ABC Test purports to measure simultaneous and successive information-processing strengths and weaknesses in children up to age twelve years. In addition to the Simultaneous and Successive Scales, a third Achievement Test Cluster is used to measure acquired knowledge and verbal learning ability. The test-user is then encouraged to formulate hypotheses regarding remediation of academic deficiencies; these hypotheses should emphasize the subject's preferred processing mode. Unique to the K-ABC remediation framework (Gunnison, 1984) is the specificity of these recommendations to academic domains—reading, arithmetic reasoning, and written language—and the well-elaborated models of intervention, which attempt to code both the learner's behavior and the tasks' demands along the simultaneous/sequential dichotomy.

Unfortunately, the usefulness of the K-ABC even for descriptive and classification purposes has not been uniformly accepted (Lyon, Moats, & Flynn, in press). For example, Sternberg (1984a) argued that the test lacks construct validity, a problem that might be related to the author's misrepresentation or misreading of the evidence supporting a simultaneous-successive processing dichotomy. Further, in equating processing style with scores on selected tasks, the test fails to assess constructs that pertain to dynamic problem-solving. Selecting and conducting remediation on the basis of K-ABC results would thereby be a questionable practice.

Empirical support for remediation based on the K-ABC, as for other neuropsychological approaches reviewed in this chapter, is sparse. Although Gunnison and her colleagues (research in press, cited in Gunnison, 1984) have shown that children taught with methods described as simultaneous or sequential in emphasis can make meaningful gains in reading, both the assumptions underlying the aptitude-treatment linkages and the data base supporting those assumptions are weak (Ayres & Cooley, 1986). The logical-intuitive classification of children's responses and teaching strategies appears to have most value in its provision of a conceptual framework for diagnostic teaching. The concept of dual processing modes might simply encourage the clinician to behave in a flexible manner when alternative representations of concepts are needed by the learner.

## Alternative Approaches

A number of researchers and clinicians attempt to assess children's neuropsychological characteristics with tasks that are not standardized in battery form (Lyon, Moats, & Flynn, in press). Generally, the tasks are selected according to their relevance to a particular theoretical model or a research question. Because the tasks included in selected assessment batteries lack a common standardization sample from which scores are derived, control groups matched on relevant variables are generally assessed along with the clinical group of interest.

In the main, studies employing this type of assessment approach are conducted for the purpose of establishing a classification scheme for children who are included in heterogeneous clinical populations (i.e., children with learning disabilities). Children are classified into different subtypes on the basis of their performances on the selected neuropsychological tasks. Once a solution is obtained, it must be internally and externally validated. To achieve internal validation, the examiner ensures that the identified subtypes are reliable, replicable, and robust enough to include most members of the clinical population of interest. To examine external validity, the examiner determines whether the classification is useful for descriptive, predictive, and clinical practice. One specific way to address external validity is to determine whether the subtypes' responses to treatment differ from one another (Lyon & Risucci, in press).

To date, a number of research programs have reported preliminary data that suggest that subtypes do respond differently to varying forms of remediation. Although all of the published investigations have been carried out with learning-disabled readers (dyslexics), the studies differ with respect to theoretical orientation, assessment tasks used to form subtypes, and classification methodology. For example, to identify subtypes, Lyon and his colleagues (Lyon, 1983; Lyon, 1985a, 1985b; Lyon, Stewart, & Freedman, 1982; Lyon & Watson, 1981) have applied empirical, multivariate, quantitative clustering methods to information-processing–task scores obtained by large samples of learning-disabled readers. External validity studies have then involved attempts to teach the disabled learners and to determine the interactions of teaching methods with various subtypes.

In contrast, Bakker (1983) has classified dyslexics into two major subtypes according to clinical criteria, the most important of which is left-ear/right-ear asymmetries in dichotic-listening tasks. External validation consisted of hemisphere-specific stimulation via presentation of words to right and left visual fields, and identification of whether subtypes responded differently to both site of presentation and type of stimulus used.

Flynn and her associates (Flynn, 1987) have concentrated on clinically identifying dyslexic subtypes on the basis of their reading and spelling error patterns. She has presented compelling pilot data showing that children with particular patterns respond well to specific methods of reading instruction.

Space limitations preclude a more comprehensive discussion of these types of alternative, neuropsychological assessment procedures. Interested readers are referred to Lyon, Moats, and Flynn (in press) and Stoddart and Knights (1986) for in-depth reviews.

## ADVANCES IN NEURODIAGNOSTIC TECHNOLOGY AND THEIR APPLICATIONS

Recent advances in neuroimaging techniques, such as Computed Tomography (CT), Brain Electrical Activity Mapping (BEAM), and Magnetic Resonance Imaging (MRI), raise the possibility of construct validity being provided for the neuropsychological assessment of children. Each of these three neurodiagnostic procedures has the potential of providing unique informa-

tion valuable to the early identification and ongoing study of exceptional children. Each in turn has limitations that require careful consideration of methodological design. In this section, the potential benefits and current limitations of each will be briefly discussed in relation to the neuropsychological assessment of exceptional children, particularly those with dyslexia. Duane (1986) has provided a more extensive review of these neurodiagnostic tools and should be consulted for greater detail.

### Computed Tomography

When this procedure is used, a special x-ray scanner and a computer produce a cross-sectional computed tomogram, called a CT scan, which provides a visualization of brain anatomy. Cerebral asymmetries, particularly in the widths of the two cerebral hemispheres, have been noted in CT studies of the general population; the left, posterior hemisphere is generally wider than the right, in right-handed individuals (Galaburda, LeMay, Kemper, & Geschwind, 1978; LeMay, 1976).

Because of the hypothesized relationship between left-handedness and dyslexia, computed tomography has been of interest in the study of dyslexia. However, because radiation is involved, CT scans are not indicated in the routine examination of dyslexic children. Therefore, few such studies have been conducted. Of the extant studies (Haslam, Dalby, Johns, & Rademaker, 1981; Hier, LeMay, Rosenberger, & Perlo, 1978; Leisman & Ashkenazi, 1980; Rosenberger & Hier, 1980), only Haslam and colleagues (1981) studied children exclusively and controlled for left- and right-handedness. CT scans of twenty-six right-handed, dyslexic males, nine to thirteen years of age, and eight normal-reading matched controls revealed no correlation of reversed asymmetry with dyslexia, history of language delay, or verbal IQ, although there was a higher incidence of hemispheric symmetry in dyslexics. The Leisman and Ashkenazi CT study of eight dyslexic children (C.A. 7-10.9) did find reversed symmetry in two children, and equal left and right parietooccipital regions in the remaining six; however, there was no mention of subject handedness. Thus, CT scans of dyslexic children have to date produced inconclusive data.

## Computerized Electroencephalograms (EEG) and Evoked Potentials (EP)

In the past two decades, the possibility of neurophysiological studies through the computerization of EEG and EP data has emerged. The most recent generation of computer programs displays colored maps of the averaged electrical activity at selected cortical sites. The colors correspond to the amplitude of a particular brain-wave frequency at each electrode site; thus, areas of relative activation and quiescence can be visualized. An advantage of this technique is that children can be studied while they are performing cognitive tasks designed to elucidate neuropsychological profiles.

This approach has yielded enough early evidence of dyslexic neurophysiology, that Duffy, Denckla, Bartels, and Sandini (1980) concluded that quantitative neurophysiology may do for learning disabilities what the clinical EEG did for the diagnosis of epilepsy. To date, a number of studies have differentiated dyslexic children from normal achievers on the basis of their brain-wave patterns while resting and while performing cognitive tasks (Ahn, Baird, Trepeptin, & Kaye, 1980; Duffy, Denckla, Bartels, & Sandini, 1980; Hanley & Sklar, 1976; Naour, 1982).

Computerized EEG's and EP's have also been used to provide evidence that dyslexic children represent a heterogeneous population with distinct subtypes (see Lyon, Moats, & Flynn, in press). The second author's laboratory has used the Boder (1971, 1973) typology in its study of dyslexic children. Boder proposed three dyslexic subtypes: dysphonetic, dyseidetic, and mixed dysphonetic-dyseidetic, each characterized by a distinctive reading-spelling pattern. Dyslexics in the dysphonetic group have "difficulty interpreting written symbols with their sounds" (Boder & Jarrico, 1982, p. 6, 7). However, they have no major difficulty with visual

gestalt function. Difficulty with the "memory of letters and whole-word configurations, or gestalts" (p. 7), characterize the dyseidetic group. The phonetic skills are intact in this group. Members of the mixed dysphonetic and dyseidetic subtype have problems in both grapheme-phoneme correspondence and the visual recall of words.

Analysis of ongoing EEG activity during performances of reading, spelling, and spatial-numerical tasks provide partially replicated evidence for a distinctly different, left-hemisphere, brain-wave activation pattern in one subtype of exceptional children (Flynn & Deering, 1987; Lyon, Moats, & Flynn, in press). Other subtyping projects using BEAM have classified children according to language characteristics; these projects have again found distinct differences in brain neurophysiology displayed during performances of cognitive tasks (Duffy & McAnulty, 1985).

## Magnetic Resonance Imaging (MRI)

MRI images, generated by radio-frequency pulses within a magnetic field, are visually similar to CT scans, but yield superior resolution. Additionally, MRI procedures do not require x-irradiation and therefore would be preferred in pediatric studies. Disadvantages of MRI procedures include cost and the closeness of the chamber, which youngsters might find frightening. It is anticipated that newer systems will correct the latter constraint.

## Combined Neuroimaging Studies

To date, no study has combined all three neuroimaging techniques in the examination of dyslexic children. Certainly, as Duane (1986) pointed out, such a study would provide some important complementary information regarding the neuroanatomical and neurophysiological substrates of dyslexia, and more importantly, of dyslexic subtypes. However, completion of such a study, and the replication necessary for validation of results, involves considerable logistical problems. The most formidable of these is the formation of homogeneous, distinct subtypes of dyslexic children; such a grouping would have to take into account such factors as handedness, activity level and attention, sex, age, socioeconomic and educational opportunities, intelligence, language profile, and type of reading disability. Because of the number and complexity of these subtyping variables and the usual attrition of at least one-third of the sample in most neurophysiology studies (Flynn & Deering, 1987; Duffy & McAnulty, 1985), such a study would need to be extraordinarily large to result in a sample size sufficient for statistical analysis. Duffy and McAnulty, for example, examined over 100 children in order to obtain a final sample of 44 children in a recent study using BEAM technology.

In addition to issues surrounding subject selection and subtyping, various constraints associated with each of the neuroimaging techniques must be addressed. Of these, the radiation used in CT scans is most problematic in the design of an integrated study. The possibility of linking brain-behavior mechanisms in dyslexia and other developmental disorders via investigations of cerebral anatomical structure, interhemispheric and lower-brain-stem activity, and ongoing cortical activity during the performance of cognitive tasks such as reading, clearly warrants the effort needed to complete such a study.

## SUMMARY AND CONCLUSIONS

Neuropsychological assessment may contribute some useful clinical information to an understanding of the learning and behavioral difficulties observed in exceptional children. These clinical contributions most likely will have an impact on the diagnosis and description of neuropathology in pediatric populations. This will be particularly true as additional advances are made in the development and application of neuroimaging procedures.

Unfortunately, the clinical utility and validity of clinical neuropsychological assessment procedures in the design of remediation programs for exceptional children remain sparse (Lyon & Moats, in press). This limitation appears to exist for several reasons. First, a large portion of the assessment tasks that comprise the most widely used, standardized neuropsychological batteries for children, are downward extensions of batteries initially developed and validated on adult clinical populations. This is particularly true of the Halstead Neuropsychological Test Battery for Children (Reitan & Davison, 1974), the Reitan-Indiana Neuropsychological Test Battery (Reitan, 1969), and the Standardized Luria-Nebraska Battery for Children-Revised (Plaisted, Gustavson, Wilkening, & Golden, 1983). Likewise, the type of stimuli (task content) used in tasks to assess specific brain-behavior relationships are downward extensions of stimulus items presented to adults.

These test-development practices could seriously compromise a battery's power in predicting which treatment methods are most efficacious for particular children because (1) the tasks employed and their content are primarily based on models of adult brain function and dysfunction that occur following a period of normal development, (2) many tasks are designed to assess the effects of focal neuropathology typically seen in adults (e.g., tumors, cerebral vascular accidents, penetrating head wounds) rather than the generalized neural disorders usually observed in children (e.g., closed head injury, anoxia, epilepsy, perinatal trauma, etc.), and, (3) the neuropsychological tasks' content might have minimal relationship to the ecological demands that the child is facing in home and school environments. For example, even though many widely used children's batteries contain tasks assessing reading, mathematics, and writing skills, such tasks rarely possess adequate content validity. Consider that the Wide Range Achievement Test, a staple of many children's neuropsychological batteries and procedures, assesses only the oral reading of single words, mathematics calculation, and spelling, and thus leaves abilities in reading comprehension, math reasoning, and written language open to question.

A second issue, related to the previous points, is that some neuropsychological assessment procedures employed with children use tasks that yield static measures of competence in neuropsychological ability structures. The data obtained from such measures reflect only a child's past and current declarative knowledge of perceptual, linguistic, cognitive, psychomotor, and academic skills, not how they use or do not use such abilities in their daily lives (Brown & Campione, 1986; Lyon, 1987; Lyon & Moats, in press; Lyon, Moats, & Flynn, in press). A notable exception is the Category Test, known for its sensitivity to abstract concept formation, mental efficiency, and the ability to assess new learning (Boll, 1981).

Third, there is increasing concern that tasks making up neuropsychological assessment batteries for children primarily assess general cognitive ability, not distinct neuropsychological processes (Hynd & Obrzut, 1986; Seidenberg, Giordani, Berent, & Boll, 1983; Tramontana, Klee, & Boyd, 1984). If this possibility is true, administering time-consuming batteries beyond administration of a WISC-R can net redundant information. Further, the consistent finding that

the WISC-R is not particularly useful for the development of instructional or remediation programs (Ysseldyke & Algozzine, 1982; Ysseldyke & Mirkin, 1982) does not bode favorably for the use of redundant neuropsychological batteries for the same purpose.

Fourth, issues related to development and brain maturation might obscure any possible benefits that accrue from the administration of standard neuropsychological batteries to children for the purpose of treatment-program design. For instance, Hynd and Obrzut (1986) reported that a number of neuropsychological tasks are simply not age appropriate and that no neuropsychological test battery has established adequate cross-sectioned norms. Further, these authors concluded that without such norms, "it becomes nearly impossible to provide any accurate appraisal of the possible impairment of developing abilities" (p. 10).

Finally, as Lyon and Toomey (1985) have stressed, describing brain-behavior relationships through the application of assessment procedures does not insure successful remediation of brain-based deficiencies. For example, neuropsychological assessment can help to clarify the physiological correlates of dyslexia, but altering the underlying neuropathology or identifying alternate intact processing routes might not be possible.

# CHAPTER 12

# Assessing Infants and Young Children

*A Developmental/Interactive Approach*

STAN SCARPATI
PATRICIA GILLESPIE-SILVER

## OUTLINE

Multidisciplinary team approach
Developmental/Interactive approach to assessment
Screening measures
Infant development and assessment
Assessment of preschool language
Intelligence testing
Assessment of motor development and disorders
Social and emotional assessment
Multidimensional developmental diagnostic tests
Multicultural preschool assessment
Summary

**T**he assessment of preschool children with special needs is based on the assumption that early identification will lead to an educational plan that will either prevent or diminish the effects of an inappropriate education. It is inappropriate to assess children without clearly recognizing the effect on interventions. Intervention must be driven by accurate diagnostics, which in turn consider the effectiveness of the intervention. Bricker and Littman (1982) suggest that assessment and evaluation are interrelated, in that they guide individual program development and generate feedback information about the success of the interventions for an individual and for groups of children. In recent years the matching of assessment methods with the goals and objectives of intervention has been stressed. History has shown that traditional assessment with young children that does not link measurement to treatment is ineffective.

This traditional conceptualization of assessment often inappropriately labels and misclassifies children. With young children in particular, there is insufficient evidence to support a total reliance on formal assessment that attempts to predict future performance from present measurement. Individual differences between young children have different implications; the younger the child the more difficult the interpretation becomes. Some special needs, such as physical or sensory disabilities, are usually easily uncovered. Others, such as cognitive and potential-learning problems, are more difficult to predict, as preschool children have had little opportunity, if any, to engage in academics. Trying to predict through assessment the success or failure of young children's future performances is less precise than determining their immediate needs. Tests of young children are notably limited for several reasons. First, test scores are unstable and will fluctuate over time. Second, scores of cohesive norm groups with which to compare test results are often lacking, especially for tests that measure the more subtle aspects of cognitive and affective development.

Although programming for children with special needs has advanced considerably since the Education of the Handicapped Act (EHA) was fully implemented during the 1970s, notable deficiencies in the law's effect on preschool children have been recognized. Behind the movement to address this concern is a judgment that early intervention programs that appear costly now will result in longterm benefits and substantial savings in services provided later. In 1986, P.L. 99-457 was enacted as an amendment to the EHA; the new legislation had the specific mandate to 1) enhance the development of handicapped infants and toddlers, and minimize delays in their development; 2) minimize the costs related to educating these children when they reach school age; and 3) minimize the likelihood of institutionalization and increase their potential to become productive citizens and to assist their parents in meeting their needs (Education of the Handicapped Act Amendments, 1986).

To qualify for particular funds, states must provide specified services, including the timely and appropriate identification, screening, and assessment of children with special needs. The law requires that a multidisciplinary team conduct a comprehensive evaluation based on the physical, cognitive, language and speech, psycho-social, and social needs of the child. This legislation has significant implications for service delivery for children with special needs, from infancy to kindergarten, and also promises to change the course of the entire special-education service-delivery system.

One of the major components of this legislation is the development of the *Individual Family Service Plan.* According to Weiner and Koppelman (1987), this law gives the parents a great deal of participation in developing programs for their young children. In keeping with the new focus on the development of young children and subsequent intervention within a family context, multidisciplinary teams need to develop assessment models that will provide useful and practical information. Furthermore, because of the nature of young children's development, multidisciplinary teams must refrain from using assessment procedures and materials that result in a primary diagnosis. In fact, P.L. 99-457 allows professionals to use a more generic label, e.g., developmental delay, for determining a subject's eligibility for services. Weiner and Koppelman (1987) explain the reason for the term's use:

> Because it is difficult to properly diagnose or label a handicapped infant or toddler as having a particular handicap, and because such diagnoses or labels can be impossible to discard even if proven incorrect or unnecessary later in the child's life, P.L. 99-457 adds the term "developmental delay" as a way to serve children from birth through age 2 without labeling them (p. 20).

Another important aspect of the legislation is the emphasis on integration of young children with special needs, aged three to five years, with other children with more typical development. Because of this attention to preschool integration, multidisciplinary teams must use assessment tools that provide information to identify those skills that will enable a young special-needs child to succeed in an integrated setting.

In this chapter we present the elements of the developmental/interactional assessment model, the areas of assessment as required by P.L. 99-457, and the specific tests for each area. We also include sections on the technical adequacy of assessment measures, the purposes of assessment, and the types of tests that will accommodate these purposes.

## MULTIDISCIPLINARY TEAM APPROACH

P.L. 94-457 explicitly states that "each handicapped infant or toddler will receive multidisciplinary assessment to unique needs" (Sec. 677, Education of the Handicapped Act Amendment of 1986). A team approach was also mandated in P.L. 94-142, the Education for All Handicapped Children's Act (1975). While these laws

mandate such an assessment approach, there is controversy concerning a multidisciplinary assessment team's effectiveness in decision-making (Courtnage & Smith-Davis, 1987; Ysseldyke, Algozzine, & Mitchell, 1982). Essentially, some researchers have found that teams of professionals might not make better decisions than individuals (e.g., Yoshida, 1983). However, a rationale for multidisciplinary input, especially in the assessment of the infant and young child, can be made. In organizational literature, for example, Drucker (1974) notes that one major advantage of the team approach is that all participants are aware of the entire process and communication among team members is enhanced. Because P.L. 99-457 requires assessment in physical, cognitive, language and speech, psycho-social, and self-help development, no one discipline can adequately assess all these areas. The preschool special-needs teacher and the early childhood teachers "should become familiar with the roles and responsibilities and the language or jargon of the professionals with whom they team" (Golightly, 1987, p. 127). If all disciplines involved in the assessment process are aware of the types of assessments used by other specialists and the basic developmental issues in each area, professionals will be able to complement their findings and to develop a common language (Golightly, 1987).

## DEVELOPMENTAL/INTERACTIVE APPROACH TO ASSESSMENT

Gathering accurate information about the performance of young, special-needs children is hampered in ways unique to this group. Early-childhood educators are faced with the predicament of knowing that early identification is crucial to the detection of developmental problems, yet also knowing that children develop according to variable patterns and that many of the instruments available have questionable reliability and validity. They are also well aware that the environment, and the ways in which children interact with the environment in purposeful ways to satisfy their needs and desires, affect development and the accurate measurement of performance.

The developmental/interactive approach makes several assumptions: (1) the development of all children results from interaction with their parents, siblings, peers, and teachers, (2) a developmental approach toward assessment and programming is more beneficial than a deficit-model approach, and (3) measurements of traits must be repeated in different settings and at different times for the development of effective treatment plans.

Developmental assessment assumes that children progress through specific patterns and that these patterns can be used in the detection of qualitative and quantitative differences between children. Developmental guidelines provide a baseline against which evaluation statements are made. These standards for normal and sequential progress offer the assessor a framework within which he or she can conduct the assessment and generate hypotheses. For example, representing a child's performance as a point on a continuum of behaviors can be a source for comparison. This approach assumes that young children learn advanced skills only after they have passed through and mastered a sequence of prerequisites. For example, walking would be achieved after a child has learned to sit, crawl, and stand. Young children are characterized by a maturing neurological system that is primarily motoric; this system eventually generates language, adaptive, and social behaviors.

In contrast, a pragmatic or functional approach to assessment and intervention would view children in terms of how well their current performance enables them to succeed in their environment. If self-feeding capabilities are the focus of an evaluation, for example, a functional approach would focus on the steps associated with the transfer of food from a plate to a child's mouth and on the child's ability to independently repeat this task over time. Little attention would be paid to assumed precursors to the "feeding process."

Although at first glance these two approaches appear to be mutually exclusive, and their differences will often divide assessment and intervention teams, the two approaches should be used in tandem. Limiting the assessment process to either one or the other could result in a restrictive and incomplete intervention. Developmental approaches alone might lead to educational plans that stress certain milestones, yet the skills associated with those milestones might be irrelevant or unimportant to the particular case. This is notably true of many gross and fine motor skills. Governing the assessment according to strict functional procedures would also present problems. This approach might prevent a teacher from training a child in prerequisite skills that are absolutely necessary for further learning. A comprehensive assessment would incorporate instruments that yield data from both perspectives. Fortunately, most assessment instruments are flexible enough to adapt to an evaluation that seeks to understand children from both perspectives. And most importantly, results from developmental and functional tests must be interpreted with a clear understanding of the role of environmental variables, and the means by which children's interacting with their environment affects their performance.

## A Combined Developmental/Interactional Approach

While development guidelines provide a baseline against which assessment statements can be made, these developmental profiles are based on the norms from groups of typical children and might not represent the growth of a child with special needs. Because the child's interactions with the environment will affect development, and conversely, we propose the use of a developmental/interactional approach to assessment. This approach, which is also called the adaptive-transactive perspective (Peterson,

1987) or the transactional approach (McClean & Snyder-McClean, 1978), has the following underlying assumptions:

1. Developmental components (e.g., motor, cognitive, language, social) cannot progress in isolation. For example, a child uses language for social purposes, and motor and cognitive development can affect language development.
2. Each child has his or her own "unique or idiosyncratic concepts, interactive strategies, and preferences" (McClean & Snyder-McClean, 1978, p. 123). An infant interacts with his/her environment "willfully" (Mahoney & Powell, 1986, p. 4); the infant's and the young child's development is a product of their own motivation to learn (Mahoney & Powell, 1986).
3. Development is a product of the complex interactions of the child with his or her environment and caregivers (Mahoney & Powell, 1986; McClean & Snyder-McClean, 1978). Development reflects the transactions that involve a "complex reciprocal relationship" between the child and the caregivers and peers. Furthermore, the quality of these transactions can affect the child's development (Mahoney & Powell, 1986). Additionally, researchers have determined that the child's unique needs and characteristics (e.g., hearing difficulties) can affect the type and quality of interactions (e.g., Stoneman, Brody, & Abbott, 1983).

## Implications for Assessment

The developmental/interactional approach has the following implications for assessment procedures:

1. Assessment must be continuous and ongoing. Because the complex interactions are continuously changing, assessment must be frequently made so that a clear description of the child's developmental needs is produced.
2. Assessment devices are not used to mandate the content of assessment (McClean & Snyder-McClean, 1978). Instead, environmental and situational questions guide the assessment process, and specific behaviors at each developmental level are targeted for assessment.
3. Assessment procedures include more than standardized norm-referenced instruments. Observational systems, rating scales, structured interviews, and other devices for assessing the child's transactions in his/her own environment are integral components of the assessment process.
4. Assessments are comprehensive. That is, the team considers all developmental areas. Because developmental areas are interrelated (e.g., cognitive and language development), assessment procedures must provide results that define these unique relationships for the child. For example, assessment must target specific behaviors in cognitive and social development that can affect the child's language development. Furthermore, environmental factors that may affect the child's total development must also be assessed.

## Role of Preschool Assessor

Professionals who work with preschool children, particularly in educational settings, must be prepared to evaluate children in all areas of growth and development. Although special education has traditionally serviced children according to categories of disabilities, this approach would seriously impede the effectiveness of evaluations of preschool children and would predispose the evaluator to search for certain conditions that might not exist or might have little relation to intervention.

Several important differences between assessing school-aged children and preschool children require the examiner to draw on a repertoire of skills. For one, very young children simply cannot be asked to perform. Controlling

the testing situation by means of the test instructions is usually not possible. Examiners must
ensure that children are cooperative and attending to the test demands; both of these conditions might require the use of creative and novel
techniques. This is particularly challenging in
assessing infants, because it has been shown
that an infant's test performance will be influenced by the presence of a strange adult
(Stevenson & Lamb, 1979). Also, the younger
the children the less regard they have for responding according to the demands of a test.
For example, the need to give a "correct" answer or to "please" the examiner plays virtually
no part in the testing of younger preschoolers, in
contrast to older children and adults. More
severe problems, such as limitations in communications or linguistic incompetence, might also
lead an examiner to consider the child untest-
able.

Examiners must take precautions not to let
test instruments dictate whether or not critical
information can be gathered from children, and
must recognize that their influence when they
are interacting with the child is a vital part of the
process. To provide trustworthy test results, special methods and routines to engage young
children must reflect the children's unique behavioral styles for interacting with adults and
responding to their environment. A systematic
way of observing young children's behavior
while they are being assessed should be employed as well; such observation is a source of
invaluable data that is matched to the actual test
results.

These observations have led psychologists
and teachers at times to "adapt" or change
either the standard way in which a test is given,
or reword or reorder the administration of a test
item or series of items. When special-needs
children are being tested, some of these
changes, such as pairing of difficult items with
easier items to ensure success or extending the
amount of time allowed for completion of a
subtest, are conditionally permissible. However,
if alterations seriously confound a test's reliabil-

ity or validity, the examiner should interpret the
results with caution and identify these changes
when reporting the outcomes.

## Observation and Recording: An Integral Component of Assessment

Direct, systematic observation should be part of
the initial and ongoing processes for assessment of infants and young children (Erickson,
1976). Erickson (1976) describes the observation process:

> Both observation and recording are important
> because they free those involved from making
> judgments or allowing philosophical views to re-
> main barriers to potential behavior changes. The
> art of observation and recording also eliminates
> bias. Child care professionals and parents learn to
> look at a child in regard to what the child does and
> says, when he moves, when he interacts, with
> whom he interacts, how often he interacts, and
> what and with whom he plays. They learn to
> observe and document precisely what a child is
> doing. They become accustomed to observing
> events, gradually obtaining a picture of the child's
> overall interactions (p. 206).

The determination of observation's technical
adequacy requires as much rigor as does the
development and use of standardized tests. The
assessment team must be able to determine
what behaviors are important for observation,
and must define these behaviors precisely and
clearly so that all team members can agree
upon them. Formal observational instruments
for use with young children are available. For
example, the Home Observation for Measurement of the Environment (Birth to Three)
(1970) is an instrument developed for observations of such factors in the home as parent-child
interactions, organization of the physical environment and the daily schedule.

Observation records may be in the form of
checklists, rating scales, anecdotal records, or
diaries. Prior planning to determine the precise
reasons for observation, the types of representative behaviors to be noted, and the means for
analysis are important factors in developing an

observation system. Guidelines for observing infants and young children may be found in Boehm and Weinberg (1977), Browder (1987), Cartwright and Cartwright (1974), Day (1983), Erickson (1976), and Peterson (1987).

## Screening: Definition, Types, Tools, and Concerns

By the time specialists identify a young child who is at risk developmentally or educationally, interactional patterns that affect the child's cognitive, social, and language developments might have already been established (Lilly & Shotel, 1987; Mahoney & Powell, 1988). Many child-development experts have emphasized the need for early identification and intervention, because the infant and young child develop so rapidly during the first three years of life (e.g., Bloom, 1964; White, 1975). Furthermore, early-childhood specialists and educators of special children have begun to note the developmental influence of the infant's and young child's interactions with his or her environment (Mahoney & Powell, 1988; Coles, 1988).

Screening is a popular procedure for identifying children who may be developmentally or educationally at risk. Screening is but one component of the overall preschool assessment process. The practice of assessing groups of children to identify those who may be at risk for school failure is routine in most school systems. Logically, not all children initially identified for screening would require an in-depth diagnostic evaluation. By definition, screening is a process to identify both the at-risk children, so that they can be provided with a more detailed evaluation, and those children who were suspected of having difficulty but who demonstrate that a true problem does not exist. At best, screening indicates that a special need might be present or that no serious developmental deviation exists. Screening instruments must be considered as gauges of future problems. In most cases it is screening data that convinces assessors to seek more detailed information (Salvia & Ysseldyke, 1985).

Screening measures therefore are not valid for diagnostics and should only be used to assist in referring a child for further testing. Although screening measures are valuable in the assessment process, they should not be used as the basis for precise evaluations or educational plans. Meisels (1985b) also cautions that screening instruments should not be used as 1) as indicators of intelligence; 2) for assignment of diagnostic labels; 3) if they are not sensitive to cultural or language differences; and 4) in isolation, but should be used as part of a comprehensive evaluation and intervention program.

As with any instrument used to determine how children perform, screening measures must meet certain guidelines. Observing and testing children, and interviewing their parents, are techniques associated with screening. The rapid and sporadic patterns in which children develop render most screening instruments technically unreliable and invalid. Meisels (1987) alerts professionals about the serious ethical and diagnostic dangers associated with using many of the undependable instruments available. Because screening is not intended to be diagnostic, comprehensive, or accurately predictive, instruments should not be expected to meet these demands. Also, low cost and efficient administration and scoring would mark a test as potentially useful. An overview of typical screening approaches and procedures and, finally, a review of the screening tests that are popular and also technically sound are presented in the following sections.

*Approaches and Procedures.* The screening approach to early identification is a two-stage process (Lichtenstein & Ireton, 1984). In the first stage, school systems typically use cost-effective, simple, and brief measures and processes, to identify the young children who might be at risk (Lichtenstein & Ireton, 1984; Meisels, 1987). In the first stage, screening procedures may be implemented by various approaches. The school system or related agency (e.g., Department of Public Health in Massachusetts) may choose to conduct a mass screening as part of their child-finding or case-finding (Peterson, 1987) process. If screening is to be effective, the outreach program must reach as many families as possible. For children from birth to two years of age, the identification process may be one of outreach/referral rather than mass screening (Lichtenstein & Ireton, 1984).

Once a child is referred by an agency or a pediatrician, the early-childhood specialists may administer developmental screening tests, e.g., the Denver Developmental Screening Test (DDST) (Frankenburg & Dodds, 1967; Frankenburg, Dodds, Fandal, Kazuk, & Cohrs, 1975). Other types of mass screening for children ranging in age from birth to two years are outreach programs operated through the school or an agency, in which public notices alert parents to opportunities for attending periodic screening services. Another approach is to use selective screening to "selectively provide direct screening for those demographic subgroups or geographic areas that have a substantial number of unidentified children with special needs" (Lichtenstein & Ireton, 1984, p. 12). In addition, what typically was known as kindergarten screening has, in many areas, been modified to preschool screening. This process is conducted annually and typically includes a review of medical histories and screening for visual and hearing impairments, and, sometimes, lead poisoning and anemia.

Screening services vary in the amount of time they require, the specialists involved, and the actual procedures used during the screening sessions. For example, one system may establish "stations" through which the child and his or her parents move in a prescribed sequence. Included in this session might be a structured interview with the parents or request for the parent to complete a developmental history questionnaire (Lichtenstein & Ireton, 1984). For comprehensive overviews of screening approaches, see Lichtenstein and Ireton (1984) and Peterson (1987). All of these screening approaches have advantages and disadvantages; we discuss issues related to screening in the summary to this section.

In the second stage, if the results from the screening indicate a potential problem, the child is referred for diagnostic assessment. Because the early years are critical developmental periods, the accuracy of screening procedures in identifying students who might need further diagnosis is vital. Specific screening tools, their components, and their degrees of technical adequacy are presented here.

## SCREENING MEASURES

Screening tests can be classified as developmental or school-readiness (Meisels, Wiske & Tivnan, 1984). Each type of screening test can be multidimensional or unidimensional (Lichtenstein & Ireton, 1984). Multidimensional instruments cover many developmental areas or functional skills, and unidimensional screening instruments focus on only one area, e.g., language. For this chapter's review, we do not include screening tests for school readiness because, typically, programs for preschoolers with special needs focus on developmental rather than pre-academic skills.

A multitude of screening instruments exist (Meisels, 1987); unfortunately few are technically adequate (Lichtenstein & Ireton, 1984; Meisels, 1985). Screening procedures can identify as at risk some children who are not at risk developmentally—a situation called an overreferral (a false-positive identification)— or can fail to identify children who are indeed at risk (a false-negative identification). Therefore, those specialists who are responsible for selecting screening instruments must consider each instrument's technical aspects. Unfortunately, at least one survey of teachers for special-needs preschoolers has shown that their rationale for selecting screening and other preschool instruments was that the instruments were "already in use" (Johnson & Beauchamp, 1987). If specialists administer tests simply because the tests are available, they might not recognize the importance of the criteria for test selection.

A thorough discussion of the psychometric characteristics of screening tests is beyond this chapter's scope. The reader is referred to the American Psychological Association's *Standards for Educational and Psychological Testing* (1985), Salvia and Ysseldyke (1985), and Lichtenstein and Ireton (1984) for more thorough presentations of technical criteria.

Two most important criteria for screening instruments are validity and reliability; these criteria can seriously affect the accuracy of the initial screening process (Flory, 1988). The American Psychological Association's *Standards for Educational and Psychological Testing* (1985) defines validity as "the most important consideration in test evaluation. The concept refers to the appropriateness, meaningfulness, and usefulness of the specific inferences made from test scores. . . . The inferences regarding uses of a test are validated, not the test itself" (p. 9).

Meisels (1987) considers reliability to be extremely important to accurate screening procedures. Reliability refers to the consistency with which the instrument performs. Early-childhood specialists note the inconsistent performance of young children and the difficulty of finding measures that yield consistent results; however, high reliability should be expected of any screening instrument used to determine early in his or her development if a child might need intervention in some particular developmental area.

Another important technical feature is the standardization of the instrument. Flory (1988) notes the importance of the sample group:

The sample group used to norm the test plays a critical role in the development of most screening instruments for two reasons. First, the sample group should represent the population at large for which the test was targeted for use. For instance, if the test was intended to screen just four year olds and normed accordingly using a sample of four

years, it would not be appropriate to use the screening measure with a group of three year olds. Likewise, if a test was normed using only English-speaking children, one would question the accuracy of the test for Spanish speaking children.

The second concern relates to the development of an appropriate scoring system and the identification of cut-off scores. Often, the initial sample group's scores are used to establish the overall scoring norms for the test, which become the standard against which the scores of all persons taking the screening test are compared.

Other features of standardized tests are qualitative (Lichtenstein & Ireton, 1984). That is, test administrators consider such factors as attractiveness, ease of administration, clarity of directions, scope, and cost effectiveness, as important selection criteria (Johnson & Beauchamp, 1987; Lichtenstein & Ireton, 1984).

Meisels (1985) indicates that few screening tests meet the essential criteria for technical adequacy. Meisels (1985b) considers that five tests do meet these essential criteria, and we provide a brief review of these five: the Revised Denver Developmental Screening Test (RDDST), the Developmental Indicators for the Assessment of Learning (DIAL-R), the Early Screening Inventory, the McCarthy Screening Test, and the Minneapolis Preschool Screening Instrument. For a more comprehensive review of these tests, see Lichtenstein and Ireton (1984) and Meisels (1985b). We provide a review of the screening tests' components, technical adequacy, and qualitative features.

### THE REVISED DENVER DEVELOPMENTAL SCREENING TEST (RDDST)

(Frankenburg, Dodds, Fandal, Kazuk, & Cohrs, 1975, Ladoca Publishing Foundation)

Frankenburg (1985) describes the RDDST:

[This test was] devised to provide a simple method of screening the development of infants and preschool children. This test was designed to be a quick, simple procedure that would be applied to a presumptively asymptomatic population to identify children highly suspect of being delayed in development (p. 135).

The RDDST is perhaps the most popular, early-childhood screening test; it is used in more than fifty-four countries and standardized in more than fifteen countries (Frankenburg, 1985). The test consists of 105 test items in four functional areas: gross motor, fine motor-adaptive, language, and personal-social. It can be administered to children aged from six weeks to six years.

Frankenburg and his associates have conducted studies of the RDDST's reliability and validity (e.g., Frankenburg, Camp, Van Natta, Demersseman, & Voorhees, 1971). Frankenburg (1985) notes that overall, the "test-retest stability of the DDST is not only satisfactory for a screening test but compares favorably with test-retest stability of diagnostic tests" (p. 137). To determine its validity, Frankenburg and his associates have compared the test to such other tests as the revised Bayley's Infant Scales (Bayley, 1984) and the Stanford-Binet, and have reported high correlations (above .83).

Another form of validity, predictive validity, is an important criterion for a screening test because its purpose is to identify children who are in need of diagnosis and early intervention. Predictive validity has also been assessed for the RDDST (Camp, van Doorninck, Frankenburg, & Lampe, 1977; Diamond, 1987). Results of these studies indicate that the RDDST is most accurate in predicting failure for the severely involved young infants and children. In Meisels' (1985b) review of the RDDST, he cautions against this interpretation of the results, in that the test "seriously underrefers" children who might be at developmental or educational risk.

Qualitative factors lend to the RDDST's attractiveness as a screening device. For example, administration time is only 20 minutes; a wide variety of specialists may administer the test; multi-media training materials are available; and cost is reasonable. In addition, Frankenburg (1985) has added a manual that encourages parental participation. "This book is to be given to parents at the time of the first health maintenance visit by the child physician, who explains that the parents are being enlisted to help monitor their child development" (Frankenburg, 1985, p. 147).

### EARLY SCREENING INVENTORY (ESI)
(Meisels & Wiske, 1983, Teacher's College Press)

This is another test that was designed to meet the essential criteria discussed earlier in this section. "The ESI is intended to identify children who may have a learning or handicapping condition that could affect their overall potential for success in school" (Meisels, Wiske, & Tivnan, 1984, p. 25).

In contrast to that of the RDDST, the age range of the ESI does not include infants to two-year-olds; instead, the age range is four to six years. The ESI consists of thirty items that cluster around three developmental areas: visual-motor/adaptive functioning, language and cognition, and gross motor/body awareness (Meisels & Wiske, 1983). A parental questionnaire, which accompanies the test, obtains basic information about the child's family, such as the child's prior school and medical history, the family's history of birth defects and illness, a review of the child's health history, and finally, the child's development (Meisels & Wiske, 1983, p. 7). Other components considered as part of this screening are a medical examination, and hearing and vision testing.

The ESI's technical adequacy has been studied (Meisels & Wiske, 1983; Meisels, Wiske, & Tivnan, 1984). The test's constructors have determined, through interscorer procedures and a test-retest reliability study, that "the scores on the ESI can be expected to show consistency when the test is administered by different examiners, when it is repeated over time, and when it is administered to different groups of children" (Meisels, Wiske, & Tivnan, 1984, p. 29). As determined by the test's constructors, tests of validity, on a short-term basis, reveal that the test overrefers more than it underrefers (Meisels,

Wiske, & Tivnan, 1984). Also, in studies of predictive validity, "the ESI is highly correlated with school success in kindergarten and moderately correlated with first- and second-grade school performance" (Meisels, Wiske, & Tivnan, 1984, p. 31). The test is normed on children primarily from white, lower-income communities, and communities are encouraged to establish their own local cutoffs for referrals.

An important feature of this screening instrument is that scores can be used in decisions to refer, to rescreen after eight to ten weeks, or to define as "OK." The test takes 15 minutes to administer, and can be administered by teachers, specialists, and paraprofessionals, if supervised. The test is inexpensive and a video-tape is available to assist in the training of prospective test administrators.

### DEVELOPMENTAL INDICATORS FOR THE ASSESSMENT OF LEARNING-REVISED (DIAL-R)

(Mardell-Czudnowski & Goldenberg, 1983, Childcraft-Educational Corporation)

This is another multidimensional screening test that includes screening for fine and gross motor, conceptual, and communications skills in children aged two to six years. This revision has several advantages: 1) identification of potentially advanced or gifted children, 2) use of separate sets of norms for different populations, 3) specific instructions for administration, including floor plans for examiners, 4) relatively short administration time (20–30 minutes), and 5) a team approach to administration (Linder, 1985). The DIAL-R is more expensive than the previously reviewed two tests. Professionals trained in the test's administration are required for appropriate implementation of the screening procedure. A behavioral observation checklist is included; also, although visual and hearing tests are not included, the test's authors recommend their inclusion.

For comprehensive reviews of the technical aspects of the DIAL-R, see Lichtenstein and Ireton (1984), and Linder (1985). In summary, the test was standardized on a large population

that was stratified (grouped) according to sex, race, socioeconomic status, and demographic setting. Linder's (1985) critique indicates that, in their manual, Mardell-Czudnowski and Goldenberg (1983) could have been more specific concerning the standardization procedure. Although data for validity and reliability are available in the manual, both Lichtenstein and Ireton (1984) and Linder (1985) agree that more research is need on both these technical aspects. In addition, the test authors have conducted no predictive-validity studies. However, Miller and Sprong (1986), in a review of the DIAL-R vis-à-vis the *Standards for Educational and Psychological Testing* (American Psychological Association (APA), 1974), noted that most of the APA's psychometric criteria are met. Lichtenstein and Ireton (1984), in their discussion of the DIAL prior to its most recent revision, noted that "the DIAL has considerable potential as a screening instrument" (p. 161).

### MINNEAPOLIS SCREENING INSTRUMENT (MSI)

(Lichtenstein, 1980, Prescriptive Instruction Center)

This test was developed as part of the early identification research project, Project Reach. "The objective was to develop a screening instrument to select out preschool children with special educational needs as part of the efforts to fulfill the mandate of Public Law 94-1422" (Lichtenstein & Ireton, 1984, p. 178). The test's age ranges are from three years, seven months to five years, four months. The fifty items include eleven subtests: building, copying shapes, providing information, matching, sentence completion, hopping and balancing, naming colors, counting, prepositions, identifying body parts, and repeating sentences. Also, a speech intelligibility rating is determined for each child. Lichtenstein and Ireton (1984) list the test's advantages: "(1) brief to administer—20 minutes at the most, (2) inexpensive—in terms of materials, consumables, and personnel requirements, and (3) simple—so that both professionals and nonprofessionals could master administration and scoring without undue difficulty" (p. 178).

The four-year-olds are the "primary target" for the test. Items are chosen such that the majority of children would pass, so that the children most at risk will be identified (Lichtenstein & Ireton, 1984).

The test appears to meet many technical criteria. Test-retest methods and inter-rater reliability studies indicate consistency in results. The author has conducted validity studies and found moderate to high correlations with other measures (Lichtenstein & Ireton, 1984). One major difficulty is that the test is limited to norms from one geographic area. Meisels' (1985b) conclusion is that "the MPSI is a well-developed test that excludes items requiring extensive examiner judgment . . . It includes a higher proportion of classroom readiness tasks than most developmental screening tests" (p. 39).

## Summary

In summary, these four multidimensional developmental screening tests are available for teams to use to determine young children who might be at risk. Early-childhood specialists must consider the limitations of screening procedures, which are not substitutes for effective referral (Lund & Duchan, 1983). Unless there is a comprehensive, coordinated network for early identification and intervention, some children can fall through the screening net. Furthermore, assessment teams must realize how critical timing is to the screening of young children (Lilly & Shotel, 1987). Moreover, follow up and reassessment of the decisions resulting from screening procedures are important. We can report statistically that a screening instrument can produce false-negatives and false-positives; however, Flory (1988) stresses the humanistic approach: "we must realize that error rates impact child and families on a social/humanistic level. An incorrect assessment of the child whether it occurs at the initial screening or at some future date places families under greater stress, either by delaying needed treatment or by falsely labeling the child as having special needs" (p. 12).

## INFANT DEVELOPMENT AND ASSESSMENT

As public institutions become more involved with younger and younger preschool children, the search for "high-risk" infants is rapidly becoming an integral part of the early-intervention team process. Assessing an infant must be viewed as an opportunity for a professional to interact with an infant, observe how his or her parents react, and develop an understanding of the infant's functioning in the environment (Brazelton & Nugent, 1987). Observing and interpreting infants' behavior in terms of a rich environment is critical when educational plans that will enable high-risk infants to compensate for their deficits are being designed. For example, longitudinal research (e.g., Sigman & Parmelee, 1979) has revealed that early, intensive visual and environmental stimulation are the best compensators for neurological deficiencies.

The newborn, or neonate, enters the world while experiencing great changes, ranging from the trauma of the birth process itself and maternal medication, to the environmental differences between intra- and extrauterine life. We now know that prenatal nutrition, drug and alcohol use, and a mother's psychological stress can affect the developing fetus. The neonate brings with it the traits and characteristics coded into its genetic makeup, as it faces the social influences of those responsible for caring for it and providing a safe environment.

Interactional assessment of infants emerges from within this context. Changes in infants' behavior result from the reciprocity of infant-caregiver involvement. Rapid growth and development quickly turn the neonate into an infant; the speed of this change adds to the complexity of gathering accurate data. Nonspecific response patterns (e.g., crying and smiling) and irregular maturation that at times can appear variant to established norms restrict effective measurement. Techniques and instruments in current practice require that the examiner maintain a sensitivity to the lack of continuous development. Also, the observer must recognize that particular behaviors that are maladaptive at one developmental stage can indeed be needed at another.

A developmental/interactive assessment focuses on the quality of responses, when a developing infant adapts to his or her environment and responds to the immediate caregivers. Infants are active participants in their own experiences. Sroufe (1979) has designed a framework comprised of features from several theoretical viewpoints. Although this framework is not specifically an assessment protocol, it is useful in the conducting of assessments of infants. Following these features would not reduce the observer's emphasis on observing behaviors, but would urge assessors to search for the meaningfulness of the behavior, in terms of its effect and its function. According to this framework, assessments should follow these guidelines (Sroufe, 1979):

1. *Focus on adaptation:* Infants are actively engaged in fitting themselves into the environment to satisfy their needs. They seek stimulation and organize their behavior in a goal seeking manner.
2. *View the infant as a coherent whole:* Infants may not exhibit the same behaviors in different situations but behavior is consistent across situations. Infants may be spontaneous and interactive in a situation that allows for their occurrence yet deliberate and purposeful when required.
3. *Consider the roles of affect and emotion:* Infants will demonstrate security when in familiar settings but will also demonstrate curiosity and attempt to explore new and novel situations. Assessment should view the balancing of inquisitiveness and wariness as predictive of emerging emotional development.
4. *Focus on individual differences:* Environmental influences on behavior play important roles in the degree to which infants develop.

Opportunities for behavioral growth and patterns in the quality of care may characterize and differentiate infants more than inherent differences.
5. *View development as a series of reorganizations:* Infants' development is not necessarily linear and incremental. Qualitative differences occur as the infant interacts and transforms its behavioral repertoire in response to situational challenges (pp. 835–836).

Data collected about mothers and their development, gestational milestones, obstetric concerns, neonatal reports, and the infant's development immediately following birth usually provide the basis of the evaluation. When a number of these variables are considered abnormal, and that number exceeds those found in the average infant population, the profile indicates a need for intervention. The presence of one specific problem might not generate concern. For example, prematurity might signal future developmental deviations, but deviations are more likely when prematurity is found in conjunction with infections, seizures, or some central-nervous-system disorders. The weight-for-gestational-age indicator becomes a predictor of psychosocial problems when an unusual indication is compounded by maternal drug or alcohol use, or psychosis. When infants are born within the average weight range, the presence of a congenital abnormality, birth trauma, hypoxia, or unfavorable psychological and social factors is used to identify high-risk children.

Systematic approaches for identifying at-risk infants itemize a variety of possible prenatal, perinatal, and postnatal factors associated with a child's physical and cognitive development. Most instruments, whether a checklist, health form, or personal interview, categorize clinical observations and accumulative scores predict whether a potential risk is likely to develop. While administering these tests, examiners should consider that many prenatal problems are transient rather than permanent and that some pregnancy and perinatal problems might not become fully evident until more complex behaviors begin to develop. Examiners should also keep in mind that some parents seem able to furnish a mildly impaired child with an experiential environment that allows the infant to compensate (Parmelee & Michaels, 1971).

### NEONATAL BEHAVIORAL ASSESSMENT SCALE (NBAS)

(Brazelton, 1973, 1984, Lippincott/Harper Publishers, Inc.)

This is one of the most popular and comprehensive infant assessment instruments. Although it was originally developed to record dimensions of reflexes, motor responses, and interactive behavior of normal infants, the NBAS is widely used to predict emotional and cognitive patterns in high-risk infants as well. The NBAS is an interactive assessment in which parents play a significant part in fostering the evolving skills of the infant. Medical professionals and paraprofessionals use this instrument, when they are working with parents, to identify the changes that the behavior and temperament of the infant are going to incur over time. The examiner must be trained in proper administration before the instrument is used, and experience in assessing normal infants is essential to scoring and interpreting the results. The NBAS is individually administered and, although untimed, usually takes 20–30 minutes to complete each measurement. Because the NBAS is dynamic in construct, repeated measurements during the first month of life are expected.

Normative data are not available because of the difficulty in defining what "normal" newborn behavior is. Because newborns are influenced by many factors, the factors constituting a normative population have not been sufficiently established for comparative purposes. Limited predictive-validity data are also available. The NBAS, in comparison to other neurological exams, seems likely to accurately predict abnormalities in infants and has less chance of falsely identifying an at-risk infant (Tronick & Brazelton, 1975).

Test reliability, typically determined by the stability of measures over time or across test forms, assumes that the traits measured are relatively stable. Most reported reliabilities for the NBAS are in the low to moderate range, and it has been suggested that the test-retest statistic might be inappropriate for this instrument (Brazelton, Nugent, & Lester, 1987). Because the NBAS measures dynamic (interactive) change, particularly that which occurs during the first ten days of life, expecting invariable performance across any two successive assessments could be counter to the instrument's purpose.

An infant's behavioral skills are evaluated by scoring twenty-eight items on a nine-point scale. These items reflect the adaptive and coping abilities of infants as they emerge into the extrauterine world and adjust to the environment's demands. These items are 1) decreasing response to light, 2) response decrement to rattle, 3) response decrement to bell, 4) response decrement to tactile stimulation of the foot, 5) orientation—inanimate, visual stimulus, 6) orientation—inanimate, auditory stimulus, 7) orientation—inanimate, visual and auditory stimulus, 8) orientation—animate visual stimulus, 9) orientation—animate, auditory stimulus, 10) orientation—animate, visual and auditory stimulus, 11) alertness, 12) general tonus, 13) motor maturity, 14) pull-to-sit, 15) cuddliness, 16) defensive movements, 17) consolability, 18) peak of excitement, 19) rapidity of buildup, 20) irritability, 21) activity, 22) tremulousness, 23) startle, 24) lability of skin color, 25) lability of states, 26) self-quieting activity, 27) hand-mouth facility, and 28) smiles. Two or three individual examinations are suggested, on days two or three and again either in one week or in two weeks to a month.

A series of neurological items that measure reflexes on a four-point scale are included. Deviation scores will identify gross abnormalities but these items are not proposed for detailed neurological purposes. Three or more abnormal scores, however, would suggest that a more specific neurological evaluation is needed. Nine supplementary items, specifically designed for high-risk infants, are particularly appropriate for premature infants. These items, which are considered optional, intend to summarize the quality of an infant's response, the responses' demands on the infant, and the amount of effort needed by the examiner to elicit those responses. The items relate to the 1) quality of alert responsiveness, 2) cost of attention, 3) examiner persistence needed, 4) general irritability, 5) robustness and endurance, 6) regulatory capacities, 7) state regulation, 8) balance of motor tone, and 9) reinforcement value of the infant's behavior.

The NBAS views infants as rapidly evolving, merging, and adapting their innate abilities to the stimulation and demands of the environment. The scale measures these changes as observed during specific interactions as well as during continuous observations occurring throughout the entire examination and scored at the conclusion. Examiners are encouraged to be flexible; that is, to modify the items or vary the assessment procedures in ways that will ensure that they are extracting the infant's best performance.

## ASSESSMENT OF PRESCHOOL LANGUAGE

Early detection of a language disorder is critical for a number of reasons. First, the child's linguistic difficulty can affect other areas of development, e.g., social/emotional development, self-help skills, and cognitive development (McClean & Snyder-McClean, 1978). Second, the child's ability to communicate affects his or her social integration within the preschool setting (Peterson, 1987). Finally, language delays can affect the child's educational and interpersonal achievements (Aram, Ekelman, & Nation, 1984).

If a screening procedure (e.g., formal screening test, observation, interview with a parent) identifies the infant or young child as having a potential language difficulty, an in-depth language assessment should be conducted. Teach-ers of preschoolers with special needs and other specialists (such as pediatrician, physical therapist) should have a basic understanding of language development and indicators of potential difficulties in language development. The reader is referred to Berry (1980) for a list of positive markers of language development and early signs of language difficulties.

Language-learning is part of the communication-learning system. Many elements comprise the whole and are "so interrelated as to be inseparable in the practical sense" (Newman, Creaghead, & Secord, 1985, p. 6). Language assessment should include the areas of form, content, and use (Cole, 1982). *Form* includes phonology (the study of the sound system), morphology (the study of basic meaningful units, e.g., plurals), and syntax (part of grammar). *Content* includes the meaning conveyed in the child's use of lexicons (vocabulary). *Use* (often referred to as functional language or pragmatics) includes the infant's and young child's ability to communicate with his or her caregivers and peers.

Evaluations of such skills as engaging in a conversation, obtaining wants and needs through gestures and words, and using augmentative communication systems (e.g., sign language, communication boards) are included in pragmatic assessment.

Traditional language assessment, which included the use of formal tests that yielded developmental age-norms and presented the child's linguistic deficits, is no longer in favor with many academicians and practitioners who use an interactionist perspective toward language development and assessment (e.g., Lund & Duchan, 1983; McClean & Synder-McClean, 1978; Newman, Creaghead, & Secord, 1985). In all areas of language, assessment in naturalistic settings is preferred by many language specialists (e.g., Berry, 1980; Lund & Duchan, 1983). Other specialists (e.g., McClean & Synder-McClean, 1978) suggest a combination of formal and informal assessment procedures. Furthermore, approaches for language analyses that yield patterns of the child performance in form, content, and use have emerged (Lund & Duchan, 1983; Newman, Creaghead, & Secord, 1985). Also, the processes that the child uses for discovering the language rules are sometimes assessed (Shriberg & Kwiatkowski, 1980).

We suggest that language assessment be conducted in natural settings, and that a combination of valid and reliable instruments and procedures be used. Checklists and observational systems can be used in the home and preschool. Formal assessment instruments can serve to validate the observations of educators and parents.

We present some of the most frequently used language assessment procedures and tests, and suggest that the reader refer to Berry (1980), Lund and Duchan (1983), McClean and Synder-McClean (1978), Miller (1981), Shriberg and Kwiatkowski (1980), and Wiig and Semel (1984) for a comprehensive review of language assessment. We provide a brief presentation of these procedures applied to all three areas—form, content, and use. Furthermore, we divide assessment instruments into receptive and expressive analysis.

Although we present these assessments as reflections of three components, we do not intend to imply that these language areas do not overlap and interact with each other. For example, the young child's inability to be intelligible to peers and caregivers can affect his or her language use. Because the child cannot easily interact with caregivers and peers, he or she will not develop the same functional skills that a more skilled communicator might develop. Furthermore, language assessment should be ongoing; it should consider the relationship of the child's linguistic development to that of other areas (e.g., social, motor, and cognitive skills). Language assessment should be conducted by a skilled, trained language therapist; the teacher of preschoolers with special needs and other therapists, however, should have an understanding of language development and the types of language assessment, and should also be able

to interpret the results in a manner that will facilitate comprehensive individual/interactive programs.

The preschool teacher or specialist who manages the infant's or young child's program might be able to detect indicators of linguistic retardation and refer the infant or young child for further assessment. For example, the REEL (Bzoch & League, 1971) and the Oliver: Parent-Administered Communication Inventory (Mac-Donald, 1978) can be used as tools in parental interviews concerning the child's linguistic development.

### Assessment of Linguistic Forms

These are formal and informal tests and procedures for the assessment of the infant's and young child's development of phonological and articulatory language, morphology, and syntax. As noted in the above section, therapists using a developmental/interactional approach prefer to make assessments of spontaneous, continuous language in natural settings. The most common type of measure of spontaneous language is the *language sample.* These samples must adhere to the same standards as formal tests—i.e., the assurances of reliability and validity. Lund and Duchan (1983) provide guidelines for conducting adequate language samples.

"A major portion of the acquisition of the phonological system of the language occurs during the first year" (Newman, Creaghead, & Secord, 1985, p. 47). With this information as a guide, preschool assessment teams should carefully consider the use of diagnostic measures of articulatory and phonological disorders, if any evidence obtained from screening, observations, or interviews with the parents, leads toward such a need. Typically, articulation, or "the actions of the organs of speech producing the sounds of speech" (Newman, Creaghead, & Secord, 1985, p. 13) is assessed concurrently with phonology.

Lund and Duchan (1983) recommend a multifaceted approach to phonological assessment that can determine irregularities in phonological development. Articulation tests and language samples can be part of the assessment. Shriberg and Kwiatkowski (1980) provide a procedure for the phonological analysis of continuous speech samples for children aged one to twelve years. They provide procedures for such analyses, information concerning the reliability and validity of the procedures, and a progression of phonological development commencing at birth. Only a trained clinician is capable of administering this procedure. The authors also recommend that the younger the child, the more samples might be needed to determine the child's phonological patterns.

Newman, Creaghead, and Secord (1985) critique the Shriberg-Kwiatkowski analysis as being a streamlined method of phonological analysis that is not extremely time-consuming; however, the procedures assess only ninety different words. For other phonological analyses made from language samples, see Ingram (1981), Lund and Duchan (1983), and Newman, Creaghead, and Secord (1985).

Other considerations made in phonological assessment are articulatory assessment and assessment of auditory discrimination (ability to distinguish between speech sounds). Newman, Creaghead, and Secord (1985) also provide suggestions for tests for stimulability, or the determination of "how readily a child can modify his/her errors when asked to imitate the examiner's correct production of them" (p. 76) and assessment of the oralfacial structures, e.g., an examination of the teeth, palatal and pharyngeal areas, and the tongue.

Popular formal tests for articulation, phonology, and auditory discrimination are the following: Goldman-Fristoe-Woodcock Auditory Skills Test Battery, Scales No. 2 & 3; Diagnostic Auditory Discrimination Test, Parts I and II (1976), which assesses discrimination of speech sounds (ages three years–adult); and the Goldman-Fristoe Test of Articulation (1972), which assesses the child's sound production. The Wepman Auditory Discrimination Test (Wepman, 1973) assesses discrimination of minimal word

pairs and can be administered to children aged five to eight years.

Morphological development can be assessed once the child begins to use words. Lund and Duchan (1983) define grammatical morphemes as "a set of words, usually little words, and a set of word endings that convey subtle meaning and serve special grammatical and pragmatic functions in language" (p. 111). According to Lund and Duchan (1983), the morphological system is the least difficult for clinical assessment. Moreover, the use of checklists is an efficient way to assess morphological development. The correct morphemes (e.g., plurals, possessives, adjective forms) can be easily detected as either apparent or missing from the child speech.

Because the clinician cannot assess the child's morphological development before the child uses words (typically, two- or three-word sentences), assessment cannot commence before the child's first birthday. Furthermore, a deficit approach to morphological assessment is not appropriate. That is, the specialist or teacher should view the child's errors as a disorder. By using error analysis, the clinician should not determine the morphological rules the child is developing. Sources for morphological analysis are Lund and Duchan (1983), Miller (1981), and Dever (1978). The clinician may use an assessment-measure such as the Berry-Talbott Test of Grammar (Berry & Talbott, 1966); however, this measure is not norm-referenced and is not helpful unless the clinician conducts a pattern analysis of the child's responses.

Morphological assessment is important in that delays in the development of morphological rules are apparent in language/learning disabled children (Wiig & Semel, 1980); however, if a young child is exhibiting difficulty with phonological development, morphological assessment should be secondary (Lund & Duchan, 1983).

*Syntax* is also included as a component of language form. Syntactical skill is the child's ability to place words into meaningful structures such as phrases, clauses, and sentences. Although syntax cannot be divorced from meaning or the child's communicative intent, analyses can determine regularities in the child's combinations of words (Lund & Duchan, 1983).

As with morphological analyses, running transcripts are the most appropriate method of gathering data for syntactic analysis. Dever (1978), Lund and Duchan (1983), and Miller (1981) offer stages of syntactic development and methods for syntactic analysis. Both Lund and Duncan (1983) and Miller (1981) discuss formal tests for syntactic analysis. A popular test is the Developmental Sentence Types (DST) (Lee, 1966), which analyzes 100 utterances and is intended for use on children aged twenty-two months to six years. The Developmental Sentence Analysis (DSS) (1974) is an analysis of 50 utterances and is intended for use on children aged three to seven years. The author's intention is to provide a tool for descriptive analysis rather than a mere reporting of scores.

The content of language is often referred to as *semantics,* or the meanings of words. Traditionally, meanings have been assessed as a component of the child's linguistic skills; however, current semantic assessment determines the child's use of relational language (i.e., expression of temporal and spatial relationships as manifested by such functional words as prepositions), use of words in context, and expression of abstract concepts. Referential meaning is one of the earliest developed components of semantics. The caregiver and the child establish "joint referents." Through joint interactions, "the child learns the specific referents or lexical tags of objects, actions, and events as specified by adults" (Lucas, 1980, p. 2). The child's relationships with caregivers and his or her environment are represented in word usage. If the environment is meaningful to the child, he or she will attempt to represent those surroundings and relationships in his or her language.

Semantic assessment is more complex and time-consuming than other types of language assessment. Lund and Duchan (1983) indicate that more than one language sample is necessary for determination of the child's representation of meaning. Lucas (1980), Lund and Duchan (1983), McClean and Snyder-McClean (1978), and Miller (1981) provide guidelines for semantic analysis.

Two formal assessment procedures for semantic analysis that include environmental analysis are the Environmental Prelanguage Battery (Horstmeier & MacDonald, 1978) and the Environmental Language Inventory (MacDonald, 1978). The prelanguage battery can be used for preschool children who function at or below the one-word level (Horstmeier & MacDonald, 1978, p. 1). The test has verbal and nonverbal sections and is based on the "development of the child meanings . . . and the social processes enabling the child to use language for its primary function, communication" (Horstmeier & MacDonald, 1978, p. 4). The Environmental Language Inventory (MacDonald, 1978) is similar to the Prelanguage Battery and includes the Oliver: Parent-Administered Communication Inventory.

The assessment of the functional use, or pragmatics, component of language is relatively new. Lund and Duchan (1983) term the 1980s as the pragmatics revolution. According to Duchan (1984), the focus on social interactions and their relationships to language has provided an impetus for the study of pragmatics. The focus on the conversation is one aspect of pragmatics. Lund and Duchan (1983) organize analysis of pragmatics around four categories: (1) situational context, (2) intentional context, (3) listener context, and (4) the linguistic context. A thorough discussion of pragmatics is beyond the scope of this chapter. For further information, refer to Cole (1982), Duchan (1984), Lucas (1980), Lund and Duchan (1983), McClean and Snyder-McClean (1978).

Language samples are sometimes used for pragmatic assessment. The communicative intent of young children has been studied by such individuals as Halliday (1975) and Dore (1974;

1979), and these findings have been used in the analysis of the pragmatics component of language. For guidelines for pragmatic analysis, see Lucas (1980), Lund and Duchan (1983), and Miller (1981).

The assessment strategies presented here are designed primarily for young children who will develop speech and functional language skills. The educator of preschoolers with special needs will also encounter children whose development does not follow the typical stages of language development and who might need radically different assessments and interventions in order to facilitate communication. For example, some children will remain nonvocal and will need to rely on alternative means of communication, e.g., manual signs, communication boards. Specialists must be prepared to decide whether or not the student will need such intervention. For help in making these types of decisions, we refer the reader to Musselwhite and St. Louis (1982) and Shane (1981).

Other patterns of language development can be influenced by the characteristics manifested by children who are often labeled as autistic. For characteristics of the emerging language in autistic children, see Fay and Schuler (1980).

## INTELLIGENCE TESTING

Intelligence testing of young children, particularly infants, mirrors the historical pattern of the study of cognitive ability during this century. Early investigators, for example, were interested only in the abilities of very young children, because they believed that severely mentally retarded individuals performed as normal two-year-old children. They assumed that by making these comparisons, they would be able to predict the future development of mentally retarded individuals and the positions they would take in society. It was not until the 1920s that theorists questioned the assumption that the intelligence of preschool children as well as school-aged children is stable over time. The notion of fixed,

or unalterable intelligence, coincided with genetic explanations of ability. Intelligence, in these terms, was a function of the structural integrity of a young child's neurological makeup.

Although widespread testing of very young children did not begin until the 1940s, the foundation was set two decades prior. One serious attempt at measuring the IQ of very young children and infants revised downward the measures of coordination, speech, recognition and imitation from Binet's test (Kuhlman, 1922). This test was rarely used but established the need for scores that were systematically normed and reliable. With the growing popularity of preschool programs and the belief that their effects could alter intelligence, the period of 1920–1940 saw the development of a plethora of tests. Although many of these tests demonstrated moderately reliable measures, it was their predictive validity that determined whether a test was successful or not. (See Brooks & Weinraub, 1976, for a detailed history of infant intelligence testing.) Of these, tests by Gessell, Bayley, and Cattell were used most for measuring intelligence in infants and remain in use today by assessment teams. (See Chapter 5 for further discussion.)

Although arguments persist today that heredity contributes the major share of the performance variance associated with intelligence (e.g., Jensen, 1969), we contend that genetics alone most likely plays a trivial part in the expression of traits, demonstrated by young children, that are associated with intelligence and cognitive ability. This expression embodies the complex interaction of inherited abilities and the environment. Attending to stimuli, storing and recalling information, and problem-solving are language-based, cognitive processes; these develop as young children find meaning in their environment. The significance of the experience (the product) influences the mechanisms with which children establish the way (the process) in which they effectively interact with their environment. Meaningfulness is contingently linked to the reinforcement provided during the interaction.

The impact of early experience on later cognitive capacity has been established, and studies have shown little if any correlation of intelligence scores of children younger than two years of age with measures taken later in life (e.g., McCall, 1979). And it is assumed by educators of young, special-needs children that early intervention produces substantial and immediate benefits (e.g., White, Bush & Casto, 1985). But whether young children possess a capacity for systematic change remains in question, because some current research is inconclusive. Intensive, early-intervention programs have produced gains in IQ scores for disadvantaged children (e.g., Ramey & Campbell, 1987; Zigler & Freedman, 1987), but unfortunately these gains do not endure for more than two or three years. Although particular factors of these programs, such as the extent of parental involvement and the age at which children enter the program, appear to be more influential than other factors, the general lack of demonstrated longterm effects has tarnished the early-intervention position. White and Casto (1985) suggest that because most studies that question the efficacy of early intervention did not include special-needs children in their sample, more intensive study is required.

To rely heavily on change in one variable (IQ score) to indicate the impact of early interventions on cognitive ability, seriously disregards the dynamic interactions in which children engage during their daily experiences, that contribute to their mental developmental. Intelligence quotients alone cannot represent children's cognitive ability because environmental factors can shape both the magnitude of an intellectual trait and its change over time.

A developmental / interactional approach to measuring the intellect of young children considers that traditional IQ measures are necessary but that they should be recognized as stable and therefore unable to disclose dynamic change. McCall (1987) suggests factors that go beyond the traditional measures in aiding our understanding of intellectual development in young children. These factors include sibling interactions, birth order and spacing (Zajonc, Markus, & Markus, 1979), illness, and the influence of nonfamily members. Research is beginning to show that these factors, along with culture, can actually contribute as much as half of the cognitive-performance variance associated with environment. While we agree with this premise, information-gathering to this extent might be unrealistic for many preschool educators, and we offer a modified data-collection protocol.

Assessing cognition in infants and young children can be facilitated by the sorting of interactional patterns into categories. These categories vary from responding to sensory stimuli, to using toys and other objects for imaginary play, and problem-solving. Placed within these categories, behaviors are observed and measured repeatedly; using this process, the examiner can generate assessment hypotheses. The essential feature of each category is a recognition that cognition in very young children changes rapidly, often in uneven patterns, and that an evaluation must take into account these changes.

Following this paragraph are categories representing young children's developmental changes that pertain to cognitive ability. Included within each category are examples of assessment questions that would be associated with these abilities and would help operationalize an interactional assessment. We have selected these categories according to our experience with young children and have adapted them to a generalized consensus about child development. Although these categories appear hierarchical, they are not presented with that notion in mind.

*Responding to environmental stimulation*: Beginning to recognize their environment, very young children attend to sounds, visual changes in light and movement, and touch. Assessment questions would evaluate the quality and quantity of ways in which the child orients himself or herself to sounds, and to visual and tactile stimuli. For example, measures may indicate response time, startle reflexes, or length of engagement with an object.

*Recognizing people and objects in the environment*: Beginning to make sense of their world, children recognize that certain events (i.e., feeding) and people are consistently available to them. Socialization is a function of these interactions. For instance, assessment questions would relate to changes in children's response patterns that occur when a primary caregiver enters and leaves their environment, when toys are given to them and then taken away, and when they are confronted with unfamiliar experiences.

*Modeling*: As their environment becomes recognized as a source of meaning, children will begin to imitate what they see and hear. Behavior modeling may involve duplicating a verbal request from a caregiver, repeating words, or imitating a motor response, such as picking up a toy block or helping to turn the pages of a book while being read to. Assessment questions would be focused on the child's ability to model or imitate a variety of verbal and motor requests.

*Play*: Using objects and people are common ways in which children begin to identify and interact with their environment. Play activities, whether with others or in isolation, can be used as a source of assessment information. Cognitive ability may be measured by analysis of the production and quality of language used by children at play. The amount of engagement, the complexity and richness of the activity and the ways children use their imaginations may indicate developmental delays or potential for future difficulties.

*Indicators of academic ability*: Academic readiness is indicated when young children exhibit knowledge about concepts that are considered to be related to later learning. The ability to categorize objects by color, size, or function, or to remember simple number facts and letter names, can be used to predict whether school tasks would eventually present problems.

*Social cognition*: Children begin to establish that there is a relationship between their actions and what happens to them as a consequence of their actions. This recognition influences future social behavior, such as causal attributions and beliefs about what occurs as a function of their action that is under either environmental or personal control. Children's parts in an interactive play activity might demonstrate whether or not they will initiate a response or whether they will allow the activity to continue. Other indices of causality could emerge from children's maneuvering of objects to obtain an unanticipated outcome.

*Problem-solving*: Being able to successfully interact with environmental demands is closely linked to adaptive behavior. Accommodation might require a child to have ready a variety of problem-solving strategies and an ability to invoke the proper plan. For many special-needs children, adaptive behavior plays a major role in the determination of intellectual ability. Asked of young children, questions such as "Does a child use more than one way to move around obstacles?" or "Does a child use objects as 'tools' to produce a desired outcome?" would help in describing problem-solving ability.

The use of standardized instruments to conduct a cognitive assessment of infants and very young children should occur in conjunction with informal observations, parental interviews, and medical- and historical-data gathering. Formal measures most commonly used with preschool children are the Stanford-Binet (Terman & Merrill, 1972), WPPSI (Weschler, 1967) and the McCarthy (1972) Scales. This section restricts its review to tests used with very young children and infants, and will describe the Uzgiris and Hunt Scales, Bayley's Scales of Infant Development, and the Cattell Infant Intelligence Scale.

## UZGIRIS AND HUNT SCALES
(Uzgiris & Hunt, 1975, University of Illinois Press)

This test is based on Piaget's theory and consists of six scales. The test is suited to measuring sensorimotor correlates to cognitive development in infants and older, developmentally delayed, and at-risk children. Cognitive performance is not considered global but a composite of (1) visual pursuit and the permanence of object—ability to recognize objects outside of the immediate perceptual field, (2) means of obtaining desired environmental events—ability to initiate actions to achieve a particular goal, (3) the development of vocal and gestural imitation—ability to differentiate and imitate sounds and gestures requiring body movements, (4) the development of operational causality—ability to anticipate and establish antecedent-consequence relationships, (5) the construction of object relations in space—ability to appreciate three-dimensional space, to track and locate objects, and (6) the development of schemes for relating to objects—ability to use toys progressively as extensions of the infant. To measure each domain, the Uzgiris and Hunt uses an ordinal scale and thereby treats the concepts or constructs as successive achievement levels. Lower-order skills must be attained before subsequent cognitive skills can be developed. A profile of strengths and weaknesses can be constructed because performance on any one scale is considered unrelated to the parallel scales.

Test reliabilities were established from small samples of infants from middle-class families. Test-retest stability measures between observers were high (over 92%), and all scales were highly correlated with age. Scale intercorrelations were also high but decreased considerably when age was partialed out. The samples were not used primarily to establish age-level normative data. Limited predictive validity has been established (Wachs, 1975).

## BAYLEY SCALES OF INFANT DEVELOPMENT
(Bayley, 1969, The Psychological Corporation)

The scales have been used with children aged two to thirty months for more than forty years and have undergone extensive restandardization during this time. The scales are divided into a Mental Scale and a Motor Scale. The mental scale contains 163 items, which determine an infant's ability to learn a task, demonstrate adaptive behavior, and attempt early communication. This scale yields a mental-development index. The motor scale, containing 81 items, measures general body control and coordination of large muscles; results are compiled into a psychomotor development index. The Bayley establishes a child's current developmental status relative to other children of the same age. Experience is required to properly administer the scales. Included is an Infant Behavior Record for noting quantitative and qualitative aspects of an infant's social and emotional behavior during the test's administration. Split-half reliabilities, using a stratified sample of white and nonwhite, urban and rural children, averaged over .86 for both scales. Correlations with intelligence tests such as the Stanford-Binet have ranged from extremely low (.02) to moderate (.53). Standardization does not include children from bilingual or non-English-speaking families.

## CATTELL INFANT INTELLIGENCE SCALE
(Cattell, 1940, 1960, The Psychological Corporation)

This test was initially designed to standardize the assessment of mental ability and to provide an objective interpretation of infants' performances. Used with children from birth to 2½ years old, the test's items were modified from those of the Gessell, Minnesota Preschool, and Merrill-Palmer Scales; the test was intended to be a downward extension of the Stanford-Binet. Each age level contains five items that are scored on a pass/fail bias. Items are related to the infant's verbalizations, motor control, and the manipulation of objects such as pencils and pegboards. Split-half reliabilities range from .56 for the three-month-old scale and increase to approximately .90 for the later ages. However, it appears that children receiving high scores at a very young age tend to remain above average after three years, but low scores at a very young age have much less predictive validity unless accompanied by other related indices of poor performance. Overall, this test should be used in conjunction with other observations gathered by experienced professionals.

## ASSESSMENT OF MOTOR DEVELOPMENT AND DISORDERS

According to P.L. 99–457, the Individual Family Service Plan is to include a statement of the child's physical development (Sec. 677, P.L. 99–457, 1986). We include motor development in this category. Assessment of motor skills requires interdisciplinary cooperation and planning (Browder, 1987). Although the preschool teacher can assist in assessing motor development (e.g., via checklists), the physical and occupational therapists, and medical specialists must be involved, especially if a difficulty is suspected.

According to Conner, Williamson, and Siepp (1978), a child's motor development is not complete until the age of five or six years; however, "many of the important components have been introduced by the end of the first year" (p. 99). As with other developmental areas, e.g., cognition and language, motor development cannot be viewed as apart from all other developmental areas (Lorton & Walley, 1979). Furthermore, the child's motor development can affect other developmental areas, e.g., cognition (Conner, Williamson, & Siepp, 1978).

Because the infant learns from movement sensations that result from motor activities, child-development experts use the term *sensorimotor development* (Conner, Williamson, & Siepp, 1978). Attention to several principles of sensorimotor development can guide the assessment team in determining the child's motor development.

First, sensorimotor development is sequential. "It occurs in a definite sequence over time, with each new acquisition based on those that went before" (Conners, Williamson, & Siepp, 1978, p. 100). Developmental milestones can be used to define the infant's, toddler's, and young child's motor development (Brazelton, 1969; Caplan, 1973; Caplan & Caplan, 1981; Dodson, 1970; White, 1975).

Motor development is also guided by other principles of maturation:

1. The stages in motor-skill development overlap. That is, an infant or young child may be experimenting with a new motor skill while he or she is mastering another one.
2. Motor-skill development progresses in the cephalo-to-caudal (head to tail) direction. The infant gains control over his head, neck, and trunk muscles before his legs.
3. Development progresses in a proximal-to-distal direction (from the midline to away from the midline, or toward the periphery).
4. Motor development is at first random and then refined; gross movements are segmented into more specific patterns (Conner, Williamson, & Siepp, 1978; Dunn, 1982).

Often, motor development is divided into gross motor skills (large-muscle movement) and fine motor skills (small-muscle movement). The fine-motor control progresses more slowly than the large-muscle control.

Early identification of motor disorders is critical for infants and preschoolers. For example, for children with cerebral palsy, handling and positioning is necessary to prevent "needless deformity or loss of function" (Kneedler, 1984, p. 259). Regular and periodic assessments of sensorimotor development and motor movements are important because all physical anomalies are not discovered during the newborn period (Erickson, 1976; Froman, 1983).

Because the parents typically interact with medical specialists first, the physician must be integrally involved in early detection of motor difficulties. If the child is referred to a team for assessment, interdisciplinary assessment is necessary. The reader is referred to Copeland, Ford, and Solon (1976), Connor, Williamson, and Siepp (1978), Cratty (1980), Erickson (1976), Froman, (1983), Gallahue (1982), and Harryman (1976), for discussions of motor development assessment from infancy through the preschool ages and for assessment of motor disorders.

## Motor Assessment Tools

Developmental checklists are beneficial in identifying potential motor problems. If a child does not fall within the range of normal motor development on these checklists, he or she should be referred to the physical and occupational therapists and related specialists for further assessments. These checklists are "snap-shots" of movement and can not substitute for continual, ongoing observations. Furthermore, they often do not include observations of such important factors as muscle tone, motivation for movement, and reflex sequences.

Two early-intervention, developmental profiles that include motor-development checklists for ages birth to six years are (1) Volume 2: Early Intervention Developmental Profile (Rogers et al., 1981) and Volume 5: Preschool Developmental Profile (Brown et al., 1981), both of the Developmental Programming for Infants and Young Children (Schafer & Moersch, 1981), and (2) the Hawaii Early Learning Profile (HELP) (Furuno et al., 1984) and Help for Special Preschoolers: Assessment Checklist: Ages 3–6 (Santa Cruz County, 1987). (Screening measures that include motor development are listed in the screening section of this chapter.)

The Early Intervention Developmental Profile (Rogers, Donovan, Eugenior, Brown, Lynch, Moersch, & Schafer, 1981) was designed to be used by a multidisciplinary team who combine their skills in the areas of motor, language, and cognitive development, and who incorporate parents as an integral part of the team process. Specific programming follows the assessment process. Gross- and fine-motor skills are assessed. Also, integration for reflexes are included. Skills are listed by chronological ages, e.g., 0–2 months.

The Hawaii Early Learning Profile is also designed for multidisciplinary team use. The gross- and fine-motor sections include 146 and 93 items, respectively, for use on an age range of 0–36 months. Reflex integration is also included. The Help for Special Preschoolers Assessment Checklist: Ages 3–6 is a criterion-referenced assessment with measures of sensory-perceptual skills (e.g., subjects are required to use tactile cues to match like objects: hot/cold, wet/dry, p. 7), fine motor/visual discrimination skills (e.g., subject is asked to string large beads, p. 8), and gross motor skills. Wheelchair skills for the nonambulatory child are also included, as well as a checklist for swimming skills. Both these checklists are used through observation and parental interview.

One individually administered, standardized motor test that is often used for preschool assessment is the Bruininks-Oseretsky Test of Motor Proficiency (Bruininks, 1978). This test's age range is 4½ to 14½ years; it therefore measures only the upper age range of preschool children. The complete battery can be administered in 45–60 minutes, and the short form in 15–20 minutes. The test includes gross motor development (running speed, balance, bilateral coordination, and strength), gross and fine motor development (upper-limb coordination), and fine motor development (response speed, visual-motor control, and upper-limb speed and dexterity). The Complete Battery includes forty-six items and the Short Form includes fourteen items that can be used for a screening measure. To use the test, the examiner must have advanced training in measurement, guidance, and individual psychological assessment.

For presentations of other standardized, motor development tests for infants and young children, see Davis (1980) and Peterson (1987).

## SOCIAL AND EMOTIONAL ASSESSMENT

Perhaps the most heterogeneous category of behaviors assessed in young at-risk and special-needs children depicts their social and emotional development. Although actual prevalence is not known, there are probably fewer preschoolers than school-aged children with social and behavioral disorders. Social and emotional behavior of young children includes sharing, cooperation, taking turns, and following rules. Behavioral disorders include aggressiveness, withdrawal, depression, attentional deficits, and hyperactivity. The problems of many preschool children do not become apparent until they enter school or other structured environments that place unexpected demands on their performance. The early experiences of children, the nature and intensity of the care provided, and the attachments made when they respond to their sensations, actions, and feelings, provide the basis for later affective ability. Positive and negative reactions to their performance in interacting with their environment will maintain or eliminate behaviors as well.

Previous opinions about the causality of behavior have led researchers to investigate parenting patterns, for example, and other single sources, as the precipitators of disorders. The derivation of emotions, i.e., whether they are innate, learned, or a drive-reduction, is not clear; moreover, no one account helps explain infants' emotional behavior in particular. Also, theory offers little assistance to assessment and planning of an intervention. We contend that a clear understanding of the social facilitation and reciprocity that occur within a child's environment best serves the assessment process. However, we caution, as Kaufmann's (1981) review demonstrates, that family relations alone cannot be directly associated with a child's behavioral disorders. Social and emotional disorders in children are more likely a matter of the interactional patterns established between the developing child and his or her environment.

What is not clear, however, is the relationship between the subsequent social and emotional difficulties and the type, magnitude, and schedule of these early episodes. A multitude of behaviors are possible when these factors confront a variant child's development patterns, and this complexity makes accurate assessment difficult. For example, a common notion is that children confront a variety of stressful situations (physiological and social) that either impel them over developmental milestones or require a need for coping strategies (e.g., Selye, 1982). Some examples are loss of a loved one, illness, problems associated with socioeconomic level, and prematurity. At one time it was thought that having a handicapped child in the family could also cause emotional problems among that child's siblings, but that has been discounted (e.g., Breslau, 1982). Because both internal and external factors can contribute to the stress it appears that children's reactions to stress are based on the meaning that they attribute to the circumstance in which it occurs. Age level, gender, and cognitive ability also seem to play a role. A multi-element assessment would require an analysis of all components; the most difficult to derive is the meaning generated by the child him- or herself.

Social and emotional problems are usually measured only after they have become serious enough to demand intervention. There are no available instruments that can accurately predict future social and emotional problems by evaluating very young children. Exacerbating the difficulty is that group and family expectations make it difficult to distinguish between what is "normal" and "deviant" behavior, particularly when cultural diversity is taken into consideration. Often, deviance (i.e., a behavior deemed unacceptable by those doing the observing) is deduced from the frequency and intensity of a behavior, and the effect that a behavior or series of behaviors has on the child or those around the child. It is often difficult to determine if a young child is truly disturbed or just disturbing to those around him or her. Additionally, immature behavior may be acceptable when a child is alone but causes difficulty when the child plays with other children. And as children grow older, excessive behaviors such as hyperactivity or inattention are more likely to cause concern than the less noticeable but equally important manifestations of depression or withdrawal.

Young children's ability to interact with adults and other young children is part of the socialization process. Social and emotional development during the preschool years is heavily influenced by changes in physiological states, cognitive ability, and language facility. They provide a child with the tools to mobilize an interaction. This occurs mainly for infants involved with their primary caregivers and for young children at play. Affect in infants (e.g., smiling, eye contact, requests to satisfy needs) constructs a familiarization process and the basis for attachment with the caregiver. Lack of attachment with one significant person within the first two years of life is related to future antisocial behavior.

Play is seen as an opportunity for children to develop independence, practice their behavior, and learn about the people, objects and events that define their world (Weisler & McCall, 1976). These situations should serve as the settings in which assessment would yield the most reliable measures. Careful arrangement of a play experience provides an evaluator with a structure in which child-centered and environment-centered variables can be assessed.

Types of play can represent social-development benchmarks. Parten's (1932) description of developmental change associated with a typical child at play is still appropriate and can be applied to the social and emotional assessments of children with special needs. *Unoccupied play* occurs when a child will observe anything of interest; if nothing of interest is available, the child is content with entertaining him- or herself. *Solitary* play occurs when a child watches from a distance other children play, or plays by him- or herself. It is most noticeable among children between the ages of twenty-four and thirty-six months. Children may take the role of *onlooker,* in which they watch other children play, might attempt to converse with them, but do not attempt to play with them. As he or she develops advancing recognition of other children, a child might venture closer to the group, play *parallel,* yet independently, might even mimic the group's activity, but is unable to maintain social engagement. No at-

tempt is made to alter or interfere with the behaviors of others. This usually occurs between thirty and forty-two months of age. Once social interactions become more involved and less self-centered, *associative play* occurs: children, usually between forty-two and fifty-four months, share activities, join in a common discourse about toys or games, etc., yet do so randomly. Advancing social and cognitive ability will enable children to play *cooperatively*—to use rules, assign roles, and expect each other to perform accordingly. Young children will also use their imaginations when at play and display egocentric, overt language. These verbalizations guide behavior, establish a sense of self-control and independence, and are useful as sources of information about behavior.

## Assessment Techniques

Observational techniques using qualitative analyses (anecdotal recordings) and behavior ratings in natural settings provide the best results. These results are valid, however, only to the extent that the recorded observations are unbiased and that the observer has not interfered with the natural interactions. Naturalistic observation ratings are time-consuming and require all participants to adjust to the observing, before typical behaviors are displayed. For instance, if a playground game is used as the assessment setting, the observer would have to take part in several games before behaviors again become characteristic. Abbreviated assessments are usually not reliable. The use of systematic procedures to identify the target behavior(s) and to collect and record data will validate the measures (see Chapter 8 for a variety of techniques). Within observational periods, the natural events can be orchestrated to disclose authentic behaviors. Also, interactional patterns (such as those in dyads or triads) are closely observed. Parent and teacher interviews, self-reports, and ratings of the behavioral traits complete the process.

Very few dependable, standardized observational/rating scales for children below kindergarten age are available (see Chapter 8 for descriptions of the Behavior Problem Checklist and the Walker Behavior Problem Identification Checklist as popular examples). Most report poor to moderate reliability and validity coefficients because of their dependence on verbal measures, lack of operational definitions of behaviors, and inconclusive theoretical construct of socioemotional development. Some multidimensional instruments that contain subparts that measure social skills and emotional disorders are described in the next section of this chapter.

Assessing a young child's social and emotional makeup to predict how that makeup will contribute to the child's developing coping behavior requires an understanding of child development and the means by which social interactions guide and shape a child's world. According to this premise, intervention plans that are based on reliable observational data are more effective than those based on scores from commercial instruments.

## MULTIDIMENSIONAL DEVELOPMENTAL DIAGNOSTIC TESTS

There are many preschool tests that purport to diagnose specific developmental needs of typical and special-needs preschoolers. (For a listing and description of many of these tests, the reader is referred to Mitchell, 1985, & Peterson, 1987.) We present a sample of these tests for discussion.

The use of developmental tests for diagnosing preschool children is controversial (Switzky, 1985; Switsky, Rotatori, Miller, & Freagon, 1979; Walker, 1985). Because these tests are either normed on typical-needs children or derived from previously determined developmental norms (e.g., Gessel, 1940; White, 1975), their usefulness in assessing behavioral domains of children with special needs (e.g., visual impairment) is diminished (Switzky, 1985). Furthermore, in many instances, we are not knowledgeable about the development of young children with special needs. As we note in the section on

the developmental-interactional model, development, for the most part, is the result of the complex interactions of the child with the environment and caregivers; moreover, these developmental areas can not be separated into discrete and separate entities. If one developmental area, e.g., language, is impaired, others will be affected. Furthermore, caregivers might act differently with the child with a special need than they would with a typical child (Mahoney & Powell, 1988); these interactions will, in turn, affect the child's development. These developmental tests can not replace interdisciplinary assessments, observations, and interactions with the infant or young child and his or her family. The tests can serve as indicators of the need for more fine-grained analyses.

Most of these tests assess the areas of motor, perceptual, language, social-emotional, cognition, and self-help skills. We present a brief discussion of some of the popular or frequently cited tests (Johnson & Beauchamp, 1987). These are the Brigance Diagnostic Inventory of Early Development (Brigance, 1978), the Battelle Developmental Inventory (Newborg, Stock, Wnek, Guidubaldi, & Suinicki, 1984), the Learning Accomplishment Profile for Infants (Lemay, Griffin, & Sanford, 1981), and the Learning Accomplishment Profile-Diagnostic Edition-Revised (Lemay, Griffin, & Sanford, 1981), the Early Intervention Developmental Profile (Rogers et al., 1981), and the Preschool Developmental Profile (Brown et al., 1981), The Hawaii Early Learning Profile (Furono, O'Reilly, Hosaka, Aleman, & Zeiloft, 1984) and the Help for Special Preschooler: Assessment Checklist: Ages 3–6 (Santa Cruz, 1987).

### BRIGANCE DIAGNOSTIC INVENTORY OF EARLY DEVELOPMENT

(Brigance, 1978, Curriculum Associates, Inc.)

For ages 0–7 years, this is a criterion-referenced test, which compares the child's performance to the mastery of a specific task or skill area. These tests are an outgrowth of the behavioristic or task-analytic approach and its attempts to individualize instruction. These tests are typically used to target behaviors that need to be addressed in intervention. One major difficulty with criterion-referenced tests is that their quality is difficult to establish (McLoughlin & Lewis, 1981).

The Brigance Diagnostic Inventory of Early Development reflects the typical difficulties of criterion-referenced measurement. The manual provides no reliability data or information concerning norms. The tasks are based on traditional developmental scales (e.g., Gessell). The final edition was field-tested for content validity on 100 developmental specialists in sixteen states. The tasks do not, however, provide a fine-grained analysis that is necessary for evaluation of the more severely involved infant or young child. Also, no detailed information of tasks exists for appropriate auditory or visual assessment (Bagnato, 1985). In addition, no social/emotional tasks are included.

The test concerns ninety-eight skills in five areas: (1) motor skills, including preambulatory motor skills and fine motor skills, (2) self-help skills, (3) speech-related skills, including prespeech, (4) general knowledge/comprehension, and (5) written language skills (readiness), basic reading skills, manuscript writing and math skills. The test is inexpensive and the manual provides suggestions for obtaining information from multiple sources and techniques. Also, suggestions for modification of the tasks are included. The test manual also provides information for the targeting of instructional objectives.

### BATTELLE DEVELOPMENTAL INVENTORY (BDI)

(Newborg, Stock, Wnek, Guidubaldi, & Suinicki, 1984, DLM Teaching Resources, Inc.)

This is a relatively new developmental test. This test was designed to assess strengths and weaknesses in children from birth to eight years in the following domains: personal-social (e.g., adult interaction), adaptive (e.g., eating, dressing, toileting), motor (including fine and gross skills), communication, and cognitive. The test takes approximately one hour to complete and

also includes a screening test. The test's authors purport that the test can be used for the planning of instruction and intervention. The test's manual includes suggestions for adaptations in administration to children with specific special needs. Observation and interviews with the parents are also included in the overall assessment.

McClean, McCormick, Bruder, and Burdg (1987), after a review of the research on the BDI, conclude "although the Battelle is a very new test, it has already been received with enthusiasm" (pp. 238–239). The technical adequacy of the test has been assessed with school-aged and younger children (see McClean, McCormick, Bruder, & Burdg, 1987); however, more research is needed to determine test-retest reliability and its use for early childhood, special-needs intervention and program evaluation.

Disadvantages of the BDI, as outlined by McClean, McCormick, Bruder, and Burdg (1987) include "administration time, training requirements for administrators, acquisition of assessment materials, and extrapolation procedures used in calculating extreme standard scores" (p. 244).

Advantages are the fact that standard scores are provided across all the domains, so that strengths and weaknesses can be determined and adaptations for sensory, motor, and behavioral disabilities can be made (McClean, McCormick, Bruder, & Burdg, 1987).

### THE EARLY LEARNING ACCOMPLISHMENT PROFILE FOR INFANTS (EARLY LAP)

(Glover, Preminger, & Sanford, 1978, Kaplan School Supply)

### LEARNING ACCOMPLISHMENT PROFILE-DIAGNOSTIC EDITION-REVISED

(Lemay, Griffen, & Sanford, 1981, Kaplan School Supply)

These are criterion-referenced tests for children aged 0–6 years. The Early LAP, for children from birth to age three years, assesses the following skills: gross and fine motor, cognitive, language, self-help, social, and emotional. The test "facilitates programming for severely handicapped young children" (Peterson, 1987, p. 305). The LAP-Revised provides information on acquired, absent, and emergent capabilities in the areas of fine and gross motor, language, cognitive, self-help, and social skills. The items for both tests, listed in behavioral terms, are drawn from other widely used instruments. Developmental age and age range are provided. A classroom teacher can use the tests to measure the young child's progress.

### EARLY INTERVENTION DEVELOPMENTAL PROFILE
(Rogers et al., 1981, University of Michigan Press)

### PRESCHOOL DEVELOPMENTAL PROFILE
(Brown et al., 1981, University of Michigan Press)

These tests are part of a series for program implementation for children aged 0–60 months (Schafer & Moersch, 1981). The intent is to combine assessment with programming. The tests were designed to be used by multidisciplinary teams who have combined skills in motor, language, and cognitive development. Parents are included as part of the team. Six areas of development are assessed: perceptual/fine-motor, cognition, language, social/emotional, self-care, and gross motor. The materials can be adapted for children with special needs. Supplemental materials are provided so that specialists can train parents to work with their child in the home environment. Behavioral objectives are provided for the items. Ongoing assessment is encouraged.

Items in the tests are arranged according to developmental age ranges and are similar to test items on other developmental tests. The cognitive component is based on Piagetian tasks, e.g., the sensori-motor stage of development. The test is not standardized; instead items are taken from other instruments and the literature. When items exist on more than one instrument, an average for the item was given. Concurrent validity has been determined with such measures as the Bayley and the REEL. Test-retest reliability measures indicate that the test has adequate reliability. Fourteen handicapped children were tested on the items and the results

compared favorably to information from multidisciplinary assessment teams. More research is needed on the technical adequacy. The items are not fine-grained for intervention for a more severely involved infant or young child; however, the stimulation activities that accompany that profiles provide additional developmental information, intervention strategies, and suggestions for modifying the tasks for the visual and hearing impaired and the motoric involved.

### HAWAII EARLY LEARNING PROFILE (HELP)
(Furuno et al., 1984, VORT Corporation)

### HELP FOR SPECIAL PRESCHOOLERS ASSESSMENT CHECKLIST: AGES 3–6
(Santa Cruz County Office of Education, 1987, VORT Corporation)

These are also criterion-referenced, developmental checklists. Items are listed by chronological age levels. Charts are provided to assist the examiners with a visual representation of the child's abilities and progress (Furuno et al., 1984). For use with children aged 0–36 months, 685 developmental skills are included in the HELP, in the following areas: cognitive, expressive language, gross motor, fine motor, social-emotional, and self-help. The test's constructors recommend the use of a multidisciplinary team, which includes an early childhood special educator, psychologist, speech/language pathologist, and physical and occupational therapist. This team should be involved in the assessment and planning for the multiply handicapped child. The authors note that special adaptations (e.g., positioning and handling) may be necessary for use on a child with physical and/or neuro-motor disabilities and for children with hearing or visual impairment. Information may be obtained from a variety of sources, e.g., observations, parent interviews, etc. A HELP Activity Guide is provided for the planning of intervention and instruction.

The Help for Special Preschoolers Assessment Checklist: Ages 3–6 assesses over 600 skill areas, which are developmentally sequenced; the age ranges represent normal developmental milestones. These items, as were those of the HELP, were selected from existing tests and literature, and were edited by field reviewers. This test is administered visually to one child at a time. Blocks and cards are used as stimuli, and administration is facilitated by the color-coding of interrelated skills into clusters. These clusters represent a lifelike way in which a child's individual developmental patterns can be interpreted. The areas for assessment are self-help; motor development, including sensory perception; fine motor/visual discrimination; gross motor skills; wheelchair; and swimming skills (see the "Motor Assessment Tools" section of this chapter for more discussion of this test in relationship to motor skills); auditory perception/listening skills; language comprehension skills; language skills; sign-language skills; speech reading skills; social skills (adaptive behaviors, responsive behaviors, inter-personal relations, personal welfare-safety, social manners); and learning/cognitive skills.

The checklist is intended to be a practical tool for the identification of needs, the setting of objectives, and monitoring, and can be used by professionals and parents. These checklists included assessments that are not typically available (e.g., wheelchair skills and sign-language skills). The items are adequate for analysis; however, more fine-grained analysis may be needed for the more severely involved. Also, some items are placed in sections that are typically included in separate sections or other areas on other developmental checklists. For example, on the HELP, receptive language is included in the cognitive section.

Other criterion-referenced profiles that have been developed for multiply handicapped children or more severely delayed are the Developmental Assessment for the Severely Handicapped (DASH) (Dykes, 1980), and the Uniform Performance Assessment System (UPAS) (White et al., 1981). Other developmental tests that assist in the development of objectives are the Portage Guide to Early Education (Shearer et al., 1976), and the Callier-Azuza (Stillman, 1982), which assesses deaf-blind and multiply

handicapped children, aged 0–9 years, in the areas of motor, perceptual, daily living, language, and socialization skills.

In summary, these developmental/diagnostic tests provide a great deal of information concerning development as determined primarily from "normal or typical" development. The items should be used only as indicators of development. Early-childhood teachers in special-education programs should not attempt to use these assessments to represent the complex developmental interactions of the special-needs child. Multidisciplinary assessment teams should include parents in these developmental assessments, should conduct observations of these behaviors in the child's natural environment, and should provide ongoing assessment and monitoring.

## MULTICULTURAL PRESCHOOL ASSESSMENT

Every member of a preschool assessment team will encounter families who represent his or her own cultural background; however, the member must be prepared to encounter families who represent cultures that vary widely from his or her own. Moreover, examiners must realize that they will work with families who are fluent only in a language other than English. By the time the preschool assessment team encounters a child from a linguistically diverse or culturally different background (other than the typical, Anglo-American, middle-class background), the family has begun to socialize the young child in the mores of its own culture. Parents unconsciously teach their children their own culture at an early age (Ogbu, 1987). Furthermore, culture can not be separated from such developmental areas as cognition. "Cognitive skills are influenced by cultural tasks" (Ogbu, 1987, p. 159).

Early-childhood educators of children with special needs must be sensitive to cultural and linguistic differences, because they are, perhaps, the first professionals with whom the family must interact to receive appropriate services for the child. According to Hall (1973) one must understand the influence of one's own culture in order to understand individuals from other cultures.

Preschool assessment teams must consciously examine possible biases, stereotypes, and assumptions concerning the culture of the family with whom they work. They should not merely aim to provide interventions that match biological factors with early experiences (e.g., health and environmental issues); instead, they must also assess the "nature and meaning of early experiences" for the young children from culturally and linguistically diverse backgrounds (Ogbu, 1987, p. 166).

### Children from Diverse Backgrounds

Linguistically diverse children may represent any of a number of different groups: children who have immigrated from another country; children living in the United States who are learning two or more languages concurrently; and second-generation children who prefer to speak English at home. Children of migrant workers are also included under the heading of linguistically and culturally different (Advisory Board of Access, 1981). Other categories include the subordinate minority children (e.g., blacks, American Indians) (Ogbu, 1987), and children from Appalachian subcultures, e.g., Scotch-Irish groups in the southern West Virginia mountainous areas.

Few of these cultural groups are represented among assessment teams, i.e., school psychologists, speech and language specialists, preschool special-needs teachers, and early-childhood educators (Nuttall, 1987; Reynolds & Jennifer, 1987; Silver, 1986). Furthermore, few professionals on interdisciplinary teams can assess a non-English-speaking child in his or her native language (Nuttall, 1987).

### Mandates

P.L.-94-142 includes a provision for nondiscriminatory assessment in Section 612 (5) (C):

> Procedures to assure that testing and evaluation materials and procedures utilized for the purpose of evaluation and placement of handicapped chil-

dren will be selected and administered so as not to be racially or culturally discriminatory. Such materials or procedures shall be provided and administered in the child's native language or mode of communication unless it clearly is not feasible to do so and no single procedure shall be the sole criterion for determining an appropriate educational program for the child.

According to Landurand (1983), nondiscriminatory assessment is a dynamic process that considers the interactions among the examiner, the tests, and the testee. Citing Plata (1982), Landurand (1983), in describing the examiner's qualifications, noted,

> Who should test linguistically/culturally different students? All things being equal, a tester who speaks the language of the child, understands the culture of the child, and is a skilled assessor will be the best choice for the child. The examiner's knowledge of the culture of the child, either through birth or training, is extremely important for understanding the examinee's behavior and perception of the testing situation (p. 13).

The majority of assessment tools represent middle-class individuals, especially the values and concepts of Euro-American, middle-class persons (Landurand, 1983; Mercer, J., 1979; Ogbu, 1987). Also, many of these tests are normed on the majority population.

Assessors have developed several approaches to eliminate or reduce test bias. We discuss these briefly. For more information on nonbiased assessment, see Ambert and Dew (1982), Bernal (1972), Chinn (1979), Coulopoulos and DeGeorge (1982), De Avila and Havassy (1974), Laosa (1977), Mercer, J. (1979), and Nuttall (1987) and Chapter 13.

The major approaches for nonbiased assessment are to use (1) test translation, (2) ethnic norms, (3) "culture-fair" tests, (4) culture-specific tests, (5) a multicultural-pluralistic approach (e.g., System of Multicultural-Pluralistic Assessment (SOMPA)—Mercer, 1979), (6) task analysis of skills and behavior related to each test item and child's response, (7) criterion-referenced tests, and (8) a global approach to test bias. All these approaches have their critics.

For a review, see Mowder (1980). All these approaches are costly, time-consuming, and do not necessarily eliminate tests' and examiners' biases. For example, a popular method is to translate a test (Nuttall, 1987). Although the words are in the child's language, they might not have the same meaning as the original intent and also might not reflect the child's dialect (Plata, 1982). Essential to all these approaches is the obligation to meet the letter and spirit of the P.L. 94-142 regulations and to most accurately assess the child's needs and competencies. The global approach to assessment holds promise, in that examiners view nonbiased assessment as a "process rather than a set of instruments" (Landurand, 1983, p. 24). Guidelines for this approach exist (Tucker, 1980). Within this approach can be the use of task analysis, criterion-referenced tests, etc.

With the advent of P.L. 99-457, which mandates that professionals involve families in the development of Individual Family Service Plans, more attention must be given to the families' cultural and linguistic differences. Such projects as LEAP (Legal Education and Advocacy Project) (Santiago, 1988) can provide parents and public school systems with assistance in the development of family service plans and can assist parents in understanding the assessment process. LEAP provides a network with other programs, community agencies, and professionals for the referral of families with bilingual/bicultural special needs and for the facilitation of the family's participation in the process (Santiago, 1988, p. 4). Such community networks are critical to the success of referral, screening, and assessment of linguistically and culturally diverse infants and young children.

## SUMMARY

The procedures and tests for assessing the special needs of preschoolers have been viewed from a developmental framework. The framework assumes that the child's performance can be measured within his or her environmental context and can be matched to his or her developmental level. In addition, the developmental/interactive model assumes that performance measures are taken repeatedly and across settings. This is best accomplished with informal, observational data-gathering. Most standardized tests lack the technical flexibility and sensitivity needed for this purpose. However, by pinpointing those developmental areas in need of further exploration, formal instruments make the assessment process more efficient, more precise, and less costly. Also, the results of these tests are readily communicated to other professionals and parents. However, these tests should not direct the process, but instead serve as tools for answering specific questions regarding the reason for referral.

# CHAPTER 13

# Issues in the Assessment of Minorities

ELOY GONZALES

## OUTLINE

The issues of discrimination and bias in intelligence testing are discussed in this chapter. These problems have their roots in inappropriate use and interpretation of tests in the making of social and educational decisions about the futures of all children, regardless of their ethnic or socioeconomic backgrounds. Although Binet (1902) developed a test that was to be used to predict academic success, the test was soon adopted for other purposes; namely, to aid in the making of educational and socioeconomic decisions about children's futures. These decisions were made for all children, regardless of ethnicity, but for minority children the decision often resulted in discriminatory placement in vocational track courses or in special-education programs. It has been further argued that IQ tests did indeed measure innate abilities and that these abilities were predetermined by heredity.

The nature/nurture debates regarding intelligence were rekindled by Jensen (1969), who argued that education could not compensate for inherited deficits. Jensen's article set the stage for most of the controversy surrounding intelligence tests and their use today.

## HISTORICAL BACKGROUND

A careful review of literature and litigation indicates that the recent increase in concern about nonbiased assessment did not originate from a sincere humanistic concern for the social consequences of biased assessment, but from critical court decisions and consequent legislation. A review of early studies dealing with psychological evaluation of minority children reveals that minorities' potential as students has been systematically shrouded by bigotry, aloofness, and insensitivity. The pattern was set in this country as early as 1916. However, potential consequences of inappropriate use of the Binet test results were noted by Binet himself, when he cautioned professionals to spare undeserving students from assignment to special schools (Mercer & Lewis, 1978).

The earliest evidence of concern about Binet's test was in 1910, when Treves and Saffiotti reported substantial differences in the test scores of students from various social strata (Blanton, 1975). Later evidence indicated that Binet's test indeed did not accurately assess the intelligence of minorities. From this evidence Blanton concluded that test interpretation must take into account cultural and racial factors related to diverse group scores. He further advocated the development of special population norms.

The orientations of the three Americans who first imported Binet's test were quite different from those who were concerned about misuse of the Binet test. Lewis Terman at Stanford, Robert Yerkes at Harvard, and Henry Goddard at Vineland, New Jersey, were to be hailed as pioneers in the American testing movement. Terman's comment (1916) about the initial use of the Stanford-Binet test with Indian and Mexican children is quoted by Kamin (1975):

> Their dullness seems to be racial, or at least inherent in the family stocks from which they come. The fact that one meets this type with such extraordinary frequency among Indians, Mexicans, and Negros suggests quite forcibly that the whole question of racial differences in mental traits will have to be taken up anew ... there will be discovered enormously significant racial differences. ... which cannot be wiped out by any scheme of mental culture. Children of this group should be segregated in special classes.... They cannot master abstractions, but they can often be made efficient workers.... There is no possibility at present of convincing society that they should not be allowed to reproduce ... they constitute a grave problem because of their unusually prolific breeding (p. 6).

Soon after the test's translation and introduction in the U.S., the U.S. Public Health Service invited Goddard to apply the translated Binet test to arriving European immigrants for the purpose of detecting feeble-minded aliens. His results indicated that 83% of Jews, 80% of Hungarians, 79% of Italians, and 87% of Russians were feeble-minded (Kamin, 1975). These results, taken as scientific fact, brought about the quota system and the deportation of many aliens.

One of the earliest studies comparing different ethnic groups was by Garth (1923). He compared differences in intelligence between "blood groups of white, Indian and Mexican children." He summarized his findings by stating, "If these groups may be taken as representative of their racial stocks, [and] the results indicate differences between their racial stocks in intelligence as here measured, one is inclined to believe that differences in mental attitude toward the white man's way of thinking and living are here made apparent" (p. 401).

At about the same time, Yerkes and Foster (1923), commenting on the interpretation of the IQ score, warned about biased interpretations of those scores:

> Never should such a diagnosis be made on the IQ alone.... We must inquire further into the subject's economic history. What is his occupation; his pay? We must learn what we can about his immediate family. What is the economic status or occupation of the parents? When ... this information has been collected ... the psychologist may be of great value in getting the subject into the most suitable place in society ... (p. 80).

The first attempt to modify language to accommodate the bilingual child was reported by Sheldon (1924). In administering group tests to Mexican-American children, he found it necessary for the students to be given the group tests by their own teachers. These teachers were able to make themselves understood by speaking to the children in a Spanish-English dialect colloquially known as "spic" or "mongrel Spanish." Paschal and Sullivan (1925) first attempted to translate the Stanford-Binet for the testing of Mexican-American children. They found that the group of 9-year-old children had lower IQ scores than the group of 12-year-old children. They speculated that the difference was the result of school intervention that enhanced the IQ scores as the Mexican-American students underwent further education.

Testing 1,004 Mexican-American children, Garth (1928) found significantly lower scores among this group than in the standardization sample. He failed to cite language as a major contributor to the lower scores. Garth, Eson, and Morton (1936) concluded that Mexican-American children were at a disadvantage when tested with verbal tests of intelligence. They administered the Pitner Non-Language Intelligence Test and found that Mexican-American children scored as well as the norm population. They concluded that "such results suggest that the Mexican-American child in the United States is handicapped when he is tested with a verbal intelligence test" (p. 55).

Sanchez (1932a, 1932b, 1934a, 1934b) conducted one of the most comprehensive studies on intelligence testing and the Mexican-American child. He identified five factors that appeared to lower the IQ scores of Mexican-American children: limitations of heredity, inferior home environment (including both socioeconomic and educational deficits), linguistic handicaps, unsuitability of tests, and lack of parallel conditions under which tests were given (1932a). Several words commonly used in intelligence tests have different meanings and concepts to Mexican-American children, thus their interpretations and uses of them were confused (1934b). He criticized the use of literal Spanish translations of tests because of lack of adequate validation (1934a). Citing the 2% completion rate of Mexican-American students in school programs, as compared with the 14% completion rate for white children (1932b), he also criticized the schools for failing to provide an adequate and comparable education for Mexican-American children in New Mexico. These sociocultural factors that were later found to affect test performance were to be systematically measured and interpreted by Mercer and Lewis (1978).

In 1937, Mitchell administered a Spanish translation of the Otis Group Intelligence Scale to a group of Spanish-speaking children. He then administered an English version and found that the subjects scored significantly higher in

Spanish (MA 13.2) than in English (MA 7.6). Using the same test, Mahakian (1939) obtained similar results. Both authors concluded that intelligence tests administered in English to Spanish-speaking children were not valid. Carlson and Henderson (1950) criticized the majority of earlier studies comparing intelligence-test results of different ethnic groups. They claimed that these studies ignored too many factors that influence scores: (1) rural versus urban environments, (2) socioeconomic level, (3) total cultural complex, (4) quantity and quality of formal education of parents and students, (5) diet, (6) examiner prejudice, (7) motivation, and (8) bilingualism.

Keston and Jimenez's (1954) results raised important questions about the previous studies cited above. They found that Mexican-American children scored lower on the Spanish versions of the Binet and WISC than on the English version. Administering Form M of the 1937 Stanford-Binet in English and, one month later, Form L in Spanish, to fifty fourth-grade children, they found a mean IQ of 86 on Form M in English, and 71.8 on Form L in Spanish. Although many methodological concerns can be raised about their study, their findings began to undermine widespread acceptance that test administration in Spanish was superior to administration in English for this population. In the majority of prior studies, degree of bilingualism rarely had been measured or considered. Control for bilingualism since that time has become a more commonly identified adjustment.

Knapp (1960) was the first to identify time as a significant variable in the performance of Mexican-American children. Testing 100 Mexican and 100 Anglo boys on the Cattell Culture Free Intelligence Test, he withdrew the time limits for the former group and found that the Mexican students scored significantly higher than the Anglo students. He also concluded that the "culture fairness of the test was suspect." However, his methodology of requiring different (i.e., timed) conditions for the Anglo subjects weakens the results' validity. Cohen (1969) investigated the conceptual styles of different cultural groups as those styles related to intelligence testing. He predicted that there would be continuous, significant differences in IQ scores as long as so-called culture-fair nonverbal tests of intelligence remain biased against groups who have different conceptual styles from those that are necessary for successful performance.

Tate (1952) investigated the Leiter International Performance Scale in regard to its cultural fairness. He tested four groups of preschool children from various socioeconomic groups. Using the Stanford-Binet, Arthur Point Scale, and Leiter Scale, Tate found the Leiter to be no more "culture-free" than the Binet or Arthur.

Comparing applications of the Leiter Scale and the Stanford-Binet on black preschool children, Costello and Dickie (1970) found a mean Binet IQ of 89 and a Leiter score of 83. Although the difference was not significant, only three of the children scored higher on the Leiter.

One of the most significant studies of the early 1970s that dealt with the identification of mental retardation and its application to minorities was by Mercer (1973). Using the two-dimensional definition of mental retardation as subaverage intellectual functioning and impaired adaptive behavior, Mercer evaluated Mexican-American, black, and white children from Riverside, California, who were classified as educable mentally retarded. She found that 60% of Mexican-American and 91% of black children passed the adaptive-behavior rating scale, but none of the white students who scored below 70 passed the adaptive-behavior rating scale. It was obvious that IQ scores were valid for white children but inappropriate for the other ethnic groups.

In a separate study, Mercer and Brown (1973) grouped black and Mexican-American children according to sociocultural characteristics typical of the middle-class white population. They found that when either black or Mexican-American children possessed certain sociocultural characteristics, their IQ scores were near the mean. The IQ scores decreased proportionately for both groups when these positive socio-cultural variables were not present.

The System of Multicultural Pluralistic Assessment (SOMPA), developed by Mercer and Lewis (1978), was the first systematic method of measuring and interpreting sociocultural variables. Through pluralistic assessment, the meaning of a particular test score or adaptive behavior score could now be evaluated in relation to the sociocultural group to which the child belonged. By evaluating the position of youngsters within the norms for their own sociocultural group, their ability to learn was assessed. Current status of the system will be discussed later.

The sudden surge for nondiscriminatory testing of minority children during the early 1970s can be attributed to litigation, consequent court mandates, and P.L. 94-142. The two most notable cases dealing specifically with the evaluation and placement of minority children are *Diana* v. *California State Board of Education* (1970) and *Larry P.* v. *Riles* (1972). In the state of California, a precipitous decline in diagnoses of mild mental retardation, from more than 50,000 to 19,000, occurred between 1970 and 1977 (Meyers, MacMillan, & Yoshida, 1978). Although the numbers declined, the proportion of minorities to white students has remained high, with 25% of this sub-group being black (Prassee & Reschly, 1986).

The *Diana* case stipulated the modified use and selection of tests that weighed heavily on language skills, and required testing in both primary and secondary languages. Work on Mexican-American norms was also mandated.

The *Larry P.* v. *Riles* case was filed on behalf of black elementary school children who allegedly were inappropriately placed in classes for students with mental retardation. In the court settlement, a preliminary injunction regarding future testing with the Wechsler Intelligence Scale for Children and Stanford-Binet was granted.

The repercussions of this case have been far-reaching and have affected minority children both positively and negatively. Most significant has been the effect on services to students. Programs for students with mild mental retardation have provided, in many cases, increasingly better services for these students. Offerings typically include smaller student-teacher ratios, individualized instruction, supportive services, and specialized methods and materials used by highly trained teachers. However, the stigma of the label associated with these programs has prompted many parents to request regular classroom placements for their children. Administrators frequently have been forced to dismantle such programs because of widespread parental concerns that their children would be stigmatized.

The result has been the removal of most students, even those who have demonstrated significant educational deficits, from classes for mild mental retardation. However, the turmoil surrounding instruction of these students may only have begun; the defendants of *Larry P.* v. *Riles* (1984) have stated their intention to appeal the appellate court verdict.

In a similar case in Illinois, *PASE* v. *Hannon* (1980), Federal District Court Judge Grady ruled that IQ tests were not biased regardless of overrepresentation and that multifactored assessment has guarded against misplacement in the category of mild retardation. Although this particular case has become moot, it did reveal judicial thinking contrary to the earlier decision in the *Larry P.* v. *Riles* case.

More recently, in *Marshall et al.* v. *Georgia* (1984), the court was asked to determine whether disproportionate classification and placement across a variety of educational programs constituted discrimination. Judge Edenfield's opinion was that mild mental retardation occurs more frequently with lower socioeconomic groups. He believed that the socioeconomic circumstances of poverty among black students in Georgia provided a sufficient explanation for their overrepresentation.

In May 1987 in California, a 14-year-old boy, the son of a Mexican-American woman and black man, was denied IQ testing as per the Peckham decision in *Larry P.* v. *Riles.* His mother, realizing her son's need for remedial intervention, has sought help in challenging the ban on IQ tests for blacks. Dr. William Allen, a member of the U.S. Commission on Civil Rights, has agreed to present the case to the commission, adding that he believes the woman's rights as a parent may have been violated and that the state should find a way to give those who want the test the option to take it (Mathew, 1987).

## TEST BIAS

P.L. 94-142, the Education of All Handicapped Children Act of 1975, attempted to set guidelines to guard against bias in testing and programming of minority children:

> Tests must be selected and administered so that they are not racially or culturally discriminatory (121a.530); tests must be provided and administered in the child's native language or other mode of communication, if feasible (121a.531); tests must have been validated for the specific purpose for which they are used (121a.532).

The issue of test bias, apart from use, selection, and interpretation of test scores, will be discussed in this section. Reynolds and Brown (1984) define *bias* as "an accepted, well-defined statistical term denoting constant or systematic error rather than random, patternless error" (p. 19). The issue, in essence, comes down to the validity of the test itself. A similar psychometric definition of test bias by Cleary and Hilton (1968) states:

> A test is biased for members of a subgroup of the population if, in the prediction of criterion for which the test was designed, consistent nonzero errors of prediction are made for members of the subgroup. In other words, the test is biased if the criterion score predicted from the common regression line is consistently too high or too low for members of the subgroup. This definition of bias may include the connotation of unfairness, particularly if the test's use produces a prediction that is too low (p. 62).

This definition has been supported by Anastasi (1982), Cronbach (1970), Einhorn and Bass (1971), and Grant and Bray (1970). Using Cleary and Hilton's definition above, Mercer (1979) compared the regression lines used in the prediction of grade-point averages (GPAs) from WISC-R verbal IQ test results for 142 black, 241 Hispanic, and 425 white elementary school children. An attempt was made to determine whether a single regression system could be used to predict GPA. The slopes were so significantly different that they crossed; the regression lines for Hispanic and black children were the closest to each other. Similar findings were demonstrated by Goldman and Hartig (1976).

A psychometric model of bias proposed by Thorndike (1971) holds that a test used for educational or employment selection is fair only if, for any given criterion of success, the test admits or selects the same proportion of minority applicants that would be admitted or selected by the criterion itself or by a perfectly valid test. This approach, based on a probability matching, can actually lead to assigning to minority students a range of expected intellectual functioning that is beyond their capability. It can also contribute to reverse discrimination, in which capable nonminority individuals might be denied educational opportunities.

Darlington (1971) proposed a third model, now referred to as the *corrected criterion model,* that would weight scores to minority students' advantage. Darlington asserted that a new model was needed to correct past discrepancies: "Any specific decision made between groups must weight importance attributed to selecting persons who score highest and to giving members of a given minority group a better opportunity" (p. 75). He proposed that bonus points be given to the predicted criterion for minority groups. Giving bonus points to veterans, a common practice employers use to help veterans obtain jobs, is an example of the application of this model.

The model commonly used by the Office of Civil Rights is referred to as the *quota model.* In this model, placement bias is defined as the placement of more minority children than non-minority children in special-education classes. The Office of Civil Rights (1972) states: "Placement of students in special education may be considered biased when there is a higher incidence of improper placement or improper nonplacement of minority children in such classes than nonminority children." In essence, the number of minority children in special education must not exceed the proportion in the general population.

These psychometric models and approaches that address the issue of test bias are somewhat questionable, although they are adequate and acceptable under some circumstances. There now appears to be no single model or approach that can satisfactorily meet all needs.

To evaluate bias in existing tests, Mercer and Lewis (1978) used the nonpsychometric definition of bias; that is, partiality, tendency to favor unfairly, and inequity. They determined that instruments were biased if they generally included questions reflecting one group's cultural heritage but excluded questions reflecting another group's cultural heritage. They cited several tests in which test items reflected the language, traditions, and skills of the dominant white culture but which contained no test items reflecting aspects of minority cultures. They found that IQ scores from such tests were highly correlated with cultural characteristics, and that minority children most assimilated into the dominant culture typically scored higher on these tests than did those less assimilated. They concluded that such tests were used unfairly when, on the basis of test scores, inferences about intelligence or potential were drawn and, in particular, when inferences were drawn by the comparison of one cultural group's performance with another's.

## BIASED TEST ITEMS

Another approach to evaluating test bias is to focus on test content. This approach contends that even though a test as whole is not biased, it can have individual items that have significant prejudicial effects on selected subgroups and these items, therefore, should be modified or dropped altogether. The subsequent test would not favor any one group over another. We must keep in mind that when tests are developed the items are selected by someone. Therefore, according to Reynolds and Brown (1984), "the means of item selection tends both to bias the tests and to negate the statistical assumption underlying most psychometric analyses, that is, that the items behave as if drawn at random" (p. 134).

According to Mercer and Lewis (1978), the items reflecting the dominant culture and thus favoring members of that culture can be identified. In other words, it is readily accepted that children from different cultures enter school with different experiences in language, motivation, and other skills that might not be relevant or conducive to success in Anglo-oriented schools. Items that children have not had an opportunity to learn or that do not reflect their daily experience should be regarded as biased. Again, bias in tests affects the tests' validity. If a child is tested in a language other than his or her native tongue or is asked questions beyond his or her experience, how can the instrument indicate that child's performance in a given area?

Including test items relevant to particular minority groups has been recommended. The idea sounds good, but in practice does not work. Special test items typically are eliminated after norming, because only test items that are neither too easy nor too difficult for the entire norming population would remain in the final item pool. However, procedures to insure the inclusion of content-appropriate items could be devised.

## MISUSE OF TESTS

Interpretations of test results are frequently misconstrued as biased when actually the test has been used for purposes other than those specified by the author. Interpretation indeed can sometimes be biased, but many times it is not; it is important that the difference between misinterpreting test results (when the interpretation reveals disappointing findings) and actually misusing test results must be made clear. The interpretation of a WISC-R IQ score is a prime example. Kaufman (1979) believes that the WISC-R items are merely samples of learned behaviors and that performance should not be interpreted as an estimate of intellectual functioning. He stated:

> The WISC-R subtests measure what the individual has learned . . . From this vantage point, the intelligence test is really a kind of achievement test . . . a measure of past accomplishments that is predictive of success in traditional school subjects. When intelligence tests are regarded as measures of prior learning, the issue of heredity versus environment becomes irrelevant. Since learning occurs within a culture, intelligence tests obviously must be considered to be culture loaded—a concept that is different from culture biased (pp. 12–13).

Test results for the WISC-R and similar tests can be misused when they are taken to indicate innate intellectual functioning rather than academic potential, which the test was specifically designed to measure. According to Reynolds and Brown (1984), such misuse that directs test results in an unfair or prejudiced manner toward any one group yields low predictive validity for everyone.

Including a sufficient number of minority students in the norming of tests has also been recommended. For example, according to the *Standards for Educational and Psychological Testing* (American Education Research Association, APA, & NCRE, 1985), the WISC-R is considered well normed because 2,200 subjects were included. The ethnic breakdowns matched the percentages in the latest U.S. Census Bureau statistics. However, further examination reveals that 330 were nonwhite children, 305 of whom were black, so only 25 "others" were Orientals and Hispanics. With such low num-

bers, it is obvious how their particular cultural experiences can be quickly screened out in final item analyses. The dichotomy is ironic; norming procedures established to ensure valid, reliable tests automatically produce bias that affects particular ethnic groups.

## CULTURE-SPECIFIC TESTS AND LOCAL NORMS

Culture-specific tests have been developed for one reason. That reason is to counter inappropriate testing of culturally and linguistically different populations within systems that traditionally have based decisions on scores normed among the dominant culture. The earliest recommendation for the development of special norms is discussed by Blanton (1975). He cites the work of Treves and Saffiotti who, in 1910, not only recommended that test interpretation take into account cultural and racial factors, but also advocated that special population norms be developed.

The development of tests specifically for particular ethnic groups receives continual discussion; it has been attempted in a few instances. The Black Intelligence Test of Cultural Homogeneity (BITCH) is one example. Items dealing mainly with black vocabulary (that is, vocabulary found within black culture, particularly in the St. Louis area) were included (Williams, 1972). When administered to two groups of students, one white and one black, white students obtained low scores, while black students obtained significantly higher scores. No significant difference was found, however, between the scores of lower-class blacks and whites (Andre, 1975). Milgram (1974) pointed out that the BITCH may be useful for building black pride but is useless as a predictor of success in the prevailing culture. Ortiz and Ball (1972) developed a 31-item multiple choice test for Mexican-American children. The so-called "Enchilada Test" was composed of items common to the Mexican-American barrio child of Los Angeles. When administered to Anglo children, testers obtained findings similar to those found in the BITCH experiment.

The development of local norms has not received much support. Local norms are considered provincial (Bailey & Harbin, 1980), and although their use in tests appears progressive and humanitarian, it actually works against a child's mobility because it confines interpretation to identified groups.

The use of locally normed tests has also met with negative comments from within the minority community itself (Bernal, 1972; Chinn, 1984; DeAvila & Havassy, 1974; Gonzales, 1982). Bernal (1972) contends that norming tests is dishonest because renorming does not involve test modification in the critical area of content. Gonzales (1982) supports development of local norms under the following conditions:

1. When a population's cultural and linguistic characteristics are significantly different from the norm population, as is the case with Navajo populations living on reservations, the practice would especially be beneficial in domains such as adaptive-behavior inventories, which traditionally measure adaptation to middle-class, metropolitan life.
2. When a local school district is interested in screening or developing programs within its own area, the practice would be useful.

In the long run, such approaches have far more negative effects than they have positive. The following conclusions about local norms are the most significant:

1. Such findings and scores encourage expectations of lower performance for the given population.
2. This norming approach assumes that the particular group is homogeneous in mental capacity and socioeconomic levels.
3. Support of such an approach would reinforce the proposal (Hernstein, 1971; Jensen, 1969) that genetics (i.e., racial heritage) determine intelligence.

4. Support of such an approach would also reinforce the assumption that lower scores are clearly indicative of lower intellectual potential.
5. Such scores would have little predictive validity within the mainstream culture in which students must compete.
6. Scores would likewise reduce the population's aspirations for academic success.

The reality is that these culturally different groups must participate in the dominant culture in order to survive. It is therefore essential and beneficial to know their level of capability in relation to the dominant culture in which they must compete.

## CULTURE-FAIR TESTS

To be culture-fair, a test should meet the following criteria:

1. It should be possible to make the same predictions from the results across cultures.
2. Language and reading should be kept at a minimum.
3. Pictures or symbols used in items must be familiar to all cultures.
4. Subjects should not be penalized by timed items.
5. Item content must be either familiar or unfamiliar to the majority of cultures.
6. Items or tasks should equally motivate (i.e., appeal to) all cultures.

The culture-fair movement had its beginning with the development of instruments that were purported to yield similar scores for any given population regardless of race or culture. The Leiter International Performance Scale (1929) and the Raven's Progressive Matrices (Raven, Court, & Raven, 1977, 1986) are the most widely used culture-fair tests.

The Leiter International Performance Scale (Leiter, 1929) was initiated in 1927 at the University of Hawaii Psychological Clinic. Funded by the Rockerfeller Foundation, the Leiter was to test IQ differences between races. Leiter, the test's developer, verified the appropriateness of the forty-nine subtests for six years, with a series of school children in Hawaii. The initial assumption was that if language is removed as part of a test's format, the test will serve as a culture-fair instrument. Even from its initial studies, results revealed significant differences between the test scores of subjects of Japanese descent and those of Chinese descent. Additional efforts ranging from work with tribes in Africa to bushmen and aborigines in Australia showed significant performance differences; some subjects were totally unable to grasp the nature of the test (Porteus, 1937).

In dealing with culturally different children in this country, Tate in 1952 tested the hypothesis that the Leiter International Performance Scale (LIPS) was relatively culture-free and unaffected by environmental factors. Basing his groups on parental work status, he used a professional preschool group (PP), a kindergarten professional group (KP), a lower socioeconomic group (KL), and an orphanage group (OL). He administered the Binet, Leiter, and the Arthur Point Scale. Results in IQ scores of 128, 121 and 105 were found respectively for the PP group; 124, 123, and 105, respectively for the KP group; 105, 109, and 82, respectively for the KL group; and 90, 92, and 73, respectively for the OL group.

Some twenty years later, Costello and Dickie (1970) compared the LIPS and Binet IQ scores of black preschool children. Only three of the children in their sample scored higher on the LIPS than on the Binet. They concluded that the "Leiter has no obvious advantage over the Binet for assessing disadvantaged preschool children; in fact, the reverse may be true" (p. 314). Johnston (1982) believes that LIPS scores for children in the lower age groups may represent primarily perceptual, rather than conceptual, ability.

Although never intended to address the deaf and hearing-impaired, the Leiter became the

tool of preference because of a total lack of clinical instruments for this population.

Because of this lack of available devices, the LIPS's critical weaknesses in norming and statistical data were disregarded, and it remains in use today. Matthews and Birch (1949) were early supporters of its use with deaf populations but clearly cautioned about its validity with handicapped populations. Ratcliffe and Ratcliffe (1979) and Sullivan and Vernon (1979) reviewed its use with hearing-impaired children; they concluded that pyschometric properties of the test leave many serious questions about its use.

Despite very inadequate 40-year-old norms, the lack of item modification since 1936, and total lack of reliability across cultures and socioeconomic groups, the Leiter today remains one of the most popular instruments included under the term "culture-fair." Salvia and Ysseldyke (1985) conclude that it is inadequately standardized; little if any reliability and validity support are given in its manual. These experts state that, until this test is made technically adequate, its use should be restricted to procurement of qualitative information by only the most experienced examiners. Furthermore, evaluation of this instrument would reveal it to be severely deficient in all categories of the Technical Standards for Test Construction and Evaluation, of the *Standards for Educational and Psychological Testing* (1985).

The Raven's Progressive Matrices (Raven, Court, & Raven, 1986), like the Leiter International Performance Scale, has been very popular as a nonverbal and, consequently, as a culture-fair test for some years. Like the Leiter, it, too, has been severely criticized for its inadequate and out-dated norming, which was completed in England and Scotland and dates back over twenty years (Orme, 1966; Peck, 1970). No norms for American children were obtained until 1986. This norming did not include test modification, so that past research has significant contributions to its current use and interpretation. There are three versions of the Ravens. Coloured Progressive Matrices (C.P.M.) are designed for younger children. Standard Progressive Matrices (S.P.M.) are for children and adolescents, and Advanced Progressive Matrices were designed for adults.

To examine the validity of the CPM, Keir (1949); Banks and Sinha (1951); and Johnson, Johnson, and Price-Williams (1967) compared the CPM with tests of their own design. Although their investigations lacked uniformity, they found correlations of .62, .54, and .42, while Raven had found a correlation of .86.

Norman and Midkiff (1955), while studying the culture-fairness of the Goodenough Draw-A-Man and Raven Progressive Matrices with ninety-six Navajo children, expected high scores because of adult Navajos' skills in sand-painting and weaving. Instead, Navajos scored only 65 IQ points on these tests. After contacting the tests' author (Leiter), who admitted to similar findings with similar groups of Africans and Maoris, the authors drew two conclusions: (1) poor performance of these children on the Raven test is consistent with findings from other psychological studies of native populations, and (2) it is apparent from other results that the Progressive Matrices Test is, for some reason, inadequate as a cross-cultural instrument for evaluating intellectual capacity (p. 136). Burke's (1958) review of the Raven's Progressive Matrices led him to conclude that the test "could and should be improved with respect to both reliability and validity, and is not a substitute in any sense for the Binet, Wechsler nor for any verbal or nonverbal group test of mental ability" (p. 222).

Norms for the Standard Progressive Matrices for the United States range in age from six years, three months to sixteen years, eight months. Norms for the Coloured Progressive Matrices range in age from five years, three months to eleven years, nine months, while the Advanced Progressive Matrices includes norms from a sample of 300 University of California at Berkeley students.

Split-half reliabilities range from .65 to .94 for the Coloured Progress Matrices. These were the only 1986 reliability figures presented in the 1986 renorming manual. Various validity studies including white, black, Mexican-American, Native American, and exceptional populations of deaf and mentally handicapped children, reveal validity coefficients of .50 to .80s when the test is compared with intelligence tests, and .30 to .60s with achievement tests (Raven, Court, & Raven, 1986; Raven & Summers, 1986).

Because the norming is so recent, only one reference addressing the new 1986 norms was located. Sattler (1988), after reviewing the new norms, made the following conclusions:

1. It is a useful measure of nonverbal reasoning ability.
2. Its ease of administration makes it a useful supplementary screening test for children with severe language, auditory or physical disabilities.
3. It is useful with children with limited command of English.
4. For English speakers it should be supplemented by a vocabulary test.
5. It provides a measure of intelligence based on figural reasoning only.
6. It should not be used as a substitute for either the WISC-R or Stanford Binet (4th ed.) (p. 310).

Because no internal changes have occurred on the Ravens other than re-norming on an American population, the content and dependence on figural reasoning skills remain. Therefore the conflicting results with culturally different populations such as those cited by Norman and Midkiff (1955) should persist. In summary, the Raven's Progressive Matrices have not shown evidence to warrant its use as a substitute for the WISC-R, Stanford-Binet, or K-ABC as a score of intelligence. Its new norms will increase its utility as a supplementary instrument in measuring nonverbal reasoning.

Existing tests, then, have been widely criticized, and several researchers have attempted to devise new culturally fair tests. The Kaufman Assessment Battery for Children (K-ABC) (1983) is one such test. The works of neuropsychology researchers Das, Kirby and Jarman (1975); Kinsbourne (1978); and Luria (1966a, 1973), and Neisser (1967), a cognitive psychologist, led the Kaufmans to define intelligence through a mental processing model. For the purpose of determining a child's preferred style of problem-solving and processing of information, two types of mental processes, sequential processing and simultaneous processing, were identified. Once the child is assessed, remediation and training utilizing this strength are advocated. Measurement of the two processes were accomplished by (a) the Sequential Processing Scale, which assesses a child's ability to mentally manipulate stimuli in serial order in order to solve problems, and (b) the Simultaneous Processing Scale, which measures a child's skill in solving problems by simultaneously organizing and integrating many stimuli. The scores of these tests can be combined to yield a Mental Processing Composite Score, which is analogous to a full scale IQ score obtained from the WISC-R. Finally, a Nonverbal Supplementary Score can be derived from the subtests that require no language for either the directions or the responses.

Hailed as the solution to the problem of cultural bias in tests, the K-ABC, specifically designed to provide nondiscriminatory assessment for minority children, was the prototype for the current generation of culturally fair tests. It attempted to provide nondiscriminatory assessment through the following strategies: (a) carefully selecting items never included in prior tests, (b) minimizing the role of language responses, (c) including supplementary sociocultural norms, and (d) including 550 minority subjects in the norming. Whether the K-ABC achieved its aims remains a matter of controversy, but to the test's credit, norming research with the K-ABC showed no significant differences between the scores of black, Mexican-American, and white children.

The controversy surrounding the K-ABC began even before its distribution in 1983 and continues to this day. One group of researchers contends that the K-ABC does not possess greater validity or less bias than other tests, while another group favoring the K-ABC says that it is indeed more valid and less biased. Jensen (1984), certainly the Kaufman's greatest critic, represents the former faction. In an article in the *Journal of Special Education,* which devoted an entire issue to the controversy soon after the test's release, Jensen argued that the reduced difference between the scores of black and white children should be attributed to the K-ABC and not to the mental capacities it attempted to measure:

> The apparently reduced difference between black and white samples, as compared with the one standard deviation difference typically found on other IQ tests, is not the result of greater validity or of less biased measurement of children's intelligence by the K-ABC. The diminished black-white difference seems to be largely the result of psychometric and statistical artifacts (p. 377).

Other noted authors, including Salvia and Hritcko (1984), Das (1984), and Gunnison (1984), also submitted articles to the special issue. Of these, three leveled criticism. Salvia and Hritcko, as well as Das, contended that the K-ABC did not adequately measure sequential and simultaneous processing. Only Gunnison wrote in favor of the test, although other authors later wrote in its support. Among these were Valencia and Rankin (1986), who administered the K-ABC to 100 Anglo and 100 Mexican-American children. They concluded that their work lends some support to the hypothesis that the K-ABC is not a biased instrument in construct validity with respect to the samples in their study. In the achievement section of the K-ABC, however, the authors found that a significant number of items reflected cultural bias against Mexican-American children.

Other authors have found additional aspects of the K-ABC to criticize. McLoughlin and Lewis (1986) questioned the efficacy of mental-process training over time and across various tasks. One of the most critical studies to date was a validity study, by Ayers and Cooley (1986), of the sequential versus simultaneous processing. A total of 208 white, first-grade children were administered the K-ABC. Fifty-one children met the criteria for having one process significantly higher than the other. The authors then used tasks that followed the recommended procedures for sequential and simultaneous instruction, which the Kaufmans presented in the manual. Analysis revealed that the results failed to support the validity hypothesis of the K-ABC, but actually supported hypotheses in the opposite direction. They concluded that the aspects of mental processing that are labeled as sequential or simultaneous on the K-ABC are quite different from the sequential and simultaneous aspects of the learning tasks used in this study. These selected tasks could be questioned in terms of their face validity; or, one could question the face validity of the description of recommended tasks presented in the Kaufman manual.

Naglieri and Anderson (1985); and McCallum, Karnes, and Edwards (1984), challenged the test's use in identifying gifted children. The contention has been that children who score in the superior ranges on highly verbal tests will be penalized on the K-ABC because of the minimal use of language. Kaufman (1986) defends the K-ABC's use in identifying gifted children. Citing a study by Barry, Klanderman, and Stipe (1983), Kaufman noted that children who qualified for gifted programs according to their Binet IQ scores obtained much higher Mental Processing Composite scores than did those who failed to qualify for the program. It is of interest that Kaufman also proposes that a child who meets criteria for gifted programs by scores from *either* the intelligence or the achievement portion of the K-ABC be allowed into the program, provided that other requirements are met. In an earlier article, however, Kaufman (1983) predicted that school-age white children who exhibited well-developed verbal or language skills would likely score lower on the K-ABC than on other standard measures of current intellectual functioning.

Two studies (McCallum, Karnes & Edwards, 1984; Naglieri & Anderson, 1985) do not support Kaufman's argument that the K-ABC is useful for identifying gifted children. In both studies, children's K-ABC Mental Composite scores were significantly lower than those on the WISC-R; in the former study, the K-ABC scores were also lower than the Binet scores. McCallum, Karnes, and Edwards (1984) concluded that conventional, IQ-test scores would better predict success in gifted programs with heavy verbal orientation than would K-ABC scores.

This author's experience as a bilingual educational diagnostician, as well as the experiences of other diagnosticians throughout the state of New Mexico, supports the findings cited above. Hispanic children consistently score significantly lower on the K-ABC than on the WISC-R Performance score; their K-ABC scores tend to fall closer to the WISC-R Verbal scores. In addition, its use is not recommended in obtaining intellectual abilities of either mentally handicapped or gifted students.

In summary, there are serious questions about the K-ABC's validity and the instructional strategies based on the K-ABC profile. Although the test may be useful when measures of nonverbal cognitive abilities are needed, or in cases when verbal rapport is limited, it should not be the sole instrument used in placement decisions when an IQ test is called for.

## PROCEDURES IN UNBIASED TESTING

### Examiner Biases

The idea of selecting an examiner with the same ethnic background as the testee was for some time a matter of controversy. If a second language is not a variable that will affect test results, the majority of recent research reveals no general tendency for minority children to score higher or lower when tested by an examiner not of their own ethnic group (Meyers, Sundstrom, & Yoshida, 1974; Sattler, 1973a; Shuey, 1966). If an examiner is technically proficient in testing, his or her greatest asset in effectively evaluating any child, regardless of the child's ethnic background and of the capacity being measured, is rapport. Ultimately, the examiner who demonstrates warmth, understanding, and good listening skills will win the child over and obtain from her or him the best performance possible.

When the child is culturally and linguistically different from the dominant culture, many professionals feel that he or she would be better served by an examiner with the same cultural and linguistic background (Chinn, 1984; Gonzales, 1982; Plata, 1986). The key factor in obtaining an accurate measure of a culturally and linguistically different child's knowledge and skills is to test the child in both the child's dominant language and in her or his second language. Testing in both languages is particularly important when a child is suspected to have a communicative disorder, because the child's cultural and linguistic differences might be perceived as the real problem when in fact they are not. By testing the child in both languages, the examiner can determine whether the child actually has a communicative disorder. Language dominance and proficiency will be discussed later in more detail.

## Use of Interpreters

The use of an interpreter should be the last resort when a child is clearly dominant in a language other than English. This author has in some instances been forced to use an interpreter in testing Native American children. The pitfalls are many and should be kept in mind:

1. Once an interpreter is used, standardization is broken and the test immediately becomes invalid.
2. Valid test procedures and terminology are not known by the majority of translators, who in many cases may be paraprofessionals.
3. Direct, on-the-spot translation in many instances loses the test's true meaning and level of complexity (i.e., the translation auto-

matically changes the vocabulary's difficulty level).
4. Many words, such as those in Native American languages, do not have a singular direct translation. For example, *turtle* in English is translated into *the one that walks slow* in Navajo. Therefore, unintended cues are provided in the test situation.
5. The interpreters lack skills in different dialects of the same language. It is very common to find different dialects among Native American speakers as well as among Spanish speakers.
6. It has been the author's experience that untrained interpreters tend to misjudge the purpose of testing and aid the child in any way possible, such as by supplying extra cues (e.g., facial expressions) or modifying the question.

Nevertheless, any interpreter is often better than no interpreter at all (Plata, 1986). Plata stated that "ultimately, however, using interpreters to try to compromise the effect of an examinee's language on test results is better than no attempt at all" (p. 4). When a school is forced to use interpreters, the district should train these interpreters before they are sent out into the field. They must be made to understand the purpose of the testing. They must learn testing procedures to ensure that rapport is established, avoid prompting, state directions and questions verbatim, and avoid giving gestures or verbal cues. They need to be familiar with terminology and directions of the instrument to be used. Moreover, questions to be used in testing should be discussed with interpreters before testing begins, so that it can be determined whether the questions are directly translatable.

## Test Translation

Translating the language of tests to a child's native tongue often seems the best means of evaluating the child's capacity. Nonetheless, translations do present some difficulties.

Sanchez (1934a) criticized literal Spanish translations because of lack of adequate empirical validation. Quay (1971); DeAvila and Havassy (1974); Sechrest, Fay, and Zaidi (1972); Samuda (1975); Mercer (1979); Gonzales (1982); Chinn (1984); and Plata (1986) have identified the following shortcomings of translating tests:

1. Not all words directly translate from one language to another.
2. The levels of vocabulary and complexity often change with translations.
3. Dialects complicate the task of translators, who might not understand unfamiliar idioms that are nonetheless part of the tongue.
4. When the test is translated, its original norms immediately become invalid.
5. Although the words of test items can be translated, the concepts in test items frequently cannot; many test items reflect American middle-class culture, which is different from the experience of many culturally and linguistically different children.
6. Tests written in a minority child's native tongue but normed in a foreign country would include test items reflecting that country's culture and would preclude an accurate assessment of the child's abilities; for example, the WISC-R normed in Mexico contains items dealing with Mexico's geography, history and culture, all or most of which would be beyond the experience of a Spanish-speaking child raised in the U.S.

In summary, the use of translated intelligence and norm-referenced achievement tests is discouraged, with certain exceptions. These exceptions might include use on recent immigrants who are familiar with the test items' content, or students for whom Spanish is the only means of communication.

## PLURALISTIC ASSESSMENT

Researchers have long held that sociocultural variables affect intelligence, at least as intelligence is measured by intelligence tests. In his work with Mexican-American children, Jensen (1961) concluded that:

> Findings of the study are consistent with the hypothesis that their distribution of basic learning abilities is not substantially different from that in the Anglo-American population of comparable socio-economic level (p. 158).

The effect of a child's socioeconomic background on his or her academic achievement has been well documented (Cohen, 1969; Davis, 1948; Mercer, 1973; Sanchez, 1932a; Sattler, 1973b; Schmidt and Hunter, 1974). However, it was not until 1978 that Mercer and Lewis statistically measured, with the System of Multicultural, Pluralistic Assessment (SOMPA), the effects that sociocultural variables can have on a child.

*Pluralistic assessment* involves the use of more than one source of information in the making of assessment decisions, such as whether a child qualifies for special class placement. The most positive aspect of the system is that it assures that the two-dimensional definition of mental retardation (i.e., subaverage intelligence as well as impaired adaptive behavior) is applied through its own Adaptive Behavior Inventory for Children (ABIC). The estimated learning potential (ELP) provides the IQ score needed to complete the two-facet definition. The ELP is derived by statistical inclusion of the sociocultural variables identified as affecting the calculation of the IQ. The result is an upward adjustment for IQ level for children who lack any of the identified sociocultural variables.

The SOMPA was immediately accepted and widely used without much question about its longterm effect. Today, after years of use, the SOMPA has been found to have significantly affected a large number of mildly handicapped black and Hispanic children placed in special-education classes (Figueroa, 1982; Fisher, 1977; Harbin, 1980; Heflinger, Cook & Thackrey, 1987; Oakland, 1979, 1983; Polloway & Smith, 1983; Reschly, 1981; Tebeleff & Oakland, 1977;

Witt & Martens, 1984). In 1981 Reschly estimated that the use of the SOMPA would result in
a prevalence figure of less than .5% for mild
mental retardation and would have a major
effect on children by making them no longer
eligible for services.

A recent study by Heflinger, Cook, and
Thackrey (1987), which used the SOMPA to
investigate the dual criteria (intelligence plus
adaptive behavior) for identification of mental
retardation, further demonstrates its effect on
Hispanic children. Analyzing archival data collected by Mercer (1979) in her standardization
of the SOMPA, Heflinger, Cook, and Thackrey
applied the dual criteria to the population.
Mixed numbers of failures were found in the
separate scores on the ABIC, WISC-R, and ELP.
However, when the dual criteria of scoring two
standard deviations below the mean on the
ABIC and ELP were used, only 3 out of 1913
children (0.2%) met the criteria to be classified
as mentally retarded. This is in contrast to an
accepted prevalence figure for mental retardation of approximately 2.5% among our nation's
school-age population.

Several major concerns have been identified
since the SOMPA's development:

1. The ABIC concerns itself primarily with behaviors outside of the school environment.
   This is in direct contradiction to the original
   concept of adaptive behavior, which requires
   observing a child in a variety of settings, and
   school is a primary environment for a school-
   aged child.
2. The system lacks inclusion of English/ Spanish
   language proficiency.
3. The ELP fails to adequately predict academic
   achievement (Oakland & Matuszek, 1977).
4. The ELP projects an intellectual level that
   might be possible if intervention occurs or if
   the ideal environment is provided. But in
   reality, few of those environments actually
   exist; therefore, the ELP becomes educationally useless for purposes of educational planning and programming (Chinn, 1984).

5. The awarding of extra IQ points on the
   surface is degrading to minority populations.
6. National norms are absent (Nuttall, 1979).

The result has been the denial of services in
special education to large numbers of blacks
and Hispanics with academic deficits, whom the
schools are unprepared to serve in regular education. It appears that many of these students
possess severe learning handicaps that warrant
special-education services. They are not qualify-
ing for such services through the SOMPA system.

## ALTERNATIVES TO NORM-REFERENCED TESTING

The courts required a complete moratorium on
all intelligence testing for blacks in the *Larry P.* v.
*Riles* case (1972). The results of the moratorium in California have been mixed and at best
have prevented large numbers of black children
from being placed in special-education classes.
As previously mentioned, the result has also
been that a large number of children with serious learning difficulties have received no services at all. Such were the events that led to the
potential court case reported by Matthews
(1987), discussed earlier in this chapter.

The moratorium on psychological testing is
not a new issue. In 1970, Messick and Anderson
concluded that the social consequences of not
testing are potentially far more harmful than any
possible adverse effects of testing. A general
feeling that still prevails today is that the outcome of a moratorium would be longer and
slower assessment processes, with most of the
responsibility for testing falling on teachers, who
in the past have been shown to systematically
rate students of minority groups lower than they
do white individuals (Mercer & Brown, 1973;
Sparks & Manese, 1970). After reviewing the
alternatives to testing, Cleary, Humphreys, Kendrick, and Wesman (1975) stated that there is as
much or more reason to expect lack of fairness
for alternative methods as for tests.

The profession strongly but cautiously advocates continued use of intellectual and educational testing, with various modifications and safeguards. Although testing has received the majority of criticism, it is evident that the discriminatory practices have not been limited to tests themselves but to the interpretations and selection of the testing instruments. Recent policies that grant the Educational Appraisal and Review Committee (EARC) responsibility for making placement decisions and for ensuring nonbiased assessment have been a tremendous step forward.

This chapter has concerned itself primarily with psychological testing used in determining qualification for special-education services. At this time and apparently for some time to come, state and federal agencies will continue to fund only children who have been labeled and categorized according to set guidelines. For this reason the author has not addressed the use of criterion-referenced assessment, which has been shown to be very effective with minority children within the classroom setting (see Plata, 1986). These processes have been designed for and shown to be very successful within programming and curriculum efforts.

## NONDISCRIMINATORY MODELS AND PRACTICES

Diagnostic evaluation models and current practices that have been proposed specifically to address the issue of nondiscriminatory testing have been in existence for some time. The practice of not including language-proficiency assessment as part of the testing battery has been lacking and has contributed significantly to biased test interpretation. In the past, determining language dominance typically consisted of simply asking parents or taking information from registration files. The result has been particularly unfortunate for the Hispanic child who shows a balance in English and Spanish or even dominant English skills, but who lacks sufficient

cognitive skills in that language to succeed academically.

By describing its development, Cummins (1984) contributed significantly to the field's recognition of the critical variable of language proficiency. He discusses two levels of language proficiency: basic interpersonal communication skills (BICS), and cognitive academic language proficiency (CALP). The BICS level includes skills characterized by visible, spoken language, and is defined as "the manifestation of language proficiency in everyday communicative contexts" (p. 137). In general, this level can be attained within a year if the child has no disabilities. CALP is conceptualized in terms of the manipulation of language in decontextualized academic situations (Cummins, 1984). Even with normal development and experiences, a child might take up to five years to develop this level.

Although these levels of proficiency are related to intelligence testing, the necessity of being able to function at the CALP level is obvious. A child must function at that level if he or she is to respond appropriately to the verbal section of tests. Any child not functioning at the CALP level simply would not have the linguistic skills that he or she needs to validly respond. The implications are significant in the current educational system. Ortiz (1986) reviewed the folders of limited English proficient (LEP) children in special-education classes and found that only 25% of the files contained evidence of current language testing. The implications are clear. Scores from verbal sections of intelligence tests for a child functioning at the BICS level in English are invalid until the child is functioning at the CALP level.

Another related concern is referrals. Research reveals that about 75% (Ortiz, 1986) of students referred by teachers for assessment for special-education services are found to be handicapped. With some districts, the percentage of placements is as high as 90% (Reynolds, 1984). Such high percentages indicate either that the teachers conduct efficient screening and referral procedures, or that many of these students are functioning at BICS levels and assumed by most school personnel to have learning handicaps.

The Implications for Policy and Practice Research Project (Ortiz, 1986), described above, issued the following recommendations for more effective evaluations of the LEP student:

1. A prereferral process, which is the responsibility of and under the jurisdiction of regular education, should be instituted.
2. Every language minority child referred to special education should receive a comprehensive language assessment in the native and the English languages.
3. Language assessments should provide evidence that the student has developed the cognitive, academic-language proficiency required for mastery of literacy skills.
4. Evaluations for the purpose of determining special-education eligibility should, except in the most unusual circumstances, be conducted by someone who is fluent in the student's language and trained in assessment of linguistically and culturally different students.
5. Practices used to assess intelligence and achievement of language minority students, including adaptations and/or deviations from standardized procedures, should be clearly documented in psychoeducational reports.
6. Eligibility criteria should require evidence that the handicapping condition exists in the primary language, not only in English.
7. When LEP students who have received native-language instruction in basic skills show significant discrepancies between intelligence and English academic achievement, appraisal personnel must provide evidence of low achievement in the primary language.
8. A bilingual individual with expertise in the education of language-minority students should participate in referral and placement committees (pp. 3–5).

## NONDISCRIMINATORY ASSESSMENT AND EVALUATION MODEL

The nondiscriminatory assessment model (Figure 13-1), described in this section, contains many familiar components and some which the reader may find unfamiliar. It provides a structure outlining key sequential steps, emphasizing a multidisciplinary *assessment team* approach, and recommending diagnostic instruments that can play an important part in ensuring nondiscriminatory assessment practices.

### Pre-Referral

Because of the large numbers of minority students who are qualified once referred (Ortiz, 1986), a pre-referral process under the jurisdiction of regular education is one of the most critical steps in the model. The primary purpose is to determine if any variables within the child's learning environment are the cause of his or her learning difficulties. Proficiency in both languages is the most critical factor to be evaluated, so it can be determined that the problem is not related to language deficiencies. Parental involvement, to include input about variables within the home setting, is critical at this point. Information necessary to eliminate variables such as vision, hearing, and health is provided at this level. Formal observational data in areas appearing to contain problems are obtained and documented. To ensure that current curricula and teacher(s) are effective in addressing individual needs, evaluations of their effectiveness are conducted. Finally, alternative interventions (i.e., bilingual education, Chapter I reading or math programs, peer tutors, varied teaching modes) should be exhausted. Before any referral decisions are made, a minimum time of one month should be spent on alternate or modified interventions.

Only when these variables have been investigated should a special education referral be initiated by the screening committee. The key member of this committee should be the bilin-

| Step 1 Pre-referral | Step 2 Referral | Step 3 Pre-evaluation data | Step 4 Differential diagnosis | Step 5 E. A. & R. | Step 6 Programming |
|---|---|---|---|---|---|
| Screening | Parental conference | Vision/hearing screening | Non-bias | Qualification | Least restrictive environment |
| Parental involvement | Consent to test | Medical history | Bilingual diagnostician | Program level | |
| Language assessment in both languages | | Educational history | Bilingual diagnosis | Supportive services | Bilingual special education classroom |
| | | Case history | Instrument selection | Bilingual representative | |
| Alternative intervention | | Adaptive behavior assessment | Pluralistic evaluation | Consent to place | Instructional component |
| Formal observation | | | | Total service plan | Bilingual speech/ language pathologist |

**Figure 13-1**
Gonzales model of nondiscriminatory assessment and evaluation model.

gual speech and language therapist who is familiar with the child's language and cultural background.

## Referral

Once the decision has been made to proceed with the referral, the special education evaluation process is initiated. Formal documentation of the referral, with information obtained in the pre-referral stage, is gathered. Parental notification and consent must include an explanation of all procedural safeguards and procedures to be followed. These should be provided to parents in a language that they understand.

## Pre-Evaluation Data

The school psychologist or educational diagnostician at this stage collects and analyzes data obtained in the pre-referral stage along with a complete educational and case history. If the child is suspected of mental retardation, the adaptive behavior scale is administered at this stage. A child passing the scale thus would not

qualify for that exceptionality; administration at this time also allows for early exploration of other disabilities.

## Differential Diagnosis

Test selection is critical at this stage and should be heavily influenced by the child's sociocultural background and language proficiency. For example, a child with a fifth-grade education, who moved to this country from Mexico this past year, would most likely have a BICS level in English with a CALP level in Spanish. For such a child, the Spanish translations would be more appropriate than tests in English. A bilingual examiner would be assigned to the student to conduct a pluralistic evaluation. Assessing an LEP student would include use of either the WISC-R or Kaufman intelligence tests. Selection of tests to evaluate academic achievement would likewise be determined by language-proficiency skills. Measures in both English and Spanish might be necessary, according to the sociocultural background of the child. Criterion-referenced tests supported by norm-referenced data should be used to determine academic skills in both languages.

### The Educational Appraisal and Review Committee

The Educational Appraisal and Review (E. A. & R.) Committee is a group of individuals directly involved with the education of the child. They are responsible for ensuring that the evaluation, placement, and programming decisions are in compliance with prescribed federal, state, and local educational standards. Such standards mandate a nonbiased assessment; therefore, the responsibility to guarantee such an assessment ultimately falls on this committee.

The key person in this committee is again a bilingual representative with expertise in educating the particular minority group of which the child is a member. Considerable knowledge about evaluation is also important. The bilingual diagnostician would be an individual possessing such knowledge. If the diagnostician were unable to participate, an individual from the evaluation team must be present. Representatives from other programs (i.e., bilingual education, ESL) should also be included.

Parental involvement as well as permission to place is obtained at this time. Parents should be reminded about their due-process rights at this point. Together with the parents, the E. A. & R. committee develops the individualized educational program (I.E.P.); a total service plan is developed. It includes a broad outline of goals and objectives, ancillary or supportive services that the child is to receive, and names of the responsible personnel. Dates of initiation and duration of services are specified at this time. If

a language disorder is identified, a bilingual speech and language therapist, as one of the related service providers, should be included in the I.E.P.

### Programming

Once a specific handicap not related to sociolinguistic background has been identified as an influence on the child's academic process, placement in the least restrictive environment is to be provided. Three models for delivery of services to the bilingual, exceptional student are presented in detail in a handbook by Ambert and Dew (1985).

## SUMMARY AND CONCLUSIONS

This chapter has highlighted the major concerns expressed by professionals dealing with the assessment of children from culturally and linguistically diverse groups. The controversial discussions present much material for debate and force those dealing with these issues to constantly question current practices. It is hoped that such ongoing debate will help practitioners and researchers develop new, improved tools and procedures. In addition, insights about better utilization of what already exists in the field are equally desirable outcomes. Ultimately, it is the examiners' and administrators' professional ethics and knowledge that will determine whether assessments are unbiased. As a guideline for those wishing to approximate fair testing practices, the nondiscriminatory assessment and evaluation model brings together the major issues, concerns, and recommendations discussed in the chapter.

# CHAPTER 14

# State of the Art and Speculations on the Future

Undoubtedly any attempt to describe the state of the art of assessment and especially to speculate on future events is bound to be deficient. Even so there is an abiding belief that on occasion a profession should look at its current position and contemplate the future. As to the future, the field of assessment is alive and well. In the past twenty years, new assessment models have risen to meet new assessment problems (for example, ecological, decision-making theories). A field that can respond to need for change with appropriate alterations is healthy. These changes have occurred in spite of and because of a body of theories and knowledge, which have competent and flexible adherents who are willing to test their assumptions.

Probably the most obvious advance in assessment from our earlier edition of this text is the influence of microcomputers in assessment. Current uses of microcomputers in assessment include scoring and interpretation, report writing, and data management. For example, a quick look at some test catalogues (e.g., *Psychware Sourcebook, 1987–1988*) shows there is a growing number of test-scoring programs available (e.g., WISC-R, Woodcock-Johnson Psychoeducational Battery, Peabody Individual Achievement Test, Kaufman-Assessment Battery for Children, Iowa Test of Basic Skills). Generally, these software programs depend on the examiner (or a clerk) to type in raw data. The computer then displays or prints out standardized scores. In some programs the standard scores are accompanied by a written analysis of the scores. In other programs, a description of what the tests measure is accompanied by a discussion of the subject's performance as compared to the norm group and as compared to himself or herself. In addition, because tests have a particular orientation that is used to analyze test scores, a number of interpretative procedures, using the Sattler, Kaufman, Lutey and other statistical methods of interpretation, are available. These analyses vary in the approach taken to interpret the data; each report is supported to

some extent by the literature. Computers are also used in report writing: editors or word processors abound in the marketplace. Typical report-writing programs contain a means by which common phrases or frequently used blocks of text can be inserted into reports. In dealing with data management, a plethora of record-keeping software is available, for use with tests scores, psychological reports, client daily contacts, IEP goals and objectives, and so on.

Despite the advantages of computer-technology applications to the assessment process (e.g., cost effectiveness, efficient generation of standardized data, efficient and accurate scoring, ease of data management) Sampson (1983) and Brown (1984) have reviewed some disadvantages of the use of computer technology in assessment practices. Some of these disadvantages are (1) inability of the computers to store mass verbal information to allow for the production of comprehensive verbal reports, (2) poorly designed software, which produce reports based on insufficient data, and (3) the confidentiality of the information collected by the computer is not guaranteed. Another disadvantage is the inability of the software program to integrate multiple pieces of information *across* standardized tests. No doubt the progressive improvement of computer software, coupled with complex forms of psychological and educational assessment, will be the norm practice of the 1990s. We anticipate, however, that many theoretical, as well as ethical and training problems, will surround the development of computerized assessment.

New theoretical concepts in the various testing domains are an omen of change. Sternberg's (e.g., 1985, 1988) work in the area of intellectual assessment is one example. Because of the comprehensive aspects of educational and psychological assessment, developments in other disciplines often give rise to changes in testing procedures. The increasing sophistication of computers, combined with electrophysiological procedures, offers the possibilty of operationalizing theoretical constructs in intelligence, language, affective, and perceptual-motor assessment.

Many aspects of the field of assessment, such as norm-referenced tests, procedures associated with item analysis, and determination of reliability and validity, have a venerable history and hence provide a strong base for future growth. Only from a clear understanding of the strengths and weaknesses of norm-referenced testing could come criterion-referenced measurements, which have become a multifaceted aspect of assessment, as demonstrated by Nitko's (1980) earlier classification system for criterion-referenced tests.

The technical aspects of norm-referenced test construction have not remained static. Earlier procedures developed by Rasch (1960) and Wright (1968) result in an interval scale of measurement, that is, a scale of equal units. Although testing measures did not have the characteristics of an interval scale, they were often treated as though they did. In addition, the development of methods for determining the reliability and validity of criterion-referenced tests has presented a new challenge to statisticians, who learned very early that the traditional procedures were inadequate.

Tests and testing have received much criticism for two reasons: (1) test authors and publishers did not live up to the high standards expected of them, and (2) the general public has assumed that tests could do things they were never intended to do. These assumptions have been fostered all too often by the individuals who interpret test results (e.g., Haney, 1984). This is a reflection on the training institutions. Because serious errors have been made, courts have played and will continue to play a significant role in the construction, use, and interpretation of tests. Many of these serious errors have occurred in the assessment of individuals from minority groups. However, the issues and options are now in much clearer focus and research can begin to sort out which variables must be given major consideration in the testing of minorities. For example, in testing a person

whose primary language is not English, one could logically assume that tests for that individual should be administered in the primary language. Some legal rulings require it. However, data now available indicate that such an assumption is not always justified.

As a result of increased research in variables affecting test performance in minority individuals, the recent models of assessment discussed in Chapter 1 are far more comprehensive than the earlier models. For example, cultural concepts and values in regard to time are a significant factor in test performance and must be considered in selection of tests and interpretation of the performance of members of those cultures.

As the demands of society for "hard" evidence of competency and performance increase, tests now include an ever-widening array of topics. Areas once assessed by "expert observers" with a "behavior checklist" now are the subject of comprehensive formal assessment, as evidenced by the fact that Part II, on testing domains, makes up the major portion of this book.

Although testing issues are a major societal concern, relatively little research is being done to evaluate many instruments being used almost daily with handicapped children, as demonstrated by the paucity of research on testing in the perceptual-motor (Chapter 6) and academic (Chapter 7) areas in contrast to the amount of research on intelligence tests (Chapter 4).

Economics will play an increasing role in the development of new tests and procedures. Because of increasing costs of test construction and a continuing demand for large representative normative samples, future tests will have to prove their worth in wide-ranging research with a variety of subjects before they undergo the expensive process of being normed on a national sample. Consequently, there should be a decrease in the number of commercial tests published and an increase in the number of new measures presented in the assessment literature. It is hoped that the increasing sophistication of educators and psychologists will result in a less lucrative market for tests that are poorly designed and constructed.

The market is now being flooded with so-called criterion-referenced tests. Most of these are of limited use because they meet few of the criteria discussed in Chapter 2 and because they are frequently only peripherally related to the curriculum content being used in a local school system. Because of the increasing number of well-trained personnel and the availability of computers, local school systems will find that they can develop criterion-referenced measures to suit their own needs at less cost than the purchase of commercially available tests that will have to be modified and supplemented to meet their needs. Development of criterion-referenced tests, such as competency examinations in the basic skills, is already occurring at the state level. By complementing their norm-referenced testing based on large representative national samples with locally relevant criterion-referenced tests, school systems should be able to obtain adequate data from which to develop optimal instructional programs.

The high cost of test construction will also result in a reexamination of some basic assumptions in test construction. Although a strong case can be made for a large representative national normative sample, what actual discrepancies arise in results if a limited sample is used? Is it possible that this country's population has become so mobile that a representative sample of any one geographical area will adequately reflect national characteristics? In regard to the representativeness of a sample, must every group be included, so that a sample with the characteristics of a national group is obtained? Obviously the answers to these questions require extensive research.

As a result of developments in the assessment of minority individuals, researchers will become increasingly aware of the variables that affect the test performances of all children. Both awareness and the technical skills needed to assess these variables will increase. In the future, for example, assumptions about test performance will not be made on the basis of general data on socioeconomic status, but the specific effects of the social-cultural-economic milieu of the child will be determined. Whether these speculations or others more awesome become reality will depend to a large extent on the ability, sensitivity, commitment, and training of the personnel who will conceptualize, construct, administer, and interpret the tests of the future.

# APPENDIX A

# Glossary of
# General Measurement Terms

**academic aptitude** Likelihood of success in mastering academic work estimated from measures of the necessary abilities.

**accomplishment quotient (AQ)** The ratio of educational age to mental age—EA:MA.

**achievement age** Estimated age from a given achievement test score (also called educational age or subject age). If the achievement age corresponding to a score of 36 on a reading test is 10 years 7 months (10-7), this means that pupils 10 years 7 months of age achieve, on the average, a score of 36 on that test.

**achievement test** A test that measures the extent to which a person has acquired certain information as a result of specific instruction.

**age norms** Values of various age groups representing typical or average performance.

**alternate-forms reliability** A measure of the extent to which two forms are consistent or reliable in measuring whatever they do measure, assuming that the subjects themselves do not change in the abilities measured between the two testings (*see* Coefficient of correlation, Reliability, Standard error).

**aptitude** Abilities and other characteristics, whether native or acquired, indicative of an individual's ability to learn in some particular area.

**arithmetic mean** A set of scores divided by the number of scores (commonly called average mean).

**assessment** A strategic or problem-solving process that may use educational and psychological tests put into some theoretical framework for collecting relevant information.

**average** Applies to measures of central tendency. The three most widely used averages are arithmetic mean, median, and mode.

**battery (static)** Several tests standardized on the same population so that their results are directly comparable; applied to any group of tests administered together, even though not standardized on the same subjects.

**ceiling** The upper limit of ability measured by a test.

**central tendency** A general term for the middle of a group of scores.

**coefficient of correlation** The degree of relationship between two scores or measures; $r$ denotes the mathematical basis of its calculation. Correlation coefficients range from .00, denoting complete absence of relationship, to 1.00, denoting perfect correspondence, and may be either positive or negative.

**completion item** Questions requiring completion (filling in) of a phrase or sentence from which one or more parts have been omitted.

**construct** Traits or abilities derived from a theoretical reference (*see* Factor).

**correlation** Relationship between two scores or measures for the same individuals.

**criterion** A standard by which a test may be judged or evaluated.

**criterion-referenced** Measurement of specific objectives to determine what a person can and cannot do.

**decile** Percentile points (scores) in a distribution that divide the distribution into 10 equal parts—the first decile is the 10th percentile, the ninth the 90th percentile.

**deviation** Score that differs from some reference value, such as mean, norm, or score on some other test.

**diagnostic test** A test to locate specific areas of weaknesses or strengths. It yields measures of the components of subparts of large bodies of information or skill.

**discriminating power** The ability of a test (item) to differentiate between individuals possessing some trait.

**distribution (frequency distribution)** A tabulation of scores from high to low or low to high.

**domain-referenced** Body of knowledge against which the performance of students is measured.

**equivalent forms** Forms of a test that are closely parallel with respect to the nature of the content and the difficulty of the items.

**extrapolation** A process of estimating values of a function beyond the range of available data. The process of extending a norm line beyond the limits of actually obtained data for the purpose of interpretation of extreme scores.

**factor** A hypothetical trait, ability, or component of an ability that underlies and influences performance; strictly refers to a theoretical variable, derived by a process of factor analysis, from a table of intercorrelations among tests.

**factor analysis** Several methods of analyzing the intercorrelations among a set of variables such as test scores. The analysis accounts for the interrelationships in terms of some underlying "factors" and reveals how much of the variation in each of the original measures arises from or is associated with each of the hypothetical factors.

**g** General factor of intelligence assumed to be related to all measures of intellectual functioning.

**grade equivalent** Grade level for which a given score is the real or estimated average score.

**grade norm** Average score obtained by pupils of given grade placement.

**group test** One that may be administered to several individuals at the same time by one examiner.

**individual test** One that can be administered to only one person at a time.

**inner language** The proverbial organization of experience.

**intelligence quotient (IQ)** The ratio of a person's mental age to his or her chronological age, or the ratio of mental age to the mental age normal for chronological age (in both cases multiplied by 100 to eliminate the decimal).

**interpolation** The process of estimating intermediate values between two known points. A procedure used in assigning interpreted values, such as grade or age equivalents, to scores between the successive average scores actually obtained in the standardization process.

**item** A single question or exercise in a test.

**item analysis** Evaluating single test items by any of several methods. It usually involves determining the difficulty value and the discriminating power of the item and often its correlation with some criterion.

**linguistics** The study of the nature and use of language.

**matching item** The correct association of each test item in one list with an entry in a second list.

**mean** *See* Arithmetic mean.

**measurement** The qualification (assignment of numbers) of behaviors.

**median** The middle score in a distribution; the 50th percentile; the point that divides the group into two equal parts. Half of the group scores fall below the median and half above it.

**mental age (MA)** The age for which a given score on an intelligence test is average or normal.

**mode** The value that occurs most frequently in a distribution.

**multiple-choice item** A test item in which the subject chooses the correct or best answer from several answers on options.

**N** The number of cases in a distribution.

**normal distribution** A distribution of scores or measures that in graphic form is bell-shaped. In a normal distribution, scores or measures are distributed symmetrically about the mean, with as many cases at various distances above the mean as at equal distances below it and with cases concentrated near the average and decreasing in frequency the farther one departs from the average, according to a precise mathematical equation.

**norm-referenced** Subject's status in relation to performance of group who has completed the test.

**norms** Norms are often assumed to be representative of some large population, such as pupils in the entire country. Norms are descriptive of average, typical, or mediocre performance; they are not to be regarded as standards or as desirable levels of attainment. Grade age and percentile are the most common types of norms.

**objective test** The scoring of a test in which there is no possibility of difference of opinion among scorers as to whether responses are to be scored right or wrong.

**percentile (P)** A point (score) in a distribution below which fall the percent of cases indicated by the given percentile; it does not relate to the percent of correct answers on a test.

**percentile rank** The percent of scores corresponding to the given rank in a distribution.

**perception** The processing of information obtained through the senses.

**personality test** A measure intended to test one or more of the nonintellectual aspects of an individual's mental or psychological makeup.

**phonology** The system of speech sounds in a language.

**pluralistic assessment** An assessment procedure that combines measures of functioning in the different systems in which the subject lives and works, such as cultural, ethnic, socioeconomic, educational, organic, or internal.

**profile** A graphic representation of the results on several tests, for either an individual or a group, when the results have been expressed in some uniform or comparable terms.

**projective technique (projective method)** A method of study in which the subject responds as he or she chooses to a series of stimuli, such as inkblots, pictures, or unfinished sentences. The Rorschach (inkblot) Technique and the Murray Thematic Apperception Test are the most commonly used projective methods.

**quartile** One of three points that divide the cases in a distribution into four equal groups. The lowest quartile, or 25th percentile, sets off the lowest fourth of the group; the middle quartile is the same as the 50th percentile, or median; and the third quartile, or 75th percentile, marks off the highest fourth.

*r* See Coefficient of correlation.

**random sample** A population drawn in such a way that every member of the population has an equal chance of being included.

**range** The lowest and the highest score differences obtained on a test by some group.

**raw score** The first quantitative result obtained in scoring a test, usually the number of right answers or number right minus some fraction of number wrong.

**readiness test** Measures the extent to which an individual has achieved a degree of maturity or acquired certain skills or information needed for successfully undertaking some new learning activity.

**reliability** The extent to which scores on a test are consistent across items (internal consistency, split-half reliability), forms (alternate- or parallel-forms reliability), and time (test-retest reliability).

*s* Specific factors that do not correlate with factors on other tests.

**semantic** The system of meaning in language.

**skewness** The tendency of a distribution to depart from symmetry or balance around the mean.

**sociometry** Measurement of the interpersonal relationships prevailing among the members of a group.

**Spearman-Brown** A formula giving the relationship between the reliability of a test and its length. Its most common application is in the estimation of reliability of an entire test from the correlation between two halves of the test (split-half reliability).

**standard deviation (SD)** The variability or dispersion of a set of scores. The more the scores cluster around the mean, the smaller the standard deviation.

**standard error (SE)** The amount by which an obtained score differs from a hypothetical true score. The standard error is an amount such that in about two-thirds of the cases the obtained score would not differ by more than one standard error from the true score.

**standard score** Any of a variety of standard deviation scores used to express raw scores.

**standardized test (standard test)** A systematic sample of performance obtained under prescribed conditions, scored according to definite rules, and capable of evaluation by reference to normative information.

**stanine** The stanine (short for standard-nine) scale has values from 1 to 9, with a mean of 5, and a standard deviation of 2.

**survey test** A test that measures general achievement in a subject or area, usually with the connotation that the test is intended to measure group status rather than yield precise measurement of individuals.

*T* **score** A standard score that has a mean of 50 and a standard deviation of 10.

**tests** Series of systematic tasks used to obtain observations on child performance.

**true-false item** An exercise in which the subject indicates whether a given statement is true or false.

**true score** The average value of an infinite series of measurements with the same or exactly equivalent tests, assuming there is no practice effect or change in the subject between the testings.

**validity** The extent to which a test measures what it says it measures. Validity has different connotations for various kinds of tests and, therefore, different kinds of validity evidence.

**variability** Extent to which test scores spread out from the average score in the group.

*Z* **score** A standard score having a mean of 0 and a standard deviation of 1.

# Test Publishers

Academic Therapy Publications, 20 Commercial Boulevard, Novato, CA 94947

Allyn & Bacon, 470 Atlantic Avenue, Boston, MA 02210

American Association on Mental Deficiency, 5101 Wisconsin Avenue, Washington, DC 20016

American Guidance Service, Inc., Publisher's Building, Circle Pines, MN 55014

Bobbs-Merrill Company, Inc., 4300 West 62nd Street, Indianapolis, IN 46208

William C. Brown Company, 2460 Kerper Boulevard, Dubuque, IA 52001

Bureau of Educational Research and Service, University of Iowa, Iowa City, IA 52240

The Callier Center for Communication Disorders, The University of Texas at Dallas, 1966 Inwood Road, Dallas, TX 75235

Childcraft Educational Corporation, 20 Kilmer Road, Edison, NJ 08818

Communication Research Associates, P. O. Box 11012, Salt Lake City, UT 84111

Consulting Psychologists Press, Inc., 577 College Avenue, Palo Alto, CA 94306

Counselor Recordings and Tests, Box 6184, Acklen Station, Nashville, TN 37212

CTB/McGraw-Hill, Del Monte Research Park, Monterey, CA 93940

Curriculum Associates, Inc., 5 Esquire Road, North Billerica, MA 08162

The Devereux Foundation Press, 19 South Waterloo Road, Devon, PA 19333

DLM Teaching Resources, Inc., 1 DLM Park, 200 Bethany Road, Allen, TX 75002

The Economy Company, 1901 North Walnut Avenue, Oklahoma City, OK 74103

Educational and Industrial Testing Service, P. O. Box 7234, San Diego, CA 92107

Educational Performance Associates, 563 Westview Avenue, Ridgefield, NJ 07657

Educational Testing Service, Princeton, NJ 08540

Educator's Publishing Service, 75 Moulton Street, Cambridge, MA 02138

Evaluation Systems, Inc., P. O. Box 5087, Chicago, IL 60610

Exceptional Resources, Inc., 7701 Cameron Road, Suite 105, Austin, TX 78766

Fearon Publishing Service, 6 Davis Drive, Belmont, CA 94002

Follett Educational Corporation, 1010 West Washington Boulevard, Chicago, IL 60607

Garrard Publishing Company, 1607 North Market Street, Champaign, IL 61820

Grune & Stratton, 111 Fifth Avenue, New York, NY 10003

Harcourt Brace Jovanovich, Inc., 757 Third Avenue, New York, NY 10017

Houghton Mifflin Company, One Beacon Street, Boston, MA 02107

Industrial Relations Center, University of Chicago, 1225 East 60th Street, Chicago, IL 60637

Institute for Personality and Ability Testing, 1602 Coronado Drive, Champaign, IL 61820

Institutional Services, ICD Rehabilitation and Research Center, 340 East 24th Street, New York, NY 10010

Jastak Associates, Inc., 1526 Gilpin Avenue, Wilmington, DE 19806

Kaplan School Supply, Winston-Salem, NC

Ladoca Publishing Foundation, Laradon Hall Training and Residential Center, East 51st Avenue and Lincoln Street, Denver, CO 80216

Language Research Associates, 175 East Delaware Place, Chicago, IL 60611

MacKeith Press, Distributed in USA by Lippincott/ Harper Publishers, Inc., Journals Division, 2350 Virginia Avenue, Hagerstown, MD 21740

McCarron-Dial System, P. O. Box 45628, Dallas, TX 75254

Minneapolis Preschool Screening Instrument, Prescriptive Instruction Center, 254 Upton Avenue South, Minneapolis, MN 55405

National Computer Systems/PAS Division, P. O. Box 1416, Minneapolis, MN 55440

The Nissonger Center, The Ohio State University, 1581 Dodd Drive, Columbus, OH 43210

Northwestern University Press, 1735 Benson Avenue, Evanston, IL 60201

Personnel Press, 191 Spring Street, Lexington, MA 02173

Prep, Inc., 1007 Whitehead Road Extension, Trenton, NJ 08638

Pro-Ed, 333 Perry Brooks Building, Austin, TX 78701

Psychological Assessment Resources, Inc., P. O. Box 98, Odessa, FL 33556

Psychological Corporation, P. O. Box 7954, San Antonio, TX 78204

Psychological Test Specialists, Box 1441, Missoula, MT 59801

Psychometric Affiliates, Box 3167, Munster, IN 46321

The Riverside Publishing Company, 8420 Bryn Mawr Avenue, Chicago, IL 60631

Scholastic Testing Service, Inc., 480 Meyer Road, Bensenville, IL 60106

Science Research Associates, Inc., 259 East Erie Street, Chicago, IL 60611

Scientific Research Associates, Inc., 155 North Wacker Drive, Chicago, IL 60606

Sheridan Psychological Services, P. O. Box 6101, Orange, CA 92667

Singer Education Division/Career Systems, 80 Commerce Drive, Rochester, NY

R.V. Skoczylas, 7649 Santa Inez Court, Gilroy, CA 95020

Slosson Educational Publications, P. O. Box 280, East Aurora, NY 14052

C. H. Stoelting Company, 424 North Homan Avenue, Chicago, IL 60624

System Design Associates, Inc., 723 Kanawha Boulevard East, Charleston, WV 25301

Talent Assessment, Inc., P. O. Box 5087, Jacksonville, FL 32207

Teachers College Press, Columbia University, 1234 Amsterdam Avenue, New York, NY 10027

Teaching Resources Corporation, 100 Boylston Street, Boston, MA 20116

United States Employment Service, Department of Labor

University of Illinois Press, Urbana, IL 61801

University of Michigan Press, Box 1104, 839 Greene Street, Ann Arbor, MI 48106

Valpar International Corporation, 3801 East 34th Street, Tucson, AZ 85713

Vocational Psychology Research, University of Minnesota, Elliot Hall, 75 East River Road, Minneapolis, MN 55455

Vocational Research Institute, 1624 Locust Street, Philadelphia, PA 19103

VORT Corporation, P. O. Box 60132, Palo Alto, CA 94306

Webster Division, McGraw-Hill, Manchester Road, Manchester, MO 63011

Western Psychological Services Corporation, 12031 Wilshire Boulevard, Los Angeles, CA 90025

Richard L. Zweig Associates, 20800 Beach Boulevard, Huntington Beach, CA 92648

# Informal Tests

The purpose of this appendix is to provide the diagnostician with informal (nonstandardized) tests that may be helpful in assessing children's educational needs. These informal tests have been gathered from several teachers and school psychologists. The appendix is divided into various sections so the reader can choose areas of interest. Before informal testing is done, some general information questions should be asked, such as:

1. Where do you live? What is your address?
2. How many people are in your family?
3. How many brothers and sisters do you have?
4. How old are you?
5. When is your birthday? In what year were you born?
6. What is your telephone number?
7. What do you like most about school?
8. What do you like least about school?
9. What are the days of the week, in order?
10. What are the months of the year, in order?
11. What is the opposite of (a) boy, (b) start, (c) his, (d) open, (e) new, (f) day, (g) tall, (h) up, (i) big, (j) under?

## Section I: Rapid survey

The purpose of this section is for the teacher to record various superficial strengths and weaknesses of the child. Information can be gathered about the child through review of cumulative folders, permanent classroom products (worksheets), and teacher observation of the child.

**Items to check**                                                    **Suggested methods**

1. Special interests and abilities                                     Observation

2. Attitudes toward self and others                                    Observation

3. Communication skills (ability to follow directions):               Observation
   ☐ Well  ☐ Imperfectly  ☐ Poorly

4. Reads at these levels: Instructional, Gr. _____                    Reading kit
                          Independent, Gr. _____

5. Needs help with these skills:
   ☐ Alphabet
   ☐ Sight words
   ☐ Word endings
   ☐ Compound words
   ☐ Consonants
   ☐ Consonants in context
   ☐ Substituting consonants
   ☐ Vowel sounds
   ☐ Vowel combinations
   ☐ Mechanical skills adequate, but lacks comprehension

6. Arithmetic:
   ☐ Can count by rote to 100
   ☐ Can count objects to 20
   ☐ Recognizes number groups to 10
   ☐ Can count by 2s
   ☐ Can write numbers below 100 from dictation
   ☐ Recognizes coins
   ☐ Can count money to $1
   ☐ Can make change to $1
   ☐ Knows addition combinations to 10
   ☐ Knows subtraction combinations to 10

7. Arithmetic: Grade level for textbook _____                         Permanent Products
                                                                      Arithmetic

8. Needs help in these computational skills:
   ☐ Addition facts
   ☐ Subtraction facts
   ☐ Multiplication facts
   ☐ Division facts
   ☐ Fractions
   ☐ Addition processes
   ☐ Subtraction processes
   ☐ Multiplication processes

**Items to check**

☐ Division processes

☐ Decimals

Can do simple problems involving practical needs of children at grade

level _____.

9. Speech before group:                                               Observation

☐ Clear and comfortable  ☐ Halting or confused  ☐ Extremely shy

10. Speech difficulty

11. Writing and spelling:                      Regular work:

☐ Does not write                               ☐ Very poor

☐ Uses manuscript                              ☐ Fair quality

☐ Uses cursive                                 ☐ Excellent

☐ Can copy a simple sentence from the board

☐ Can write a simple sentence from dictation

☐ Can write one or more original sentences

☐ Can do regular work in spelling for grade _____

12. Spells successfully at grade level _____                         Written language

Can write from dictation at level _____                              skills sheets

13. Can write original ideas:                                         Writing assignment

☐ Not at all

☐ Simple sentence

☐ Short paragraph

☐ Fluently

☐ In good form

☐ Readable, but with errors

☐ Unreadable

14. Health problems needing special consideration:                    Records, nurse,

☐ Energy level                                                        observation

☐ Vision

☐ Limited activity

☐ Hearing

☐ Seizures

☐ Other _____

## Section II: Reading checklist

The purpose of this section is to informally test the child's skill in letter and word recognition, sentence closure, syllabication, definitions, classifications, and context clues. Questions in each area represent a span from second-grade to fifth-grade skills.

1. Do you know these letters?

   b  w  c  r  p  d  e  t  L  S  F  G  M  Y  Q

2. What are the names of these letters?

   d  p  t  a  w  r  n  j  b  v  A  W  R  T  N  P  J

3. Recites alphabet orally

4. Names alphabet letters from visual presentation

5. Writes letters from name dictation

6. Writes letters from sound dictation

7. Can give the sound of each letter

8. Long vowels

9. Short vowels

10. Read these words:

    | boy | call | look | help |
    |-----|------|------|------|
    | boys | called | looks | helping |

11. Can you read these words?

    | call | swim | want | cry |
    |------|------|------|-----|
    | calls | swimming | wanted | crying |
    | called | swims | wants | cried |

12. Can you read these words?

    | maybe | sometimes | hilltop |
    |-------|-----------|---------|
    | playground | wallpaper | bedtime |

13. Do you know these words?

    | just | what | clean | which |
    |------|------|-------|-------|
    | please | walk | under | around |
    | laugh | this | never | write |
    | help | went | buy | here |
    | will | after | small | about |
    | said | because | together | always |

14. Do you know these words?

    into    someone    playground    anywhere    downhill

15. I am going to say some words. Point to the first letter of each word:

    m  b  s  p  r  f  l  c  n  d

16. Do these the same way:

    sh  bl  sp  cr  cl  dr  sl

17. I am going to read several words. Point to the first letter or letters of each word.

    m  s  l  r  b  d  bl  cr  pl  dr  sh  ph

18. Digraphs: Gives sounds from written stimuli:  sh  th  ch  wh

    Pairs with pictures _____

    Isolated digraphs _____

19. Blends: Gives sounds from written stimuli:

    wr  squ  sk  fr  tw  spr  scr  fl  tr  sp  sc  dr  thr  sp

    pr  cr  sw  sn  pl  cl  kn  str  sm  gr  br  qu  st  sl  gl  bl

    Pairs with pictures _____

    Isolated blends _____

20. Sound blending from nonsense pattern (C-V-C) from written stimuli:

    dac  pog  ris  tuv  lem  pab  jox  vig  fuf  hef

21. I will read the first word. Can you read the word under it?

    send     round     teach     bone

    bend     pound     reach     stone

22. Can you read these words?

    bake  pin  can  pole  tune  fun  hot  mile

23. Try these:

    coal  seed  proud  paw  fail  spoil  gown

24. Do you know these words?

    all      have     many     where     that     how

    laugh    today    away     never     before   just

25. Can you read these words?

    pen     blow     road     bun     hop

    pan     blew     read     bin     hope

26. Read these words as fast as you can—HURRY! (word and letter reversals)

    pal _____     even _____     no _____     saw _____

    raw _____     ten _____      tar _____    won _____

    pot _____     rats _____     keep _____   naps _____

    tops _____    read _____     meat _____   lap _____

    never _____

27. Write each word under one of the headings given below. (If the student does not know a word, tell him.)

    work       peas       coat       talk

    peaches    ham        pie        sing

    hat        grapes     mittens    socks

    jacket     oranges    smile      jump

    apples     skip       beans      gloves

    **Things to wear**               **Things to eat**               **Things to do**

28. Number these words so they will be in alphabetical order in each column. (If the student does not know a word, tell him.)

| _____ day | _____ girl | _____ when |
|---|---|---|
| _____ been | _____ book | _____ all |
| _____ all | _____ mother | _____ they |
| _____ cow | _____ people | _____ good |
| _____ fat | _____ house | _____ tree |
| | | _____ any |
| | | _____ very |
| | | _____ window |

29. What do these words mean? (Pronounce the words for the student.)

uncle _____

coward _____

chunky _____

sprout _____

balance _____

whirling _____

30. Which word does not belong? (Say the words for the student.)

knife, fork, cup, spoon _____

man, woman, army, child _____

fall, June, spring, winter _____

31. Can you read and complete these sentences?

a. Mother said, "It is time to go to b_____."

b. Dick hit his f_____ with the hammer.

c. Mary likes to drink m_____.

32. This story has some words missing. Try to read the story by guessing the missing words.

"Tim," _____ Mother, "will you go to the store for me?"

"Sure, _____," said _____. "What shall I get?"

"I need a _____ of butter, a loaf of _____, and a _____ eggs," said _____. "Hurry!" _____ ran to the _____ and was soon back.

"That's a good _____," said _____. "Thank _____ very much."

"You're welcome, Mom," said _____, and he ran off to _____ ball with his _____.

33. Can you divide these words and sound them?

| cabbage | reply |
|---|---|
| complain | shelter |
| porcupine | melody |

34. Story sequencing: Have the student read the story and answer the questions following it.

> After supper that evening, we found another dead bird. A few days later, my father brought in the third robin. It was dead.
>
> "The last one is a strong fellow," Father said later. "He may try out his wings soon. But this little one will have a hard job. There is no one to teach him to fly. Perhaps he is weak from too little food."
>
> One day we found the little robin rocking on a twig. I so much wanted this bird to fly! His wings fluttered. He was off the branch. For a second his wings beat the air. Then he fell to the ground. His legs kicked once, and he was dead.
>
> "Poor little fellow," father said. "He didn't have much of a chance, did he?"
>
> Sadly I cried out, "Oh, Dad, it's all my fault! I killed his mother."
>
> "I know, son. I saw you do it. It was a thing that many boys have done. But I just wanted you to see that you cannot hurt anything or anybody without hurting others. Perhaps you may hurt even the ones who love you. And so often you yourself are the one who is hurt most."

The sentences below tell what happened in the story. Write 1 before what happened first, write 2 before what happened next, and so on.

_____ Father showed Harry four young birds in a nest.

_____ Father gave Harry an air gun.

_____ Three baby birds died in a few days.

_____ Harry shot a robin.

_____ One of the baby birds tried to fly.

_____ One baby bird fell to the ground and died.

## Section III: Mathematics

The purpose of this section is to provide an estimate of starting places from grade 1 to grade 8. The place of instruction is the level at which the child cannot solve the problems.

**Arithmetic**

*Level 1*

$$5 \atop +2$$  $$\begin{matrix} 4 \\ 2 \\ +3 \end{matrix}$$  $$5 \atop -3$$  $$7 - 1 =$$

*Level 2*

$$5 \atop +8$$  $$\begin{matrix} 3 \\ 5 \\ 8 \\ +2 \end{matrix}$$  $$11 \atop -8$$  $$17 \atop -10$$

*Level 3*

$$35 \atop +42$$  $$116 \atop -81$$  $$42 \atop \times 2$$  $$3\overline{)669}$$

| | | | |
|---|---|---|---|
| *Level 4* | $6.50<br>+3.25 | 6)762 | 25<br>42<br>+37 | 692<br>×6 |

| | | | |
|---|---|---|---|
| *Level 5* | 421<br>×53 | 62)3560 | 6¼<br>+3 | 4.8<br>5.2<br>6.7<br>+4.9 |

*Level 6*     98.7 + 6.4 + 297.5 + .8 =

729     39)874     13½
×405                72¼
                  + 6½

*Level 7*     125 + 43751 =     .76)4.408

15% of 60 gallons =

Find the area of a rectangle 26.2 inches long and 14.8 inches wide.

## Word problems

*Level 3*
1. Sam bought a pencil for 5¢. He gave the man at the store a quarter. How much change did he get?
2. There are 28 children in the third grade. Only 25 are here today. How many are absent?
3. Sam has 8 marbles. Jack has 6 marbles. John has 4 marbles. How many marbles do the boys have all together?

*Level 4*
1. Mary, Sally, and Jane each pumped up 4 balls. How many balls did they fix?
2. The class is having a cookie sale. The children put 6 cookies in each paper bag. They have 96 cookies left. How many bags will this make?
3. Ray bought an airplane for 65 cents. He gave the man at the store a $5 bill. How much change did he get?

*Level 5*
1. Tom's mother bought 4 toothbrushes for 39¢ each. She bought 2 tubes of toothpaste for 63¢ each. How much did she spend?
2. Paul and his father are going to Los Angeles. If they drive at an average speed of 50 miles an hour, how long will it take them to go the 225 miles?
3. Jack bought a $35 bicycle on sale for $27.50. How much did he save?

*Level 6*
1. A man can earn $12.40 a day picking cotton. He has been offered a job at the railroad at $1.75 an hour. On which job can he make more money if he works 8 hours a day? How much more?
2. The class took a 3-minute reading test to measure reading speed. Mary read 720 words and Catherine read 675 words. How many more words a minute did Mary read?
3. A used car costs $325 with $35 down and the rest to be paid in 20 monthly installments. How much will each monthly payment be?

*Level 7*    1. A $25 coat is offered for sale at 35% off. How much will it cost?
2. At one store canned milk was for sale at 3 cans for 29¢. At another store the same brand was priced at 4 cans for 43¢. Find the difference in price per can.
3. Mike's father took a trip of 2136 miles and used 118 gallons of gas. To the nearest tenth of a mile, what was his average mileage for each gallon of gasoline?

## Section IV: Written language

The purpose of this section is to informally assess spelling, writing, and expressing ideas.

1. Print or write the following words:

| | | |
|---|---|---|
| found | court | squatting |
| bonus | examine | purpose |
| stampede | innocent | troubled |

2. Dictate the following spelling words to the pupil. Stop when he is unable to go further.

**Grade levels**

| Second | Third | Fourth | Fifth | Sixth | Seventh | Eighth |
|---|---|---|---|---|---|---|
| dog | spend | besides | notice | decide | stranger | subscription |
| play | south | inch | empty | signal | attractive | describe |
| want | middle | paid | machine | natural | vacant | alcohol |
| fish | climb | talked | button | groceries | suggestion | permanent |
| show | glass | wrong | chocolate | success | delicious | poultry |
| keep | pick | fresh | neighbor | growth | religion | witness |

3. Dictate the following sentences to find out approximately how well the pupil spells when he is writing sentences.

*Grade 2*    I have a big dog.

*Grade 3*    We rode to town on the truck.

*Grade 4*    I drink a glass of milk with each meal.

*Grade 5*    Last summer I visited a big ranch in the mountains. We rode across several thousand acres on our horses.

*Grade 6*    We stopped at a garage after the accident. It was a stormy night for traveling, and we were afraid to go on until someone examined the car.

*Grade 7*    I think it would be exciting to correspond with a student in a foreign country. Can you suggest how to make arrangements?

*Grade 8*    Our cafeteria has the most modern and efficient equipment available. We certainly appreciate its convenience.

4. *Written expression:* Show the student a picture. Have him write a story about the picture. Encourage him by telling him to write more.

## Section V: Interests and self-concept

This section has two parts. The first part, through questioning of the child, determines interests. The second part seeks, through informal questioning, to determine how the child views himself.

**Interests**

1. I like to do these things in school: _____
2. I think this is what I do best at school: _____
3. This is what I liked best about my last class (or school): _____
4. I like to do these things at home: _____
5. I like these games best: _____
6. I like stories about: _____
7. My favorite person is: _____ because: _____.
8. I have the most fun when I: _____.
9. Have you ever earned money? _____ How? _____
10. From this class, whom would you invite to go home with you? _____
11. If you had the opportunity to work with someone else in this class, whom would you choose?
12. Write the name of a good friend in this class: _____
13. If you could have a wish, what would it be? _____

**Self-concept**

Which sentence is most like me?

1. (a) Nothing gets me too mad.
   (b) I get mad easily and explode.
2. (a) I don't stay with things and finish them.
   (b) I stay with things and finish them.
3. (a) I don't like to work on projects with other people.
   (b) I like to work with others.
4. (a) I wish I were smaller (taller).
   (b) I'm just the right height.
5. (a) I worry a lot.
   (b) I don't worry much.
6. (a) I don't like the way my hair looks.
   (b) My hair is nice looking.
7. (a) Teachers like me.
   (b) Teachers don't like me.
8. (a) I have lots of energy.
   (b) I don't have much energy.
9. (a) I don't play games very well.
   (b) I play games very well.
10. (a) I'm just the right weight.
    (b) I wish I were heavier (lighter).
11. (a) The girls don't like me, leave me out.
    (b) The girls like me a lot, choose me.
12. (a) I'm very good at speaking before a group.
    (b) I'm not much good at speaking before a group.

13. (a) My face is pretty (good looking).
    (b) I wish I were prettier (better looking).

14. (a) I like teachers very much.
    (b) I don't like teachers very much.

15. (a) I don't feel at ease, comfortable, most of the time.
    (b) I feel very at ease, comfortable, most of the time.

16. (a) I get along well with teachers.
    (b) I don't get along with teachers.

17. (a) I don't like to try new things.
    (b) I like to try new things.

18. (a) I do well in school.
    (b) I don't do well in school.

19. (a) I don't think I am a good person.
    (b) I think I am a good person.

20. (a) I have trouble controlling my feelings.
    (b) I can handle my feelings.

21. (a) I don't like the way I look.
    (b) I like the way I look.

22. (a) I'm not much good at making things with my hands.
    (b) I'm very good at making things with my hands.

23. (a) I wish I could do something about my skin.
    (b) My skin is nice looking.

24. (a) I'm very healthy.
    (b) I get sick a lot.

25. (a) I write well.
    (b) I don't write well.

26. (a) School isn't interesting to me.
    (b) School is very interesting to me.

27. (a) I use my time well.
    (b) I don't know how to plan.

28. (a) I don't do arithmetic well.
    (b) I'm really good in arithmetic.

29. (a) The boys like me a lot, choose me.
    (b) The boys don't like me, leave me out.

30. (a) I like school.
    (b) I don't like school.

31. (a) I'm smarter than most of the others.
    (b) I'm not as smart as the others.

32. (a) I wish I were built like the others.
    (b) I'm happy with the way I'm built.

33. (a) I read well.
    (b) I don't read well.

34. (a) I don't learn new things easily.
    (b) I learn new things easily.

35. (a) I like my name.
    (b) I wish I could change my name.

## Section VI: Supplementary checklist during testing

The purpose of this section is to provide a checklist in which informal comments can be made during the administration of standardized or informal testing.

Name _____ Date _____

Age _____ Test _____

**Appearance**
- ☐ Neat
- ☐ Untidy
- ☐ Physical handicaps

**Sensory abilities**
- ☐ Inadequate hearing
- ☐ Inadequate vision
- ☐ No problems noted

**Medication**
- ☐ No sedation
- ☐ Light sedation
- ☐ Moderate sedation
- ☐ Heavy sedation

**Language usage**
- ☐ Speech difficulty
- ☐ Facility in verbalizing
- ☐ Difficulty in verbalizing
- ☐ Overtalkative
- ☐ Undertalkative
- ☐ Circumlocution
- ☐ Egocentric responses
- ☐ Irrelevant speech
- ☐ Bizarreness
- ☐ Incoherent speech
- ☐ Flight of ideas
- ☐ Verbal perseveration
- ☐ Self-deprecatory remarks

**Anxiety signs (apprehension)**
- ☐ Excessive questioning
- ☐ Expressions of inadequacy
- ☐ Excessive concern with correctness

**Test behavior (approach)**
*Following directions*
- ☐ Directions were given only once per item
- ☐ Directions had to be repeated occasionally
- ☐ Directions had to be repeated frequently
- ☐ Responds quickly
- ☐ Responds slowly, deliberates

**Test behavior (approach)—cont'd**
- ☐ Continues looking at model
- ☐ Insufficient attention to model
- ☐ Verbalizes criticism of work without correction
- ☐ Systematic work
- ☐ Painstaking worker
- ☐ Impulsive careless worker
- ☐ Impulsive careful worker
- ☐ Loose worker
- ☐ Blocking

**Distractibility**
- ☐ Attention to irrelevant material
- ☐ Attention to external stimuli

**Somatic complaints** (*check things such as physical condition, use of drugs*)
- ☐ Complains of headaches
- ☐ Blurred vision

**Physical signs**
- ☐ Flushing
- ☐ Excessive perspiration
- ☐ Excessive swallowing
- ☐ Uneven respiration
- ☐ Gross tremulousness, tenseness

**Reaction to failure**
- ☐ Gives up easily
- ☐ Persists
- ☐ Rationalizes
- ☐ Easily upset

**Compensatory psychomotor activity**
- ☐ Fidgets, squirms, shifts position
- ☐ Purposeless hand movements
- ☐ Excessive laughing
- ☐ Laughing
- ☐ Whistling
- ☐ Making vague exclamatory noises
- ☐ Toying with test materials
- ☐ Drumming or tapping

**General attitude**
- ☐ Alert
- ☐ Antagonistic
- ☐ Apathetic
- ☐ Bored
- ☐ Calm
- ☐ Cocky
- ☐ Complains
- ☐ Depressed
- ☐ Elated
- ☐ Evasive
- ☐ Friendly
- ☐ Hesitant
- ☐ Inhibited
- ☐ Preoccupied
- ☐ Self-confident
- ☐ Silly
- ☐ Stares into space
- ☐ Sullen
- ☐ Surly
- ☐ Tearful
- ☐ Timid
- ☐ Well poised
- ☐ Whiny
- ☐ Worried

**Motor ability**
- ☐ Quick motor execution
- ☐ Much trial and error
- ☐ Fumbling with test material
- ☐ Slow motor execution
- ☐ Poor motor execution

**Cooperativeness**
- ☐ Responsive
- ☐ Eager to make good impression
- ☐ Actively cooperative
- ☐ Passively cooperative
- ☐ Needs reassurance
- ☐ Uncooperative

Comments: _____
_____
_____
_____

# APPENDIX D

# Developmental History Form

The following provides a format for gathering developmental and medical information. Information pertaining to family and general development can be supplied by parents or guardians of the child. Medical information is to be supplied by the family physician, gynecologist, and pediatrician.

## FAMILY INFORMATION

Child's name _____ What name does child prefer to be

called? _____ Child's sex _____ Date of birth _____

Age _____ School attending _____

Grade _____ Principal _____

### Family history

Father's name _____ Major language _____ Birth date _____

    Address _____ ZIP _____

    Phone (Home) _____ (Business) _____

Mother's name _____ Major language _____ Birth date _____

    Address _____ ZIP _____

    Phone (Home) _____ (Business) _____

Church preference: Father _____ Mother _____

Father's occupation _____ Employed by _____

Mother's occupation _____ Employed by _____

Was father in service? ☐ Yes ☐ No    If so, date _____ to _____

Highest grade completed: Mother _____ Father _____

Physician _____ Address _____ Phone _____

Present marital status of parents: Married _____ Divorced _____ Separated _____

Other _____

Date of marriage _____

Are both parents the child's natural parents? ☐ Yes ☐ No  If not, explain briefly _____

_____

List all the children in the family, including the child described on p. 1.

| Name | Birth date | Grade in school |
|------|-----------|-----------------|
| | | |
| | | |
| | | |
| | | |
| | | |
| | | |

Other persons living in the home (grandparents, in-laws, etc.)

| Name | Age | Relationship to child | Major language |
|------|-----|----------------------|----------------|
| | | | |
| | | | |
| | | | |

## MEDICAL INFORMATION

### Pregnancy and delivery information

Was the pregnancy trouble free? ☐ Yes ☐ No  If no, explain _____

_____

Was the delivery trouble free? ☐ Yes ☐ No  If no, explain _____

_____

Length of pregnancy in weeks _____ What medications did the mother take during pregnancy? _____

_____

Is there a history of difficult pregnancies? _____

Any difficulties in delivery? _____

Child's condition at birth: Weight _____ Length _____ General health (APGAR) _____

Are normal immunizations completed or up-to-date? ☐ Yes ☐ No  If the child has had the following diseases or conditions, please check. List approximate dates, if known.

□ Pertusis          □ Chickenpox          □ Swollen glands          □ Constipation

□ Measles (rubeola)   □ Scarlet fever      □ Otitis                 □ Head injuries

□ Rubella           □ Diphtheria          □ Colds (frequent)        □ Convulsions (describe)

□ Mumps             □ Rheumatic fever     □ Tonsillitis             □ Allergies (describe)

Is there a history of fractures or surgery? _____

Is or has the child been on medication or drugs? Type _____ Date _____

Present medications and dosages _____

**Physical examination**

Sex:  □ Male  □ Female

Race:  □ Caucasian  □ Negro  □ Oriental  □ Other _____

Height: _____ Head circumference: _____

Weight: _____ Blood pressure: _____ Pulse: _____

General appearance:  □ Bright  □ Average  □ Dull

Posture:  □ Good  □ Fair  □ Scoliosis  □ Lordosis  □ Kyphosis

Gait:  □ Normal  □ Abnormal

Skin:  □ Normal  □ Abnormal  □ Moist  □ Rash

Head:  □ Symmetrical  □ Asymmetrical

Hair:  □ Fine  □ Coarse  □ Dry

Eyes:  □ Normal  □ Nystagmus  □ Strabismus  □ Exophthalmos  □ Enophthalmos

    □ Other diseases or anomalies: _____

Eardrums:  □ Normal  □ Injected  □ Dull  □ Perforation

Nose:  □ Normal  □ Abnormal

Tonsils:  □ Present  □ Absent  □ Enlarged  □ Scarred  □ Infected

Lymph nodes:  □ Normal  □ Enlarged

Neck:  □ Supple  □ Resistant to flexion

Thyroid:  □ Palpable  □ Not palpable

Chest:  □ Clear  □ Rhonchi  □ Wheezing

Heart:  □ Normal  □ Enlarged  □ Murmurs  □ Type and location: _____

Hernia:  □ Absent  □ Present   Location: _____

Abdomen:  □ Normal  □ Abnormal

Genitalia:  □ Normal  □ Anomalies

Extremities:  □ Movement symmetrical  □ Limited  □ Paralysis

Neurological:

| Reflexes | Right | Left |
|---|---|---|
| Patellar | □ | □ |
| Achilles | □ | □ |
| Abdominal | □ | □ |
| Biceps | □ | □ |
| Supinators | □ | □ |
| Cremasteric | □ | □ |

|  | Present | Absent |
|---|---|---|
| Kernig's | ☐ | ☐ |
| Brudzinski | ☐ | ☐ |
| Babinski | ☐ | ☐ |
| Romberg | ☐ | ☐ |

| **Cranial nerves** | **Normal** | **Abnormal** |
|---|---|---|
| Olfactory (smell) | ☐ | ☐ |
| Optic (sight) | ☐ | ☐ |
| Oculomotor (loss of pupil movement; eye turned outward) | ☐ | ☐ |
| Trochlear (eye turned up and in) | ☐ | ☐ |
| Trigeminal (muscles of mastication) | ☐ | ☐ |
| Abducens (internal strabismus) | ☐ | ☐ |
| Facial (wrinkling forehead, closing lips) | ☐ | ☐ |
| Auditory (hearing) | ☐ | ☐ |
| Glossopharyngeal (difficulty swallowing; control of palate) | ☐ | ☐ |
| Vagus (vocal cords) | ☐ | ☐ |
| Spinal accessory (shrugging shoulders, rotating head) | ☐ | ☐ |
| Hypoglossal (tongue deviation) | ☐ | ☐ |

Are you the family physician:  ☐ Yes  ☐ No

Do you see this patient:  ☐ Regularly  ☐ Seldom  ☐ Not at all

**Developmental information (to be filled out by parent)**

Age at which child sat up alone: _____ months

Age at which child walked: _____ months

Was there any difficulty in any of the above?  ☐ Yes  ☐ No    If yes, please explain _____

_____

Age at which child toilet trained: _____ months. Was there any difficulty?  ☐ Yes  ☐ No    If yes, please explain _____

_____

Have you noticed any sudden personality or behavior changes in your child?  ☐ Yes  ☐ No    If yes, please explain (use reverse side if necessary) _____

_____

_____

_____

Signature of person completing this form

_____

Position

# APPENDIX E

# School History Form

The following provides a format for collecting important school-related information.

**PERSONAL IDENTIFICATION**

1. Name of child: _____
                  Last                  First             Middle

2. Sex: ☐ M ☐ F

3. Parent or guardian's name: _____
                                 Last           First          Middle

4. Parent or guardian's address: _____
                                    Number               Street

   _____
             City       State       County      Zip Code

5. Date of birth: _____
             Month             Day            Year

6. Place of birth: _____
           City            County          State

**EDUCATIONAL STATUS**

7. Has the child ever attended any type of school? ☐ Yes ☐ No

8. Last school attended:
   Name: _____ Location: _____ Date: _____

9. For what reason is the child not attending school:
   ☐ Child is institutionalized; if so, where? _____
   ☐ Child is blind or otherwise visually impaired
   ☐ Child is deaf or otherwise aurally impaired

- ☐ Child is mentally retarded
- ☐ Child is physically handicapped (crippled)
- ☐ Child has serious health problem
- ☐ Child is disadvantaged or from migrant family
- ☐ Child has dropped out
- ☐ Religious conflict
- ☐ Other _____
- ☐ Other _____
- ☐ Other _____

*If the child is attending school, answer the questions below:*

10. Child's immediate difficulties (What do you believe to be his problem?)


11. Major contributing factors (What do you believe to be the major factors contributing to this problem?)


12. Current grades (Are these typical of the child's performance?)


13. Special abilities:


14. Special handicaps (physical, social, emotional)


**SCHOOL HISTORY**

15. Attendance (check one)
    - ☐ Regular
    - ☐ Frequently absent; erratic
    - ☐ Occasionally absent for a day or two
    - ☐ Occasionally absent for longer periods

16. Interest level in class
    - ☐ Far above average
    - ☐ Above average
    - ☐ Average
    - ☐ Below average
    - ☐ Far below average

17. Attitude toward school
    - ☐ Very positive
    - ☐ Positive
    - ☐ Above average
    - ☐ Average
    - ☐ Below average
    - ☐ Far below average

18. Relationships with peers
    - ☐ Very good
    - ☐ Good
    - ☐ Average
    - ☐ Poor
    - ☐ Very poor
19. Activity level
    - ☐ Hyperactive
    - ☐ Above average
    - ☐ Average
    - ☐ Below average
    - ☐ Very withdrawn
20. Amount of supervision required for control
    - ☐ Far more than average
    - ☐ More than average
    - ☐ Average
    - ☐ Less than average
    - ☐ Much less than average
21. Amount of assistance required from teacher
    - ☐ Far more than average
    - ☐ More than average
    - ☐ Average
    - ☐ Less than average
    - ☐ Much less than average

22. Child's leadership ability
    - ☐ Far above average
    - ☐ Above average
    - ☐ Average
    - ☐ Below average
    - ☐ Far below average
23. Child's general adjustment in school
    - ☐ Far above average
    - ☐ Above average
    - ☐ Average
    - ☐ Below average
    - ☐ Far below average
24. Child's interaction on the playground
    - ☐ Far above average
    - ☐ Above average
    - ☐ Average
    - ☐ Below average
    - ☐ Far below average
25. Parent-school relationship (please comment)

26. School history
    a. Date student began at present school: _____
    b. Schools attended previously:

| Name of school | Location | Grades attended |
|---|---|---|
| _____ | _____ | _____ |
| _____ | _____ | _____ |
| _____ | _____ | _____ |
| _____ | _____ | _____ |

    c. Age at entrance into grade one: _____
    d. Has pupil repeated any grades?  ☐ Yes  ☐ No   If so, which ones? _____ Why was
       repetition considered necessary?

27. Classroom information
    a. How many students are in this child's classroom? _____
    b. What is the range of ability in this child's class? _____
    _____
    c. What is the range of achievement in this child's class? _____
    _____
    d. What is this child's rank in this class:
    In ability? _____
    In achievement? _____

28. Standardized test results
    a. Intelligence tests (group administered paper-and-pencil tests)

| Name of test | Date given | IQ |
|---|---|---|
|  |  |  |
|  |  |  |
|  |  |  |
|  |  |  |
|  |  |  |
|  |  |  |

    b. Achievement tests (please list subtest, e.g., arithmetic, reading)

| Name of test | Subtest | Date given | Norm group | Results percentile grade level |
|---|---|---|---|---|
|  |  |  |  |  |
|  |  |  |  |  |
|  |  |  |  |  |
|  |  |  |  |  |
|  |  |  |  |  |

    c. Individual intelligence test results

| Name of test | Date given | Examiner | Results |
|---|---|---|---|
|  |  |  |  |
|  |  |  |  |
|  |  |  |  |

29. Previous special help (Has the child had any special help with school work including tutoring? If so, of what type?)

_____
Signature of person completing this form

_____
Position

How much time per day does your child spend doing the following:

Reading (other than school work) _____

Reading (for school) _____

Homework for school _____

Playing outside the house: Alone _____ With others _____

Playing inside the house: Alone _____ With others _____

Listening to radio _____

Watching television _____

Sleeping _____

Does your child have an easy time making friends?  ☐ Yes  ☐ No

What is your child's favorite subject in school? _____

In what school subject does your child do best? _____

# APPENDIX F

# Assessment Forms*

Past litigation (see Chapters 4 and 13) and P.L. 94-142 have provided two implications in the area of assessment. First, P.L. 94-142 authorizes an evaluation by the state educational administration on IEPs in accordance with criteria established with the U.S. Commissioner of Education. A comprehensive assessment is necessary. In addition, the state educational agency ensures that procedural safeguards are observed in child placement. Parents have the right to examine all relevant records that pertain to the child's identification, evaluation, and placement and to an independent evaluation of the child. Procedures designed to protect the rights of the child include dissemination of information regarding parents' rights and steps that may be taken should aggrieved persons wish to initiate action. The state ensures that nondiscriminatory testing practices are in force. Culturally biased tests will not be considered valid. Also, states, and more specifically teachers, must have procedures and policies to ensure the confidentiality of records of handicapped individuals.

Second, an IEP must be developed for each handicapped child served within a given state. The IEP is developed in consultation with school staff and parents. A written IEP must include the child's present level of educational performance, annual goals and short-term objectives, and specific educational services to be provided. This appendix provides an example of classroom format for IEP compliance. Administrators must ensure that individualized programs will be established at the beginning of each school year and reviewed at least once annually. Assessment must determine the child's level of functioning, determine instructional priorities, and set up annual goals and short-term objectives. State services must also indicate to what extent the child is being served in the "least restrictive" environment. Program development should emphasize mainstreaming the child into the

*We are indebted to Dr. Stan Scarpati for the development of the majority of these forms, which are adapted from the Demonstration Classroom for Severe Emotionally Disturbed, Project Director H.L. Swanson, University of Northern Colorado (Department of Education Grant Number 6008001002).

regular classroom to the maximum extent appropriate. Other aspects of P.L. 94-142 require projected dates of services, criteria for evaluation, and schedules involved in meeting instructional objectives.

The forms provided in this appendix include assessed abilities and current function to be done at the beginning of the school year. This information is to be further developed into a specific identification of needs (Section II). Section III converts those needs into annual goals and objectives. Section IV provides an annual review form. The reader is reminded that the basis of an IEP is not assessment strategy or theory but child protection and program efficiency. Mere completion of these forms *does not constitute* an assessment process (Chapter 1).

## ASSESSED ABILITIES AND CURRENT FUNCTIONING

☐ IEP conference        ☐ Review        ☐ Direct

Student _____ Date of birth _____ Age _____ Sex _____

Mother _____ Address _____ Phone _____

Father _____ Address _____ Phone _____

Lives with _____

School year _____ Grade _____ Attendance _____

|  | **Date** |  | **Date** |  | **Date** |
|---|---|---|---|---|---|
| Referral | _____ | Initial assessment | _____ | Parent permission | _____ |
| Vision screening | _____ | Hearing screening | _____ | Health history | _____ |
| Developmental history | _____ | Health status | _____ | Physical assessment | _____ |
| Educational assessment | _____ | Psychological | _____ | Speech/language | _____ |
| Adaptive behavioral | _____ | assessment |  | assessment |  |
| assessment |  | Social history | _____ | Initial staffing | _____ |
| First IEP | _____ |  |  |  |  |

Vision _____

Hearing _____

Present school performance _____

Present health status/motor/medication _____

_____

_____

Intelligence _____ Test _____ Date _____

Cognitive strengths _____

Cognitive weaknesses _____

Perceptual strengths _____

Perceptual weaknesses _____

### Achievement levels—G.E. (reading and math)

| **Reading** | **G.E.** | **Test** | **Date** |
|---|---|---|---|
| Silent comprehension | _____ | _____ | _____ |
| Oral comprehension | _____ | _____ | _____ |

**Math**

Calculation          _____    _____    _____

Reasoning           _____    _____    _____

Concept comprehension   _____    _____    _____

Oral communication skills _____
_____
_____

Written communication skills _____
_____
_____

Emotional status/self-feelings _____
_____
_____

Social skills _____
_____
_____


## NEED IDENTIFICATION

Student _____ Grade _____ Date _____

1. Curricular needs (List necessary changes or adjustments to regular curriculum)



2. Physical/environmental needs (List necessary changes/adjustments)



3. Social/emotional needs (List provisions/conditions)



4. Communicative needs



5. Educational needs

6. Special needs (avocational/vocational, transportation, etc.)

Modifications/adaptation to regular classroom

Special program considerations

Individual educational program
(complete one of these for each goal statement)

Date of program entry _____     Educational goal statement _____     Project ending date _____

_____ (includes general statement) _____

| Short-term instructional objective | | | | | | |

| Written as a behavioral objective that includes four criteria | Task analysis for teaching objective | Time sequence | Criteria for mastery | Procedure/ techniques | Materials | Comments |
|---|---|---|---|---|---|---|
| Performance terms Conditions for behavior Criteria of acceptance Measurement procedure | A _____ B (includes hierarchy of instructional steps) C _____ D _____ E | A — B C — D — | A Criteria must include statements of qualification B (e.g., percentage, rate proportion) C _____ D _____ | A Includes statements related to motivation (e.g., verbal reinforcement) methodology (e.g., B Fernald approach), and supportive (e.g., counselor) C Activities D _____ | A List materials for each B Task analysis objective C _____ D _____ | A _____ B _____ C _____ D _____ |
| | | List assessment dates | | | | |
| | X _____ Y _____ Z _____ | X — Y — Z — | X _____ Y _____ Z _____ | X _____ Y _____ Z _____ | X _____ Y _____ Z _____ | X _____ Y _____ Z _____ |

_____
(Child's name)

Parent-child conference date

Reschedule date

Regular classroom objective _____

(State procedures for meeting requirements of least restrictive environment)

_____

Child's teacher _____

Regular classroom teacher _____

Long-term annual instructional objective _____

(State goal for academic year in behavioral objective format)

_____

Assessment date and procedure for evaluation of instructional objective

_____

(e.g., criterion-referenced test, standardized achievement test)

_____

| | | | |
|---|---|---|---|
| Spec. Ed. admin/student | Date | Parent | Date |
| Teacher | Date | Parent | Date |
| Principal | Date | Other (title) | Date |
| Other (title) | Date | Spec. Ed. teacher | Date |

Person responsible for completion of this form

## ANNUAL REVIEW

A. Review of annual goals/instructional objectives

B. Recommendations:
  - ☐ Continue in same program
  - ☐ Transfer to other school: _____
  - ☐ Consider for additional services
  - ☐ Refer for reevaluation
  - ☐ Explore other alternatives
  - ☐ Other: _____
    _____
    _____

### Annual review committee

Spec. Ed. Admin./student _____

Parent _____  Speech therapist _____

Parent _____  Occupational therapist _____

Principal _____  Nurse _____

Social worker _____  Psychologist _____

Teacher _____  Other _____

Date of review _____

Chairperson          Person responsible for completion of this form

# References

Achenbach, T. M., & Edelbrock, C. S. (1979). The child behavior profile: II, Boys aged 12–16 and girls aged 6–11 and 12–16. *Journal of Consulting and Clinical Psychology, 47,* 223–233.

Adams, J. (1973). Clinical neuropsychology and the study of learning disorders. In H. Grossman (Ed.), *Pediatric clinics of North America* (Vol. 20, pp. 587–598). Philadelphia: W. B. Saunders.

Adelman, H. (1979). Diagnostic classification of LD: A practical necessity and a procedure problem. *Learning Disability Quarterly, 3,* 56–62.

Adelman, H., & Taylor, L. (1979). Initial psychoeducational assessment and related consultation. *Learning Disability Quarterly, 2,* 52–63.

Adler, S. & Birdsong, S. (1983). Reliability and validity of standardized testing tools used with poor children. *Topics in Language Disorders, 3*(3), 76–88.

Advisory Board of Access. (1981). *National task-oriented seminar in bilingual special-education personnel preparation.* Unpublished paper.

Ahn, H., Baird, H., Trepeptin, M., & Kaye, H. (1980). Developmental equations reflect brain dysfunctions. *Science, 12,* 1259–1262.

Alfano, D. P., & Finlayson, M. A. J. (1987). Clinical neuropsychology in rehabilitation. *The Clinical Neuropsychologist, 1,* 105–123.

Algozzine, B., Mercer, C., & Counteronine, T. (1977). The effects of labels and behavior on teacher expectations. *Exceptional Children, 44,* 131–132.

Alkin, M. C. (1974). Criterion-referenced measurement and other such terms. In C. W. Harris, M. C. Alkin, & W. J. Popham (Eds.), *CSE monograph series in evaluation: (No. 3). Problems in criterion-referenced measurement.* Los Angeles: Center for the Study of Evaluation, University of California at Los Angeles.

Alper, A. E. (1958). A comparison of the WISC and the Arthur adaptation of the Leiter International Performance Scale with mental defectives. *American Journal of Mental Deficiency, 63,* 312–316.

Alper, T. G., & Borgin, E. G. (1944). Intelligence test scores of northern and southern White and Negro recruits in 1918. *Journal of Abnormal and Social Psychology, 39,* 471–474.

Altus, W. D. (1949). The effect of adjustment patterns on the intercorrelation of intelligence subtest variables. *Journal of Social Psychology, 30,* 39–48.

Ambert, A., & Dew, N. (1982). *Special education for exceptional bilingual students: A handbook for educators.* University of Wisconsin-Milwaukee: Midwest National Origin Desegregation Assistance Center.

Ambert, A., & Dew, N. (1985). *Special education for exceptional bilingual students: A handbook for educators* (p. 85). Milwaukee, WI: Midwest National Origin Desegregation Assistance Center.

American Educational Research Association, American Psychological Association, and National Council on Measurement in Education, [AERA, APA, and NCRE]. (1985). *Standard for educational and psychological testing.* Washington, D.C.: American Psychological Association.

American Psychiatric Association. (1968). *Diagnostic and statistic manual of mental disorders* (2nd ed.). Washington, D.C.: Author.

American Psychological Association. (1972). *Casebook on ethical standards of psychologists.* Washington, D.C.: Author.

American Psychological Association. (1985). *Standards for educational and psychological tests.* Washington, D.C.: Author.

Ammons, R. B., & Aguero, A. (1950). The full-range picture vocabulary test: VII. Results for a Spanish-American school-age population. *Journal of Social Psychology, 32,* 3–10.

Anastasi, A. (1961). Psychological tests: Uses and abuses. *Teacher's College Record, 62,* 389–393.

Anastasi, A. (1967). Psychology, psychologists, and psychological testing. *American Psychologist, 22,* 297–306.

Anastasi, A. (1968). *Psychological testing* (3rd ed.). New York: Macmillan.

Anastasi, A. (1976). *Psychological testing* (4th ed.). New York: Macmillan.

Anastasi, A. (1982). *Psychological testing* (5th ed.). New York: Macmillan.

Andre, J. (1975). Bicultural socialization and the measurement of intelligence. *Dissertation Abstracts International, 36y,* 3675B–36786B. (University Microfilms No. 75–29, 904)

Aram, D. M., Ekelman, B. L., & Nation, J. E. (1984). Preschoolers with language disorders: 10 years later. *Journal of Speech & Hearing Research, 27,* 232–244.

Armstrong, C. P., & Heisler, F. (1945). Some comparisons of Negro and White delinquent boys. *Journal of Genetic Psychology, 67,* 81–84.

Arndt, S. (1981). A general measure of adaptive behavior. *American Journal of Mental Deficiency, 85,* 554–556.

Aronson, E., & Rosenbloom, S. (1971). Space perception in early infancy: Perception within a common auditory-visual space. *Science, 172,* 1161–1163.

*Arreola v. Santa Ana Board of Education* (Orange County, Calif.). No. 160-577, 1968.

Arthur, G. (1949). The Arthur adaptation of the Leiter International Performance Scale. *Journal of Clinical Psychology, 5,* 345–349.

*Aspira of New York, Inc. v. New York Board of Education,* 72 Civ. 4002 (S.D.N.Y., filed September 20, 1972).

Atkinson, R. C., & Shiffrin, R. M. (1968). Human memory: A proposed system and its control processes. In K. W. Spence & J. T. Spence (Eds.), *The Psychology of Learning and Motivation: Vol. 2.* New York: Academic Press.

Ausebel, D. (1952). *Ego development and personality disorders.* New York: Grune & Stratton.

Axelrod, S. (1977). *Behavior modification for classroom teachers.* New York: Macmillan.

Aylward, E. H. & Schmidt, S. (1986). An examination of three tests of visual-motor integration. *Journal of Learning Disabilities, 19.* 328–335.

Ayres, A. J. (1964). *Southern California motor accuracy test manual.* Los Angeles: Western Psychological Services.

Ayres, R. R. & Cooley, E. J. (1986). Sequential versus simultaneous processing on the K-ABC: Validity in predicting learning success. *Journal of Psychoeducational Assessment. 4,* 211–220.

Bachor, D. (1979). Using work samples as diagnostic information. *Learning Disability Quarterly, 2,* 45–52.

Baddeley, A. (1978). The trouble with levels: A reexamination of Craik and Lockhart's framework for memory research. *Psychological Review, 85,* 139–152.

Bagnato, S. J. (1985). Review of the Brigance Diagnostic Inventory of Early Development. In J. V. Mitchell (Ed.), *The 9th mental measurement yearbook.* Lincoln, NE: University of Nebraska Press.

Bailey, D. B., & Harbin, G. L. (1980). Nondiscriminatory evaluation. *Exceptional Children, 46,* 590–596.

Bailey, E. J., & Bricker, D. (1986). A psychometric study of a criterion-referenced assessment instrument designed for infants and young children. *Journal of the Division for Early Childhood, 10,* 124–134.

Baker, E. L., & Herman, J. L. (1983). Task structure design: Beyond linkage. *Journal of Educational Measurement, 20,* 149–164.

Baker, R., & Dryer, R. (1977). The preschool behavioral classification project. *Journal of Abnormal Child Psychology, 5,* 241.

Bakker, D. (1983). Hemispheric specialization and specific reading retardation. In M. Rutter (Ed.), *Developmental neuropsychiatry* (pp. 203–232). New York: Guilford Press.

Ball, W., & Tronick, E. (1971). Infant responses to impending collision: Optical and real. *Science, 171,* 818–820.

Balthazar, E. E. (1973). *The Balthazar scales of adaptive behavior, II: The scales of social adaptation.* Palo Alto, CA: Consulting Psychologists Press.

Banks, C., & Sinha, U. (1951). An item-analysis of the Progressive Matrices Test and Binet. *British Journal of Psychology, Statistical Section, 4,* 91–94.

Baran, J. & Gengel, R. (1984). Test-retest reliability of three GFW subtests. *Language, Speech and Hearing Services in Schools, 15,* 199–204.

Barker, R. (1968). *Ecological psychology: Concepts and methods for studying the environment of human behavior.* Stanford, CA: Stanford University Press, 1968.

Barry, B., Klanderman, J., & Stipe, D. (1983). In A. S. Kaufman & N. L. Kaufman (Eds.), *Kaufman Assessment Battery for Children: Interpretive Manual* (p. 94). Minneapolis: American Guidance Service.

Bartlett, F. (1932). *Remembering.* Cambridge, Mass.: Harvard University Press.

Bateman, B. (1974). Educational implications of minimal brain dysfunction. *The Reading Teacher, 27,* 662–667.

Bates, E. (1976). Pragmatics and sociolinguistics in child language. In D. Morehead & A. Morehead (Eds.), *Language deficiency in children.* Baltimore: University Park Press.

Bauer, R. (1982). Information processing as a way of understanding and diagnosing learning disabilities. *Topics in Learning and Language Disabilities, 2(2),* 33–45.

Baum, D. (1975). A comparison of the WRAT and the PIAT with learning disabled children. *Educational and Psychological Measurement, 35,* 487–493.

Bayley, N. (1969). *Bayley Scales of Infant Development.* New York: Psychological Corporation.

Bayley, N. (1984). *Bayley Scales of Infant Development.* New York: Psychological Corporation.

Beatty, L. S., Madden, R., Gardner, E. F., and Karlsen, B. (1983, 1984). *Stanford diagnostic mathematics tests (3rd ed.)* San Antonio, TX: Psychological Corporation.

Becker, H. (1963). *Studies in the sociology of deviance.* New York: Free Press.

Becker, J. T. (1970). Spatial orientation and visual discrimination. *Perceptual and Motor Skills, 31,* 943–946.

Becker, J. T. & Sabatino, D. A. (1973). Frostig revisited. *Journal of Learning Disabilities, 6,* 180–184.

Becker, W., and others. (1967). The contingent use of teacher attention and praise in the reduction of classroom behavior problems. *Journal of Special Education, 1,* 287–307.

Beery, K. D. (1982). *Revised administration, scoring, and teaching manual for the developmental test of visual-motor integration.* Chicago: Follett.

Behor, L. (1977). The preschool behavior questionnaire. *Journal of Abnormal Child Psychology, 5,* 265–275.

Beitchman, J., Nair, R., Clegg, M. & Patel, P. (1986). Prevalence of speech and language disorders in 5-year-old kindergarten children in the Ottowa-Carleton region. *Journal of Speech and Hearing Disorders, 51,* 98–110.

Bellack, A. S., Hersen, M., & Lampmarski, D. (1979). Roleplay tests for assessing social skills: Are they valid? Are they useful? *Journal of Consulting and Clinical Psychology, 47,* 335–342.

Belmont, J., & Butterfield, E. (1971). Learning strategies as determinants of memory deficiencies. *Cognitive Psychology, 3,* 411–420.

Belmont, J. M. (1978). Individual differences in memory: The cases of normal and retarded development. In M. M. Gruneberg & P. Morris (Eds.), *Practical aspects of memory* (pp. 153–185). London: Methuen.

Belmont, J. M., Ferretti, R. P., & Mitchell, D. W. (1982). Memorizing: A test of untrained retarded children's problem solving. *American Journal of Mental Deficiency, 87,* 197–210.

Bender, L. (1938). A visual motor Gestalt test and its clinical use. New York: *American Orthopsychiatric Association Research Monograph,* No. 3.

Benton, A. L. (1963). *The revised visual retention test* (3rd ed.). New York: Psychological Corporation.

Benton, A. L. (1974). *The revised visual retention test* (4th ed.). New York: Psychological Corporation.

Berdine, W. H. and Meyer, S. A. (1987). *Assessment in special education.* Boston: Little, Brown.

Berk, R. A. (Ed.). (1980). *Criterion-referenced measurement: The state of the art.* Baltimore: Johns Hopkins.

Berk, R. A. (1986). A consumer's guide to setting performance standards on criterion-referenced tests. *Review of Educational Research, 56,* 137–172.

Berko, J. (1958). The child's learning of English morphology. *Word, 14,* 150–177.

Bernal, E. M. (1972). *Assessing assessment instruments: A Chicano perspective.* Paper prepared for the regional training program to serve the bilingual/bicultural exceptional child. Sacramento, CA: Montal Educational Associates.

Berry, M. F. (1980). *Teaching linguistically handicapped children.* Englewood Cliffs, N.J.: Prentice-Hall.

Berry, M., & Talbott, R. (1966). *Exploratory Test of Grammar.* Rockford, IL.

Bersoff, D. N. (1973). Silk purses into sow's ears: The decline of psychological testing and a suggestion for its redemption. *American Psychologist, 10,* 892–899.

Bervin, N. L. (1980). Psychometric assessment in rehabilitation. In M. B. Bolton & D. Cook (Eds.), *Rehabilitation client assessment.* Baltimore: University Park Press.

Best, F. (1984). Technology and the changing world of work. *The Futurist, 18,* 61–66.

Bijou, S. (1968). Child behavior and development. *International Journal of Psychology, 3,* 221–238.

Bijou, S., Peterson, D., & Ault, M. (1968). A method to integrate descriptive and experimental field studies at the level of data and empirical concepts. *Journal of Applied Behavior Analysis, 1,* 179–180.

Binet, A. (1902). *L'Etude experimentale de l'intelligence.* (An experimental study of intelligence). Paris: Ancienne Librairie Schleicher.

Binet, A. & Henri, V. (1985). La memoire des phrases. *L'Annee Psychologique, 1,* 24–59.

Birch, H. G., & Bortner, M. (1960). Perceptual and perceptual-motor dissociation in brain-damaged patients. *Journal of Nervous and Mental Diseases, 130,* 49–53.

Birch, H. G., & Walker, H. A. (1966). Perceptual and perceptual-motor dissociation. *Archives of General Psychology, 14,* 113–118.

Bitter, J. (1979). *Introduction to rehabilitation.* St. Louis: C. V. Mosby.

Bitter, J. A. (1967). Using employer job-sites in evaluation of mentally retarded for employability. *Mental Retardation, 5,* 21–22.

Bitter, J. A., & Bolanovich, D. J. (1970). WARF: A scale for measuring job-readiness behaviors. *American Journal of Mental Deficiency, 54,* 616–621.

Blair, F. (1980). *Language evaluation scale.* Unpublished manuscript, University of Wisconsin–Milwaukee, Department of Special Education.

Blanton, R. L. (1975). Historical perspective on classification of mental retardation. In N. Hobbs (Ed.), *Issues in the classification of children.* San Francisco: Jossey-Bass.

Bliss, L. (1985). A symptom approach to the intervention of childhood language disorders. *Journal of Communication Disorders, 18,* 91–108.

Bloom, B. S. (1964). *Stability and child in human characteristics.* New York: John Wiley & Sons.

Bloom, L. (1975). *Language development: Form and function in emerging grammars.* Cambridge, MA: MIT Press.

Bobele, R. M. (1976). Efficacy of the Visual Retention Test as a group-administered instrument for young children. *Perceptual and Motor Skills, 43,* 267–272.

Boder, E. (1971). Developmental dyslexia: Prevailing diagnostic concepts and a new diagnostic approach. In H. Mykelbust (Ed.), *Progress in Learning Disabilities.* (Vol. 2, 60–81). New York: Grune and Stratton.

Boder, E. (1973). Developmental dyslexia: A diagnostic approach based on three atypical reading-spelling patterns. *Developmental Medicine and Child Neurology, 15,* 663–687.

Boder, E. & Jarrico, S. (1982). *The Boder Test of Reading-Spelling Patterns.* New York: Grune and Stratton.

Boehm, A. E. (1986). *Boehm test of basic concepts-revised-manual.* San Antonio, TX: Psychological Corporation.

Boehm, A. E., & Weinberg, R. A. (1977). *The classroom observer: A guide for developing observation skills.* New York: Grune and Stratton.

Boll, T. J. (1981). The Halstead-Reitan neuropsychological test battery. In S. B. Filskov & T. J. Boll (Eds.), *Handbook of Clinical Neuropsychology* (pp. 577–607). New York: John Wiley and Sons.

Boll, T. J. & Reitan, R. M. (1970, May). *Motor and sensory-perceptual deficits in brain-damaged children.* Paper presented at the Midwestern Psychological Association meeting.

Boll, T. J., & Reitan, R. M. (1972). Comparative ability interrelationships in normal and brain-damaged children. *Journal of Clinical Psychology, 28,* 152–156.

Bolton, B. (Ed.). (1982). *Vocational Adjustment of Disabled Persons.* University Park Press, Baltimore.

Bornstein, R. A., King, G., & Carroll, A. (1983). Neuropsychological abnormalities in Gilles de la Tourette's Syndrome. *Journal of Nervous and Mental Disease, 171,* 497–502.

Bossard, M. D., & Galusha, R. (1979). The utility of the Stanford-Binet in predicting WRAT performance. *Psychology in the Schools, 16,* 488–490.

Botterbusch, K. F. (1976). *A comparison of seven vocational evaluation systems.* Menomonie, WI: Materials Development Center.

Botterbusch, K. F. (1978). *Psychological testing in vocational evaluation.* Menomonie, WI: Materials Development Center.

Botterbusch, K. F. (1983). Computers and vocational evaluation. *Vocational Evaluation and Work Adjustment Bulletin, 16,* 79–81.

Botterbusch, K. F. (1984). *A Comparison of Computerized Job Matching Systems.* Menomonie, WI: Materials Development Center—Stout Vocational Rehabilitation Institute, University of Wisconsin-Stout.

Bountress, N. G. & Laderberg, C. M. (1981). A comparison of two tests of speech-sound discrimination. *Journal of Communication Disorders, 14,* 149–156.

Bountress, N. G. (1984). A second look at tests of speech-sound discrimination. *Journal of Communication Disorders, 17,* 349–359.

Bower, E. (1960). *Early identification of emotionally handicapped children in school.* Springfield, IL: Thomas.

Bower, T. G. R. (1966). The visual world of infants. *Scientific American, 215,* 80–92.

Bower, T. G. R. (1971). The object in the world of the infant. *Scientific American, 255,* 30–38.

Bower, T. G. R. (1977). Comment on Yonas et al.: Development of sensitivity to information for impending collision. *Perception and Psychophysics, 21,* 281–282.

Bower, T. G. R., Broughton, J. M., & Moore, M. K. (1970). Infant response to approaching objects:

An indicator of responses to distal variables. *Perception and Psychophysics, 9,* 193–196.

Bowerman, M. (1973). Structural relationships in children's utterances: Syntactic or semantic. In T. Moore (Ed.), *Cognitive development and language acquisition.* New York: Academic Press.

Bowerman, M. (1976). Semantic factors in the acquistion of rules for word use and sentence construction. In D. Morehead & A. Morehead (Eds.), *Normal and deficient child language.* Baltimore: University Park Press.

Braine, M. (1976). Children's first word combination. *Monographs of the Society for Research in Child Development* (Serial N. 164), *41.*

Brazelton, T. B. *Infants and mothers.* (1969). New York: Dell Publishing Company.

Brazelton, T. B. (1984). *The neonatal behavioral assessment scale.* Hagerstown, MD: Lippincott/Harper Publishers, Inc.

Brazelton, T. B. & Nugent, J. K. (1987). Assessment as an intervention. In H. Raugh and C. F. Steinhausen (Eds.), Amsterdam, The Netherlands: Elsevier.

Brazelton, T. B., Nugent, J. K., & Lester, B. M. (1987). Neonatal behavioral assessment scale. In J. Osofsky (Ed.), *Handbook of infant development,* (2nd Ed). New York: John Wiley and Sons.

Breen, M. J., Carlson, M., & Lehman, J. (1985). The revised developmental test of visual-motor integration: Its relation to the VMI, WISC-R, and Bender Gestalt for a group of elementary aged learning disabled students. *Journal of Learning Disabilities, 18,* 136–138.

Breen, M. J., Lehman, J., & Carlson, M. (1984). Achievement correlation of the Woodcock-Johnson Reading and Mathematics subtests, Key-Math, and Woodcock Reading in an elementary aged learning disabled population. *Journal of Learning Disabilities, 17,* 258–261.

Breslau, N. (1982). Siblings of disabled children: Birth order and spacing effects. *Journal of Abnormal Child Psychology, 10,* 85–96.

Bricker, D. & Littman, D. (1982). Intervention and evaluation: The inseparable mix. *Topics in Early Childhood Special Education, 1,* 23–33.

Brigance, A. (1978). *Brigance Diagnostic Inventory of Early Development.* Billerica, MA: Curriculum Associates, Inc.

Brilliant, P. J. & Gynther, M. D. (1963). Relationships between performance on three tests of organicity and selected patient variables. *Journal of Consulting Psychology, 27,* 474–479.

Brock, H. (1982). Factor structure of intellectual and achievement measures for learning disabled children. *Psychology in the Schools, 19,* 297–304.

Brolin, D. (1973). Vocational assessment: What can be gained from it? In *Vocational assessment systems: Application in programs serving special needs populations.* Des Moines: Iowa Department of Public Instruction.

Bronfenbrenner, U. (1979). *The ecology of human development.* Cambridge, MA: Harvard University.

Brook, R. M. (1975). Visual Retention Test: Local norms and impact of short-term memory. *Perceptual and Motor Skills, 40,* 967–970.

Brooks, J. & Weinraub, M. (1976). A history of infant intelligence testing. In M. Lewis (Ed.), *Origins of intelligence* (pp. 19–57). New York: Plenum.

Browder, D. M. (1987). *Assessment of individuals with severe handicaps: An applied approach to life skills assessment.* Baltimore, MD: Paul H. Brookes Publishing Co.

Brown, A. (1978). Knowing when, where and how to remember: A problem of mental cognition. In R. Glaser (Ed.), *Advances in instructional psychology* (Vol. 1). Hillsdale, NJ: Erlbaum Associates.

Brown, D. (1984). Automated assessment systems in school and clinical psychology: Present status and future direction. *School Psychology Review, 13,* 455–460.

Brown, R. (1973). *A first language.* Cambridge, MA: Harvard University Press.

Brown, A., & French, L. (1979). The zone of potential development: Implications for intelligence testing in the year 2000. In R. Sternberg & D. Detterman (Eds.), *Human intelligence: Perspectives on its theory and measurement* (pp. 217–235). Norwood, NJ: Ablex.

Brown, A. L., & Campione, J. C. (1986). Psychological theory and the study of learning disabilities. *American Psychologist, 14,* 1059–1068.

Brown, L., & Hammill, D. (1978). *Behavior rating profile.* Austin, TX: PRO-ED.

Brown, A. L., & Palinscar, A. S. (1987). Reciprocal teaching of comprehension strategies: A natural history of one program for enhancing learning. In J. Borkowski & J. P. Das (Eds.), *Intelligence and cognition in special children: Comparative studies of giftedness, mental retardation, and learning disabilities.* New York: Ablex.

Brown, S. L. et al. (1981). Preschool developmental profile, volume 5, in D. D'Eugenio & M. S. Moersch (Eds.), *Developmental Programming for Infants and Young Children.* Ann Arbor, MI: University of Michigan Press.

Brown, W., & McGuire, J. (1976). Current assessment practices. *Professional Psychology, 7,* 475–484.

Bruininks, R. H. (1978). *Bruininks-Oseretsky test of motor deficiency.* Circle Pines, MN: American Guidance Service.

Bruner, J. (1983). *Child's talk: Learning to use language.* New York: W. W. Norton & Company.

Bruner, J., Goodnow, J., & Austin, G. (1956). *A study of thinking.* New York: Wiley, 1956.

Bruner, J. S. (1957). On perceptual readiness. *Psychological Review, 64,* 123–152.

Bryan, Q. R. (1964). Relative importance of intelligence and visual perception in predicting reading achievement. *California Journal of Educational Research, 15,* 44–48.

Buktenica, N. A. (1968). Perceptual mode dominance: An approach to assessment of first grade reading and spelling. *Proceedings of the annual convention of the American Psychological Association, vol. 3.* Washington, D.C.: American Psychological Association.

Buktenica, N. A. (1975). *Test of nonverbal auditory discrimination.* Chicago: Follett Publishing Co..

Bureau of the Census, U.S. Department of Commerce. Washington, D.C., 1967.

Bureau of the Census, U.S. Department of Commerce. (July 1975). *Language usage in the United States.* Current Population Studies, July 1976.

Burke, H. R. (1958). Raven's progressive matrices: A review and critical evaluation. *The Journal of Genetic Psychology, 93,* 199–228.

Burks, H. (1968). *Manual for Burks' behavior rating scales.* El Monte, Calif.: Arden Press, 1968.

Buros, O. K. (Ed.). (1938). *The nineteen thirty-eight mental measurements yearbook.* New Brunswick, NJ: Rutgers University Press.

Buros, O. K. (Ed.). (1941). *The nineteen-forty mental measurements yearbook.* Highland Park, NJ: Mental Measurements Yearbook.

Buros, O. K. (Ed). (1949). *The third mental measurements yearbook.* New Brunswick, NJ: Rutgers University Press.

Buros, O. K. (Ed.). (1953). *The fourth mental measurements yearbook.* Highland Park, NJ: Gryphon Press.

Buros, O. K. (Ed.). (1959). *The fifth mental measurements yearbook.* Highland Park, NJ: Gryphon Press.

Buros, O. K. (Ed.). (1965). *The sixth mental measurements yearbook.* Highland Park, NJ: Gryphon Press.

Buros, O. K. (Ed.). (1972). *The seventh mental measurements yearbook* (2 vols.). Highland Park, NJ: Gryphon Press.

Buros, O. K. (Ed.). (1978). *The eighth annual mental measurements yearbook* (Vols. 1 & 2). Highland Park, NJ: Gryphon Press.

Burt, C. (1958). The inheritance of mental ability. *American Psychologist, 13,* 1–15.

Bush, W., & Waugh, K. (1976). *Diagnosing learning disabilities.* Columbus, OH: Merrill.

Butterfield, E. C., & Belmont, J. M. (1977). Assessing and improving the executive cognitive functions of mentally retarded people. In I. Bialer & M. Sternlicht (Eds.), *Psychological issues in mental retardation* (pp. 277–318). New York: Psychological Dimensions.

Butterfield, E., Wambold, C., & Belmont, E. (1973). On the theory and practice of improving short-term memory. *American Journal of Mental Deficiency, 77,* 654–669.

Byrne, J. M. and Horowitz, F. D. (1984). The perception of stimulus shape: The influence of velocity of stimulus movement. *Child Development, 55,* 1625–1629.

Bzoch, K., & League, R. (1971). *Receptive-Expressive Language Scale.* Gainesville, FL: The Tree of Life Press.

Cain, L., Levine, S., & Elzey, F. (1963). *Manual for the Cain-Levine Social Competency Scale.* Palo Alto: Consulting Psychologists Press.

Caldwell, B. M., & Bradley R. (1978). *Home observation for measurement of the environment.* Little Rock: University of Arkansas, Center for Child Development & Education.

California achievement tests, forms C and D. (1977, 1978). Monterey, CA: CTB–McGraw-Hill.

Camp, B. W., van Doornick, W. J., Frankenburg, W. J., & Lampe, J. (1977). Preschool developmental testing in prediction of school problems. *Clinical Pediatrics, 16,* 257–263.

Campione, J. C., & Brown, A. L. (1977). Memory and metamemory development in educable retarded children. In R. V. Kail, Jr. & J. W. Hagen (Eds.), *Perspectives on the development of memory and cognition* (pp. 367–406). Hillsdale, NJ: Erlbaum.

Caplan, F. (Ed.). (1973). *The first twelve months of life.* New York: Grosett & Dunlap.

Caplan, F., & Caplan, T. (1981). *The second twelve months of life.* New York: Bantam Books.

Carew, J. (1981). Experience and the development of intelligence in young children at home and in day care. *Monograph of the Society for Research in Child Development,* Nos. 6–7, *45.*

Carey, S. and Diamond, R. (1977). From piecemeal to configurational representation of faces. *Science, 195,* 312–314.

Carlson, C., Scott, M., & Elclund, S. (1980). Ecological theory and method for behavioral assessment. *School Psychology Review, 9,* 75–82.

Carlson, H. B., & Henderson, N. (1950). The intelligence of American children of Mexican parentage. *Journal of Abnormal and Social Psychology, 45,* 544–551.

Carroll, J. (1978). How shall we study individual differences in cognitive abilities? *Intelligence, 2,* 87–115.

Carroll, J., & Maxwell, S. (1979). Individual differences in cognitive abilities. *Annual Review of Psychology, 30,* 603–640.

Carroll, J. A., Fuller, C. G., & Carroll, J. (1979). Comparison of culturally deprived school achievers and underachievers on memory function and perception. *Perceptual and Motor Skills, 48,* 59–62.

Carrow-Woolfolk, E. & Lynch, J. (1982). *An integrative approach to language disorders in children.* New York: Grune & Stratton, Inc.

Carrow, S. E. (1968). The development of auditory comprehension of language structure in children. *Journal of Speech and Hearing Disorders, 33,* 99–111.

Carrow, S. E. (1974). A test using elicited imitations in assessing grammatical structure in children. *Journal of Speech and Hearing Disorders, 39,* 437–444.

Cartwright, C. A., & Cartwright, G. P. (1974). *Developing observation skills.* New York: McGraw-Hill.

Caskey, W. E., Jr. (1985). The use of the Peabody Individual Achievement Test and the Woodcock Reading Mastery Tests in the diagnosis of a learning disability in reading: A caveat. *Diagnostique, 11,* 14–20.

Caskey, W. E., Jr. & Larson, G. L. (1983). Relationship between selected predictors and first and fourth grade achievement test scores. *Perceptual and Motor Skills, 56,* 815–822.

Cassell, R. (1972). *The child behavior rating scale.* Beverly Hills, CA: Western Psychological Services.

Cattell, J. M. (1980). Mental tests and measurements. *Mind, 14,* 373–381.

Cattell, R. (1940). *The measurement of intelligence of infants and young children.* New York: Psychological Corporation.

Cattell, R. (1971). *Abilities: Their structure, growth, and action.* Boston: Houghton Mifflin.

Cattell, R. B. (1950). *Culture Fair Intelligence Test.* Champaign, IL: Institute for Personality and Ability Testing.

Cautela, J., & Upper, D. (1973). *A behavioral coding system.* Unpublished manuscript, Boston College.

Cautela, J., & Upper, D. (1976, December). *A behavior coding system.* Presidential address presented at the annual meeting of the Association for Advancement of Behavior Therapy, Miami.

Ceci, S., Ringstrom, M., & Lea, S. (1981). Do language-learning disabled children have impaired memories? *Journal of Learning Disabilities, 14,* 159–162.

Cermack, L. (1972). *Human memory.* New York: Ronald Press.

Chalfant, J. C., & Scheffelin, M. A. (1969). *Central processing dysfunctions* (NINDS Monograph No. 9). Washington, D.C.: U.S. Government Printing Office.

Chapman, R., & Miller, J. (1975). Word order in early two and three word utterances. *Journal of Speech and Hearing Disorders, 18,* 355–371.

Chase, J. B. (1985). Assessment of developmentally disabled children. *School Psychology Review, 14,* 150–154.

Chinn, P. (1979, April). The exceptional minority child: Issues and some answers. *Exceptional Children,* 532–536.

Chinn, P. C. (1984). *Education of culturally and linguistically different exceptional children.* Reston, VA: Council for Exceptional Children.

Chomsky, C. (1969). *The acquisition of syntax in children from 5 to 10.* Cambridge, Mass.: MIT Press.

Chomsky, N. (1965). *Aspects of the theory of syntax.* Cambridge, Mass.: MIT Press.

Chomsky, N. (1968). *Language and mind.* New York: Harcourt Brace Jovanovich.

Choong, J. & McMahon, J. (1983). Comparison of scores obtained on the PPVT and the PPVT-R. *Journal of Speech and Hearing Disorders, 48,* 36–40.

Clark, E. (1973). What's in a word? On the child's acquisition of semantics in his first language. In L. T. Moore (Ed.), *Cognitive development and language acquisition.* New York: Academic Press.

Clark E. (1975). Knowledge, context, strategy in the acquisition of meaning. In D. Dato (Ed.), *Georgetown University round table on languages and linguistics 1975.* Washington, D.C.: Georgetown University Press, 77–98.

Clark, H., & Clark, E. (1977). *Psychology and language.* New York: Harcourt Brace Jovanovich.

Clawson, A. (1962). *The Bender Visual-Motor Gestalt Test for children.* Los Angeles: Western Psychological Services.

Cleary, A. T., & Hilton, T. L. (1968). An investigation of bias. *Educational and Psychological Measurement, 28,* 61–75.

Cleary, T. A., Humphreys, L. G., Kendrick, S. A., & Wesman, A. G. (1975). Educational uses of tests with disadvantaged students. *American Psychologist, 30,* 15–41.

Cobb, R., & Larkin, D. (1985). Assessment and placement of handicapped pupils into secondary vocational education programs. *Focus on Exceptional Children, 17,* 1–14.

Cochran, W. G., & Cox, G. M. (1957). *Experimental design* (2nd ed.). New York: John Wiley and Sons.

Coers, W. C. (1935). Comparative achievement of White and Mexican junior high school pupils. *Peabody Journal of Education, 12,* 157–162.

Cohen, E. (1965). Examiner differences with individual intelligence tests. *Perceptual and Motor Skills, 20,* 1324.

Cohen, J. S., & DeYoung, H. (1973). The role of litigation in the improving of programming for the handicapped. In L. Mann & D. Sabatino (Eds.), *The first review of special education,* (86–108). Philadelphia: JSE Press.

Cohen, R., & Nealon, J. (1979). An analysis of short-term memory differences between retardates and nonretardates. *Intelligence, 3,* 65–73.

Cohen, R. A. (1969). Conceptual styles, culture conflict, and nonverbal tests. *American Anthropologist, 71,* 828–856.

Colarusso, R., & Hammill, D. (1972). *The Motor-Free Test of Visual Perception.* San Rafael, Calif.: Academic Therapy Publications.

Cole, P. (1982). *Language disorders in preschool children.* Englewood Cliffs, New Jersey: Prentice-Hall, Inc.

Coles, G. (1978). The learning disabilities test battery: Empirical and social issues. *Harvard Educational Review, 48,* 313–340.

Coles, G. (1988). *The learning mystique: A critical look at learning disabilities.* New York: Panthenon Books.

*Comprehensive Test of Basic Skills Forms U and V.* (1981, 1982, 1983). Monterey, CA: CTB–McGraw-Hill.

Compton, A. (1976). Generative studies of children's phonological disorders: Clinical ramifications. In D. Morehead & A. Morehead (Eds.), *Normal and deficient language.* Baltimore: University Park Press.

Conner, F. P., Williamson, G., & Siepp, J. (1978). *Guide for infants and toddlers with neuromotor and other developmental disabilities.* New York: Teacher's College Press.

Connolly, A. G., Nachtman, W., & Pritchett, E. M. (1976). *Key math diagnostic arithmetic test manual.* Circle Pines, Minn.: American Guidance Service.

Conrad, F. & Rips, L. (1986). Conceptual combination and the given/new distinction. *Journal of Memory and Language, 25,* 255–278.

Cook, J. M., & Arthur, B. (1951). Intelligence ratings for 97 Mexican children in St. Paul, Minn. *Exceptional Children, 18,* 14–15.

Cooper, J. G. (1958). Predicting school achievement in bilingual pupils. *Journal of Educational Psychology, 48,* 31–36.

Copeland, M., Ford, L., & Solon, N. (1976). *Occupational therapy for mentally retarded children.* Baltimore, MD: University Park Press.

Corach, N. L., & Powell, B. L. (1963). A factor analytic study of the Frostig Developmental Test of Visual Perception. *Perceptual and Motor Skills, 16,* 39–63.

Costello, C. T. (1976). A factor analytic comparison of three tests of visual perception for children. *Dissertation Abstracts International, 37,* 1892.

Costello, J., & Dickie, J. (1970). Leiter and Stanford-Binet IQ's of preschool disadvantaged children. *Developmental Psychology, 2,* 314.

Coulopoulos, D., & De George, G. (1982). *Current methods and practices of school psychologists in the assessment of linguistic minority children.* Quincy, MA.: Massachusetts Department of Education, Division of Special Education.

Coulter, W. (1980). Adaptive behavior and professional disfavor. *School Psychology Review, 9,* 67–73.

Courtnage, L., & Smith-Davis, J. (1982). Interdisciplinary team training: A national survey of special education teacher training programs. *Exceptional Children, 53,* 451–460.

*Covarrubias v. San Diego Unified School District (Southern California).* No. 70-394-T, (S.D., Cal. February, 1971).

Covington, M., et al. (1973). *The productive thinking program.* Columbus, Ohio: Merrill.

Cowen, E., et al. (1973). The AML: The quick screening device for early identification of school adaptation. *American Journal of Community Psychology, 1,* 12–35.

Cox, R. C., & Graham, G. T. (1966). The development of a sequentially scaled achievement test. *Journal of Educational Measurement, 3,* 147–150.

Cox, R. C. & Vargas, J. S. (1966, Feb.). *A comparison of item selection techniques for norm-referenced and criterion-referenced tests.* Paper presented at the meeting of the National Council on Measurement in Education, Chicago.

Craig, A. L. (1938). A study of the performance of Mexican children on the L.I.P.S. Master's thesis, University of Southern California, Los Angeles.

Craigheid, W., Kazdin, A., & Mahoney, M. (1981). Assessment and treatment strategies. In W. Craigheid, A. Kazdin, & M. Mahoney (Eds.), *Behavior Modification.* Boston: Houghton Mifflin.

Craik, F., & Lockhart, R. (1972). Level of processing: A framework for memory research. *Journal of Verbal Learning and Verbal Behavior, 11,* 671–684.

Cratty, B. J. (1980). Motor development for special populations: Issues, problems, and operations. *Focus on Exceptional Children, 213,* 2–11.

Crawford, C. (1979). George Washington, Abraham Lincoln and Arthur Jenson: Are they compatible? *American Psychologist, 34,* 664–672.

Croft, S. B., & Franco, J. N. (1983). Effects of a bilingual education program on academic achievement and self-concept. *Perceptual and Motor Skills, 57,* 583–586.

Cromwell, R., Blashfield, R., & Strauss, J. (1975). Criteria for classification systems. In N. Hobbs (Ed.), *The futures of children.* San Francisco: Jossey-Bass.

Cronbach, L. (1951). Coefficient alpha and the internal structure of tests. *Psychometrika, 16,* 297–334.

Cronbach, L. J. (1970). *Essentials of psychological testing* (3rd ed.). New York: Harper & Row.

Cronbach, L. (1975). Five decades of public controversy over mental testing. *American Psychology, 30,* 1–14.

Cronbach, L., & Gleser, B. (1965). *Psychological tests and personnel decisions* (2nd ed.). Urbana: University of Illinois Press.

Crowell, D. C., Hu-pei Au, K., and Blake, K. M. (1983). Comprehension questions: Differences among standardized tests. *Journal of Reading, 26,* 314–319.

Crudeck, R. (1980). A comparative study of indices for internal consistency. *Journal of Educational Measurement, 17,* 117–130.

Cummins, J. (1984). *Bilingualism and special education.* San Diego: College-Hill Press.

Cummings, J. A., Huebner, E. S., & McLeskey, J. (1986). Psychoeducational decision making: Reason for referral versus test data. *Professional School Psychology, 2,* 249–256.

*Curriculum Referenced Tests of Mastery.* (1983–1984). San Antonio, TX: The Psychological Corporation.

Daines, D., & Mason, L. G. (1972). A comparison of placement tests and readability graphs. *Journal of Reading, 15,* 597–603.

Dale, E., & Chall, J. (1948). A formula for predicting readability. Columbus: Bureau of Educational Research, Ohio State University.

Darakjian, G. L., & Michael, W. B. (1983). The long-term comparative predictive validities of standardized measures of achievement and academic self-concept for a sample of secondary school students. *Educational and Psychological Measurement, 43,* 251–260.

Darby, H. (1940). *The general intelligence of American-born Japanese children in California as measured by the Leiter International Performance Scale.* Master's thesis. University of Southern California, Los Angeles.

Darcy, N. T. (1952). The performance of bilingual Puerto Rican children on verbal and non-verbal language tests of intelligence. *Journal of Educational Research, 45,* 499–506.

Darlington, R. B. (1971). Another look at culture fairness. *Journal of Educational Measurement, 8,* 71–82.

Das, J. (1984). Simultaneous and successive process and the K-ABC. *The Journal of Special Education, 18,* 230–238.

Das, J., Kirby, J., & Jarman, R. (1975). Simultaneous and successive syntheses: An alternative model for cognitive abilities. *Psychological Bulletin, 82,* 87–103.

Davenport, B. M. (1976). A comparison of the Peabody Individual Achievement Test, the Metropolitan Achievement Test, and the Otis-Lennon Mental Ability Test. *Psychology in the Schools, 13,* 291–297.

Davis, A. (1948). *Social class influences upon learning.* Cambridge, MA: Harvard University Press.

Davis, F. (1974). *Standards for educational and psychological tests.* Washington, D.C.: American Psychological Association.

Davis, W. E. (1980). *Educator's resource guide to special education: Terms, laws, tests, organizations.* Boston: Allyn and Bacon.

Dawson, G. (1983). Lateralized brain dysfunction in autism: Evidence from the Halstead-Reitan Neuropsychological Battery. *Journal of Autism and Developmental Disorders, 13,* 268–286.

Day, D. (1983). *Early childhood education: A human ecological approach.* Glenview, IL: Scott, Foresman and Company.

Day, K. C., & Day, H. D. (1983). Ability to imitate language in kindergarten predicts later school achievement. *Perceptual and Motor Skills, 57,* 883–890.

Dean, R. S. (1976). *Comparison of PIAT validity with Anglo and Mexican-American children.* University of Arizona, ERIC Document Reproduction Service, *133,* 638.

Dean, R. S. (1977). Internal consistency of the PIAT with Mexican-American children. *Psychology in the Schools, 14,* 167–168.

De Avila, E. A., & Havassy, B. (1974). The testing of minority children: A neo-Piagetian approach. *Today's Education, 63,* 71–75.

De Avila, E. & Havassy, B. (1974). Piagetian alternative to I.Q.: Mexican-American study. In N. Hobbs (Ed.), *Issues in the classification of exceptional children.* San Francisco: Jossey-Bass Publishers.

De Gruijter, D. N. M., & Hambleton, R. K. (1984). On problems encountered using decision theory to set cutoff scores. *Applied Psychological Measurement, 8,* 1–8.

Deemer, B. (1985). Review of school psychological software. *Journal of School Psychology, 23,* 388–390.

De Hirsch, K., Jansky, J. J., & Langford, W. S. (1966). *Predicting reading failure.* New York: Harper & Row.

Deno, S. L. (1985). Curriculum-based assessment: The emerging alternative. *Exceptional Children, 52,* 219–232.

Deno, S. L. (1986). Formative evaluation of individual programs: A new role for school psychologists. *School Psychology Review, 16,* 290–305.

Dever, R. B. (1978). *TALK: Teaching the American language to kids.* Columbus, Ohio: Merrill.

deVilliers, J., & deVilliers, P. (1973). A cross-sectional study of the acquisition of grammatical morphemes in child speech. *Journal of Psycholinguistic Research, 2,* 267–278.

deVilliers, P. & deVilliers, J. (1979). *Early language.* Cambridge: Harvard University Press.

Diamond, K. (1987). Predicting school problems from preschool developmental screening: A four-year follow-up of the Revised Denver Developmental Screening Test and the role of the parent report. *Journal of the Division for Early Childhood, 11,* 247–253.

*Diana v. California State Board of Education.* No. C-70 37 RFP, District Court of Northern California (February, 1970).

Dihoff, R. E., & Chapman, R. S. (1977). First words: Their origins in action. Stanford University, *Papers and Reports on Child Language Development, 13,* 1–7.

Diller, L., & Gordon, W. A. (1981a). Intervention for cognitive deficits in brain-injured adults. *Journal of Consulting and Clinical Psychology, 49,* 822–839.

Diller, L., & Gordon, W. A. (1981b). Rehabilitation and clinical neuropsychology. In S. B. Filskov & T. J. Boll (Eds.). *Handbook of clinical neuropsychology* (pp. 702–733). New York: Wiley and Sons.

Diller, L., & Weinberg, J. (1977). Hemi-inattention in rehabilitation: The evolution of a rational remediation program. In E. A. Weinstein & R. P. Friedland (Eds.), *Advances in neurology* (Vol. 18, pp. 62–82). New York: Raven Press.

Dillon, R. (1980). Matching students to their preferred testing conditions: Improving the validity of cognitive assessment. *Educational & Psychological Measurement, 40,* 999–1004.

Dodge, K. A., Pettit, C. L., & Brown, M. M. (1986). Social competence in children. *Monographs of the Society for Research in Child Development.* (Serial no. 213).

Dodson, F. (1970). *How to parent.* New York: Signet Books, The New American Library.

Doll, E. A. (1953). *Measurement of social competence.* Circle Pines, MN: American Guidance Service.

Doll, E. A. (1965). *Vineland social maturity scale.* Circle Pines, MN: American Guidance Service.

Dore, J. A. (1978). Description of early language development. *Journal of Psycholinguistic Research, 4,* 423–30.

Dore, J. (1978). Conversational and preschool language development. In P. Fletcher & M. Garman (Eds.), *Language acquisition* (pp. 337–362). Cambridge, England: Cambridge University Press.

Doris, J., & Cooper, L. (1966). Brightness discrimination in infancy. *Journal of Experimental Child Psychology, 3,* 31–39.

Douglas, V., Parry, P., Norton, P. & Gerson, D. (1976). Assessment of a cognitive training program for hyperactive children. *Journal of Abnormal Child Psychology, 4,* 389–410.

Drucker, P. F. (1974). *Management: Tasks, responsibilities, practice.* New York: Harper & Row.

Duane, D. (1986). Neurodiagnostic tools in dyslexic syndromes in children: Pitfalls and proposed comparative study of computed tomography, nuclear magnetic resonance, and brain electrical activity mapping. In G. Pavlidis & D. Fisher (Eds.), *Dyslexia: Its neuropsychology and treatment* (pp. 65–86). New York: John Wiley & Sons.

DuBois, P. H. (1970). *A history of psychological testing.* Boston: Allyn & Bacon.

Duchan, J. (1984). Language assessment: The pragmatics revolution. In R. C. Naremore (Ed.), *Language science* (pp. 147–180). San Diego, CA: College-Hill Press.

Duffy, F. H., Denckla, M. B., Bartels, R. H., & Sandini, G. (1980). Dyslexia: Regional differences in brain electrical activity by topographic mapping. *Annals of Neurology, 5,* 412–420.

Duffy, F. H., & McAnulty, G. B. (1985). Brain electrical activity in mapping (BEAM): The search for a physiological signature of dyslexia. In Duffy, F. H., & N. Geschwind (Eds.), *Dyslexia: A neuroscientific approach to clinical evaluation* (pp. 105–122). Boston: Little Brown and Co.

Dunleavy, R. A., & Baade, L. A. (1980). Neuropsychological correlates of severe asthma in children 9–14 years old. *Journal of Consulting and Clinical Psychology, 48,* 564–577.

Dunn, D. J. (1973). Recording observations. *Consumer Brief, 1,* 1–3. Menomonie, WI: Research & Training Center, University of Wisconsin—Stout.

Dunn, L. M., & Markwardt, F. C. (1970a). *Peabody Individual Achievement Test.* Circle Pines, MN: American Guidance Service.

Dunn, L. M., & Markwardt, F. C. (1970b). Manual for the Peabody Individual Achievement Test. Circle Pines, MN: American Guidance Service.

Dunn, L. M., & Markwardt, F. C., Jr. (1988). Peabody Individual Achievement Test. Circle Pines, MN: American Guidance Service.

Dunn, L. & Smith, J. (1968). *Peabody Language Development Kits.* Circle Pines, MN: American Guidance Service.

Dunn, M. L. (1982). *Pre-sign language motor skills.* Tucson, AZ: Communication Skill Builders.

Dworkin, N. E. (1977). Public Law 94-142: A focus on assessment. *Diagnostique, 2,* 38–44.

Dykes, M. (1980). *Developmental assessment for the severely handicapped.* Seattle, WA: Exceptional Resources.

D'Zurilla, T., & Goldfried, M. (1971). Problem solving and behavior modification. *Journal of Abnormal Psychology, 78,* 107–126.

Eagle, N., & Harris, A. S. (1968). Interaction of race and test on reading performance scores. *Journal of Educational Measurement, 6,* 131–135.

Eaves, R., & McLaughlin, P. (1977). A systems approach for the assessment of the child and his environment: Getting back to basics. *Journal of Special Education, 11,* 99–111.

Ebel R. (1971). Criterion-referenced measurements: Limitations. *School Review, 79,* 282–288.

Ebel R. (1975). Educational tests: Valid? biased? useful? *Phi Delta Kappan, 57,* 83–88.

Ebel, R. L. (1962). Content standard test scores. *Educational and Psychological Measurement, 22,* 15–25.

Ebel, R. L. (1963). The social consequences of educational testing. *Proceedings of the 1963 Invitational Conference on Testing Problems.* Princeton, N.J.: Educational Testing Service, 130–143.

Ebel, R. L. (1972). *Essentials of educational measurement.* Englewood Cliffs, N.J.: Prentice-Hall.

Edelman, M. (1981). Who is for children? *American Psychologist, 36,* 109–116.

Eells, K. (1951). *Intelligence and cultural differences.* Chicago: University of Chicago Press.

Einhorn, H. J., & Bass, A. R. (1971). Methodological considerations relevant to discrimination in employment testing. *Psychological Bulletin, 75,* 261–269.

Eisenberg, N., & Harris, J. D. (1984). Social competence. *The School Psychology Review, 13,* 267–277.

Ellis, N. (1970). Memory processes in retardates and normals. In N. Ellis (Ed.), *International review of research in mental retardation* (Vol. 4). New York: Academic Press.

Ellis, R. (1980). Analysis of social skills: The behavior analysis approach. In W. Singleton, P. Spurgeon, & R. Stamers (Eds.), *The analysis of social skill.* New York: Plenum.

Elsasser, N., & John-Steiner, V. (1977). An interactionist approach to advancing literacy. *Harvard Educational Review, 47,* 355–369.

Engelman, S., & Osborn, J. (1970). *Distar: An instructional system.* Chicago: Science Research Associates.

Enright, B. E. (1983). *ENRIGHT diagnostic inventory of basic arithmetic skills.* North Billerica, MA: Curriculum Associates.

Ensminger, E. E. (1970). A proposed model for selecting, modifying or developing instructional materials for handicapped children. *Focus on Exceptional Children, 1,* 1–9.

Erickson, E. (1963). *Childhood and society.* New York: W. W. Norton and Co.

Erickson, E. (1968). *Identity, youth and crisis.* New York: W. W. Norton and Co.

Erickson, M. L. (1976). *Assessment and management of developmental changes in children.* Saint Louis: C. V. Mosby Company.

Ericson, K. (1975). *Instructions to verbalize as a means to study problem-solving processes with the 8-puzzle: A preliminary study.* Stockholm: University of Stockholm, Department of Psychology.

Estabrook, G. (1983). Test review. *Journal of Psychoeducational Assessment, 1,* 315–318.

Ewing, N., & Brecht, R. (1977). Diagnostic prescriptive instruction: A reconsideration of some issues. *Journal of Special Education, 11,* 323–327.

Exner, J. E. (1966). Variations in WISC performances as influenced by differences in pretest rapport. *Journal of General Psychology, 74,* 299–306.

Eyberg, S. M. (1980). Eyberg child behavior inventory. *Journal of Clinical Child Psychology, 9,* 29.

Fantz, R. L. (1970). Visual perception and experience in infancy. In F. A. Young & D. B. Lindsley (Eds.), *Early experience and visual information processing in perceptual and reading disorders.* Washington, D.C.: National Academy of Sciences.

Fantz, R. L., & Miranda, S. B. (1975). Newborn infant attention to form or contour. *Child Development, 46,* 224–228.

Fantz, R. L., & Nevis, S. (1967). Pattern preferences and perceptual-cognitive development in early infancy. *Merrill-Palmer Quarterly, 13,* 77–108.

Fay, W. H., & Schuler, A. (1980). *Emerging language in autistic children.* Baltimore, MD: University Park Press.

Feingold, S. N. (1984). Emerging careers: Occupations for a post-industrial society. *The Futurists, 18,* 9–16.

Feurstein, R. (1979). *The dynamic assessment of retarded performers: The learning potential device theory, instruments, and techniques.* Baltimore: University Park Press.

Fewell, R. R. and Langley, M. B. (1984). *Developmental activities screening inventory (DAS I–II).* Austin, TX: Pro-Ed.

Figueroa, R. (1982). SOMPA and the psychological testing of Hispanic children. *Metas, 2,* 1–16.

Finch-Williams, A. (1984). The developmental relationship between cognition and communication: Implications for assessment. *Topics in Language Disorders, 4,* 1–14.

Findley, W. (1956). A rationale for evaluation of item discrimination statistics. *Education and Psychological Measurement, 16,* 175–180.

Finlayson, M. A. J., Gowland, C., & Basmajian, J. V. (1986). Neuropsychological predictors of treatment response following stroke. *Journal of Clinical and Experimental Neuropsychology, 7,* 647 (abstract).

Finlayson, M. A. J., Johnson, K. A., & Reitan, R. M. (1977). Relationship of level of education to neuropsychological measures in brain-damaged and non brain-damaged adults. *Journal of Consulting and Clinical Psychology, 45,* 536–542.

Fisher, A. (1977). *Adaptive behavior in non-biased assessment: Effects on special education.* Paper presented at the annual meeting of the American Psychological Association, San Francisco.

Flavell, J. (1963). *The developmental psychology of Jean Piaget.* New York: Van Nostrand Reinhold Co.

Flavell, J. (1970). Developmental studies of mediated memory. In H. Reese & L. Lipsitt (Eds.), *Advances in child development and behavior* (Vol. 5). New York: Academic Press.

Flavell, J. (1974). The development of inferences about others. In T. Mischell (Ed.), *Understanding other persons.* Totowa, N.J.: Rowman & Littlefield.

Flavell, J., & Wellman, H. (1977). Metamemory. In I. R. Kail & I. Hogen (Eds.), *Perspectives on the development of memory and cognition.* Hillsdale, N.J.: Erlbaum Associates.

Floden, R. E., Porter, A. C., Schmidt, W. H., & Freeman, L. J. (1980). In E. L. Baker & E. S. Zuellmalz (Eds.), *Educational testing and evaluation* (pp. 109–120). Beverly Hills, CA: Sage.

Flory, K. (1988). *Preschool Screening.* Unpublished manuscript. Amherst, Massachusetts: University of Massachusetts.

Flynn, J. (1987). *Neurophysiologic characteristics of dyslexic subtypes and response to remediation.* Grant awarded by the Initial Teaching Alphabet Foundation. Roslyn, New York.

Flynn, J. & Deering, W. (1987). *Subtypes of dyslexia: Investigation of Boder's system for identification and classification of dyslexic children using quantitative neurophysiology.* Manuscript submitted for publication.

Forness, S., & Cantwell, D. (1982). DSM-III psychiatric and special education categories. *Journal of Special Education, 16,* 49–63.

Fox, W., et al. (1973). An introduction to a regular classroom approach to special education. In E. Deno (Ed.), *Instructional alternatives for exceptional children* (13–28). Arlington, VA: Council for Exceptional Children.

Frank, D. (1972). Ethnic and social status characteristics of children in EMR and LD classes. *Exceptional Children, 37,* 537–538.

Frankenburg, W. K. (1985). The Denver approach to early case finding: A review of the Denver Developmental Screening Test and a brief training program in developmental diagnosis. In W. Frankenburg, R. Emde, & J. Sullivan (Eds.), *Early Identification of children at risk.* New York: Plenum Press.

Frankenburg, W., Camp, B. W., Van Nett, P. A., Demersseman, J. A., & Voorhesses, S. F. (1971). Reliability and stability of the Denver Developmental Screening Test. *Child Development, 42,* 1315–1325.

Frankenburg, W. K., & Dodds, J. B. (1967). The Denver Developmental Screening Test. *Journal of Pediatrics, 71,* 181–191.

Frankenburg, W., Dodds, J., Fandal, A., Kazuk, E., & Cohrs, M. (1975). *Denver developmental screening test: Reference manual.* Denver, CO: Ladoca Project and Publishing Foundation.

French, J., & Michael, W. (1966). *Standards for educational and psychological tests and manuals.* Washington, D.C.: American Psychological Association.

Friedman, A., & Polson, M. (1981). Hemispheres as independent resource systems: Limited-capacity processing and cerebral specialization. *Journal of Experimental Psychology: Human Perception and Performance, 7,* 1031–1058.

Friedman, P. (1973). *Mental retardation and the law.* Washington, D.C.: U.S. Department of Health, Education and Welfare, Office of Mental Retardation.

Friedrich, F., Fuller, G. B., & Hawkins, W. F. (1969). Relationships between perception (input) and execution (output). *Perceptual and Motor Skills, 29,* 923–924.

Fristoe, M., & Blanton, R. L. (1970). *Like and cross-modality recognition at two levels of meaningfulness of a short-term memory task.* Proceedings of the 78th Annual Convention of the American Psychological Association, New York, 85–86.

Froman, K. (1983). *The chance to grow.* New York: Everest House.

Fromkin, V., & Rodman, R. (1974). *An introduction to language.* New York: Holt, Rinehart, & Winston.

Frostig, M., Lefever, W., & Whittlesey, J. R. B. (1966). *Administration and scoring manual for the Marianne Frostig Developmental Test of Visual Perception.* Palo Alto, CA: Consulting Psychologists Press.

Fuchs, L. S., & Fuchs, D. (Eds.). (1986a). Linking assessment to instructional interventions: An overview. *School Psychology Review, 15,* 318–323.

Fuchs, D. & Fuchs, L. S. (1986b). Test procedure bias: a meta-analysis of examiner familiarity effects. *Review of Educational Research, 56,* 243–262.

Fuchs, D., Fuchs, L. S., Benowitz, S. and Barringer, K. (1987). Norm-referenced tests: Are they valid for use with handicapped students? *Exceptional Children, 54,* 263–271.

Fuchs, L. S., Fuchs, D., and Deno, S. L. (1982). Reliability and validity of curriculum-based informal reading inventories. *Reading Research Quarterly, 18,* 6–26.

Furman, W. (1980). Promoting social development: Developmental implications for treatment. In B. Lohey & A. Kazdin (Eds.), *Advances in clinical child psychology,* (pp. 1–33). New York: Plenum.

Furuno, S. et al. (1984). *Vocational training test.* Palo Alto, CA.: VORT Corporation.

Gaddes, W. H. (1980). *Learning disabilities and brain function: A neuropsychological approach.* New York: Springer-Verlag.

Gaffner, D., et al. (1978). Speech and language assessment scale of deaf children. *Journal of Communication Disorders, 11,* 215–226.

Gagné, A. (1977). *The conditions of learning.* New York: Holt, Rinehart & Winston.

Gagné, R. J. (1970). Instructional variables and learning outcomes. In M. C. Wittroch & D. Wiley (Eds.), *Evaluation of instruction.* New York: Holt, Rinehart & Winston.

Gagné, R. M. (1968). Learning hierarchies. *Educational Psychologist, 6,* 1–9.

Galaburda, A. M., LeMay, M., Kemper, T. L., & Geschwind, N. (1978). Right-left asymmetries in the brain: Structural differences between the hemispheres may underline cerebral dominance. *Science, 199,* 852–856.

Galen, J. (1980). Behavioral observation for the school psychologist. *School Psychology Review, 9,* 31–45.

Gallagher, T. (1977). Revision behaviors in the speed of normal children developing language. *Journal of Speech and Hearing Research, 20,* 303–318.

Gallahue, D. (1982). *Developmental movement experiences for children.* New York: John Wiley & Sons.

Galton, F. (1892). *Hereditary genius* (2nd ed.). New York: Macmillan.

Galton, S. F. (1883). *Inquiries into human faculty and its development.* New York: E. P. Dutton.

Galvin, R. R. (1981). *Bilingualism as it relates to intelligence test scores and school achievement among culturally deprived Spanish-American children.* New York: Arno Press.

Garbarino, J., & Kapadia, S. (1986). Ecological assessment procedures. In H. M. Knoff (Ed.), *The assessment of child and adolescent personality.* New York: Guilford Press.

Gardner, E. F., Ludman, H. D., Karlsen, B., and Mervin, J. C. (1986). *Stanford Achievement Test Series*

(7th ed.) San Antonio, TX: Psychological Corporation.

Garth, T. R. (1923). A comparison of the intelligence of Mexican and mixed and full-blood Indian children. *Psychological Review, 30,* 388–401.

Garth, T. R. (1928). The intelligence of Mexican school children. *School and Society, 27,* 791–794.

Garth, T. R. (1933). The intelligence and achievement of mixed blood Indians. *Journal of Social Psychology, 4,* 234–237.

Garth, T. R., Eson, T. H., & Morton, M. M. (1936). The administration of non-language intelligence tests to Mexicans. *Journal of Abnormal and Social Psychology, 31,* 53–58.

Garth, T. R., & Johnson, H. D. (1934). The intelligence and achievement of Mexican children in the United States. *Journal of Abnormal and Social Psychology, 29,* 222–229.

Garvin, A. (1976). A simple, accurate approximate of the standard error of measurement. *Journal of Educational Measurement, 13,* 101–105.

Geary, D. C., & Gilger, J. W. (1984). The Luria-Nebraska Neuropsychological Battery-Children's Revision: Comparison of learning disabled and normal children matched on Full Scale IQ. *Perceptual and Motor Skills, 58,* 115–118.

Gellman, W. (1968). The principles of vocational evaluation. *Rehabilitation Literature, 29,* 102.

Gellman, W. & Soloff, A. (1976). Vocational evaluation. In M. B. Bolton (Ed.), *Handbook of measurement and evaluation in rehabilitation.* Baltimore: University Park Press.

Gerber, A. & Bryen, D. (1981). *Language and Learning Disabilities.* Baltimore: University Park Press.

Gesell, A., & Amatruda, C. (1941). *Developmental diagnosis: Normal and abnormal child development.* New York: Hoeber.

Gesell, A. & Ilg, F. L. (1954). *Child Development.* New York: Harper & Row Publishers.

Getzel, J. (1974). Images of the classroom and visions of the learner. *School Review, 82,* 527–540.

Gibson, E., & Levin, H. (1975). *The psychology of reading.* Cambridge, MA: MIT Press.

Gibson, E. J. (1969). *Principles of perceptual learning and development.* New York: Appleton-Century-Crofts.

Gibson, E. J., Gibson, J. J., Pick, A. D., & Osser, H. (1962). A developmental study of letterlike forms. *Journal of Comparative and Physiological Psychology, 55,* 897–906.

Gibson, E. J., Owsley, C. G., Walker, A., & Megaw-Myce, J. (1979). Development of perception of invariants: Substance and shape. *Perception, 8,* 609–619.

Gibson, J. J. (1966). *The senses considered as perceptual systems.* New York: Houghton Mifflin.

Gibson, J. J., & Yonas, P. M. (1968). A new theory of scribbling and drawing in children. In J. J. Gibson & P. M. Yonas (Eds.), *The analysis of reading skill: A program of basic and applied research.* Report number 5-1213. Ithaca, N.Y.: Cornell University and United States Office of Education Final.

Gickling, E. E., & Thompson, V. P. (1985). A personal view of curriculum-based assessment. *Exceptional Children, 52,* 205–218.

Gillung, T., & Rucker, C. (1977). Labels and teacher expectations. *Exceptional Children, 7,* 464–465.

Ginsburg, H. (1972). *The myth of the deprived child.* Englewood Cliffs, N.J.: Prentice-Hall.

Glaser, R. (1963). Instructional technology and the measurement of learning outcomes. *American Psychologist, 18,* 519–521.

Glaser, R. (1970). Evaluation of instruction and changing educational models. In M. C. Wittrock & D. E. Wiley (Eds., pp. 16–44), *The evaluation of instruction.* New York: Holt, Rinehart, & Winston.

Glaser, R., & Klaus, D. J. (1962). Proficiency measurement: Assessing human performance. In R. Gagné (Ed.), *Psychological principles in systems development.* New York: Holt, Rinehart, & Winston.

Glass, G. (1977). Integrative findings: The meta-analysis of research. In L. Shulman (Ed.), *Review of research in education* (vol. 5). (pp. 351–379). Itasca, IL: E. E. Peacock.

Glass, G. (1983). Effectiveness of special education. *Policy Studies Review, 2 (1),* 65–78.

Glass, G. V. (1978). Standards and criteria. *Journal of Educational Measurement, 15,* 237–261.

Glasser, A. J., & Zimmerman, I. L. (1967). *Clinical interpretation of the Wechsler Intelligence Scale for Children.* New York: Grune and Stratton.

Goddard, H. (1910). Four hundred feebleminded children classified by the Binet method. *Pedagogical Seminary, 17,* 387–399.

Goins, J. T. (1958). Visual perceptual abilities and early reading progress. (University of Chicago Supplementary Educational Monographs, No. 87). Chicago: University of Chicago Press.

Goldberg, I. (1971). Human rights for the mentally retarded in the school system. *Mental Retardation, 9,* 3–7.

Golden, C. J. (1987). *Luria-Nebraska neuropsychological battery: children's revision.* Los Angeles: Western Psychological Services.

Golden, C. J., Hammeke, T., & Purische, H. (1978). Diagnostic validity of a standardized neuropsychological battery derived from Luria's neuropsychological tests. *Journal of Consulting and Clinical Psychology, 46,* 1258–1265.

Goldfried, M. (1977). Behavioral assessment. In N. Sundberg (Ed.), *Assessment of persons* (pp. 66–75). Englewood Cliffs, N.J.: Prentice-Hall.

Goldfried, M., & D'Zurilla, T. (1969). A behavioral-analytic model for assessing competence. In C. D. Spielberger (Ed.), *Current topics in clinical and community psychology.* New York: Academic Press.

Goldfried, M., & Kent, R. (1972). Traditional versus behavior of personality assessment. *Psychological Bulletin, 77,* 409–420.

Goldfried, M., & Sprafkin, J. (1976). Behavioral personality assessment. In J. T. Spence, R. C. Carson, & J. W. Thibaut (Eds.), *Behavioral approaches to therapy.* Morristown, N.J.: General Learning Press, 1976.

Goldman, R., & Fristoe, M. (1972). *Goldman-Fristoe test of articulation.* Circle Pines, MN: American Guidance Service.

Goldman, R., Fristoe, M., & Woodcock, R. (1970). *The Goldman-Fristoe-Woodcock test of auditory discrimination.* Circle Pines, MN: American Guidance Service.

Goldman, R., Fristoe, M., & Woodcock, R. (1974). *Goldman-Fristoe-Woodcock auditory skills test battery.* Circle Pines, MN: American Guidance Service.

Goldman, R. D., & Hartig, L. K. (1976). The WISC may not be a valid predictor of school performance of primary-grade minority children. *American Journal of Mental Deficiency, 80,* 583–587.

Golightly, C. J. (1987). Transdisciplinary training: A step forward in special education teacher preparation. *Teacher Education and Special Education, 10,* 126–130.

Gonzales, E. (1982). Issues in assessment of minorities. In H. L. Swanson & B. L. Watson (Eds.), *Educational and psychological assessment of exceptional children* (pp. 375–388). St. Louis: C. V. Mosby.

Gonzales, E. (1981). *Renorming and translation of existing tests.* Paper presented at the Council for Exceptional Children, Bilingual Special Education Conference, New Orleans.

Goodenough, F. L. (1926). *Measurement of intelligence by drawings.* New York: Harcourt, Brace, & World.

Goodman, J. (1977). The diagnostic fallacy: A critique of Jane Mercer's concept of mental retardation. *Journal of School Psychology, 15,* 197–206.

Goodstein, H. A., Kahn, H., & Cawley, J. F. (1976). The achievement of educable mentally retarded children on the Key Math Diagnostic Arithmetic Test. *Journal of Special Education, 10,* 61–70.

Goslin, D. (1970). *Guidelines for the collection, maintenance, and dissemination of pupil records.* New York: Russell Sage.

Gottlieb, J., Semmel, M. I., & Veldman, D. J. (1978). Correlates of social status among mainstreamed mentally retarded children. *Journal of Educational Psychology, 70,* 396–405.

Goulard, L. J. (1949). *A study of the intelligence of eleven and twelve year old Mexicans by means of the Leiter International Performance Scale.* Master's thesis, University of Southern California, Los Angeles.

Goulard, S. E. (1940). *The general intelligence of American-born Japanese children in California measured by the Leiter International Performance Scale.* Master's thesis, University of Southern California, Los Angeles.

Gove, W. (1975). *The labeling process.* New York: Russell Sage.

Graham, F. K., & Kendall, B. S. (1960). Memory for designs test: Revised general manual (monograph supplement 2-VII Vol. 11). Missoula, MT: Test Specialists, 147–188.

Grant, D. L., & Bray, D. W. (1970). Validation of employment tests for telephone company installation and repair occupation. *Journal of Applied Psychology, 54,* 7–14.

Grassman, F. M. and Johnson, K. M. (1982) WISC-R factor scores as predictors of WRAT performance: A multivariate analysis. *Psychology in the Schools, 19,* 465–468.

Gray, B., & Ryan, B. (1973). *A language program for the nonlanguage child.* Champaign, Ill.: Research Press.

Gray, W. A. (1978). A comparison of Piagetian theory and criterion-referenced measurement. *Review of Educational Research, 48,* 223–249.

Graziano, W. G., Varca, P. E., & Levy, J. C. (1982). Race of examiner effects and the validity of intelligence test. *Review of Educational Research, 52,* 469–498.

Green, R. F. (1964). Desarrollo y estandarización de una escala individual de inteligencia para adultos en español [The development and standardization of an individual intelligence scale for adults in Spanish]. *Revista Mexicana de Psicología, 1,* 231–244.

Greenspan, S. (1982). *Personal competence profile.* Unpublished manuscript.

Greenstein, J., & Strain, P. S. (1977). The utility of the Key Math Diagnostic Arithmetic Test for adolescent learning disabled students. *Psychology in the Schools, 14,* 275–282.

Greenwood, C., Delquadri, J., & Hall, R. (1984). Opportunity to respond and student academic performance. In W. Heward, T. Heron, D. Hill, & J. Trap-Porter (Eds.), *Focus on behavior analysis in education* (pp. 58–88). Columbus, OH: Merrill.

Greenwood, C., et al. (1979). Selecting cost effective screening device for the assessment of preschool social withdrawal. *Journal of Applied Behavioral Analysis, 12,* 639–652.

Gregg, N. (1982). *An investigation of the breakdown in certain aspects of the writing process with college age learning disabled, normal and basic writers.* Unpublished doctoral dissertation, Northwestern University, Evanston, IL.

Gresham, F. (1984). Behavioral interviews in school psychology: Issues in psychometric adequacy and research. *School Psychology Review, 13,* 17–25.

Gresham, F. & Elliot, S. N. (1987). The relationship between adaptive behavior and social skills. *Journal of Special Education, 21,* 149–166.

Gresham, F. M., & Elliot, T. N. (1984). Assessment and classification of children's social skills: A review of methods and issues. *School Psychology Review, 13,* 292–301.

Grossman, F. M., & Johnson, K. M. (1982). WISC-R factor scores as predictors of WRAT performance: A multivariate analysis. *Psychology in the Schools, 19,* 465–468.

Grossman, H. (1983). *Manual on terminology and classification in mental retardation* (revision). Washington, D.C.: American Association on Mental Deficiency.

Group for the Advancement of Psychiatry. (1966). *Psychopathological disorder in childhood: Theoretical considerations and a proposed classification.* (GAP Report No. 62). Washington, D.C.: author.

Gruenewald, L., & Pollak, S. (1984). *Language interaction in teaching and learning.* Baltimore, MD: University Park Press.

*Guadalupe Organization Inc. v. Tempe Elementary School District,* No. CIV 71-435, Phoenix, (D. Arizona, January 24, 1972).

Guilford, J. (1967). *The nature of human intelligence.* New York: McGraw-Hill.

Guilford, J. (1980). Cognitive styles: What are they? *Educational & Psychological Measurement, 40,* 715–738.

Gulliksen, H. (1950). *Theory of mental tests.* New York: John Wiley & Sons.

Gunnison, J. (1984). Developing educational intervention from assessments involving the K-ABC. *The Journal of Special Education, 18,* 325–343.

Haertel, E. (1985). Construct validity and criterion-referenced testing. *Review of Educational Research, 55,* 23–46.

Haeusserman, E. (1958). *Developmental potential of preschool children.* New York: Grune & Stratton.

Hagen, E. (1961). Analyzing test results. *National Elementary Principal, 12,* 11–18.

Haladyna, T. M., & Roid, G. H. (1983). *Journal of Educational Measurement, 20,* 271–282.

Halahan, C., & Saegart, S. (1973). Behavioral and attitudinal effects of large-scale variation in the physical environment of psychiatric wards. *Journal of Abnormal Psychology, 82,* 455–462.

Hall, E. T. (1973). *The silent language.* Garden City, N.Y.: Doubleday Anchor Books.

Hall, R. J., Reeve, R. E., & Zakreski, J. R. (1984). Validity of the Woodcock-Johnson Tests of Achievement for learning-disabled students. *Journal of School Psychology, 22,* 193–200.

Hall, V. (1974). *Behavior modification: Measurement of behavior.* Lawrence, KS: H & H Enterprises.

Hall, V., et al. The effective use of punishment to modify behavior in the classroom. In K. O'Leary & S. O'Leary (Eds.), *Classroom management: The successful use of behavior modification (2nd ed.).* New York: Pergamon.

Hallahan, D. P. (1975). Comparative research studies on the psychological characteristics of learning disabled children. In W. Cruickshank & D. P. Hallahan (Eds.), *Perceptual and learning disabilities in children* (pp. 40–65). New York: Syracuse University Press.

Hallahan, D. P., & Cruickshank, W. M. (1973). *Psycho-educational foundations of learning disabilities.* Englewood Cliffs, N.J.: Prentice-Hall, Inc.

Halliday, M. A. (1975). *Learning how to mean: Explorations in the development of language.* New York: Elsevier-North Holland.

Hambleton, R., & Cook, L. L. (1977). Latent trait models and their use in the analysis of educational test data. *Journal of Educational Measurement, 14,* 75–96.

Hambleton, R. K., & Eignor, D. R. (1978). Guidelines for evaluating criterion-referenced tests and test manuals. *Journal of Educational Measurement, 15,* 321–327.

Hammill, D. (1972). Training visual perceptual processes. *Journal of Learning Disabilities, 5,* 552–559.

Hammill, D. D., & Larsen, S. C. (1974a). The effectiveness of psycholinguistic training. *Exceptional Children, 41,* 5–14.

Hammill, D. D., & Larsen, S. C. (1974b). The relationship of selected auditory perceptual skills and reading ability. *Journal of Learning Disabilities, 7,* 429–435.

Hammill, D. D., Leigh, J. E., McNutt, G., & Larsen, S., (1981). A new definition of learning disabilities. *Learning Disability Quarterly, 4,* 336–420.

Haney, W. (1984). Testing reasoning and reasoning about testing. *Review of Educational Research, 54,* 597–654.

Hanley, J. & Sklar, B. (1976). Electroencephalographic correlates of developmental reading dyslexias: Computer analysis of recordings from normal and dyslexic children. In G. Leisman (Ed.). *Basic visual processes in learning disabilities.* Springfield: Charles C. Thomas.

Harber, J. R. (1979). Measures of visual closure. *Perceptual and Motor Skills, 48,* 206.

Harbin, G. L. (1980). *Comparison of the use of single versus dual criteria in the classification of the EMR Black child.* Unpublished paper.

Hargreaves, D., Hester, S., & Mellar, F. (1975). *Deviance in classrooms.* London: Routledge & Kegan Paul.

Haring, N., & Bateman, B. (1977). *Teaching the learning disabled child.* Englewood Cliffs, N.J.: Prentice-Hall.

Haring, N., & Gentry, N. (1976). Direct and individualized instructional procedures. In N. Haring & R.

Schiefelbusch (Eds.), *Teaching special children* (pp. 112–128). New York: McGraw-Hill.

Haring, N. G., & Phillips, E. (1972). *Analysis and modification of classroom behavior.* Englewood Cliffs, N.J.: Prentice-Hall.

Haring, N., & Ridgeway, R. (1967). Early detection of children with learning disabilities. *Exceptional Children, 33,* 38–39.

Harmer, W. R., & Williams, F. (1978). The Wide Range Achievement Test and the Peabody Individual Achievement Test: A comparative study. *Journal of Learning Disabilities, 11,* 63–66.

Harmon, L. W., Sharma, V., & Trotter, A. B. (1976). Vocational inventories. In B. Bolton (Ed.), *Handbook of measurement and evaluation in rehabilitation.* Baltimore: University Park Press.

Harris, C. W. (1974). Problems of objectives based measurement. In C. W. Harris, M. C. Alkin, & W. J. Popham (Eds.), *Problems in criterion-referenced measurement,* CSE Monograph Series in Evaluation (No. 3). Los Angeles: Center for the Study of Evaluation, University of California.

Harris, D. J. and Subkoviak, M. J. (1986). Item analysis: A short-cut statistic for Mastery tests. *Educational and Psychological Measurement, 46,* 495–507.

Harrison, P. (1987). Research with adaptive behavior scales. *Journal of Special Education, 21,* 39–68.

Harryman, S. F. (1976). Physical therapy. In R. B. & P. R. Magrab (Eds.). *Developmental Disorders: Assessment, Treatment, Education.* Baltimore, MD: University Park Press.

Harter, S. (1982). A cognitive-developmental approach to children's understanding of affect and trait labels. In F. Serafica (Ed.), *Social-cognitive development in context.* New York: Guilford Press.

Harter, S. (1980). *Perceived competence scale for children.* Denver: University of Denver.

Hartlage, L. C., & Hartlage, P. L. (1977). Application of neuropsychological principles in the diagnosis of learning disabilities. In L. Tarnapol and H. Tarnapol (Eds.)., *Brain function and reading disabilities.* Baltimore: University Park Press.

Hartlage, L., & Lucas, D. (1973). Group screening for reading disability in first grade children. *Journal of Learning Disabilities, 6,* 317–321.

Hartlage, L. C., & Telzrow, K. F. (1983). The neuropsychological basis of educational intervention. *Journal of Learning Disabilities, 16,* 521–526.

Hasazi, S. B., Gordon, L. R., & Roe, C. A. (1985). Factors associated with the employment status of handicapped youth exiting high school from 1979 to 1983. *Exceptional Children, 51,* 455–469.

Haslam, R. H. A., Dalby, J. T., Johns, R. D., & Rademaker, A. W. (1981). Cerebral asymmetry in developmental dyslexia. *Archives of Neurology, 38,* 679–682.

Haught, B. F. (1934). Mental growth of southwestern Indians. *Journal of Applied Psychology, 18,* 137–142.

Hawkins, R. (1979). The functions of assessment: Implications for selection and development of devices for assessing repertoires in clinical, educational, and other settings. *Journal of Applied Behavior Analysis, 12,* 501–516.

Hayes-Roth, B., & Thorndyke, P. (1979). *Decision making during the planning process.* Santa Monica: Rand Corporation.

Haynes, S. (1978). Principles of behavior assessment. New York: Gardner Press.

Heflinger, C., Cook, V., & Thackrey, M. (1987). Identification of mental retardation by the system of multicultural pluralistic assessment: Nondiscriminatory or nonexistent? *Journal of School Psychology, 25,* 177–183.

Herman, B. P. (1982). Neuropsychological function and psychopathology in children with epilepsy. *Epilepsia, 23,* 545–654.

Hernstein, R. (1971). I.Q. *The Atlantic Monthly, 228,* 43.

Hessler, G. L. (1984). *Use and interpretation of the Woodcock-Johnson Psycho-educational Battery.* Allen, TX: DLM-Teaching Resources.

Hessler, G. & Kitchen, D. (1980). Language characteristics of a purposive sample of early elementary learning disabled students. *Learning Disabilities Quarterly, 3,* 36–41.

Hier, D. B., LeMay, M., Rosenberger, P. B., & Perlo, V. P. (1978). Developmental dyslexia: Evidence for a subgroup with a reversal of cerebral asymmetry. *Archives of Neurology, 35,* 90–92.

Hieronymus, A. N., Lindquist, E. F., & Hoover, H. D. (1982). *Iowa test of basic skills.* Chicago: Riverside.

Higgins, C., & Silvers, C. H. (1958). A comparison of Stanford-Binet and Raven Coloured Progressive Matrices IQ's for children with low socioeconomic status. *Journal of Consulting Psychology, 22,* 465–468.

Hildreth, G. H., Griffiths, N. L., & McGauvra, M. E. (1965). *Manual of directions, Metropolitan Readiness Tests, Form A.* New York: Harcourt Brace Jovanovich.

Hitchcock, D. C., & Pinder, G. D. (1974). *Reading and arithmetic achievement among youths 12–17 years as measured by the Wide Range Achievement Test* (National Center for Health Statistics, Series 11, No. 136). Washington, D.C.: U.S. Government Printing Office.

Hively, W. (1966). *A test-item pool for MINNEMAST science unit 2.1: Measuring weight.* MINNEMAST Project, University of Minnesota.

Hively, W., et al. (1973). *Domain-referenced curriculum evaluation: A technical handbook and a case study from the MINNEMAST project.* (CSE Monograph Series in Evaluation, No. 1). Los Angeles: Center for the Study of Evaluation, University of California.

Hively, W., Patterson, H. L., & Page, S. (1968). A "universe defined" system of arithmetic achievement tests. *Journal of Educational Measurement, 5,* 275–290.

*Hobson v. Hansen.* 269 F. Suppl. 401 (1967).

Hochberg, J. E. (1964). *Perception.* Englewood Cliffs, N.J.: Prentice-Hall.

Hodge, R. (1985). The validity of direct observation measures of pupil classroom behavior. *Review of Educational Research, 55,* 469–484.

Hoepfner, R., Stern, C., & Nunmedal, S. G. (Eds.). (1971). *CSE-ECRC preschool/kindergarten test evaluations.* Los Angeles: University of California, Center for the Study of Evaluation—Early Childhood Research Center.

Hoepfner, R. (Ed.). (1974). *CSE secondary school test evaluation* (Vols. 1, 2, 3). Los Angeles: University of California, Center for the Study of Evaluation.

Hoepfner, R. (Ed.). (1976). *CSE elementary school test evaluations.* Los Angeles: University of California, Center for the Study of Evaluation.

Hogan, R., DeSoto, C., & Solano, C. (1977). Traits test and personality research. *American Psychologist, 32,* 255–264.

Holahan, C., & Saegert, S. (1973). Behavioral and attitudinal effects of large-scale variation in the physical environment of psychiatric wards. *Journal of Abnormal Psychology, 82,* 454–562.

Holman, J. (1977). The moral risk and high cost of ecological concern in applied behavior analysis. In A. Warren & S. Warren (Eds.), *Ecological perspec-*

*tives in behavior analysis.* Baltimore: University Park Press.

Holtzman, T., Glaser, R., & Pellegrino, J. (1975). Process training derived from computer simulation theory. *Memory and Cognition, 4,* 349–356.

Holtzman, W. H. (1971). The changing world of mental measurement and its social significance. *American Psychologist, 26,* 546–553.

Honig, B. (1985, May 29). Jobs and education. *Education Week, 4,* 23.

Hooper, I. R., & Hynd, G. W. (1986). Performance of normal and dyslexic readers on the Kaufman Assessment Battery for Children (K-ABC): A discriminant analysis. *Journal of Learning Disabilities, 19,* 206–210.

Hoover, H. D. and Kolen, M. J. (1984). The reliability of six item biases indices. *Applied Psychological Measurement, 8,* 173–181.

Horodezky, B., and Lebercane, G. (1983) Criterion-referenced tests as predictors of reading performance. *Educational and Psychological Measurement, 43,* 657–662.

Horst, P. (1966). *Psychological measurement and prediction.* Belmont, CA: Wadsworth.

Horstmeir, D., & MacDonald, J. (1978). *Environmental pre-language battery.* Columbus, OH: Merrill.

Howard, A., & Shoemaker, D. J. (1954). An evaluation of the Memory for Designs Test. *Journal of Consulting Psychology, 18,* 266.

Howell, K., Kaplan, J., & O'Connell, C. (1979). *Evaluating exceptional children.* Columbus, OH: Merrill.

Howell, L. (1986). Direct assessment of academic performance. *School Psychology Review, 15,* 324–335.

Howell, R. J., Evans, L., & Downing, L. M. (1958). A comparison of test scores for the 16–17 year age group of Navaho Indians with standardized norms for the Wechsler Adult Intelligence Scale (Arizona and New Mexico). *Journal of Social Psychology, 47,* 355–359.

Hsu, T. C., & Carlson, M. (1972). *Computer assisted testing.* Unpublished manuscript, University of Pittsburgh, Learning Research and Development Center, 1972.

Hudgins, A. L. (1977). Assessment of visual-motor disabilities in young children: Toward differential diagnosis. *Psychology in the Schools, 14,* 252–260.

Huelsman, C. B. (1970). The WISC subtest syndrome for disabled readers. *Perceptual and Motor Skills, 30,* 535–550.

Humphreys, L. (1979). The construct of general intelligence. *Intelligence, 3,* 105–120.

Humphreys, L. L., & Ciminero, A. R. (1979). Parent report measures of child behavior: A review. *Journal of Clinical Child Psychology, 8,* 56–63.

Humphreys, M. S., & Revelle, W. (1984). Personality, motivation, and performance: A theory of the relationship between individual differences and information processing. *Psychological Review, 91,* 153–184.

Hunt, E. (1974). Quote the Raven? Nevermore. In L. W. Gregg (Ed.), *Knowledge and cognition* (pp. 60–73). Hillsdale, N.J.: Erlbaum Associates.

Hunt, J. (1961). *Intelligence and experience.* New York: Ronald Press.

Hunt, J., & Kirk, G. E. (1974). Criterion-referenced tests of school readiness: A paradigm of illustrations. *Genetic Psychology Monographs, 90,* 143–182.

Hunt, J. McV. (1969). Has compensatory education failed? *Harvard Educational Review, 39,* 278–300.

Hunter, W. S., & Sumermier, E. (1922). The relation of degree of Indian blood to score on the Otis Intelligence Test. *Journal of Comparative Psychology, 2,* 257–277.

Hutt, M. (1977). *The Hutt adaptation of the Bender-Gestalt* (3rd ed.). New York: Grune & Stratton.

Hynd, G. W., & Obrzut, J. E. (1986). Clinical child neuropsychology: Issues and perspectives. In J. E. Obrzut & G. W. Hynd (Eds.), *Child neuropsychology,* Volume 2, (pp. 3–14). New York: Grune & Stratton.

Idol, L., Nevin, A., & Paolucci-Whitcomb, L. (1986). *Models of curriculum-based assessment.* Rockville, MD: Aspen.

Idol-Maestas, L. (1980). Oral language responses of children with reading difficulties. *Journal of Speech Education, 14,* 366–404.

Illerbrun, D., Haines, L., & Greenough, P. (1985). Language identification screening test for kindergarten: A comparison with four screening and three diagnostic language tests. *Language, Speech and Hearing Services in Schools, 16,* 280–292.

Ingram, D. (1976a). Current issues in child phonology. In D. Morehead & A. Morehead (Eds.), *Normal* and deficient child language. Baltimore: University Park Press.

Ingram, D. (1976b). *Phonological disability in children.* New York: Elsevier.

Ingram D. (1981). *Procedures for the phonological analysis of children's language.* Baltimore, MD: University Park Press.

Ingram, T. (1975). Speech disorders in childhood. In E. Lenneberg & E. Lenneberg (Eds.), *Foundation of language development.* New York: Academic Press.

Inhelder, B. (1976). Observations on the operational and figurative aspects of thought dysphasic children. In D. Morehead & A. Morehead (Eds.), *Normal and deficient child language.* Baltimore: University Park Press.

Irwin, J., Moore, J., & Rampp, D. (1972). Non-medical diagnosis and evaluation. In J. Irwin & M. Marge (Eds.), *Principles of childhood language disabilities.* Englewood Cliffs, N.J.: Prentice-Hall.

Jackson, D., & Pavnonen, J. (1980). Personality structure and assessment. In M. Rosenweig & L. Porter (Eds.), *Annual Review of Psychology,* (pp. 200–287). Palo Alto, CA: Annual Review.

Jakobson, R. (1968). *Child language, aphasia and phonological universals.* The Hague, Holland: Mouton.

Jakobson, R., Fant, C., & Halle, M. (1963). *Preliminaries to speech analysis: The distinctive features and their correlates.* Cambridge, MA: MIT Press.

Jansky, J. J., & de Hirsch, D. (1972). *Preventing reading failure.* New York: Harper & Row.

Jastak, J. J., & Jastak, S. (1978). *Manual: The Wide Range Achievement Test.* Wilmington, DE: Jastak Associates.

Jastak, S., & Wilkinson, G. S. (1984). *Wide range achievement test-revised.* Wilmington, DE: Jastak Associates.

Jeffrey, W. E. (1968). The orienting reflex and attention in cognitive development. *Psychological Review, 75,* 323–324.

Jenkins, J., & Pany, D. (1978). Standardized achievement test: How useful for special education? *Exceptional Children, 44,* 448–453.

Jenkins, M. D. (1939). The intelligence of Negro children. *Educational Methods, 19,* 106–112.

Jensen, A. (1984). The black-white difference on the K-ABC: Implications for future tests. *The Journal of Special Education, 18,* 377–408.

Jensen, A. R. (1961). Learning abilities in Mexican-American and Anglo-American children. *California Journal of Educational Research, 12,* 147–159.

Jensen, A. R. (1969). How much can we boost IQ and scholastic achievement? *Harvard Educational Review, 39,* 1–123.

Johnson, D., Johnson, C., & Price-Williams, D. (1967). The Draw-A-Man Test and Raven Progressive Matrices Performance of Guatemalan boys and Latino children. *Revista Interamericana de Psicologia 1:* 143–157.

Johnson, D. & Myklebust, H. (1967). *Learning Disabilities Educational Principles and Practices.* New York: Grune & Stratton.

Johnson, D. L. (1984). Comparison of three intelligence tests as predictors of academic achievement and classroom behaviors of Mexican-American children. *Journal of Psychoeducational Assessment, 2,* 345–352.

Johnson, L. J., & Beauchamp, K. D. F. (1987). Preschool assessment measures: What are teachers using? *Journal of the Division of Early Childhood, 12,* 70–76.

Johnston, C. W., & Lanak, B. (1985). Comparison of the Koppitz and Walkins scoring systems for the Bender Gestalt test. *Journal of Learning Disabilities, 18,* 377–383.

Johnston, J. R. (1982). Interpreting the Leiter IQ: Performance profiles of young normal and language disturbed children. *Journal of Speech and Hearing Research, 25,* 291–296.

Jones, P. (1976). Causative factors and prevention of childhood deafness. *Volta Review, 78,* 268–275.

Jones, R., Reed, J., & Patterson, G. (1975). Naturalistic observation in clinical assessments. In P. McReynolds (Ed.), *Advances in psychological assessment* (Vol. 3). San Francisco: Jossey-Bass.

Kagen, J. (1969). Inadequate evidence and illogical conclusions. *Harvard Educational Review, 39,* 126–129.

Kagen, J., Pearson, W., & Welch, L. (1966). Modifiability of an impulsive tempo. *Journal of Educational Psychology, 57,* 359–365.

Kamhi, A. (1984). Problem solving in child language disorders: The clinician as clinical scientist. *Language, Speech and Hearing Services in Schools, 15,* 226–234.

Kamhi, A. & Catts, H. (1986). Toward an understanding of developmental language and reading disorders. *Journal of Speech and Hearing Disorders, 51,* 337–347.

Kamin, L. J. (1974). *The science and politics of I.Q.* Hillsdale, N.J.: Erlbaum Associates.

Kamin, L. J. (1975). Social and legal consequences of I.Q. tests as classification instruments: Some warnings from our past. *Journal of School Psychology, 13,* 317–323.

Kamphaus, R. W. (1985). Review of Curriculum Referenced Tests of Mastery. In J. V. Mitchell, Jr. (Ed.), *The ninth mental measurements yearbook* (Vols. 1–2), (pp. 426–427). Lincoln, NE: Buros Institute of Mental Measurement of the University of Nebraska-Lincoln.

Kampus, R. (1987). Conceptual and psychometric issue in the assessment of adaptive behavior. *Journal of Special Education, 21,* 27–36.

Kanfer, F., & Grimm, L. (1977). Behavior analysis: Selecting target behaviors in the interview. *Behavior Modification, 1,* 7–28.

Kanfer, F. H., & Nay, W. R. (1982). Behavioral assessment. In G. T. Wilson & C. M. Franks (Eds.). *Contemporary behavior therapy: Conceptual and empirical foundations* (pp. 34–55). New York: Guilford.

Kanfer, F., & Saslow, G. (1969). Behavior of diagnosis. In C. Franks (Ed.), *Behavior therapy: Appraisal and status.* New York: McGraw-Hill.

Karlsen, B., Madden, R., & Gardner, E. F. (1974). *Stanford Diagnostic Reading Test, Level III.* New York: Harcourt Brace Jovanovich.

Karlsen, B., Madden, R., & Gardner, E. F. (1977). *Stanford Diagnostic Reading Test, Level III.* New York: Harcourt Brace Jovanovich.

Karlsen, B., Madden, R., & Gardner, E. F. (1983, 1944). *Stanford Diagnostic Reading Tests.* San Antonio, TX: Psychological Corporation.

Kass, C. (1966). Psycholinguistic disabilities of children with reading problems. *Exceptional Children, 32,* 533–539.

Katz, B., & McSweeney, M. (1980). Error of misclassification in neo-Piagetian research. *Educational & Psychological Measurement, 40,* 845–858.

Katz, J. (1966). *The philosophy of language.* New York: Harper & Row.

Katz, J., & Fodor, J. (1963). The structure of a semantic theory. *Language, 39,* 170–210.

Katz, M. (1969). *Selecting an achievement test: Principles and procedures.* Princeton, N.J.: Educational Testing Service.

Kaufman, A., (1980). Issues in psychological assessment: Interpreting the WISC-R intelligently. In B. Lagey & A. Kazdin (Eds.), *Advances in child psychology* (pp. 177–209). New York: Plenum.

Kaufman, A. S. (1979). *Intelligence testing with the WISC-R.* New York: John Wiley & Sons.

Kaufman, A. S. (1983). Some questions and answers about the Kaufman Assessment Battery for Children (K-ABC). *Journal of Psychoeducational Assessment, 2,* 205–218.

Kaufman, A. S. (1986). The K-ABC and giftedness. *Assessment Information Exchange* (American Guidance Service Newsletter), *2,* 1–2.

Kaufman, A. S., & Kaufman, N. L. (1983). *Kaufman assessment battery for children: Interpretive Manual.* Circle Pines, MN: American Guidance Service.

Kaufman, A. S., & McLean, J. E. (1986). K-ABC/WISC-R factor analysis for learning disabled population. *Journal of Learning Disabilities, 19,* 145–153.

Kaufman, A. S., & McLean, J. E. (1987). Joint factor analysis of the K-ABC and WISC-R with normal children. *Journal of School Psychology, 25,* 105–118.

Kaufmann, J. M. (1981). *Characteristics of children's behavior disorders.* Columbus, OH: Merrill.

Kavale, K. (1981). The relationship between auditory perceptual skills and reading ability: A meta-analysis. *Journal of Learning Disabilities, 14,* 539–546.

Kavale, K. (1982). Meta-analysis of the relationship between visual perceptual skills and reading achievement. *Journal of Learning Disabilities, 15,* 40–51.

Kavale, K. A., & Forness, S. R. (1985). *The science of learning disabilities.* San Diego: College-Hill Press.

Kazdin, A. (1979). Unobtrusive measures in behavior assessment. *Journal of Applied Behavioral Analysis, 12,* 713–724.

Keir, G. (1949). The progressive matrices as applied to school children. *British Journal of Psychology, 2,* 140–150.

Keith, T. Z. (1986). Factor structure of the K-ABC for referred school children. *Psychology in the Schools, 23,* 241–246.

Keith, T. Z. (1987). Assessment research: An assessment and recommended interventions. *School Psychology Review, 16,* 290–305.

Keller, H. R. (1986). Behavioral observation approaches to personality assessment. In H. M. Knoff (Ed.), *The Assessment of Child and Adolescent Personality.* New York: Guilford Press.

Kelley, H., & Michela, J. (1980). Attribution theory and research. In M. R. Rosenzweig and L. W. Porter (Eds.), *Annual Review of Psychology,* (Vol. 31, pp. 302–336). Palo Alto, CA: Annual Review.

Kendell, R. (1975). *The role of diagnosis in psychiatry.* New York: Oxford University Press.

Keogh, B. K. (1965). School achievement associated with successful performance on the Bender Gestalt Test. *Journal of School Psychology, 3,* 37–40.

Keogh, B. K. (1969). The Bender Gestalt with children: Research implications. *Journal of Special Education, 3,* 15–22.

Keogh, B. K. (1971). A compensatory model for psychoeducational evaluation of children with learning disorders. *Journal of Learning Disabilities, 4,* 544–548.

Keogh, B. K., & Smith, C. E. (1961). Group techniques and proposed scoring system for the Bender Gestalt test with children. *Journal of Clinical Psychology, 17,* 172–175.

Keogh, B. K., & Smith, S. E. (1967). Visuo-motor ability for school prediction: A seven-year study. *Perceptual and Motor Skills, 25,* 101–110.

Keogh, B. K., & Vormeland, O. (1970). Performance of Norwegian children on the Bender Gestalt and Draw-a-Person Tests. *Scandinavian Journal of Educational Research, 14,* 105–111.

Keston, J., & Jimenez, C. (1954). A study of the performance on English and Spanish editions of the Stanford-Binet Intelligence Test by Spanish-American children. *Journal of Genetic Psychology, 85,* 263–269.

Kidd, A. H. (1962). The culture fair aspects of Cattell's test of g: Culture free. *Journal of Genetic Psychology, 101,* 343–363.

Killian, L. R. (1971). WISC-Illinois Test of Psycholinguistic Abilities and Bender, Visual-Motor Gestalt Test performance of Spanish-American kindergarten and first-grade school children. *Journal of Consulting and Clinical Psychology, 37,* 38–42.

Kinsbourne, M. (Ed.) (1978). *Asymmetrical function of the brain.* Cambridge, MA: Cambridge University Press.

Kirchner, D. & Klatzky, R. (1985). Verbal rehearsal and memory in language-disordered children. *Journal of Speech and Hearing Research, 28,* 556–565.

Kirchner, D. & Skarakis-Doyle, E. (1983). Developmental language disorders: A theoretical perspective. In T. Gallagher & C. Prutting (Eds.), *Pragmatic Assessment and Intervention Issues in Language* (pp. 215–246). San Diego, CA: College-Hill Press.

Kirk, S. (1972). *Educating exceptional children* (2nd ed.). Boston: Houghton Mifflin.

Kirk, S., & Kirk, W. (1971). *Psycholinguistic learning disabilities: Diagnosis and remediation.* Urbana, IL: University of Illinois Press.

Kirk, S. A., Klieban, J. M., & Lerner, J. W. (1978). *Teaching reading to slow and disabled learners.* Boston: Houghton Mifflin.

Kirk, S. A., McCarthy, J. J., & Kirk, N. D. (1968). *Illinois test of psycholinguistic abilities* (rev. ed.). Urbana: University of Illinois Press.

Klick, R. (1979). Syntactic and phonological influences on children's articulation. *Journal of Speech and Hearing Research, 22,* 841–848.

Knapp, Robert R. (1960). The effects of time limits on the intelligence test performance of Mexican and American subjects. *Journal of Educational Psychology, 51,* 14–20.

Kneedler, R. D. (1984). *Special education for today.* Englewood Cliffs, NJ: Prentice-Hall.

Knuckle, E. P., & Asbury, C. A. (1986). Benton Revised Visual Retention Test performance of black adolescents according to age, sex, and ethnic identity. *Perceptual and Motor Skills, 63,* 319–327.

Kochnower, J., Richardson, E., & Di Bennedetto, B. A. (1983). A comparison of phonic decoding ability of normal and learning disabled children. *Journal of Learning Disabilities, 16,* 348–351.

Kohlberg, L. (1958). The developments of modes of moral thinking and choice in the years two to sixteen. Unpublished doctoral dissertation, University of Chicago. Chicago, IL.

Kohlberg, L. (1964). Development of word character and moral ideology. In M. Hoffman (Ed.), *Review of child development research* (Vol. 1). New York: Russell Sage.

Kohn, M. (1977). The Kohn Social Competence Scale and Kohn Symptom Checklist for the preschool child: A follow-up report. *Journal of Abnormal Child Psychology, 5,* 249–263.

Kohn, M., Parnes, B., & Rosman, B. L., (1979). *Kohn Social Competence Scale.* New York: Martin Kohn Publisher.

Kohs, S. (1923). *Intelligence measurements.* New York: Macmillan.

Konfer, F., & Grimm, F. (1977). Behavioral analysis: Selecting target behaviors in the interview. *Behavior Modification, 1,* 7–29.

Koppitz, E. M. (1964). *The Bender-Gestalt Test for young children.* New York: Grune & Stratton.

Koppitz, E. M. (1970). Brain damage, reading disability and the Bender Gestalt Test. *Journal of Learning Disabilities, 3,* 6–10.

Koppitz, E. M. (1975). *The Bender Gestalt Test for young children* (Vol. II). New York: Grune & Stratton.

Korman, M. A., & Blumberg, S. (1963). Comparative efficiency of some tests of cerebral damage. *Journal of Consulting Psychology, 27,* 303–309.

Krathwohl, D., Bloom, B., & Masia, B. (1964). *Taxonomy of educational objectives: Affective domain.* New York: McKay.

Kratochwill, T. (1977). The movement of psychological extras into ability assessment. *Journal of Special Education, 11,* 299–311.

Kratochwill, T. (1978). *Single subject research.* New York: Academic Press.

Kratochwill, T. R., & Demuth, D. M. (1976). An examination of the predictive validity of the Key Math Diagnostic Arithmetic Test and the Wide Range Achievement Test in exceptional children. *Psychology in the Schools, 13,* 404–406.

Kreutzer, M., Leonard, C., & Flavell, J. (1975). An interview study of children's knowledge about memory. *Monographs of the Society for Research in Child Development, 40* (1, Serial no. 159).

Kruel, E. J., Bell, D. W., & Nixon, J. C. (1969). Factors affecting speech discrimination test difficulty. *Journal of Speech and Hearing Research, 12,* 281–287.

Krug, S. E. (1987). *Psychware sourcebook.* Kansas City, MO: Test Corporation of America.

Krug, S. E. (1988). *Psychware sourcebook, 1987–1988.* Kansas City, MO: Test Corporation of America.

Kuaraceus, W. (1966). *Anxious youth: Dynamics of delinquency.* Columbus, Ohio: Merrill.

Kubzansky, P. E., Rebelsky, F., & Dorman, L. (1971). A developmental study of size constancy for two versus three-dimensional stimuli. *Child Development, 42,* 633–635.

Kuder, G., & Richardson, M. (1927). The theory of the estimation of test reliability. *Psychometrika, 3,* 151–160.

Kuhlman, F. (1922). *A Handbook of infant assessment.* Baltimore: Warwick & York, Inc.

Kulman, H., et al. (1975). The tools of vocational evaluation (Report of Task Force No. 2, Vocational Evaluation Project). *Vocational Evaluation and Work Adjustment Bulletin, 8,* 49–64.

Laffey, J. L., & Kelley, D. (1979). Test review—Woodcock Reading Mastery Tests. *The Reading Teacher, 33,* 335–339.

Lambert, N. M. (1964). Present status of the culture fair testing movement. *Psychology in the Schools, 1,* 318–330.

Lambert, N. M., Hartsough, C. S., & Bower, E. M. (1979). A process for the assessment of effective student functioning. Monterey, CA: Publishers Test Service.

Lambert, N., & Windmiller, M. (1981). *AAMD adaptive behavior scale, school edition.* Monterey, CA: Publishers Test Service.

Landurand, P. (1983). *A critical look at testing and evaluation from a cross cultural perspective.* Unpublished manuscript. Amherst: University of Massachusetts.

Langsam, R. S. (1941). A factorial analysis of reading ability. *Journal of Experimental Education, 10,* 57–63.

Laosa, L. (1976). *Historical antecedents and current issues in nondiscriminatory assessments of children's abilities.* In *Non-biased assessment of minority group children.* Lexington, Ky.: Coordinating Office for Regional Resource Centers.

Laosa, L. (1977). Nonbiased assessment of children's abilities: Historical antecedents and current issues. In T. Oakland (Ed.), *Psychological and Educational Assessment of Minority Children.* New York: Brunner/Mazel.

Laosa, L. M. (1975). Bilingualism in three United States Hispanic groups: Contextual use of language by children and adults in their families. *Journal of Educational Psychology, 67,* 617–627.

*Larry P. v. Riles.* 343 F. Suppl. 1306 (1972).

*Larry P. v. Riles.* C-71-2270 RFP, Opinion, October 10, 1979.

*Larry P. v. Riles,* 495 F. Supp. 96 (N.D. Cal. 1979). Aff'r (9th Cir. 1984), 1983–84 EHLR DEC. 555:304.

Larsen, S. C. (1977). The educational evaluation of handicapped students. In R. D. Kneedler & S. G. Tarver (Eds.), *Changing Perspectives in Special Education.* Columbus, Ohio: Merrill.

Larsen, S. C. & Hammill, D. D. (1974). The relationship of selected visual perceptual abilities to school learning. *The Journal of Special Education, 9,* 281–291.

Larsen, S., Rogers, D., & Sowell, V. (1976). The use of selected perceptual tests in differentiating between normal and learning disabled children. *Journal of Learning Disabilities, 9,* 85–90.

Lee, L. L. (1977). Developmental sentence types: A method for comparing normal and deviant syntactic development. *Journal of Speech and Hearing Disorders, 42,* 323–27.

Lee, L. L. (1974). *Developmental sentence analysis.* Evanston, IL: Northwestern University Press.

Leisman, G. & Ashkenazi, M. (1980). Aetiological factors in dyslexia: IV. Cerebral hemispheres are functionally equivalent. *Neuroscience, 11,* 13–28.

Leiter, R. G. (1929). *The Leiter International Performance Scale.* Chicago: Stoelting Co.

Leiter, R. G. (1949). Part II of the manual for the 1948 Revision of the Leiter International Performance Scale. *The Psychological Service Center Journal, 1,* 136–138.

Lemay, D., Griffin, P., & Sanford, A. (1981). *Learning accomplishment profile: Diagnostic edition (Revised).* Winston-Salem, NC: Kaplan School Supply.

LeMay, M. (1976). Morphological cerebral asymmetries of modern man, fossil man, and nonhuman primate. *Annals of the New York Academy of Sciences, 280,* 349–366.

Lenneberg, E. (1975). The concept of language differentiation. In E. Lenneberg & E. Lenneberg (Eds.), *Foundations of language development.* New York: Academic Press.

Lenneberg, E., Nichols, I., & Rosenberger, E. (1966). Primitive stages of language development in mongolism. *Disorders of Communication, 42,* 119–137.

Lentz, F. E., & Shapiro, E. S. (1986). Functional assessment of the academic environment, *School Psychology Review, 15,* 346–355.

Leonard, L., & Reid, L. (1979). Children's judgments of utterance appropriateness. *Journal of Speech and Hearing Research, 22,* 500–517.

Leonard, L. & Weiss, A. (1983). Application of non-standardized assessment procedures to diversive linguistic populations. *Topics in Language Disorders, 3,*(3), 35–45.

Levine, M. (1963). Mediating processes in humans at the outset of discrimination learning. *Psychological Review.*

Levine, M. (1974). The development of hypothesis testing. In T. R. Liebert, R. Poulus & C. Strauss (Eds.), *Development at psychology,* Englewood Cliffs, N.J.: Prentice-Hall.

Levinson, P. J., & Kunze, L. H. (1973). Verbal analogies in the ITPA. *Psychology in the Schools, 10,* 354–359.

Lewis, M., & Brooks, G. J. (1980). *Social cognition and the acquisition of self.* New York: Plenum.

Lezak, M. D. (1976). *Neuropsychological assessment.* New York: Oxford University Press.

Lichtenstein, R. (1980). *Minneapolis preschool screening instrument.* Minneapolis, MN: Minneapolis Public Schools.

Lichtenstein, R. & Ireton, H. (1984). *Preschool screening.* Orlando, FL: Grune & Stratton, Inc.

Lieberman, R. G., Moore, S. P., & Hutchinson, E. C. (1984). *What's the difference between language impaired and learning disabled children?* Paper presented at the American Speech, Language, Hearing Association, San Francisco.

Ligon, G. (1985). Review of curriculum referenced tests of mastery. In J.V. Mitchell, Jr. (Ed.), *The ninth mental measurements yearbook* (Vols. 1–2) (pp. 427–428). Lincoln, NE: Buros Institute of Mental Measurements of the University of Nebraska, Lincoln.

Lilly, T. J., & Shotel, J. R. (1987). Legal issues and the handicapped infant: From policy to reality. *Journal of the Division for Early Childhood, 12,* 4–12.

Limber, J. (1973). The genesis of complex sentences. In T. Moore (Ed.), *Cognitive development and the acquisition of language.* New York: Academic Press.

Linder, T. (1985). Developmental indicators for the assessment of learning—revised. In D. Keyser & R. Sweetland (Eds.), *Test critiques* (Vol. IV.). Kansas City, MO: Test Corporation of America.

Lindsley, O. (1964). Direct measurement and prosthesis of retarded behavior. *Journal of Education, 147,* 62–81.

Lindsley, O. (1971). Precision teaching perspective: An interview with Ogden R. Lindsley. *Teaching Exceptional Children, 3,* 111–119.

Linn, R. L. (1983). Testing and instruction: Links and distinctions. *Journal of Educational Measurement, 20,* 179–189.

Lipsitt, L. P. (1970). Pattern perception and information seeking in early infancy. In F. A. Young & D. B. Lindsley (Eds.), *Early experience and visual information processing in perceptual and reading disorders.* Washington, D.C.: National Academy of Sciences.

Locke, J., & Kutz, K. (1975). Memory for speech and speech for meaning. *Journal of Speech and Hearing Research, 18,* 176–191.

Lord, F. (1969). A theoretical study of two-stage testing. *Educational Testing Service Research Bulletin, 69–*95.

Lord, F. M. (1977). A study of item bias using item characteristic curve theory. In N. H. Poortinga (Ed.), *Basic problems in cross-cultural psychology.* Amsterdam: Swits and Vitlinger.

Lorton, J. W., & Walley, B. (1979). *Introduction to early childhood education.* New York: D. Van Nostrand Company.

Lovitt, T. (1967). Assessment of children with learning disabilities. *Exceptional Children, 34,* 233–242.

Lovitt, T. (1973). Self-management projects with children with behavioral disabilities. *Journal of Learning Disabilities, 6,* 138–147.

Lovitt, T. (1974). Applied behavior analysis and learning disabilities: Curriculum research recommendation. In S. G. Brainard (Ed.), *Learning disabilities: Issues and recommendations for research.* Washington, D.C.: U.S. Department of Health, Education and Welfare.

Lovitt, T. (1975). Applied behavior analysis and learning disabilities: Part I. *Journal of Learning Disabilities, 8,* 432–443.

Lovitt, T. (1977). *In spite of my resistance I've learned from children.* Columbus, Ohio: Merrill.

Lovitt, T., & Hansen, C. (1976). Round one—Placing the child in the right reader. *Journal of Learning Disabilities, 9,* 347–353.

Lucas, E. V. (1980). *Semantic and pragmatic language disorders: Assessment and remediation.* Rockville, MD: Aspen Publications.

Lund, N. J., & Duchan, J. F. (1983). *Assessing children's language in naturalistic contexts.* Englewood Cliffs, N.J.: Prentice-Hall, Inc.

Luria, A. (1961). *The role of speech in the regulation of normal and abnormal behavior.* New York: Liveright.

Luria, A. R. (1963). *Restoration of function after brain injury.* New York: Macmillan.

Luria, A. R. (1966a). *Higher cortical functions in man.* New York: Basic Books.

Luria, A. R. (1966b). *Human brain and psychological processes.* New York: Harper & Row.

Luria, A. R. (1973). *The working brain: An introduction to neuropsychology.* New York: Basic Books.

Luria, A. (1975). Basic problems of language in light of psychology and neurolinguistics. In E. H. Lenneberg & E. Lenneberg (Eds.), *Foundations of Language Development* (Vol. 2). New York: Academic Press.

Luria, A. R. (1980). *Higher cortical functions in man (2nd Ed.).* New York: Basic Books.

Luria, A. R., & Tzetkova, L. S. (1968). The re-education of brain-damaged patients and its psychopedagogical application. In J. Hellmuth (Ed.), *Learning disorders* (pp. 139–154). Seattle: Special Child Publications.

Lutey, C. (1977). *Individual intelligence testing.* Greeley, CO: Lutey Publishing.

Lyon, G. R. (1974). *The relationship of auditory discrimination and reading achievement at first and fourth grade levels.* Unpublished master's thesis, University of New Mexico, Albuquerque, N.M.

Lyon, G. R. (1983). Subgroups of learning disabled readers: Clinical and empirical identification. In H. R. Mykelbust (Ed.), *Progress in learning disabilities* (Vol. 5, pp. 103–134). New York: Grune and Stratton.

Lyon, G. R. (1985a). Educational validation of learning disability subtypes. In B. P. Rourke (Ed.), *Neuropsychology of learning disabilities: Essentials of subtype analysis* (pp. 228–256). New York: Guilford Press.

Lyon, G. R. (1985b). Identification and remediation of learning disability subtypes: Preliminary findings. *Learning Disabilities Focus, 1,* 21–35.

Lyon, G. R. (1987). Learning disabilities research: False starts and broken promises. In S. Vaughn & C. Bos (Eds.), *Research in learning disabilities: Issues and future directions* (pp. 69–85). San Diego: College-Hill Press.

Lyon, G. R., & Moats, L. C. (in press). Critical issues in the instruction of the learning disabled. *Journal of Consulting and Clinical Psychology.*

Lyon, G. R., Moats, L. E., & Elynn, J. M. (in press). From assessment to treatment: Linkage to interventions with children. In M. Tramontana & S. Hooper (Eds.). *Issues in child neuropsychology: From assessment to treatment.* New York: Plenum Press.

Lyon, G. R., Rietta, S., Watson, B., & Rhodes, J. (1981). Selected linguistic and perceptual abilities of empirically derived subgroups of learning disabled readers. *Journal of School Psychology, 19,* 152–166.

Lyon, G. R., & Risucci, D. (in press). Classification issues in learning disabilities. In K. A. Kavale (Ed.), *Learning disabilities: State of the art and practice.* San Diego: College-Hill Press.

Lyon, G. R., Stewart, N., & Freedman, D. (1982). Neuropsychological characteristics of empirically derived subgroups of learning disabled readers. *Journal of Clinical Neuropsychology, 4,* 343–365.

Lyon, G. R., & Toomey, F. (1985). Neurological, neuropsychological, and cognitive-developmental approaches to learning disabilities. *Topics in Learning Disabilities, 2,* 1–15.

Lyon, G. R., & Watson, B. (1981). Empirically derived subgroups of learning disabled readers: Diagnostic characteristics. *Journal of Learning Disabilities, 14,* 256–261.

Lyon, R. (1977). Auditory-perceptual training: The state of the art. *Journal of Learning Disabilities, 10,* 564–572.

Lyon, R. (1978). The neuropsychological characteristics of subgroups of learning disabled readers. Unpublished doctoral dissertation, The University of New Mexico, Albuquerque, N.M.

MacDonald, J. D. (1978). *The Environmental Language Inventory.* San Antonio, TX: The Psychological Corporation.

Mackey, S. (1965). Bilingual interference: Its analysis and measurement. *Journal of Communication, 15,* 239–249.

MacWhinney, B. (1978). The acquisition of Morphophonology. *Monograph of the Society for Research in Child Development* (Serial No. 174), *43,* 1–2.

Magliacca, L. et al. (1977). Early identification of handicapped children through a frequency sampling technique. *Exceptional Children, 7,* 414–420.

Mager, R. (1972). *Preparing instructional objectives.* Palo Alto, CA: Reardon Publishers.

Mahakian, C. (1939). Measuring the intelligence and reading capacity of Spanish-speaking children. *Elementary School Journal, 39,* 760–768.

Mahoney, G., & Powell, A. (1986). *Transactional intervention program.* Farmington, CT: University of Connecticut School of Medicine.

Mahoney, G., & Powell, A. (1988). Modifying parent-child interaction: Enhancing the development of handicapped children. *Journal of Special Education* (In press for 1988).

Mahoney, G., & Seeley, P. (1986). A comparison of conversational patterns between mothers and their Down's Syndrome and normal infants. *Journal of the Division for Early Childhood, 10,* 172–180.

Maier, A. (1980). The effect of focusing on the cognitive processes of learning disabled children. *Journal of Learning Disabilities, 13,* 34–38.

Maier, H. W. (1965). *Three theories of child development.* New York: Harper & Row.

Malgady, R. S., Barcher, P. R., Davis, J., & Towner, G. (1980). Validity of the Vocational Adaptation Rating Scale: Prediction of mentally retarded workers' placement in sheltered workshops. *American Journal of Mental Deficiency, 84,* 633–640.

Mandler, G. (1980). Organization and repetition. In L. Nilsson (Ed.), *Perspective on memory research.* Hillsdale, N.J.: Erlbaum Associates.

Mann, L. (1971). Psychometric phrenology and the new faculty psychology: The case against ability assessment and training. *Journal of Special Education, 5,* 3–14.

Mann, L. (1979). *On the trail of process.* New York: Grune & Stratton.

Mann, L., & Sabatino, D. A. (1985). *Foundations of cognitive process in remedial and special education.* Rockville, MD: Aspen.

Manuel, H. T. (1935). *Spanish and English editions of the Stanford-Binet in relation to the abilities of Mexican children.* Austin, TX: University of Texas Bulletin, No. 3532.

Mardell-Czudnowski, C., & Goldenberg, D. (1983). *Developmental Indicators for the Assessment for Learning-Revised: Manual.* Edison, N.J.: Childcraft.

Marge, M. (1972). The general problem of language disabilities in children. In J. Irwin & M. Marge

(Eds.), *Principles of childhood language disabilities.* Englewood Cliffs, N.J.: Prentice-Hall.

Marquart, D. I., & Bailey, L. L. (1955). An evaluation of the culture free test of intelligence. *Journal of Genetic Psychology, 86,* 353–358.

*Marshall, et al. v. Georgia.* U.S. District Court for the Southern District of Georgia, CV482-233, June 28, 1984.

Mash, E., & Terdal, L. (1976). *Behavior therapy assessment.* New York: Springer, Verlag.

Masling, J. M. (1959). The effects of warm and cold interaction on the administration and scoring of an intelligence test. *Journal of Consulting Psychology, 23,* 336–341.

Masling, J. M. (1960). The influence of situational and interpersonal variables in projective testing. *Psychological Bulletin, 57,* 65–85.

Masling, J. M. (1965). Differential indoctrination of examiners and Rorschach responses. *Journal of Consulting Psychology, 29,* 198–201.

Maslow, P., Frostig, M., Lefever, W., & Whittlesey, J. R. B., (1964). The Marianne Frostig developmental test of visual perception, 1963 standardization. *Perceptual and Motor Skills, 19,* 463–499.

Materials Development Center. (1974). *MDC Behavior identification format.* Menomonie, WI: Materials Development Center, University of Wisconsin-Stout.

Mathews, J. (1987). A mother challenges California ban on IQ tests for blacks. *Washington Post National Weekly Edition,* p. 34.

Matluck, J. H., & Mace, B. J. (1973). Language characteristics of Mexican-American children: Implications for assessment. *Journal of School Psychology, 11,* 365–386.

Matson, J., Esveldt-Dawson, L., & Kazdin, A. E. (1983). Validation of methods of assessing social skills in children. *Journal of Clinical Child Psychology, 12,* 174–180.

Matthews, J., & Birch, J. W. (1949). The Leiter international performance scale: A suggested instrument for psychological testing of speech and hearing clinic cases. *Journal of Speech and Hearing Disorders, 14,* 318–321.

Mattis, S. (1979). Dyslexia syndromes: A working hypothesis that works. In A. L. Benton & D. Pearl, (Eds.), *Dyslexia.* New York: Oxford University Press.

Mattis, S., French, J. H., & Rapin, S. (1975). Dyslexia in children and young adults: Three independent

neuropsychological syndromes. *Developmental Medicine and Child Neurology, 17,* 150–163.

May, A. E., Urquhart, A., & Watts, R. E. (1970). Memory for Designs Test: A follow-up study. *Perceptual and Motor Skills, 30,* 753–754.

McCall, R. B. (1979). The development of intellectual functioning in infancy and the prediction of low IQ. In J. Osofsky (Ed.), *Handbook of infant development* (pp. 707–741). New York: J. Wiley & Sons.

McCall, R. B. (1987). Developmental function, individual differences, and the plasticity of intelligence. In James J. Gallagher and Craig T. Ramey (Eds.), (pp. 25–35). *The malleability of children.* Baltimore: Paul H. Brookes.

McCallum, R., Karnes, F., & Edwards, R. (1984). The test of choice for assessment of gifted children: A comparison of the K-ABC, WISC-R, and Stanford-Binet. *Journal of Psychoeducational Assessment, 2,* 57–63.

McCarthy, J., & Paraskevopoulos, J. (1969). Behavior patterns of learning disabled, emotionally disturbed, and average children. *Exceptional Children, 36,* 69–74.

McClean, J. E., & Synder-McClean, L. K. (1978). *A transactional approach to early language learning.* Columbus, OH: Merrill.

McClean, M., McCormick, K., Bruder, M. B., & Burdig, N. B. (1987). An investigation of the validity and reliability of the Battelle Developmental Inventory with a population of children younger than 30 months with identified handicapping conditions. *Journal of the Division for Early Childhood, 11,* 238–246.

McDaniel, E. L. (1973). *Inferred self-concept scale.* Los Angeles: Western Psychological Services.

McKenna, B. (1977). What's wrong with standardized testing? *Today's Education, 66,* 34–38.

McLoughlin, J. A., & Lewis, R. B. (1981). *Assessing special students.* Columbus, Ohio: Merrill.

McLoughlin, J. A. & Lewis, R. B. (1986). *Assessing special students* (2nd. ed.). Columbus, OH: Merrill.

McNeill, D. (1966). Developmental psycholinguistics. In F. Smith & G. Miller (Eds.), *The genesis of language.* Cambridge, Mass.: MIT Press.

McNeill, D. (1970). *The acquisition of language: The study of developmental psycholinguistics.* New York: Harper & Row.

McNemar, Q. (1964). Lost our intelligence? Why? *American Psychologist, 19,* 871–883.

McReynolds, P. (1971). *Advances in psychological assessment* (Vol. II). Palo Alto, CA: Science and Behavior Books.

Meeker, M., & Meeker, R. (1973). Strategies for assessing intellectual patterns in Black, Anglo, and Mexican-American boys or any other children, and implications for education. *Journal of School Psychology, 11*, 341–350.

Mehrens, W. A. and Phillips, S. E. (1986). Detecting impacts of curricular differences in achievement test data. *Journal of Educational Measurement, 23*, 185–196.

Meichenbaum, D. (1976). Cognitive-functional approach to cognitive factors as determinants of learning disabilities. In R. T. Knight & D. Baker (Eds.), *The Neuropsychology of learning disorders*. Baltimore: University Park Press.

Meichenbaum, D. (1977). *Cognitive-behavior modification: An integrative approach.* New York: Plenum.

Meisels, S., & Wiske, S. (1983). *Early Screening Inventory.* Hagerstown, MD: Teachers College Press.

Meisels, S., Wiske, M. S., & Tivnan, T. (1984). Predicting school performance with the Early Screening Inventory. *Psychology in the Schools, 21*, 25–33.

Meisels, S. J. (1985a). *Developmental screening in early childhood: A guide,* revised edition. Washington, DC: NAEYC.

Meisels, S. J. (1985b, January). Uses and abuses of developmental screening and school readiness testing. *Young Children, 12*, 4–9.

Meisels, S. J. (1987, January). Uses and abuses of developmental screening and school readiness testing. *Young Children, 14*, 68–73.

Meisels-Brion, S., & Selman, R. L. (1984). Early adolescent development of new interpersonal strategies: A review of methods and issues. *School Psychology Review, 13*, 278–292.

Meister, R. K. (1976). Diagnostic assessment in rehabilitation. In M. B. Bolton (Ed.), *Handbook of Measurement and Evaluation in Rehabilitation.* Baltimore: University Park Press.

Mellman, J. (1972). *Determining test length.* Los Angeles: International Objectives Exchange.

Memory, D., Powell, G., & Callaway, B. (1980). A study of the assessment characteristics of Woodcock Reading Mastery Tests. *Reading Improvement, 17*, 48–52.

Menyuk, P. (1971). *The acquisition and development of language.* Englewood Cliffs, N.J.: Prentice-Hall.

Menyuk P., & Looney, P. (1972). Relationship among components of the grammar in language disorders. *Journal of Speech and Hearing Research, 15*, 395–406.

Mercer, C. D. (1979). *Children and adolescents with learning disabilities.* Columbus, OH: Merrill.

Mercer, J. R. (1972). IQ: The lethal label. *Psychology Today, 6*, 44–47, 95–97.

Mercer, J. R. (1973). *Labeling the mentally retarded.* Berkeley: University of California Press.

Mercer, J. R. (1974). A policy statement on assessment procedures and the rights of children. *Harvard Educational Review, 44*, 125–141.

Mercer, J. R. (1979). *SOMPA: System of Multicultural Pluralistic Assessment. Technical Manual.* New York: Psychological Corporation.

Mercer, J. R., & Brown, W. C. (1973). Racial differences in IQ: Fact or artifact? In C. Senna (Ed.), *The Fallacy of IQ.* New York: Third Press.

Mercer, J. R., & Lewis, J. (1978). *SOMPA: System of Multicultural Pluralistic Assessment.* New York: Psychological Corporation.

Mercer, J., & Ysseldyke, J. (1976). *Designing diagnostic intervention programs in coordinating office for regional development: Non-biased assessment of minority group children with bias toward none.* Lexington: University of Kentucky Press.

Merz, W. R. (1976, April). *Estimating bias in test items utilizing principle component analysis and general linear solution.* Paper presented at the annual meeting of the American Educational Research Association, San Francisco.

Merz, W. R. (1978). Test fairness and test bias: A review of procedures. In M. Wargo & D. R. Green (Eds.), *Achievement testing of disadvantaged and minority students for educational program evaluation.* New York: McGraw-Hill.

Messick, S. (1980). Test validity and the ethics of assessment. *American Psychologist, 35*, 1012–1027.

Messick, S. (1984). The psychology of educational measurement. *Journal of Educational Measurement, 21*, 215–237.

Messick, S., & Anderson, S. (1970). Educational testing, individual development and social responsibility. *The Counseling Psychologist, 2*, 80–88.

Meyen, E. L., & White, W. J. (1980). Career Education and P.L. 94-142: Some views. In G. Clark & W. White (Eds.), *Career education and the hand-*

*icapped: Current perspectives for teachers.* Boothwyn, CA: Educational Resources Center.

Meyer, L. A., Gersten, R. M., & Gutkin, J. (1984). Direct instruction: A project follow through success story in an inner-city school. *The Elementary School Journal, 84,* 241-252.

Meyers, C. A. E., Sundstrom, P., & Yoshida, R. (1974). The school psychologist and assessment in special education. *School Psychology Monograph, 2.*

Meyers, C., MacMillan, D., & Yoshida, R. (1978). Validity of psychologists' identification of EMR students in the perspective of the California decertification experience. *Journal of School Psychology, 16,* 3–15.

Michaelson, L., & Wood., R. R. (1980). A group assertive training program for elementary school children. *Child Behavior Therapy, 2,* 2–10.

Milgram, N. A. (1974). Danger: Chauvinism, scapegoatism, and euphemism. In G. J. Williams & S. Gordon (Eds.), *Clinical child psychology: Current practices and future perspectives.* New York: Behavioral Publications.

Miller, G. (1956). The magic number seven, plus or minus two. *Psychological Review, 63,* 81–97.

Miller, J. (1981). *Assessing language production in children: Experimental procedures.* Baltimore, MD: University Park Press.

Miller, J. F., Chapman, R. S., Branston, M. B., & Reichle, J. (1980). Language comprehension in sensorimotor stages V and VI. *Journal of Speech and Hearing Research, 23,* 284–311.

Miller, J. & Yoder, D. (1972). A syntax teaching program. In J. McLean, D. Yoder, & J. R. Schiefelbusch (Eds.), *Language intervention with the retarded.* Baltimore: University Park Press.

Miller, L. J., & Sprong, T. A. (1986). Psychometric and qualitative comparison of four preschool screening instruments. *Journal of Learning Disabilities, 19,* 480–484.

Milliam, J. (1974). Criterion-referenced measurement. In W. J. Popham (Ed.), *Evaluation in education: Current applications.* Berkeley, CA: McCutchan.

Mischel, W. (1968). *Personality and assessment.* New York: John Wiley & Sons.

Mitchell, A. J. (1937). The effect of bilingualism on the measurement of intelligence. *Elementary School Journal, 38,* 29–37.

Mitchell, J. V., Jr. (Ed.). (1985). *The ninth mental measurements yearbook* (Vols. 1–2). Lincoln, NE: Buros Institute of Mental Measurement of the University of Nebraska-Lincoln.

Mitchell, V., & Nelson, R. (1978). Personality. In M. Rosenzweig & L. Porter (Eds.), *Annual Review of Psychology.* Palo Alto, CA: Annual Review.

Molino, H. (1939). *The Leiter International Performance Scale as a contribution to educational anthropology.* Master's thesis. University of Southern California, Los Angeles.

Mooney, R. L. & Gordon, L. V. (1950). *Mooney Problem Check Lists.* New York: Psychological Corporation.

Moore, O. (1965). Autotelic responsive environment and the deaf. *American Annual for the Deaf, 110,* 604–614.

Moore, O., & Anderson, A. (1975). Some principles for the design of clarifying educational environments. In C. Greenblat & R. Duke (Eds.), *Game simulation: Rationale, design, and applications.* New York: John Wiley & Sons.

Moore, T. (1973). *Cognitive development and the acquisition of language.* New York: Academic Press.

Morehead, D., & Ingram, D. (1976). The development of base syntax in normal and linguistically deviant children. In D. Morehead & A. Morehead (Eds.), *Normal and deficient child language.* Baltimore: University Park Press.

Morency, A., & Wepman, J. W. (1973). Early perceptual ability and later school achievement. *The Elementary School Journal, 73,* 323–327.

Mowder, B. (1980). A strategy for the assessment of bilingual handicapped children. *Psychology in the Schools, 17,* 36–41.

Moweder, B. A. (1979). Assessing the bilingual handicapped student. *Psychology in the Schools, 16,* 43–50.

Mowrer, H. (1980). *Psychology of language and learning.* New York: Plenum.

Moyer, S., & Newcomer, P. (1977). Reversals in reading: Diagnosis and remediation. *Exceptional Children, 7,* 424–430.

Mueller, J. (1948). The specific energies in nerves. In W. Dennis (Ed.), *Readings in the history of psychology.* Englewood Cliffs, N.J.: Prentice-Hall.

Mulliken, R. K., & Buckley, J. J. (1983). Assessment of multihandicapped and developmentally disabled children. Rockville, MD: Aspen.

Muma, J. & Pierce, S. (1981). Language intervention: Data or evidence. *Topics in Learning and Learning Disabilities, 1* (2), 1–12.

Muma, J., Pierce, S., & Muma, D. (1983, June). Language training in speech-language pathology: Substantive domains. *Journal of the American Speech-Language-Hearing Association,* pp. 35–40.

Murray, A. & Bracken, B. A. (1984). Eleven-month predictive validity of the Kaufman Assessment Battery for Children. *Journal of Psychoeducational Assessment, 2,* 225–232.

Murray, H. (1943). *Thematic apperception test.* Cambridge, MA: Harvard University Press.

Musgrove, W. J., & Counts, L. (1975). Leiter and Raven Performance and Teacher Ranking: A correlation study with deaf children. *Journal of Rehabilitation of the Deaf, 8,* 19–22.

Musselwhite, C. R., & St. Louis, K. W. (1982). *Communication programming for the severely handicapped: Vocal and non-vocal strategies.* San Diego, CA.: College-Hill Press.

Myklebust, H. (Ed.) (1968). *Progress in learning disabilities,* vol. I. New York: Grune & Stratton.

Myklebust, H. R. (1954). *Auditory disorders in children: A manual for differential diagnosis.* New York: Grune & Stratton.

Nadolsky, J. (1973). *Vocational evaluation of the culturally disadvantaged: A comparative investigation of the JEVS system and a model-based system, final report.* Auburn, AL: Auburn University, School of Education, Department of Vocational and Adult Education.

Nadolsky, J. (1985). Achieving unity in special education and rehabilitation. *Journal of Rehabilitation, 51,* 22–23.

Nadolsky, J. M. (1971). *Development of a model for vocational evaluation of disadvantaged.* Auburn, AL: Auburn University.

Naglieri, J. A. (1985). Normal children's performance on the McCarthy scales, Kaufman Assessment Battery, and Peabody Individual Achievement Test. *Journal of Psychoeducational Assessment, 3,* 123–129.

Naglieri, J., & Anderson, D. (1985). Comparison of the WISC-R and K-ABC with gifted students. *Journal of Psychoeducational Assessment, 3,* 175–179.

Naglieri, J. A., & Haddad, F. A. (1984). Learning disabled children's performance on the Kaufman Assessment Battery for Children: A concurrent

validity study. *Journal of Psychoeducational Assessment, 2,* 49–56.

Naour, P. J. (1982). *Developmental components in cognitive processing: An EEG and eye movement study of learning disabled and normal boys in the third and sixth grade.* Unpublished doctoral dissertation, Ohio State University, Columbus, Ohio.

Naslund, R. A., Thorpe, L. P., Lefever, D. N. (1978). *SRA Achievement Series.* Chicago: Science Research Association.

National Association of State Directors of Special Education. (1976). *Functions of the placement committee in special education: A resource manual.* Washington, D.C.: Author.

Neff, W. S. (1968). *Work and human behavior.* New York: Alberton Press.

Neisser, U. (1967). *Cognitive psychology.* New York: Appleton-Century-Crofts.

Neisser, U. (1979). The concept of intelligence. *Intelligence,* 217–227.

Neisworth, J. T., & Bagnato, S. J. (1986). Curriculum-based developmental assessment: Congruence of testing and teaching. *School Psychology Review, 15,* 180–199.

Nelson, N. (1986). Individual processing in classroom settings. *Topics in Language Disorders, 6,*(2), 13–27.

Nelson, D., Walling, J., & Evoy, C. (1979). Doubts about depth. *Journal of Experimental Psychology: Human Learning and Memory, 4,* 24–44.

Nelson, R., & Hayes, S. (1979). The nature of behavioral assessment: A commentary. *Journal of Applied Behavior Analysis, 12,* 49–50.

Nelson, R., & Mitchell, V. (1976). Personality. In M. R. Rosenzweis & L. W. Porter (Eds.), *Annual Review of Psychology.* Palo Alto, CA: Annual Review.

Nelson, R. O., & Hayes, S. C. (1981). An overview of behavioral assessment. In M. Hersen and A. Bellack (Eds.), *Behavioral assessment, A practical handbook* (2nd edition). New York: Pergamon.

Nesbit, M. Y. (1966). The CHILD program: Computer Help in Learning Diagnosis of arithmetic scores. *Curriculum Bulletin 7-E-B,* Miami, FL: Dade County Board of Public Instruction.

Neville, D. (1970). *The development of an instrument to predict modality preference for learning to read.* Unpublished manuscript, Institute of Mental Retardation and Intellectual Development (IM-

RID), George Peabody College for Teachers, Nashville.

Newborg, J., Stock, J., Wnek, L., Guidubaldi, J., & Suinicki, J. (1984). *Battelle developmental inventory.* Allen, TX: DLM Teaching Resources.

Newcomer, P. (1977). Special education services for the mildly handicapped: Beyond a diagnostic and remedial model. *Journal of Special Education, 11,* 153–165.

Newcomer, P., & Hammill, D. (1973). Visual perception of motor-impaired children: Implications for assessment. *Exceptional Children, 39,* 335–336.

Newcomer, P., & Hammill, D. (1976). *Psycholinguistic training in the classroom.* Columbus, OH: Merrill.

Newell, A., Shaw, F., & Simon, H. (1958). Elements of a theory of human problem solving. *Psychological Review, 65,* 151–166.

Newell, A., & Simon, H. (1972). *Human problem solving.* Englewood Cliffs, N.J.: Prentice-Hall.

Newland, T. E. (1963). Psychological assessment of exceptional children and youth. In W. Cruickshank (Ed.), *Psychology of exceptional children and youth.* Englewood Cliffs, N.J.: Prentice-Hall.

Newland, T. E. (1973). Assumptions underlying psychological testing. *Journal of School Psychology, 11,* 316–322.

Newman, P. A., Creaghead, N. A., & Secord, W. (1985). *Assessment and remediation of articulatory and phonological disorders.* Columbus, OH: Merrill.

Newman, R. & Hagen, J. (1981). Memory strategies in children with learning disabilities. *Journal of Applied Developmental Psychology, 1,* 297–312.

Nevo, D. (1983). The conceptualization of educational evaluation: An analytical review, *Review of Educational Research, 53,* 117–128.

*New Mexico Association for Retarded Citizens et al. v. The State of New Mexico* #75633-M-Civil. The United States District Court for District of New Mexico, 1956.

Nihira, K., Foster, R., Shellhaas, M., & Leland, H. (1974). *AAMD Adaptive Behavior Scale.* Washington, D.C.: American Association on Mental Deficiency.

Nitko, A. J. (1974). Problems in the development of criterion-referenced tests: The IPI Pittsburgh experience. In C. W. Harris, M. C. Alkin, & W. J. Popham (Eds.), *Problems in criterion-referenced measurement,* CSE Monograph Series. Los Angeles:

Center for the Study of Evaluation, University of California.

Nitko, A. J. (1980). Distinguishing the many varieties of criterion-referenced tests. *Review of Educational Research, 50,* 461–485. © 1980, American Educational Research Association, Washington, D.C.

Noland, D. R., Hammeke, T. A., & Barkley, R. A. (1983). A comparison of the neuropsychological performance in two groups of learning disabled children. *Journal of Clinical Child Psychology, 12,* 13–21.

Norman, R. D. & Midkiff, J. L. (1955). Navaho children on Raven Progressive Matrices and Goodenough Draw-A-Man Tests. *Southwestern Journal of Anthropology, 11,* 129–136.

Noton, D., & Stark, L. (1971). Eye movements and visual perception. *Scientific American, 224,* 34–43.

Novick, M., & Lewis, C. (1967). Coefficient alpha and the reliability of component measurement. *Psychometricka, 32,* 1–13.

Novick, M. R., & Lewis, C. (1974). Prescribing test length for criterion-referenced measurement. In C. W. Harris, M. C. Alkin, & W. J. Popham (Eds.), *Problems in criterion-referenced measurement,* CSE Monograph Series in Evaluation No. 3. Center for the Study of Evaluation, University of California, Los Angeles.

Nowicki, S., & Strickland, B. (1973). A locus of control scale for children. *Journal of Consulting and Clinical Psychology, 40,* 148–154.

Nuttall, E. V. (1979). Test reviews: System of multipluralistic assessment. *Journal of Educational Measurement, 16*(4) 285–289.

Nuttall, E. (1987). Survey of current practices in the psychological assessment of limited English-proficiency handicapped children. *Journal of School Psychology, 25,* 53–61.

Oakland, T. (1978). *Psychological and educational assessment of minority children.* New York: Brunner/Mazel.

Oakland, T. (1979). Research on the Adaptive Behavior Inventory for Children and the estimated learning potential. *School Psychology Digest, 8,* 63–70.

Oakland, T. (1983). Joint use of adaptive behavior and IQ to predict achievement. *Journal of Consulting and Clinical Psychology, 51,* 293–301.

Oakland, T., & Laosa, L. (1977). Professional, legislative, and judicial influences on psychoeducational assessment practices in schools. In T. Oakland (Ed.), *Psychological and educational assessment of minority children.* New York: Brunner/Mazel.

Oakland, T., & Matuszek, P. (1977). Using tests in nondiscriminatory assessment. In T. Oakland (Ed.), *Psychological and educational assessment of minority children.* New York: Brunner/Mazel.

Obrzut, J. E., & Hynd, G. W. (1986). *Child neuropsychology,* Vol. 2. Orlando, FL: Academic Press.

Office of Civil Rights. Elimination of discrimination in the assignment of children to special education classes for the mentally retarded. Memorandum, 11/28/72.

Ogbu, J. (1987). Cultural influences on plasticity in human development. In J. J. Gallagher & C. T. Ramey (Eds.), *The malleability of children* (pp. 155–170). Baltimore, MD: Paul H. Brookes.

O'Leary, K., & O'Leary, S. (1977). *Classroom management: The successful use of behavior modification* (2nd ed.). New York: Pergamon.

Ollendick, T. H., & Hersen, M. (1984a). An overview of child behavioral assessment. In T. H. Ollendick and M. Hersen (Eds.), *Child behavioral assessment: Principles and procedures.* Elmsford, NY: Pergamon.

Ollendick, T. H., & Hersen, M. (1984b) *Child behavior assessment.* New York: Pergamon Press.

Olson, A. (1966). Relation of achievement test scores and specific reading abilities to the Frostig Developmental Test of Visual Perception. *Perceptual and Motor Skills, 22,* 179–184.

Olson, A. V. (1968). Factor analytic studies of the Frostig Developmental Test of Visual Perception. *Journal of Special Education, 2,* 429–433.

Omer, J. L. (1976). *Evaluating the audiogram.* Danville, IL: Institute Printers & Publishers.

Orgel, A., & Dreger, R. (1955). A comparative study of the Arthur-Leiter and Stanford-Binet Intelligence Scales. *Journal of Genetic Psychology, 86,* 359–365.

Orme, J. E. (1966). Hypothetically true norms for the Progressive Matrices Tests. *Human Development, 9,* 222–230.

Ortiz, A. A. (1986). Characteristics of limited English proficient Hispanic students served in programs for the learning disabled. *Bilingual Special Education Newsletter, 4,* University of Texas at Austin.

Ortiz, C. A., & Ball, G. (1972). *The Enchilada Test.* Institute for Personal Effectiveness in Children.

Oslerger, M., et al. (1978). The evaluation of a model speech training program for deaf children. *Journal of Communication Disorders, 11,* 292–313.

Otis, A. S., & Lennon, R. T. (1976a). *Manual for administration of the Otis-Lennon Mental Ability Test, Primary II level, Form J.* New York: Harcourt Brace Jovanovich.

Otis, A. S., & Lennon, R. T. (1967b). *Manual for administration for the Otis-Lennon Mental Ability Test, Elementary II, Intermediate, and Advanced Levels, Forms J & K.* New York: Harcourt Brace Jovanovich.

Paget, K. D. & Nagle, R. J. (1986). A conceptual model of preschool assessment. *School Psychology Review, 15,* 154–165.

Paivio, A. (1971). *Imagery and verbal processes.* New York: Holt, Rinehart & Winston.

Palincsar, A. S., & Brown, A. L. (1984). Reciprocal teaching of comprehensions fostering and monitoring activities. *Cognition and Instruction, 1:* 177–185.

Palmer, J. O. (1970). *The psychological assessment of children.* New York: John Wiley & Sons.

Panagos, J. (1978). Abstract phonology, grammatical reduction, and delayed speech development. *Acta Symbolica, 79,* 2–12.

Panagos, J., Quine, M., & Lkick, R. (1979). Syntactic and phonological influence on children's articulation. *Journal of Speech and Hearing Research, 22,* 841–848.

Parker, L., & Harrison, J. (1974). *Critique of the Goodenough-Harris Drawing Test as related to standards for educational and psychological tests.* Unpublished manuscript, University of South Carolina—Columbia.

Parker, R. M., & Hansen, C. E. (1976). Aptitude and achievement test. In B. Bolton (Ed.), *Handbook of measurement and evaluation in rehabilitation.* Baltimore: University Park Press.

Parmelee, A. H. & Michaels, R. (1971). Neurological examination of the newborn. In J. Hellmuth (Ed.), *Exceptional Infant, Vol 2: Studies in Abnormalities* (page 290). New York: Brunner/Mazel.

Parten, M. (1932). Social play among preschool children. *Journal of Abnormal and Social Psychology, 27,* 243–269.

Pasamanick, B. (1951). The intelligence of American children of Mexican parentage: A discussion of uncontrolled variables. *Journal of Abnormal and Social Psychology, 46,* 598–602.

Pascal, G., & Suttell, B. (1964). *The Bender-Gestalt Test: Qualification and validity for adults.* New York: Grune and Stratton.

Paschal, F. C., & Sullivan, L. R. (1925). Racial differences in the mental and psychological development of Mexican children. *Comparative Psychology Monographs, 3,*(2).

Pascual-Leone, J. (1973). *Cognitive development and cognitive style.* Lexington, Mass.: Heath.

*PASE v. Hannon,* 506 F. Supp. 831 (N.D. Ill. 1980).

Peck, D. F. (1970). The conversion of progressive matrices and Mill Hill Vocabulary Raw scores into deviation IQs. *Journal of Clinical Psychology, 26,* 67–70.

Pecyna, P. M., & Sommers, R. K. (1985). Testing the receptive language skills of severely handicapped preschool children. *Language, Speech, and Hearing Services in Schools, 16,* 41–52.

Perez, F. M. (1980). Performance of bilingual children on the Spanish version of the ITPA. *Exceptional Children, 46,* 536–541.

Perkins, W. M. (1978). *Human perspectives in speech and language disorders.* St. Louis: The C. V. Mosby Co.

Peterson, D. R. (1968). *The clinical study of social behavior.* New York: Appleton-Century-Crofts.

Peterson, M. (1985). Trends in vocational assessment in schools: A national survey. *Vocational Evaluation and Work Adjustment Bulletin, 18,* 114–119.

Peterson, N. L. (1987). *Early intervention for handicapped and at-risk children: An introduction to early childhood special education.* Denver, CO: Love Publishing Co.

Phelan, B. M. (1940). Visual perception in relation to variance in reading and spelling. *Catholic University of America Educational Monographs, 12,* No. 3.

Piaget, J. (1926). *The language and thought of the child.* New York: Harcourt Brace Jovanovich.

Piaget, J. (1928). *Judgement and reasoning in the child.* New York: Harcourt Brace Jovanovich.

Piaget, J. (1952). *The origins of intelligence.* New York: International University Press.

Piaget, J. (1967). *Six psychological studies.* New York: Random House.

Piaget, J. (1970). Piaget's theory. In P. Mussed (Ed.), *Carmichael's manual of child psychology* (3rd ed.). New York: John Wiley & Sons.

Piaget, J. (1971). *Biology and knowledge.* Chicago: University of Chicago Press.

Piaget, J., & Inhelder, B. (1969). *The psychology of the child.* New York: Basic Books.

Plaisted, J. R., Gustavson, J. L., Wilkening, G. N., & Golden, C. J. (1983). The Luria-Nebraska Neuropsychological Battery-Children's Revision: Theory and current research findings. *Journal of Clinical Child Psychology, 12,* 13–21.

Plata, M. (1986). *Assessment, placement and programming of bilingual exceptional pupils: A practical approach.* Reston, VA: The Council for Exceptional Children.

Plue, W. V. (1984). Employment patterns of the mildly retarded. *The Journal for Vocational Special Needs Education, 7,* 23–28.

Polloway, E. A. & Smith, J. D. (1983). Changes in mild retardation: Population, programs, and perspectives. *Exceptional Children, 50,* 149–159.

Poor, C., et al. (1975). Vocational assessment potential. *Archives of Physical Medicine and Rehabilitation, 56,* 33–36.

Popham, W. J. (1974). An approaching peril: Cloud-referenced tests. *Phi Delta Kappan, 56,* 614–615.

Popham, W. J. (1978). *Criterion-referenced measurement.* Englewood Cliffs, N.J.: Prentice-Hall.

Popham, W. J., & Husek, T. R. (1969). Implications of criterion-referenced measurements. *Journal of Educational Measurement, 6,* 1–9.

Popham, W. J., & Sirotnik, K. A. (1973). *Educational statistics—use and interpretation.* New York: Harper & Row.

Porteus, S. (1937). *Primitive intelligence and environment.* New York: Macmillan Publishing Co.

Powers, D. A., & Pace, T. J. (1976). A concurrent validity study of the Key Math Diagnostic Arithmetic Test. *Mental Retardation, 4,* 48.

Powers, M. D. (1984). Behavioral assessment and the planning and evaluation of interventions for developmentally disabled children. *School Psychology Review, 14,* 155–161.

Prasse, D., & Reschly, D. (1986). Larry P.: A case of segregation, testing, or program efficacy? *Exceptional Children, 52,* 333–346.

Prasse, D. P., Siewert, J. C., & Breen, M. J. (1983). An analysis of performance in reading subtests from the 1978 Wide Range Achievement Test and Woodcock Reading Mastery Test with the WISC-R for learning disabled and regular education students. *Journal of Learning Disability, 16,* 458–460.

Prather, P. A., & Bacon, J. (1986). Developmental differences in part/whole identification. *Child Development, 57,* 549–558.

Premack, D., & Premack, A. (1974). Teaching visual language to apes and language-deficient persons. In R. Schiefelbusch & L. Lloyd (Eds.), *Language perspectives, acquisition, retardations and intervention.* Baltimore: University Park Press.

Prescott, G. A., Balow, I. H., Hogan, Q. P., & Farr, R. A. (1985). *Metropolitan achievement test: Sixth edition (MAT 6)—survey battery.* San Antonio, TX: Psychological Corporation.

Price, P. A. (1984). A comparative study of the California Achievement Test (Forms C and D) and the Key Math Diagnostic Arithmetic Test with secondary LH students. *Psychology in the Schools, 17,* 392–396.

Prichard, C., Tekieli, M., & Kozup, J. (1979). Developmental apraxia: Diagnostic considerations. *Journal of Communication Disorders, 12,* 337–348.

Pronovost, W. (1974). *The Boston University Speech Sound Discrimination Test.* Cedar Falls, IA: Go-Mo Products.

Prutting, C., & Lowell, E. (1979). Pragmatic and semantic development in young children with impaired hearing. *Journal of Speech and Hearing Research, 22,* 534–552.

Quattlebaum, L. F. (1968). A brief note on the relationship of two psychomotor tests. *Journal of Clinical Psychology, 24,* 198–199.

Quay, A. (1975). Classification in the treatment of delinquency and antisocial behavior. In N. Hobbs (Ed.), *Issues in the classification of children* (Vol. 1). San Francisco: Jossey-Bass.

Quay, H., & Peterson, D. (1967). *Manual for the behavior problem checklist* (mimeographed). Urbana: University of Illinois Press.

Quay, H. C. (1973). Special education: Assumptions, techniques, and evaluation criteria. *Exceptional Children, 40,* 165–170.

Quay, L. (1971). Language, dialect, reinforcement and the intelligence test performance of Negro children. *Child Development, 42,* 5–15.

Rabinovitch, R. (1959). Reading and learning disabilities. In S. Arieti (Ed.), *American handbook of psychiatry* (Vol. 1). New York: Basic Books.

Ramey, C., & Campbell, F. A. (1987). The Carolina Abecedarian Project: An educational experiment concerning human malleability. In James J. Gallagher and Craig T. Ramey (Eds.), *The Malleability of Children* (pp. 85–96). Baltimore: Paul H. Brookes.

Rao, S. M., & Bieliauskas, L. A. (1983). Cognitive rehabilitation two and one-half years post right temporal lobectomy. *Journal of Clinical Neuropsychology, 5,* 313–320.

Rasch, G. (1960). *Probabilistic models for some intelligence and attainment tests.* Copenhagen: Danish Institute for Educational Research.

Rasch, G. (1966). An individualistic approach to item analysis. In P. Z. Laqarfeld and N. W. Henry. (Eds.). *Readings in mathematical social sciences* (pp. 87–107). Chicago: Science Research Associates.

Raschke, D., & Young, A. (1976). The dialectic teaching system: A comprehensive model derived from two educational approaches. *Education and Training of the Mentally Retarded, 11,* 323–346.

Ratcliffe, K. J., & Ratcliffe, M. W. (1979). The Leiter Scales: A review of validity findings. *American Annuals of the Deaf, 124.*

Ratusnik, D., Klee, T. & Ratusnik, C. (1980). Northwestern syntax screening test: A short form. *Journal of Speech and Hearing Disorders, 45,* 200–208.

Raven, J. C. (1963). *Raven progressive matrices.* Los Angeles: Western Psychological Services.

Raven, J. C., Court, J. H., & Raven, J. (1977). *Coloured progressive matrices.* London: Lewis.

Raven, J. C., Court, J. H., & Raven, J. (1986). *Manual for Raven's Progressive Matrices and Vocabulary Scales,* Section 2-Coloured Progressive Matrices (1986 edition with U.S. norms). London: Lewis.

Raven, J. C., & Summers, B. (1986). *Manual for Raven's Progressive Matrices and Vocabulary Scales-research supplement no. 3.* London: Lewis.

Reed, H. B. C., Reitan, R. M., & Klove, H. (1965). Influence of cerebral lesions in psychological test performance of older children. *Journal of Consulting Psychology, 29,* 247–251.

Reitan, R. M. (1966). A research program on the psychological effects of brain lesions in human beings. In R. M. Ellis (Ed.), *International review of research in mental retardation* (pp. 153–218). New York: Academic Press.

Reitan, R. M. (1969). *Manual for administration of neuropsychological test batteries for adults and children*. Indianapolis, IN: Author.

Reitan, R. M. (1979). *Neuropsychology and rehabilitation*. Tucson: Author.

Reitan, R. M. (1980). *REHABIT—Reitan evaluation of hemispheric abilities and brain improvement training*. Tucson: Reitan Neuropsychological Laboratory and University of Arizona.

Reitan, R. M., & Boll, T. J. (1973). Neuropsychological correlates of minimal brain dysfunction. *Annals of the New York Academy of Sciences, 205,* 65–88.

Reitan, R. M., & Davison, L. A. (1974). *Clinical neuropsychology: Current status and applications*. Washington, D.C.: V. H. Winston and Sons.

Reitan, R. M., & Wolfson, D. (1985). *The Halstead-Reitan neuropsychological test battery: Theory and clinical interpretation*. Tucson: Neuropsychology Press.

Rentz, R. R. (1982, March). *Using the Rasch Model to develop a curriculum-referenced norm*. Paper presented at the meeting of the National Council on Measurement in Education. New York.

Reschly, D. (1978). *Comparisons of bias in assessment with conventional and pluralistic measures*. Paper presented at the annual convention of the Council for Exceptional Children, Kansas City, Mo.

Reschly, D. J. (1981). Evaluation of the effects of SOMPA measures on classification of students as mildly mentally retarded. *American Journal of Mental Deficiency, 86,* 16–20.

Resnick, L. (1973). Hierarchies in children's learning: A symposium. *Instructional Science, 2,* 311–349.

Resnick, L. B., Wang, M. C., & Kaplan, J. (1973). Task analysis in curriculum design: A hierarchically sequenced introductory mathematics curriculum. *Journal of Applied Behavior Analysis, 6,* 679–710.

Reynolds, C. R. (1979). Factor structure of the Peabody Individual Achievement Test at five grade levels between grades one and 12. *Journal of School Psychology, 17,* 270–274.

Reynolds, C. R. (1984). Perspectives on bias in mental testing. In C. R. Reynolds & R. T. Brown (Eds.), *Perspectives on individual differences.* New York: Plenum Press.

Reynolds, C. R., & Brown, R. T. (1984). *Perspectives on bias in mental testing.* New York: Plenum Press.

Reynolds, C. R., & Gutkin, T. B. (1980). Statistics related to profile interpretation of the Peabody Individual Achievement Test. *Psychology in the Schools, 17,* 316–319.

Reynolds, C. R., Gutkin, T. B., Elliott, S. N., & Witt, J. C. (1984). *School psychology: Essential of theory and practice.* NY: John Wiley & Sons.

Reynolds, H., & Jennifer, R. (1987). *The joint task force of teacher education.* Quincy, MA.: Massachusetts Department of Education.

Reynolds, M. (1975). Trends in special education: Implications for measurement. In W. Hively and M. Reynolds (Eds.), *Domain-referenced testing in special education.* Minneapolis: Leadership Training Institute/Special Education, University of Minnesota.

Reynolds, W. M. (1987). *Auditory discrimination test* (2nd ed.). Los Angeles: Western Psychological Services.

Rhodes, W. (1970). A community participation analysis of emotional disturbance. *Exceptional Children, 36,* 309–314.

Rice, J. A. (1978). Developmental Test of Visual-Motor Interpretation. In O. K. Buros (Ed.), *The eighth annual mental measurements yearbook.* Highland Park, N.J.: Gryphon Press.

Rice, W. (1975). Effects of discipline techniques on children's personality trait inferences. *Journal of Educational Psychology, 67,* 570–575.

Richberg, E., Parke, R., & Hetherington, E. (1971). Modification of impulsive and reflective cognitive style through observation of film mediated models. *Developmental Psychology, 5,* 369–377.

Richmond, B. O., & Aliotti, N. C. (1977). Developmental skills of advantaged and disadvantaged children in perceptual tasks. *Psychology in the Schools, 14,* 461–466.

Richmond, B. O., & Kicklighter, R. H. (1980). *Children's adaptive behavior scale.* Atlanta, GA: Humanics Limited.

Rindler, S. (1980). The effects of skipping over more difficult items on time-limited tests: Implications for test validity. *Educational and Psychological Measurement, 40,* 989–998.

Roberts, C. L. (July, 1969). Definitions, objectives and goals in work evaluation. In W. A. Pruitt & R. N. Pacinelli (Eds.), *Work evaluation in rehabilitation.* Education guide developed from an institute held in Denver, Colorado, Washington, D.C.: The Association of Rehabilitation Centers.

Rochester, S., & Martin, J. (1980). Crazy talk: A study of the discourse of a schizophrenic speaker. New York: Plenum.

Rodney Scheels v. Albuquerque Public Schools. United States District Court, New Mexico, C-79 488 M, 1979.

Roessler, R. & Bolton, B. (1985). The work personality profile: An experimental rating instrument for assessing job maintenance skills. Vocational Evaluation and Work Adjustment Bulletin, 18, 8–11.

Rogers, S. J. et al. (1981). Early intervention developmental profile, vol. 2. In D. S. Schafer & M. S. Moersch, (Eds.), Developmental programming for infants and young children. Ann Arbor: The University of Michigan Press.

Rohrer, J. H. (1942). The test intelligence of Osage Indians. Journal of Social Psychology, 16, 99–105.

Roid, G. H., & Haladyna, T. M. (1982). A technology of test-item writing. New York: Academic Press.

Rose, S. A., & Wallace, I. F. (1985). Visual recognition memory: A predictor of later cognitive functioning. Child Development, 56, 843–852.

Rosen, C. L. (1966). An experimental study of visual perceptual training and reading achievement in first grade. Perceptual and Motor Skills, 22, 978–986.

Rosenberger, P. B., & Hier, D. B. (1980). Cerebral asymmetry and verbal intellectual deficits. Annals of Neurology, 8, 300–304.

Rosenhan, D. (1973). On being sane in a sane place. Science, 180, 365–369.

Rosenhan, D. (1975). The contextual nature of psychiatric diagnosis. Journal of Abnormal Child Psychology, 84, 462–474.

Rosenthal, R. (1966). Experimenter effects in behavior research. New York: Appleton-Century-Crofts.

Ross, S. L., DeYoung, H. G., & Cohen, J. S. (1971). Confrontations: Special education placement and the law. Exceptional Children, 38, 5–12.

Rourke, B. P. (1975). Brain-behavior relationships in children with learning disabilities: A research program. American Psychologist, 30, 911–920.

Rourke, B. P. (1981). Neuropsychological assessment of children with learning disabilities. In S. B. Filskov & T. J. Boll (Eds.), Handbook of clinical neuropsychology (pp. 453–478). New York: John Wiley & Sons.

Rourke, B P., Bakker, D., Fisk, J. L., & Strang, J. D. (1983). Child neuropsychology: An introduction to theory, research, and clinical practice. New York: Guilford Press.

Rourke, B. P., Fisk, J. L., & Strang, J. D. (1986). The neuropsychological assessment of children: A treatment-oriented approach. New York: The Guilford Press.

Rovee, C. K., & Rovee, D. T. (1969). Conjugate reinforcement of infant exploratory behavior. Journal of Experimental Child Psychology, 8, 33–39.

Ruble, D., & Boggiano, A. (1980). Optimizing motivation in an achievement context. In B. Keogh (Ed.), Advances in special education (Vol. 1). Basic Constructs. Greenwich, Conn.: JAI Press.

Rudner, L. M. (1977). An evaluation of selected approaches for biased item identification. Unpublished doctoral dissertation, Catholic University of America, Washington, D.C.

Ruff, H. A. (1980). The development of perception and recognition of objects. Child Development, 51, 981–992.

Rumberger, R. W. (1984). How much "tech" do high-tech workers need. VOCED, 59, 32–34.

Rumelhart, D. (1976). Toward an interactive model of reading. Technical Report SG. Center for Human Information Processing, University of California—San Diego.

Sailor, W., & Horner, D. (1976). Educational assessment strategies for the severely handicapped. In N. Haring & L. Brown (Eds.), Teaching the severely handicapped (Vol. 1). New York: Grune & Stratton.

Salvia, J., & Hritcko, T. (1984). The K-ABC and ability training. The Journal of Special Education, 18, 345–356.

Salvia, J. & Ysseldyke, J. E. (1985). Assessment in special and remedial education. Boston: Houghton Mifflin.

Sampson, J. P. (1983). Computer-assisted testing and assessment: Current status and implication for the future. Management and Evaluation in Guidance, 15, 293–298.

Samuda, R. S. (1975). Psychological testing of American minorities: Issues and consequences. New York: Dodd, Mead.

Sanchez, G. I. (1932a). Group differences in Spanish-speaking children: A critical review. Journal of Applied Psychology, 16, 549–558.

Sanchez, G. I. (1932b). Scores of Spanish-speaking children on repeated tests. Journal of Genetic Psychology, 40, 223–231.

Sanchez, G. I. (1934a). Bilingualism and mental measures. *Journal of Applied Psychology, 18,* 765–772.

Sanchez, G. I. (1934b). The implications of a basal vocabulary to the measurement of the abilities of bilingual children. *Journal of Social Psychology, 5,* 395–402.

Sanders, J. (1978). School professionals and the evaluation function. *Journal of School Psychology, 16,* 301–311.

Sanford, A. (1981). *Learning accomplishment profile for infants (Early LAP).* Winston-Salem, N.C.: Kaplan School Supply.

Sanger, D., Keith, R., & Maher, B. (1987). An assessment technique for children with auditory-language processing problems. *Journal of Communication Disorders, 13,* 265–280.

Santa Cruz County Office of Education. (1987). *Help for special preschoolers assessment checklist: Ages 3–6.* Palo Alto, CA.: VORT Corporation.

Santiago, J. (1988). *Legal education and advocacy project (LEAP).* Amherst: University of Massachusetts, Everywoman's Center.

Sattler, J. (1965). Analysis of functions of the 1960 Stanford-Binet Intelligence Scale, form L-M. *Journal of Clinical Psychology, 21,* 173–179.

Sattler, J. (1973a). Examiner's scoring style, accuracy, ability and personality scores. *Journal of Clinical Psychology, 29,* 38–39.

Sattler, J. (1973b). Intelligence testing of ethnic minority group and culturally disadvantaged children. In L. Mann & D. Sabatino (Eds.), *The first review of special education* (Vol. 2). Philadelphia: JSE Press.

Sattler, J. (1973c). Racial experimenter effects. In K. S. Miller & R. M. Dreger (Eds.), *Comparative studies of Blacks and Whites in the United States.* New York: Seminar Press.

Sattler, J. (1974). *Assessment of children's intelligence.* Philadelphia: Saunders.

Sattler, J. (1988). *Assessment of children* (3rd ed.) San Diego: J. M. Sattler.

Sax, G. (1974). *Principles of educational measurement and evaluation.* Belmont, CA: Wadsworth.

Scarr, S. (1979). From evolution to Larry P. or what shall we do about IQ tests. *Intelligence, 2,* 325–342.

Scarr, S., & Carter-Saltzman, L. (1982). Genetics and intelligence. In R. J. Sternberg (Ed.), *Handbook of human intelligence.* New York: Cambridge University Press.

Schaefer, D. S., & Moersch, M. S. (Eds.) (1977). *Developmental programming for infants and young children* (Vol 1–3). Ann Arbor: University of Michigan Press.

Schaie, K. W., & Roberts, J. (1970). *School achievement of children 6–11 years as measured by the Reading and Arithmetic subtests of the Wide Range Achievement Test* (National Center for Health Statistics, Series II, No. 103). Washington, D.C.: U.S. Government Printing Office.

Schery, T. (1981). Selecting assessment strategies for language-disordered children. *Topics in Language Disorders, 1*(3), 59–74.

Schetz, K. (1985). Comparison of the Compton speech and language screening evaluation with the Fluharty preschool speech and language screening test. *Journal of the American Speech-Language-Hearing Association, 16,* 16–24.

Scheuneman, J. (1979). A method of assessing bias in test items. *Journal of Educational Measurement, 16,* 143–152.

Schiefelbusch, R., Ruder, K., & Bricker, W. (1976). Training strategies for language-deficient children: An overview. In N. Haring and R. Schiefelbusch (Eds.), *Teaching special children.* New York: McGraw-Hill Book Co.

Schmeiser, C. G., & Ferguson, R. L. (1978). Performance of Black and White students on test materials containing content based on Black and White cultures. *Journal of Educational Measurement, 15,* 102.

Schmidt, F. L., & Hunter, J. E. (1974). Racial and ethnic bias in psychological tests: Divergent implications of two definitions of test bias. *American Psychologist, 29,* 1–8.

Schneider, M. A., & Spivack, G. (1979). An investigative study of the Bender-Gestalt: Clinical validation of its use with a reading disabled population. *Journal of Clinical Psychology, 2,* 346–351.

Scholastic Testing Service. (1971). *STS youth inventory.* Bensenville, IL: Scholastic Testing Services.

School, G., & Schnur, R. (1975). Measures of psychological, vocational and educational functioning in the blind and visually handicapped. *New Outlook for the Blind, 69,* 365–370.

Schur, E. (1976). Labeling deviant behavior: Its sociological implications. New York: Harper & Row.

Schwartz, A., & Daly, D. (1978). Elicited limitation in language assessment. *Journal of Communication Disorders, 11,* 25–35.

Schwartz, B. J., Allen, R. M., & Cortazzo, A. D. (1974). Factors in the adaptive behavior checklists revisited and revised. *The Training School Bulletin, 70,* 248–254.

Schwartz, P. O. (1963). Adapting tests to the cultural setting. *Educational and Psychological Measurement, 23,* 673–686.

Sciberg, L. D., & Kwiatowski, J. (1980). *Natural process analysis: A procedure for phonological analysis of continuous speech samples.* New York: John Wiley & Sons.

Scott, M. (1980). Ecological theory and methods for research in special education. *Journal of Special Education, 14,* 279–294.

Scriver, M. (1973). The methodology of evaluation. In B. R. Worther & J. R. Sanders (Eds.), *Educational evaluation: Theory and practice.* Worthington, OH: Charles A. Jones.

Scull, J. W., & Branch, L. H. (1980). The WRAT and the PIAT with learning disabled children. *Journal of Learning Disabilities, 13,* 64–66.

Sechrest, L., Fay, T. L., & Zaida, S. M. (1972). Problems of translations in cross-cultural research. *Journal of Cross-Cultural Psychology, 3,* 41–56.

Seidenberg, M., Giordani, B., Berent, S., & Boll, T. J. (1983). IQ level and performance on the Halstead-Reitan Neuropsychological Test Battery for Older Children. *Journal of Consulting and Clinical Psychology, 51,* 406–413.

Selye, H. (1982). History and present status of the stress concept. In L. Goldberg & S. Breznitz (Eds.), *Handbook of stress: Theoretical and clinical aspects.* New York: The Free Press.

Selz, M. J., & Reitan, R. M. (1979). Rules for neuropsychological diagnosis: Classification of brain function in older children. *Journal of Consulting and Clinical Psychology, 47,* 258–264.

*Serna v. Portales Municipal Schools,* 351 F. Supp. 1279 (D. N.M., 1973).

Sexton, L. C. (1977). Auditory and visual perception, sex, and academic aptitude as predictors of achievement for first grade children. *Dissertation Abstracts International, 37,* 6162A. (University Microfilms No. 77-7316).

Shane, H. (1981). Decision making in early augmentative communication system use. In R. L. Schiefelbusch, & D. D. Bricker (Eds.), *Early language: Acquisition and intervention* (pp. 389–426). Baltimore, MD: University Park Press.

Shapiro, E. D. & Lentz, F. E. (1985). Assessing academic behavior: A behavioral approach. *School Psychology Review, 14,* 325–338.

Sharp, H. C. (1957). A note on the reliability of the L.I.P.S. 1948 revision. *Journal of Consulting Psychology, 22,* 320.

Shearer, D. E., Billingsley, J., Froman, A., Hilliard, J., Johnson, F., & Shearer, M. (1976). *Portage guide to early education-revised.* Portage, WI: Portage Project.

Sheldon, W. H. (1924). The intelligence of Mexican children. *School and Society, 19,* 129–142.

Shepard, L. A. (1985). Review of the Stanford Diagnostic Mathematics Test. In J. V. Mitchell, Jr. (Ed.), *The Ninth Mental Measurements Yearbook (Vol 1–2)* (pp. 1460–1462). Lincoln, NE: Buros Institute of Mental Measurement at the University of Nebraska.

Sherrer, C., & Sherrer, M. (1972). Professional or legal standards for academic psychologists and counselors. *Journal of Law-Education, 1,* 289–302.

Shriberg, L. D., & Kwiatowski, J. (1980). *Natural process analysis: A procedure for phonological analysis of continuous speech samples.* New York: John Wiley and Sons.

Shuachkin, N. (1973). Razuitye Fouematicheskoyo Vospriyatiya rechi v. vannem vozraste (1948). In T. Moore (Ed.), *Cognitive development and the acquisition of language.* New York: Academic Press.

Shuey, A. (1966). *The testing of Negro intelligence.* New York: Social Science Press.

Siebel, C. C., Faust, W. L., & Faust, M. S. (1971). Administration of design copying tests to large groups of children. *Perceptual and Motor Skills, 32,* 355–360.

Siewert, J. C., & Breen, M. J. (1983). The Revised Test of Visual-Motor Integration: Its relation to the Test of Visual-Motor Integration and the Bender Visual-Motor Gestalt Test for regular education students. *Psychology in the Schools, 20,* 304–306.

Sigman, M., & Parmelee, A. H. (1979). Longitudinal evaluation of the preterm infant. In T. M. Field, A. M. Sostek, S. Goldberg, & H. H. Shuman (Eds.), *Infants Born at Risk.* New York: Spectrum.

Silliphant, V. M. (1983). Kindergarten reasoning and achievement in grades K–3. *Psychology in the Schools, 20,* 289–294.

Silver, P. G. (1986). *Early childhood special needs training of bilingual teachers,* Unpublished document. Amherst: University of Massachusetts.

Silverstein, A. R. (1978). Note on the norms for the WRAT. *Psychology in the Schools, 14,* 152–153.

Silverstein, A. R. (1980). A comparison of the 1976 and 1978 norms for the WRAT. *Psychology in the Schools, 17,* 313–315.

Silversten, A. B. (1981). Pattern analysis on the PIAT. *Psychology in the Schools, 19,* 13–14.

Simensen, R. J., (1974). Correlations among Bender-Gestalt, WISC Block Design, Memory for Designs, and Pupil Rating Scale. *Perceptual and Motor Skills, 38,* 1249–1250.

Simon, C. (1986). *Communicative competence: A functional-pragmatic approach to language therapy.* Tucson, AZ: Communication Skill Builders, Inc.

Simon, H., & Lea, G. (1974). Problem solving and rule induction: A unified view. In L. Gregg (Ed.), *Knowledge and cognition.* Hillsdale, N.J.: Erlbaum Associates.

Sinclair, H. (1973). Language acquisition and cognitive development. In T. E. Moore (Ed.), *Cognitive development and the acquisition of language.* New York: Academic Press.

Singleton, W., Spurgeon, P., & Stammers, R. (Eds.). (1980). *The analysis of social skill.* New York: Plenum.

Sitlington, P. L. (1979). Vocational assessment and training of the handicapped. *Focus on Exceptional Children, 12,* 1–11.

Sitlington, P. L. (1980). The assessment process as a component of career education. In G. M. Clark & W. J. White (Eds.), *Career education for the handicapped: Current perspectives for teachers.* Boothwyn, PA: Educational Resources.

Sitlington, P. L., & Wimmer, D. (1978). Vocational assessment techniques for the handicapped adolescent. *Career Development for Exceptional Individuals, 1,* 74–87.

Skaggs, G., & Lissitz, R. (1986). IRT test equating: Relevant issues and a review of recent research. *Review of Educational Research, 56,* 495–529.

Skinner, B. F. (1957). *Verbal behavior.* New York: Appleton-Century-Crofts.

Slavin, R. E., Leavey, M. B., & Madden, N. (1984). Combining cooperative learning and individualized instruction: Effects on student mathematics achievement, attitudes, and behaviors. *Elementary School Journal, 84,* 409–422.

Slobin D. (1975). The more it changes ... an understanding of language by watching it move through time. *Papers and Reports on Child Language Development* (Stanford University), *10,* 1–30.

Slobin, D. (1979). *Psycholinguistics* (2nd ed.). Glenview, IL: Scott Foresman.

Slosson, R. (1971). *Slosson Intelligence Test.* East Aurora, N.Y.: Slosson Educational Publications.

Smead, V. S. (1977). Ability training and task analysis in diagnostic/perspective teaching. *The Journal of Special Education, 11,* 113–125.

Smith, C., & Knoff, H. (1981). School psychology and special education students' placement decisions: IQ still tips the scale. *Journal of Special Education, 15,* 55–64.

Smith, C. E., & Keogh, B. K. (1962). The group Bender Gestalt as a readiness screening instrument. *Perceptual and Motor Skills, 15,* 639–645.

Smith, D., & Snell, M. (1978). Classroom management and instructional planning. In M. Snell (Ed.), *Systematic instruction of the moderately and severely handicapped.* Columbus, OH: Merrill.

Smith, H. W., & May, W. T. (1967). Individual differences among inexperienced psychological examiners. *Psychological Reports, 20,* 759–762.

Smith, L. (1979). Perceptual development and category generalization. *Child Development, 50,* 705–715.

Smith, M. (1926). An investigation of the development of the sentence and the extent of vocabulary in young children. *University of Iowa Studies on Child Welfare, 3,* (5).

Smyth, N. (1979). Speech and reception in the presence of classroom noise. *Language Speech and Hearing Services in Schools, 10,* 221–230.

Snow, R. (1980). Intelligence for the year 2001. *Intelligence, 4,* 185–199.

Sokolov, E. N. (1963). *Perception and the conditioned reflex.* New York: Macmillan.

Spache, G. (1953). A new readability formula for primary grade materials. *Elementary School Journal, 1953, 53,* 410–413.

Spache, G. D. (1957). Personality patterns of retarded readers. *Journal of Educational Research, 50,* 461–469.

Spache, G. D. (1972). *Diagnostic Reading Scales, revised edition: Examiners manual.* Monterey, CA: CTB/McGraw-Hill.

Spache, G. D. (1981). *Diagnostic reading scales* (rev. ed.). Monterey, CA: CTB/McGraw-Hill.

Spache, G. D. (1982). *Diagnostic reading scales: Technical report.* Monterey, CA: CTB/McGraw-Hill.

*Spanger v. Pasadena Board of Education.* 311 F. Supp. 501 (1970).

Sparks, C. P., & Manese, W. R. (1970). Interview ratings with and without knowledge of pre-employment test scores. *The Experimental Publication System,* 1–10.

Sparrow, S. S., Balla, D. A., & Cicchetti, D. V. (1984a). *Vineland adaptive behavior scales, interview edition, survey form.* Circle Pines, MN: American Guidance Service.

Sparrow, S. S., Balla, D. A., & Cicchetti, D. V. (1984b). *Vineland adaptive behavior scales, interview edition, expanded form.* Circle Pines, MN: American Guidance Service.

Spear, L. C., & Sternberg, R. J. (1987). An information-processing framework for understanding learning disabilities. In S. Ceci (Ed.), *Handbook of cognitive, social, and neuropsychological aspects of learning disabilities* (Vol. 2, pp. 2–30). Hillsdale, N.J.: Erlbaum.

Spearman, C. (1927). *The abilities of man.* New York: Macmillan.

Sperling, G. (1967). Successive approximations to a model for short-term memory. *Acta Psychologica, 27,* 385–392.

Spivack, G., & Swift, H. (1973). The classroom behavior of children: A critical review of teacher-administered rating scales. *Journal of Special Education, 7,* 55–89.

Spivack, G., & Swift, M. (1977). The Hahnman high school behavior. *Journal of Abnormal Child Psychology, 5,* 299–307.

Sprafkin, R. (1980). The assessment of skills. *The School Psychology Review, 9,* 14–20.

Sroufe, L. A. (1979). The coherence of individual development. Early care, attachment, and subsequent developmental issues. *American Psychologist, 34,* 834–841.

Staats, A. (1971). Linguistic-mentalistic theory versus an explanatory S-R learning theory of language development. In D. I. Slabin (Ed.), *The ontogenesis of grammar: A theoretical symposium.* New York: Academic Press.

Staats, A. (1974). Behaviorism and cognitive theory in the study of language. In R. Schiefelbusch & L. Lloyd (Eds.), *Language perspectives, acquisition, retardation and intervention.* Baltimore: University Park Press.

Stafford, J. (1974). Reflections on the Diagnostic Reading Scales. *Reading Teacher, 14,* 5–8.

Stake, R. (1970). Comments on Professor Glaser's paper. In M. C. Withrock & D. E. Wiley (Eds.), *The evaluation of instruction.* New York: Holt, Rinehart, & Winston.

*The Standards for Educational and Psychological Testing* (1985). American Educational Research Association, American Psychological Association, & National Council on Measurement in Education. Washington, DC: American Psychological Association, Inc.

Stark, J. (1981). Reading: What needs to be assessed? *Topics in Language Disorders. 1*(3), 87–94.

Stephens, T. M. (1979). *Social behavior assessment.* Columbus, OH: Cedars Press.

Stephens, T. (1977). *Teaching skills to children with learning and behavior disorders.* Columbus, OH: Merrill.

Sternberg, R. (1977). *Intelligence, information processing, and analogical reasoning.* Hillsdale, N.J.: Erlbaum Associates.

Sternberg, R. (1978). Isolating components of intelligence. *Intelligence, 2,* 117–128.

Sternberg, R. (1979). The nature of mental abilities. *American Psychologist, 34,* 214–230.

Sternberg, R. J. (1981). Testing and cognitive psychology. *American Psychologist, 36,* 1181–1189.

Sternberg, R. J. (1984a). An information processing analysis and critique. *The Journal of Special Education, 18,* 269–279.

Sternberg, R. J. (1984b). Toward a triarchic theory of human intelligence. *Behavioral and Brain Sciences, 7,* 269–315.

Sternberg, R. J. (1985). *Beyond IQ: A triarchic theory of human intelligence.* New York: Cambridge University Press.

Sternberg, R. J. (1988). A unified theory of intellectual exceptionality. In J. G. Borkowski & J. Day (Eds.), *Cognition and intelligence in special children: Comparative approaches to retardation, learning disabilities, and giftedness* (pp. 135–174). Norwood, NJ: Ablex.

Sternberg, R. J., & Suben, J. (1986). The socialization of intelligence. In M. Perlmutter (Ed.), *Perspectives on intellectual development: Minnesota symposia on child psychology* (Vol. 19, pp. 201–235). Hillsdale, NJ: Erlbaum.

Stevenson, H. W., Parker, Wilkinson, Hegion, & Fish. (1976). Longitudinal study of individual differences in cognitive development and scholastic achievement. *Journal of Educational Psychology, 68,* 377–400.

Stevenson, H. W., & Newman, R. S. (1986). Long-term prediction of achievement and attitudes in mathematics and reading. *Child Development, 57,* 649–659.

Stevenson, M. B., & Lamb, M. E. (1979). Effects of infant sociability and the caretaking environment on infant cognitive development. *Child Development, 50,* 340–349.

*Stewart et al. v. Phillips et al.* Civil Action No. 70-1199F, October, 1970.

Stillman, R. (1982). *Callier-Azua scale.* Dallas, TX: Callier Center for Communication Disorders.

Stoddart, C., & Knights, R. M. (1986). Neuropsychological assessment of children: Alternative approaches. In J. E. Obrzut & G. W. Hynd (Eds.), *Child neuropsychology, Vol. II,* (pp. 229–244). Orlando, FL: Academic Press.

Stoneman, A., Brody, G., & Abbott, D. (1983). In-home observations of young Down's syndrome children with their mothers and fathers. *American Journal of Mental Deficiency, 87,* 591–600.

Strag, G. A., & Richmond, B. O. (1973). Auditory discrimination techniques for young children. *The Elementary School Journal, 73,* 447–454.

Strand, K. E. (1982). *The interconnections between metamemory and memory performance in normal and language-impaired children: A developmental study.* Unpublished doctoral dissertation, Boston University.

Stroud, J. B., Hieronymus, A. N., & McKee, P. (1968a). *Teacher's Manual, Primary Reading Profiles, Level I.* Boston: Houghton Mifflin.

Stroud, J. B., Hieronymus, A. N., & McKee, P. (1968b). *Teacher's Manual, Primary Reading Profiles, Level II.* Boston: Houghton Mifflin.

Sullivan, P. M., & Vernon, C. (1979). Psychological assessment of hearing impaired children. *School Psychology Digest, 8,* 271–290.

Sultzer-Azaroff, B., & Mayer, G. (1977). *Applying behavior-analysis procedures with children and youth.* New York: Holt, Rinehart, & Winston.

Sundberg, N. (1977). *Assessment of persons.* Englewood Cliffs, N.J.: Prentice-Hall.

Swanson, H. L. (1982). A multidirectional model for assessing learning disabled children's intelligence: An information processing framework, *Learning Disability Quarterly, 5,* 323–326.

Swanson, H. L. (1986). Verbal coding deficits in learning disabled readers. In S. Ceci (Ed.), *Hand-book of cognitive, social and neuropsychological aspects of learning disabilities* (pp. 203–228). Hillsdale, NJ: Lawrence Erlbaum Associates, Vol. 1.

Swanson, E. N., & Deblassie, R. R. (1979). Interpreter and Spanish administration effects on the WISC performance of Mexican-American children. *Journal of School Psychology, 17,* 231–236.

Swanson, H. L., Minifie, D., & Minifie, E. (1979). Conservation development in partially sighted children. *Psychology in the Schools, 16,* 309–313.

Swanson, H. L., & Reinert, H. R. (1979). *Teaching strategies for children in conflict.* St. Louis: Mosby.

Swap, S. (1973). An ecological study of disruptive encounters between pupils and teachers. *Proceedings of the 81st Annual Convention of the American Psychological Association, 8,* 521–522.

Swap, S. (1974). Disturbing classroom behaviors: A developmental and ecological view. *Exceptional Children, 41,* 163–172.

Swartz, J. P., & Walker, D. K. (1984). The relationship between teacher ratings of kindergarten classroom skills and second-grade achievement scores: An analysis of gender differences. *Journal of School Psychology, 22,* 209–217.

Switzky, H. (1985). Review of the Developmental Assessment for Severely Handicapped. In J. V. Mitchell (Ed.), *The 9th Mental Measurement Year Book (Vol 1)* (pp. 463–464). Lincoln, NE: The University of Nebraska Press.

Switzky, H. N., Rotatori, A. F., Miller, T., & Freagon, S. (1979). The developmental model and its implications for assessment and instruction for the severely/profoundly handicapped. *Mental Retardation, 17,* 167–170.

Synderman, M., & Rothman, S. (1987). Survey of expert opinion on intelligence and aptitude testing. *American Psychologist, 42,* 137–144.

Szaz, T. (1970). *Manufacture of madness.* New York: Harper & Row.

Tate, M. E. (1952). The influence of cultural factors on the Leiter International Performance Scale. *Journal of Abnormal and Social Psychology, 47,* 497–501.

Taylor, F., & Soloway, M. (1973). The Madison School Plan. In E. Deno (Ed.), *Instructional alternatives for exceptional children.* Reston, VA: Council for Exceptional Children.

Taylor, R. L., Kauffman, D., & Partenio, I. (1984). The Koppitz developmental scoring system for the

Bender-Gestalt: Is it developmental? *Psychology in the Schools, 21,* 425–428.

Tebeleff, M., & Oakland T. (1977). *Relationship between the ABIC, WISC-R and Achievement.* Paper presented at the annual meeting of the American Psychological Association, San Francisco.

Teeter, P. A. (1986). Standard neuropsychological test batteries for children. In J. E. Obrzut & G. W. Hynd (Eds.), *Child neuropsychology, Vol. 2* (pp. 187–227). Orlando, FL: Academic Press.

Telford, C. W. (1938). Comparative studies of full and mixed blood North Dakota Indians. *Psychological Monographs, 5,* 116–129.

Templin, M. (1957). *Certain language skills in children: Their development and interrelationships.* Institute of Child Welfare Monograph 26. Minneapolis: University of Minnesota Press.

Terman, L. (1921). Intelligence and its measurement. *Journal of Educational Psychology, 12,* 127–133.

Terman, L., & Merrill, M. (1960). *Stanford-Binet Intelligence Scale.* Boston: Houghton-Mifflin.

Terman, L. M. (1916). *The measurement of intelligence.* Boston: Houghton Mifflin.

Terrell, S., & Terrell, F. (1983). Distinguishing linguistic differences from disorders: The past, present and future of nonbiased assessment. *Topics in Language Disorders, 3*(3).

Thibaut, J., & Riecken, H. (1955). Some determinants and consequences of the perception of social causably. *Journal of Personality, 24,* 113–133.

Thorndike, E. (1927). *The measurement of intelligence.* New York: Teachers College Press.

Thorndike, E. L. (1910). Handwriting. *Teacher's College Record, 11,* 1–93.

Thorndike, E. L., & Lorge, I. (1944). *Teachers word book of 30,000 words.* New York: Columbia University Press.

Thorndike, R. L. (1971). Concepts of culture fairness. *Journal of Educational Measurement, 8,* 63–70.

Thorndike, R. L., & Hagen, E. (1969). *Measurement and evaluation in psychology and education* (3rd ed.). New York: John Wiley & Sons.

Thurman, S. (1977). Congruence of behavioral ecologies: A model for special education programming. *Journal of Special Education, 11,* 329–334.

Thurstone, L. L. (1938a). The perceptual factor. *Psychometrika, 3,* 1–17.

Thurstone, L. L. (1938b). Primary mental abilities. *Psychometric Monographs* (No. 1).

Thurstone, L. L. (1944). A factorial study of perception. *Psychometric Monographs* (No. 4).

Thurstone, L. L. (1949). Mechanical aptitude III: Analysis of group tests. *Psychometric Laboratory Report* (No. 55).

Tinney, F. A. (1975). A comparison of the Key Math Diagnostic Arithmetic Test and the California Arithmetic Test with learning disabled students. *Journal of Learning Disabilities, 8,* 57–59.

Tolar, A. (1978). Assessment myths and current fads: A rejoinder to a position paper on nonbiased assessment. *Psychology in the Schools, 15,* 205–209.

Tomlan, P. (1986). *The Psycholinguistic Analyses of Learning Disabled Adolescents' Written Language Abilities.* Unpublished doctoral dissertation, University of New Mexico, Albuquerque, N.M.

Torgeson, J. (1979). Factors related to poor performance on memory tasks in reading disabled children. *Learning Disabilities Quarterly, 2,* 17–23.

Torgeson, S., & Houck, G. (1980). Processing deficiencies of learning disabled children who perform poorly on the Digit Span Test. *Journal of Educational Psychology, 72,* 141–160.

Torrance, E. (1970). *Torrance Tests of Creative Thinking.* Princeton, N.J.: Personnel Press.

Tramontana, M. G., & Hooper, S. (in press). *Issues in child neuropsychology: From assessment to treatment.* New York: Plenum Press.

Tramontana, M. G., Klee, S. N., & Boyd, T. A. (1984). WISC-R interrelationships with the Halstead-Reitan and Children's Luria Neuropsychological Batteries. *Clinical Neuropsychology, 6,* 1–8.

Tronick, E., & Brazelton, T. B. (1975). Clinical uses of the Brazelton Neonatal Behavioral Assessment. In B. Z. Friedlander and L. Rosenblum (Eds.), *Exceptional Infant* (Vol III). New York: Brunner/Mazel.

Tucker, J. A., (1980). *Nineteen steps for assuring nonbiased placement of students in special education.* Reston, VA: ERIC Clearinghouse of Handicapped and Gifted Children.

Tucker, J. A. (1985). Curriculum-based assessment: An introduction. *Exceptional Children, 52,* 199–204.

Tulving, E. Episodic and semantic memory. (1972). In E. Tulving & W. Donaldson (Eds.), *Organization of memory.* New York: Academic Press.

Tulving, E. (1986). Précis of elements of episodic memory. *The Behavioral and Brain Sciences, 7,* 223–268.

Tuma, J., & Appelbaum. (1980). Reliability and practice effects of WISC-R IQ estimates in a normal population. *Educational & Psychological Measurements, 40,* 671–678.

Turaids, D., Wepman, J. M., & Morency, A. (1972). A perceptual test battery: Development and standardization. *Elementary School Journal, 72,* 351–361.

Ulman, J., & Sultzer-Azaroff, B. (1975). Multi-element baseline design in educational research. In E. Romp & G. Semb (Eds.), *Behavior analysis.* Englewood Cliffs, N.J.: Prentice-Hall, 1975.

U.S. Department of Health, Education and Welfare. (1971). *Public Health Service Vision Screening of Children.* PHS Document #2042. Washington, D.C.: Author.

U.S. Department of Labor. (1965). *Dictionary of occupational titles. Definition of titles (Vol. 1); Occupational classification* (Vol. 2) (3rd ed.). Washington, D.C.: U.S. Government Printing Office.

U.S. Department of Labor Manpower Administration. (1972). *Handbook for analyzing jobs.* Menomonie, WI: Materials Development Center.

Uzigiris, I. C., & Hunt, J. (1975). *Toward ordinal scales of psychological developmental in infancy.* Champaign, IL: University of Illinois.

Valencia, R., & Rankin, R. (1986). Factor analysis of the K-ABC for groups of Anglo and Mexican American children. *Journal of Educational Measurement, 23,* 209–219.

Valian, R., & Caplan, J. (1979). What children say when asked what? A study of the use of syntactic knowledge. *Journal of Experimental Child Psychology, 28,* 424–444.

Van der Linden, W. J. (1981). A latent trait look at pretest-posttest validation of criterion-referenced test items. *Review of Educational Research, 51,* 379–402.

Van der Linden, W. J. (1984). Some thoughts on the use of decision theory to set cutoff scores. Comment on de Gruijter and Hambleton. *Applied Psychological Measurement, 8,* 9–17.

Van Etten, C., & Van Etten, G. (1976). The measurement of pupil progress and selecting instructional materials. *Journal of Learning Disabilities, 9,* 469–480.

Van Kleeck, A. (1984). Metalinguistic skills: Cutting across spoken and written language and problem-solving abilities. In G. Wallach & K. Butler (Eds.), *Language learning disabilities in school-aged children* (pp. 128–153). Baltimore, MD: Williams & Wilkins.

Vellutino, F., et al. (1975). Reading disability: Age differences and the perceptual-deficit hypothesis. *Child Development, 46,* 487–493.

Vernon, P. (1960). *Intelligence and attainment tests.* New York: Philosophical Library.

Vocational Evaluation and Work Adjustment Association. (1975). The tools of vocational evaluation. *Vocational Evaluation and Work Adjustment Bulletin, 8,* 49–64.

Voeltz, L. M. (1983). Effects of structured interaction with severely handicapped peers on children's attitudes. *American Journal of Mental Deficiency, 86,* 380–390.

Vygotsky, L. (1962). *Thought and language.* Cambridge, MA: MIT Press.

Vygotsky, L. (1978). *Mind in society: The development of higher psychological process.* Cambridge, MA: Harvard University Press.

Vygotsky, L. (1979). *Mind in society.* M. Cole, V. John-Steiner, S. Scribner, & E. Souberman (Eds.). Cambridge, MA: Harvard University Press.

Wachs, T. D. (1975). Relation of infant's performance on Piaget scales between twelve and twenty-four months and their Stanford-Binet performance at thirty-one months. *Child Development, 46,* 929–935.

Wade, J., & Kass, C. (1987). Component deficit and academic remediation of learning disabilities, *Journal of Learning Disabilities, 20,* 441–447.

Wagner, R., & Sternberg, R. J. (1984). Alternative conceptions of intelligence and their implications for education. *Review of Educational Research, 72,* 32–38.

Wahler, R., House, A., & Stambough, E. (1976). *Ecological assessment of child problem behavior: A clinical package for home, school, and institutional settings.* New York: Pergamon.

Walden, J., Jr. (1979). A comparison of the PIAT and WRAT: A closer look. *Psychology in the Schools, 16,* 342–346.

Walker, D. (1985). Review of the developmental assessment for the severely handicapped. In J. V. Mitchell (Ed.), *The 9th mental measurement yearbook* (p. 464). Lincoln, NE: University of Nebraska Press.

Walker, H. (1969). Empirical assessment of deviant behavior in children. *Psychology in the Schools, 6,* 93–97.

Walker, L. (1980). Cognitive and perspective taking prerequisites for word development. *Child Development, 51,* 131–141.

Wallace, G., & Larsen, S. (1978). *Educational assessment of learning problems: Testing for teaching.* Boston: Allyn & Bacon.

Wallach, G., & Liebergott, J. (1984). Who shall be called 'learning disabled': Some new directions. In G. Wallach & K. Butler (Eds.), *Language-learning disabilities in school aged children.* (pp. 1–14). Baltimore: Williams & Wilkins.

Wallbrown, J. D., & Wallbrown, F. H. (1974). The relative importance of mental age and selected assessors of auditory and visual perception in the Metropolitan Readiness Test. *Psychology in the Schools, 11,* 135–143.

Walls, R., Werner, T., & Bacon, A. (1977). Behavior checklist. In J. D. Cane & R. Hawkins (Eds.), *Behavioral assessment: New directions in clinical psychology.* New York: Brunner/Mazel.

Wardrop, J. (1976). *Standardized testing in the schools: Uses and roles.* Monterey, CA: Brooks/ Cole.

Warren, A., & Warren, S. (1977). The developing ecobehavioral psychology. In A. Warren & S. Warren (Eds.), *Ecological perspectives in behavior analysis.* Baltimore: University Park Press.

Watkins, E. O. (1976). *The Watkins Bender-Gestalt scoring system.* Novato, CA: Academic Therapy.

Watson, B. L. (1970). Field dependence and early reading achievement. *Catalog of Selected Documents in Psychology, 2,* 82.

Webster, R. E., McInnis, E. D., & Carver, L. (1986). Curriculum basing effects in standardized and criterion-referenced reading achievement tests. *Psychology in the Schools, 23,* 205–213.

Wechsler, D. (1958). *The measurement and appraisal of adult intelligence* (4th ed). Baltimore: Williams & Wilkins.

Wedell, K. (1970). Diagnosing learning difficulties: A sequential strategy. *Journal of Learning Disabilities, 3,* 311–317.

Weiner, B. (1974). *Achieving motivation and attribution theory.* Morristown, N.J.: General Learning Press.

Weiner, R., & Koppelman, J. (1987). *From birth to 5: Serving the youngest handicapped children.* Alexandria, VA: Capitol Publications.

Weisler, A., & McCall, R. B. (1976). Exploration and play: Resume and redirection. *American Psychologist, 31,* 492–508.

Weller, C., & Strawser, S. (1981). *Weller-Strawser scales of adaptive behavior.* Novato, CA: Academic Therapy Publications.

Wepman, J. (1973). *Auditory discrimination test* (rev. ed). Palm Springs: Language Research Association.

Wepman, J. M. (1975). *Auditory discrimination test.* (rev. 1973). Palm Springs, CA: Research Associates.

Wepman, J. W. (1973). *Manual of administration, scoring and interpretation: Auditory Discrimination Test.* Chicago: Author.

Wepman, J., et al. (1975). Learning disabilities. In H. Hobbs (Ed.), *Issues in the Classification of Children* (Vol. 1). San Francisco: Jossey-Bass.

Werner, O., & Campbell, D. T. (1973). Translating working through interpreters and the problem of decentering. In R. Caroll & R. Cohen (Eds.), *A handbook of method in cultural anthropology.* New York: Natural History Press.

Wertheimer, M. (1923). Studies in the theory of Gestalt psychology. *Psychology Forsch, 4,* 300.

Wertheimer, M. (1958). Principles of perceptual organization. In D.C. Beardsless & M. Wertheimer (Eds.), *Readings in perception.* New York: Van Nostrand.

Wesman, A. G. (1968). Intelligent testing. *American Psychologist, 23,* 267–274.

Wesson, C., King, R. P., & Deno, S. L. (1984). Direct and frequent assessment of student performance: If it's good for us, why don't we do it? *Learning Disability Quarterly, 7,* 45–48.

Wettler, J., & French, R. W. (1973). Comparison of the Peabody Individual Achievement Test and the Wide Range Achievement Test in a learning disability clinic. *Psychology in the Schools, 10,* 285–286.

White, B. L. (1975). *The first three years of life.* New York: Avon Books.

White, K. R., Bush, D., & Casto, G. (1985). Learning from previous reviews of early intervent research. *Journal of Special Education, 19,* 417–428.

White, K. R., & Casto, G. (1985). An integrative review of early intervention efficacy studies with at risk children: Implications for the handicapped. *Analysis and Intervention in Developmental Disabilities, 5,* 7–31.

White, O., et al. (1981). *Uniform performance assessment system (UPAS).* Columbus, OH: Merrill.

White, O., & Haring, N. (1976). *Exceptional teaching.* Columbus, OH: Merrill.

White, R. (1973). Learning hierarchies. *Review of Educational Research, 43,* 361–375.

White, T. H. (1979). Correlations among the WISC-R, PIAT, and DAM. *Psychology in the Schools, 16,* 497–501.

Whitehead, A., & Russell, B. (1925). Principia mathematica (2nd ed.), vol. 1. New York: Cambridge University Press.

Whitely, S. (1977). Information-processing on intelligence test items: Some response components. *Applied Psychological Measurement, 1,* 465–476.

Whitely, S. E. (1971). Domain-referenced testing: An alternative model for test construction. *Proceedings of the 79th annual convention of the American Psychological Association, 6,* 515–516.

Wicker, A. (1979). *An introduction to ecological psychology.* Monterey, CA: Brooks/Cole.

Wiig, E., Becker-Redding, V. & Semel, E. (1986). A cross cultural, cross linguistic comparison of language abilities of 7 to 8 and 12 to 13 year old children with learning disabilities. *Journal of Learning Disabilities, 16,* 38–46.

Wiig, E., Lapointe, C. & Semel, E. (1977). Relationships among language processing and production abilities of learning disabled adolescents. *Journal of Learning Disabilities, 10,* 38–46.

Wiig, E., & Semel E. (1976). *Language disabilities in children and adolescents.* Columbus, OH: Merrill.

Wiig, E., & Semel, E. (1984). *Language assessment and intervention for the learning disabled* (2nd ed.). Columbus, OH: Merrill.

Wikoff, R. L. (1979). Determining basals for the Peabody Individual Achievement Test. *Psychology in the Schools, 16,* 172–174.

Willems, E. (1974). Behavioral technology and behavioral ecology. *Journal of Applied Behavior Analysis, 7,* 151–165.

Willems, E. (1977). Steps toward an ecobehavioral technology. In A. Warren & S. Warren (Eds.), *Ecological perspectives in behavioral analysis.* Baltimore: University Park Press.

Williams, R. (1972, September). *The Bitch-100: A culture specific test.* Paper presented at the 30th annual convention of the American Psychological Association.

Williams, R. L. (1970). Black pride, academic relevance, and individual achievement. *The Counseling Psychologist, 21,* 18–22.

Williams, R. L. (1971). Abuses and misuses in testing black children. *The Counseling Psychologist, 2,* 62–73.

Wissink, J., Kass, C., & Ferrell, W. (1975). A Bayesian approach to the identification of children with learning disabilities. *Journal of Learning Disabilities, 8,* 158–160.

Witkin H., Oltman, P., Raskin, E., & Karp, S. (1971). *A manual for the Embedded Figures Tests.* Palo Alto, CA: Consulting Psychologist Press.

Witkin, H., et al. (1977). Field-dependent and field-independent cognitive styles and their educational implications. *Review of Educational Research, 47,* 1–64.

Witt, J. C. (1986). Review of the Wide Range Achievement Test-Revised. *Journal of Psychoeducational Assessment, 4,* 87–90.

Witt, J. C., & Martens, B. K. (1984). Adaptive behavior: Tests and assessment issues. *School Psychology Review, 13,* 478–484.

Wong, B. (1987). How do the results of metacognitive research impact on the learning disabled individual? *Learning Disability Quarterly, 10,* (3), 189–195.

Wood, B. (1976). *Children and communication: Verbal and nonverbal language development.* Englewood Cliffs, N.J.: Prentice-Hall.

Woodcock, R. W. (1973). *Woodcock Reading Mastery Tests.* Circle Pines, MN: American Guidance Service.

Woodcock, R. W. (1976). *Goldman-Fristoe-Woodcock Auditory Skills Test Battery, Technical Manual.* Circle Pines, MN: American Guidance Service.

Woodcock, R. W. (1978). *Development and standardization of the Woodcock-Johnson Psychoeducational Battery.* Allen, TX: DLM Teaching Resources.

Woodcock, R. W. (1982). *Interpretation of the Rasch Ability and Difficulty Scales for educational purposes.* Paper presented at the meeting of the National Council on Measurement in Education, New York, March, 1982.

Woodcock, R. W. (1987). *Woodcock reading mastery tests-revised.* Circle Pines, MN: American Guidance Services.

Woodcock, R. W. (1987). *Examiners manual, woodcock reading mastery test-Revised.* Circle Pines, MN: American Guidance Services.

Wright, B. D. (1968). *Sample-free test calibration and person measurement.* Proceedings of the 1967 Invitational Conference on Testing Problems. Princeton: Educational Testing Service.

Wright, B. D., & Stone, M. H. (1979). *Bert test design.* Chicago: MESA Press.

Wright, D. (1987). Intelligence and achievement: A factor analytic and canonical correlational study. *Journal of Psychoeducational Assessment, 23,* 237–247.

Wright, D., & DeMers, S. T. (1982). Comparison of the relationship between two measures of visual-motor coordination and academic achievement. *Psychology in the Schools, 19,* 473–477.

Yerkes, R. M., & Foster, J. C. (1923). *A point scale for measuring mental ability.* Baltimore: Warwick and York.

Yonas, A. et al. (1977) Development of sensitivity to information for impending collision. *Perception and Psychophysics, 21,* 97–104.

Yonas, A., & Pick, H. L., Jr. (1975). An approach to the study of infant space perception. In L. B. Cohen & P. Salapatik (Eds.), *Infant perception: From sensation to cognition* (Vol. II). New York: Academic Press.

Yoshida, R. K. (1983). Are multidisciplinary teams worth the investment? *School Psychology Review, 12,* 137–143.

Yoss, K., & Darley F. (1974). Developmental appraxia of speech in children with defective articulation. *Journal of Speech and Hearing Research, 17,* 399–416.

Ysseldyke, J. (1973). Diagnostic-prescriptive teaching: The search for aptitude-treatment interactions. In L. Mann & D. Sabatino (Eds.), *The first review of special education.* Philadelphia: JSE Press.

Ysseldyke, J. E. (1985). Review of the Stanford Diagnostic Reading Test. In J. V. Mitchell, Jr., (Ed.), *The Ninth Mental Measurements Yearbook* (Vols 1–2) (pp. 1464–1465). Lincoln, NE: Buros Institute of Mental Measurements at the University of Nebraska-Lincoln.

Ysseldyke, J. E., & Algozzine, B. (1982). *Critical issues in special and remediation education.* Boston: Houghton Mifflin Co.

Ysseldyke, J., & Algozzine, B. (1979). Perspective on assessment of learning disabled students. *Learning Disability Quarterly, 2,* 3–13.

Ysseldyke, J. E., Algozzine, B., & Mitchell, J. (1982). Special education team decision making: An analysis of current practice. *The Personnel and Guidance Journal, 60,* 308–313.

Ysseldyke, J., & Mirkin, P. (1982). Assessment information to plan instructional interventions: A review of the research. In C. Reynolds & T. Gutkin (Eds.), *The handbook of school psychology* (pp. 395–409). New York: John Wiley & Sons.

Ysseldyke, J. E., Sabatino, D. A., & La Manna, J. (1973). Convergent and discriminant validity of the Peabody Individual Achievement Test with educable mentally retarded children. *Psychology in the Schools, 10,* 200–204.

Ysseldyke, J. E., & Salvia, J. (1984). Diagnostic-prescriptive teaching: Two models. *Exceptional Children, 41,* 181–185.

Zach, L. (1966). Current thought on intelligence tests. *Psychology in the Schools, 3,* 116–123.

Zach, L., & Kaufman, J. (1962). The effect of verbal labeling on visual-motor performance. *Journal of Learning Disabilities, 2,* 44–48.

Zach, L., & Kaufman, J. (1969). How adequate is the concept of perceptual deficit for education? *Journal of Learning Disabilities, 5,* 36–41.

Zajonc, R. B., Markus, H., & Markus, G. B. (1979). The birth order puzzle. *Journal of Personality and Social Psychology, 37,* 1325–1341.

Zakreski, R. (1982). *Effect of content and training on the generalization of a cognitive strategy by normally achieving and learning disabled boys.* Unpublished doctoral dissertation, University of Virginia, Charlottesville, VA.

Zeaman, D. (1978). Some relations of general intelligence and selected attention. *Intelligence, 2,* 55–73.

Zelniker, T., & Oppenheimer, L. (1976). Effect of different training methods on perceptual learning in impulsive children. *Child Development, 47,* 492–497.

Zigler, E. (1971). The retarded child as a whole person. In H. Adams & W. Boardman, III (Eds.), *Advances in experimental clinical psychology* (Vol. 1). New York: Pergamon.

Zigler, E., & Balla, D. (1979). Personality development in retarded individuals. In N. Ellis (Ed.), *Handbook of mental deficiency* (2nd ed.). Hillsdale, N.J.: Erlbaum Associates.

Zigler, E. & Freedman, J. (1987). Early experience, malleability and Head Start. In James J. Gallagher & Craig T. Ramey (Eds.), *The malleability of children* (pp. 85–96). Baltimore: Paul H. Brookes.

Zins, J. E., & Barnett, D. W. (1983). The Kaufman Assessment Battery for Children and for school achievement: A validity study. *Journal of Psychoeducational Assessment, 1,* 235–241.

Zuelzer, M. B., & Stedman, J. M. (1976). Koppitz Bender Gestalt scores in first grade children as related to ethnocultural background, socioeconomic class and sex factors. *Journal of Consulting and Clinical Psychology, 44,* 873.

# Name Index

# Subject Index

# Test Index

## WE VALUE YOUR OPINION—PLEASE SHARE IT WITH US

Merrill Publishing and our authors are most interested in your reactions to this textbook. Did it serve you well in the course? If it did, what aspects of the text were most helpful? If not, what didn't you like about it? Your comments will help us to write and develop better textbooks. We value your opinions and thank you for your help.

Text Title _____ Edition _____

Author(s) _____

Your Name (optional) _____

Address _____

City _____ State _____ Zip _____

School _____

Course Title _____

Instructor's Name _____

Your Major _____

Your Class Rank  _____ Freshman  _____ Sophomore  _____Junior  _____ Senior

_____ Graduate Student

Were you required to take this course? _____ Required  _____Elective

Length of Course? _____ Quarter  _____ Semester

1. Overall, how does this text compare to other texts you've used?

_____ Superior  _____Better Than Most  _____ Average  _____Poor

2. Please rate the text in the following areas:

|  | Superior | Better Than Most | Average | Poor |
|---|---|---|---|---|
| Author's Writing Style | _____ | _____ | _____ | _____ |
| Readability | _____ | _____ | _____ | _____ |
| Organization | _____ | _____ | _____ | _____ |
| Accuracy | _____ | _____ | _____ | _____ |
| Layout and Design | _____ | _____ | _____ | _____ |
| Illustrations/Photos/Tables | _____ | _____ | _____ | _____ |
| Examples | _____ | _____ | _____ | _____ |
| Problems/Exercises | _____ | _____ | _____ | _____ |
| Topic Selection | _____ | _____ | _____ | _____ |
| Currentness of Coverage | _____ | _____ | _____ | _____ |
| Explanation of Difficult Concepts | _____ | _____ | _____ | _____ |
| Match-up with Course Coverage | _____ | _____ | _____ | _____ |
| Applications to Real Life | _____ | _____ | _____ | _____ |

3. Circle those chapters you especially liked:
   1   2   3   4   5   6   7   8   9   10   11   12   13   14   15   16   17   18   19   20
   What was your favorite chapter? _____
   Comments:

4. Circle those chapters you liked least:
   1   2   3   4   5   6   7   8   9   10   11   12   13   14   15   16   17   18   19   20
   What was your least favorite chapter? _____
   Comments:

5. List any chapters your instructor did not assign. _____

6. What topics did your instructor discuss that were not covered in the text?_____

   _____

7. Were you required to buy this book? _____ Yes   _____ No

   Did you buy this book new or used? _____ New   _____ Used

   If used, how much did you pay? _____

   Do you plan to keep or sell this book? _____ Keep   _____ Sell

   If you plan to sell the book, how much do you expect to receive? _____

   Should the instructor continue to assign this book? _____ Yes   _____ No

8. Please list any other learning materials you purchased to help you in this course (e.g., study guide, lab manual).

   _____

9. What did you like most about this text? _____

   _____

10. What did you like least about this text? _____

   _____

11. General comments:

   May we quote you in our advertising? _____ Yes   _____ No

   Please mail to:   Boyd Lane
                     College Division, Research Department
                     Box 508
                     1300 Alum Creek Drive
                     Columbus, Ohio 43216

   Thank you!